BASIC AND CLINICAL

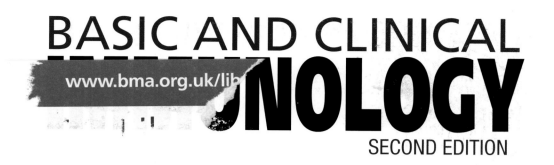

IMMUNOLOGY

SECOND EDITION

D1380087

Commissioning Editor: Timothy Horne
Development Editor: Ailsa Laing
Project Manager: Emma Riley
Designer: Sarah Russell/Kirsteen Wright
Illustration Manager: Kirsteen Wright/Gillian Richards

BASIC AND CLINICAL
IMMUNOLOGY

SECOND EDITION

Mark Peakman MBBS PhD FRCPath

Professor of Clinical Immunology,
King's College London;
Honorary Consultant Immunologist,
King's College Hospital,
London

Diego Vergani MD PhD FRCPath FRCP

Professor of Liver Immunopathology,
King's College London;
Honorary Consultant Immunologist,
King's College Hospital,
London

Illustrated by

Danny J. Pyne and Martin Woodward

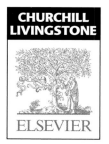

CHURCHILL
LIVINGSTONE

ELSEVIER

EDINBURGH LONDON NEW YORK OXFORD PHILADELPHIA ST LOUIS SYDNEY TORONTO 2009

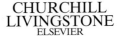

CHURCHILL LIVINGSTONE
ELSEVIER

First Edition © 1997, Elsevier Limited.
Second Edition © 2009, Elsevier Limited. All rights reserved.

ISBN: 978 0 443 10082 6
Reprinted 2009

British Library Cataloguing in Publication Data
A catalogue record for this book is available from the British Library

Library of Congress Cataloging in Publication Data
A catalog record for this book is available from the Library of Congress

Notice
Knowledge and best practice in this field are constantly changing. As new research
and experience broaden our knowledge, changes in practice, treatment and drug
therapy may become necessary or appropriate. Readers are advised to check the most
current information provided (i) on procedures featured or (ii) by the manufacturer
of each product to be administered, to verify the recommended dose or formula, the
method and duration of administration, and contraindications. It is the responsibility
of the practitioner, relying on their own experience and knowledge of the patient, to
make diagnoses, to determine dosages and the best treatment for each individual
patient, and to take all appropriate safety precautions. To the fullest extent of the law,
neither the Publisher nor the Authors assume any liability for any injury and/or
damage to persons or property arising out or related to any use of the material
contained in this book.

The Publisher

Printed in China

Preface to the second edition

Since the publication of the first edition of *Basic and Clinical Immunology*, there have been two main forces driving us inexorably towards this new edition. The first has been the continuous, and very much appreciated, commentary from our students and peers that *Basic and Clinical* was an impressive first effort. It clearly filled a gap, as we had intended, between the basic and theoretical immunology found in many textbooks, and the advanced clinical immunology found in others. By combining the main elements of both, we had created a single text that was usable in biomedical, medical and health schools. The second driver was the emergence of landmark discoveries in the understanding of immunity and its application to medicine, which began to date our first book all too quickly.

In 1997 we had devoted just a few lines to dendritic cells; they are now viewed as the master controllers of adaptive immunity. This potency is achieved through expression of an array of receptors for pathogens, the discovery of which has changed the way we think about interactions between the immune system and the environment. We speculated in the first edition about the potential for 'magic bullet' monoclonal antibody therapy, but could not have dreamt of the benefit now being realised in a number of mainstream clinical settings, that include rheumatoid arthritis, lymphoma and breast cancer. The tools have evolved too — technology for the investigation and imaging of the immune system now allows single immune cells to be tracked *in vivo*. And, inevitably, there is a new T helper cell on the block, along with the reincarnation of the suppressor T cell (only it is called a regulator). One has the sense that much has happened and much will happen hence.

London   M.P.
2009   D.V.

Preface to the first edition

'Immunology is an invention of the devil.'

From the outset, this book was intended as a text combining the basic science components required to understand the role of immunity in disease with an account of the major diseases classified under the umbrella of clinical immunology. The book would thus naturally span the curricula of most medical or paramedical courses, from basic to applied. From technical, medical, dental and science students at all levels, we had both perceived a glaring need for such a text. But as if any stimulus was required for us to see the project to completion, an article appeared in a popular news magazine for doctors whilst the book was being planned, asking several regular contributors for their most hated words. 'Immunology' made its appearance as 'an invention of the devil, who is making it up as he goes along because he is not too clear about this stuff either'. The article went on to compare immunology to a Rube Goldberg or Heath Robinson cartoon: for example, the light is turned on when you trip over a chair, startling the cat, who leaps against the door, which swings shut, knocking a picture off the wall, which strikes the light switch as it falls. And as a final evi-dence that immunology was truly demonic, a conversation with an expert physician, encountered at an international conference, was recounted in the same article. 'I hope you understand all this stuff', he had said to the journalist, 'they didn't teach it when I was in medical school and I never figured it out.' We hope that this book goes some way towards redressing the balance.

It would have been impossible to be authoritative about every aspect of clinical immunology. For this reason, we have consulted friends and colleagues with the relevant expertise to advise us, and to these we are indebted: Fred Dische, Adrian Eddleston, John Fabre, Jonathan Frankel, Elizabeth Higgins, Rob Higgins, William Hirst, Giorgina Mieli-Vergani, Lindsay Nicholson and Anton Pozniak. We are also grateful to colleagues who provided photographic material for illus-trations, notably Nat Cary, Fred Dische and Magnus Norman, Jane Evanson, Stella Knight, Jonathan Frankel, Elizabeth Higgins, Patrick O'Donnell, Bernard Portmann and John Salisbury.

London   M.P.
1997   D.V.

Contents

Symbols used in the diagrams

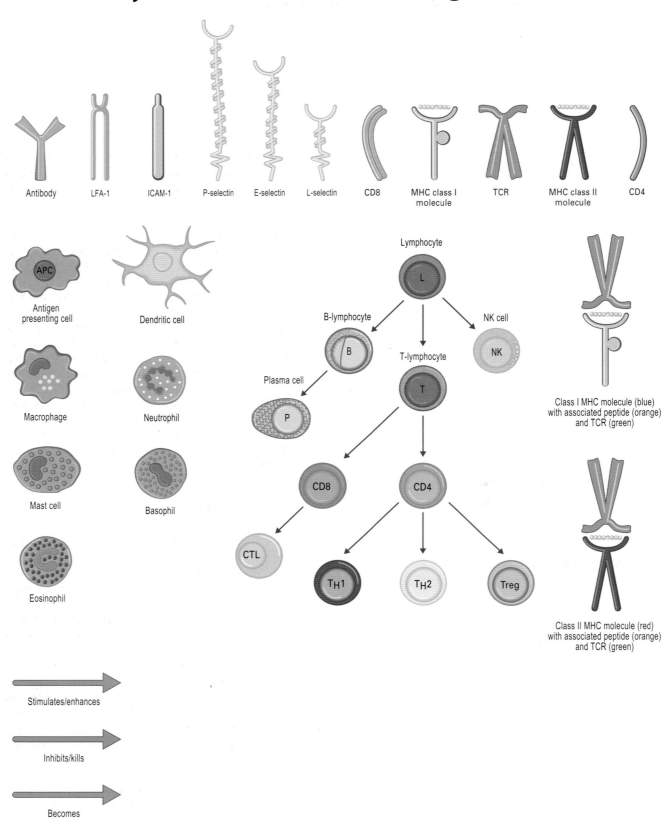

Antibody LFA-1 ICAM-1 P-selectin E-selectin L-selectin CD8 MHC class I molecule TCR MHC class II molecule CD4

Antigen presenting cell

Dendritic cell

Macrophage

Neutrophil

Mast cell

Basophil

Eosinophil

Lymphocyte

B-lymphocyte

NK cell

Plasma cell

T-lymphocyte

CD8

CD4

CTL

T_H1

T_H2

Treg

Class I MHC molecule (blue) with associated peptide (orange) and TCR (green)

Class II MHC molecule (red) with associated peptide (orange) and TCR (green)

Stimulates/enhances

Inhibits/kills

Becomes

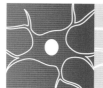

Anatomy and cells of the immune system

The immune system is like any other organ of mammalian physiology — the liver, kidney, thyroid — in being composed of specialised cells that function within discrete, organised anatomical structures. To understand its role in host defence, it is necessary first to become familiar with the cells and anatomy of the immune system.

Cells of the immune system

The bone marrow is the source of the precursor cells that ultimately give rise to the cellular constituents of the immune system, save for one brief period during foetal life when the liver is also a site of immune cell development. The production of immune cells is one component of **haemopoiesis**, the process by which all cells that circulate in the blood arise and mature. An important underlying principle of haemopoiesis is that there is a single precursor cell that is capable of giving rise to all blood cell lineages, ranging from platelets to lymphocytes (Fig. 1.1). This cell is known as the **pluripotent haemopoietic stem cell**: it is to the bone marrow what the queen bee is to the hive (Science Box 1.1). Immunology concentrates upon the roles of white blood cells in host defence: these include the granulocytes (neutrophils, eosinophils and basophils), monocytes and dendritic cells, and lymphocytes.

Granulocytes

The granulocyte/monocyte lineage gives rise to precursors that mature within the bone marrow and are released into the blood. The granulocytes constitute approximately 65% of all white cells and derive their name from the large numbers of granules found in their cytoplasm. The appearance of these granules under the light microscope following conventional staining provides a further subdivision. Granules with intense blue staining are found in basophils, which make up 0.5–1% of granulocytes; red-staining granules are present in eosinophils (3–5%); while neutrophils (90–95%) have granules that remain relatively unstained (Fig. 1.2a–c). The term '**polymorphonuclear cell**', describing the multilobed nuclei of granulocytes, has become synonymous with neutrophils, which constitute by far the majority of granulocytes, but eosinophil nuclei may have a similar appearance. Granulocytes circulate in the blood and migrate into the tissues particularly during inflammatory responses. The exception to this rule is the **mast cell**, which is fixed in the tissues. Mast cells and basophils share many common features, yet their derivation is different: the basophil is of the same lineage as neutrophils and eosinophils, whilst mast cells arise from an as yet unidentified precursor possibly in the spleen, thymus or lymph node.

Monocytes and dendritic cells

Monocytes form between 5 and 10% of circulating white blood cells and have a short half-life, spending approximately 24 hours in the blood. They enter the extravascular pool and become resident in the tissues, where they are termed **macrophages**. Whilst each macrophage was thought to derive from a single monocyte, there is now evidence that macrophages may also arise following division of immature forms of monocytes. Monocyte and macrophage morphology is highly variable, but in broad terms they are larger than neutrophils and lymphocytes, have a single nucleus and abundant granular cytoplasm (Fig. 1.2d). Several specialised forms of the mature cell exist, including **alveolar macrophages** in the lung, **Kupffer cells** in the liver, **mesangial cells** in the kidney, **microglial cells** in the brain, **osteoclasts** in bone, and other macrophages lining channels in the spleen and lymph nodes.

There is an additional very small population of immune cells in the peripheral blood, lymph nodes, bone marrow and tissues that have a characteristic appearance of numerous

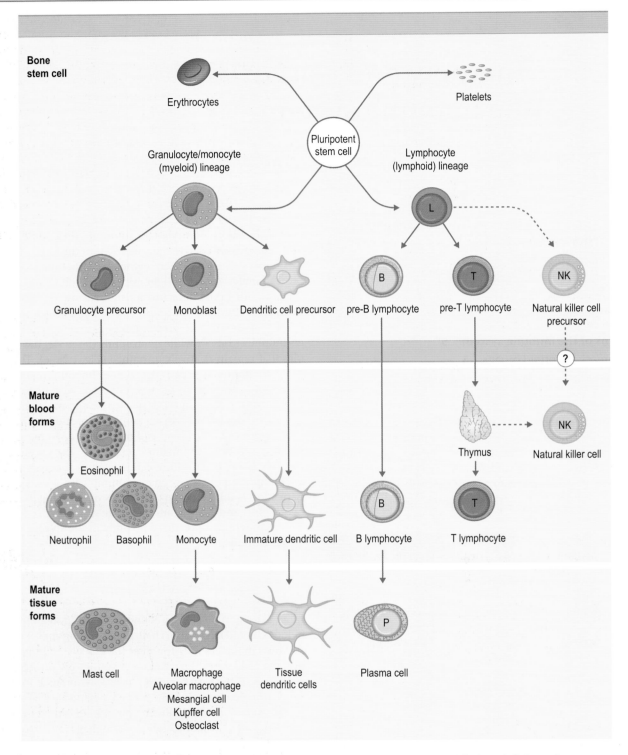

Fig. 1.1 The development of white blood cells from pluripotent stem cell to mature circulating and tissue forms.
Although mast cells are granular cells, it is not yet clear whether tissue mast cells mature from the common granulocyte precursor.

cytoplasmic processes. These are termed **dendritic cells** (**DCs**) (Fig. 1.2e). DCs are bone-marrow derived, come in many forms, and have a highly specialised function in the activation and priming of lymphocytes. DCs therefore occupy a pre-eminent position in immunology. Some specialised DC forms of these cells exist: for example, follicular dendritic cells in the lymph nodes.

Lymphocytes

Lymphocytes make up the final 25–35% of white cells and derive their name from a close association with the lymphatic system. This is illustrated by the fact that inserting a needle into the thoracic duct, the major channel leading from the lymphatics into the blood, and allowing it to drain

Pluripotent haemopoietic stem cells

The concept that there are stem cells that are capable of providing a source of regeneration of any tissue is of course an area of highly important research effort throughout the world. The pluripotent haemopoietic stem cell (HSC) provides some hope that this strategy will bear fruit, since HSCs have already been used in the clinic. It was discovered that HSCs are occasionally present in the blood, and are at their highest levels in the cord blood of newborn babies. HSCs have a distinctive surface molecule and can therefore be purified from the blood. The first cord blood transplantation was performed in 1988. The patient was a child with an inherited blood disease and was destined to die. The patient's mother became pregnant again, carrying an unborn child that was both free of the blood disease and tissue-compatible with the patient. The cord blood was duly collected and cells injected into the sick patient. Years later the child is still alive and has a cellular immune system entirely composed of the sibling's cells.

Umbilical cord blood banks have been established (for more information see http://stemcells.nih.gov) and HSCs are now used in the treatment of a variety of diseases in which new blood and immune cell precursors are required.

ing the numbers of lymphocytes in circulation and leaving the mice prone to death from infection. In addition, neonatally thymectomised mice were tolerant of skin grafts from mice of unrelated strains, whereas intact mice would vigorously destroy such grafts. Antibody production was reduced but not completely. Several conclusions were drawn about T lymphocytes from the results of these studies. First, their involvement with the thymus takes place in early life and is critical to their development. During this period, they acquire the ability to recognise and bring about the death of transplanted foreign tissues in a process termed **graft rejection**, which implies an ability to distinguish self and non-self. In the absence of T lymphocytes, protection against infection is fatally impaired. Although not capable of producing antibody themselves, T lymphocytes make a telling contribution to B lymphocyte function.

Natural killer cells

In recent years, the edges of the lymphocyte lineage have become blurred as the laboratory techniques used to identify them have become more sophisticated. Small populations of cells have been identified that resemble T lymphocytes but remain distinct. The term natural killer (NK) cell is a functional definition: cells with this activity are capable of lysing virus-infected cells and tumour cells. Unlike T lymphocytes, they do not need an education in the thymus to do this, hence the term 'natural'. Like lymphocytes, NK cells are best identified by the presence of specialised surface glycoproteins (see Science Box 2.3 (p. 20) and Ch. 7) and also typically have a very granular cytoplasm. A population of cells with characteristics of both NK and T cells also exists, termed NKT cells.

SUMMARY BOX 1.1

Cells of the immune system

- White blood cells are produced from a single precursor cell, the pluripotent haemopoietic stem cell (haemopoiesis).
- Granulocytes (65%), eosinophils, neutrophils and basophils circulate in blood and are involved in inflammatory responses.
- Monocytes (5–10%) migrate rapidly from the blood to give rise to the tissue form, termed a macrophage. Special macrophages exist in different tissues, e.g. Kupffer cells in liver.
- Dendritic cells are derived from bone marrow and are critical in activation and priming of lymphocytes.
- Lymphocytes (25–35%) divide into two main subtypes: B and T (1:5).
- B lymphocytes: antigen recognition by antibody. May become plasma cells, which are antibody 'factories'.
- T lymphocytes: pivotal cell in immune response, able to recognise and destroy infectious agents and foreign tissues.

continuously will selectively deplete the blood of circulating lymphocytes. Lymphocytes are divided into two subtypes, B and T, present in blood in a ratio of approximately 1:5. These have quite distinct functions and, though they are indistinguishable by conventional light microscopy, appear different on electron microscopy (Fig. 1.2f,g); they can be differentiated by the presence of highly specialised glycoprotein molecules on their surface (Chs 6 & 7). Lymphocytes are found in the blood, lymphoid organs or tissues and also at sites of **chronic inflammation**. Their precursors arise in the bone marrow and mature through one of two pathways.

B lymphocytes differentiate within the bone marrow before being released into the circulation. During foetal life, the liver is also an important site of B lymphocyte development. The primary role of these cells is the recognition of macromolecules (termed **antigens**) through surface receptors (called **antibodies**). B lymphocytes may mature into **plasma cells**, in which form they remain fixed in the tissues and function as secretors of soluble antibody. The B lymphocyte obtained its name from early studies on antibody production in birds, showing that removal of a lymphoid organ known as the bursa of Fabricius from near the hindgut of a chick resulted in a complete inability to produce antibody. These antibody-producing cells then became known as bursa-derived, or B lymphocytes.

The role of **T lymphocytes**, or thymus-derived lymphocytes, was studied in similar experiments. A different lymphoid organ, the **thymus**, was removed from mice. Removal of the thymus from adult mice appeared to have little effect on the animals or their lymphocytes, but thymectomy performed soon after birth had profound consequences, reduc-

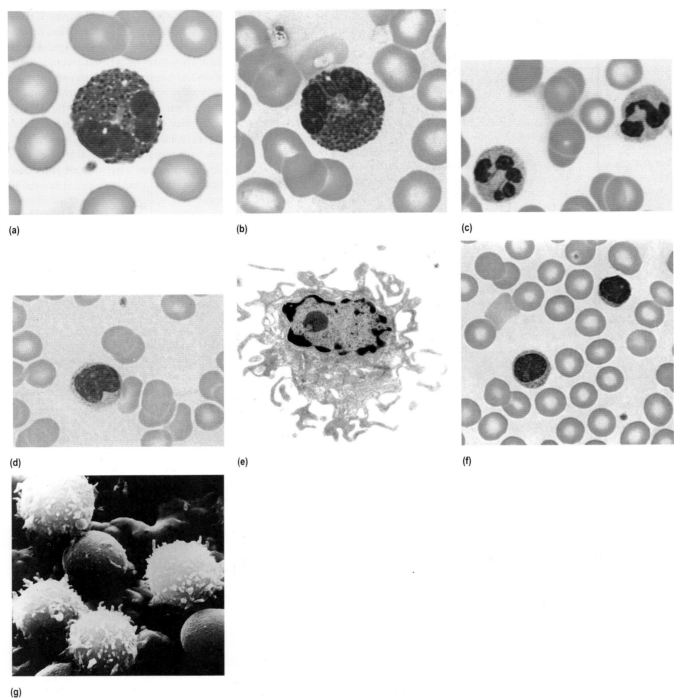

Fig. 1.2 **White blood cells.**
(**a**) Basophils have blue-staining granules seen here as dark cytoplasmic structures. (**b**) Eosinophils have characteristic red-staining granules. (**c**) Neutrophils have relatively unstained granules and characteristic polymorphic nucleus. (**d**) Monocyte with clear cytoplasm and large nucleus. (**e**) EM photomicrograph of a dendritic cell, showing the characteristic and numerous dendritic processes (courtesy of Professor Stella Knight and Dr Nick English). (**f**) Lymphocyte with scanty, clear cytoplasm. (**g**) Scanning electron microscopic appearance of T and B lymphocytes, with B lymphocytes having the slightly 'hairy' external appearance (reproduced with permission from Upjohn Inc.). (Parts (a)–(d) of this figure, and part (f), from Young B, Lowe JS, Stevens A, Heath JW 2006 Wheater's functional histology: A text and colour atlas, 5th edn. Elsevier: Edinburgh, with permission.)

Organs of the immune system

The total number of lymphocytes in a healthy adult is about 10^{12}, of which 0.1% are renewed daily. Collectively they weigh almost half as much as the liver, yet they do not reside in any single organ. Instead, lymphocytes have the distinctive feature of **recirculation**, between the blood, tissues and lymphoid organs (Fig. 1.3). Recirculation times vary from cell to cell, depending upon what is encountered during the journey, but, on average, a lymphocyte will complete a cycle in 1–2 days. Rather than being random, recirculation is a highly regulated process of **immune surveillance**, controlled according to cell type and anatomy: B lymphocytes have a greater tendency to migrate to mucosal lymphoid tissue than do T lymphocytes, for example. Cell migration is controlled by specialised lymphocyte surface receptors, binding to complementary receptors on the vessel walls of the tissues they enter.

Organs of the lymphoid system are divided into primary and secondary organs (Fig. 1.4). The **primary** lymphoid organs in humans are the bone marrow and thymus, since they are the sites of development and maturation of the lymphocytes (in birds, the bursa of Fabricius would also be included). By definition, removal of these organs removes the capacity for immune cell generation. **Secondary** lymphoid organs (lymph nodes and spleen) are not essential for the generation of lymphocytes but have a key role in the maturation of these cells and the development of immunity. Lymph nodes in particular anatomical sites are highly specialised, those surrounding the upper and lower respiratory tracts being known as the mucosa-associated lymphoid tissue (MALT) and those in the gut, the gut-associated lymphoid tissue (GALT).

Primary lymphoid organs

The precise mechanism by which a pluripotent stem cell in the bone marrow matures into any one of the immune cells remains unclear. What is known is that both the

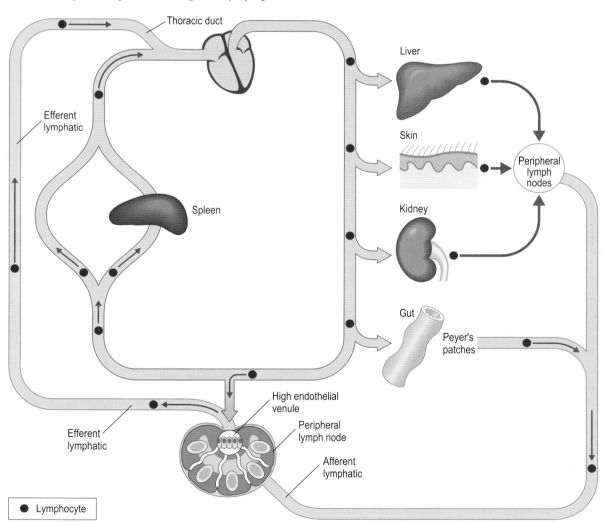

Fig. 1.3 **Lymphocyte recirculation.**
Lymphocytes returning to the blood via the thoracic duct can re-enter the lymphatics either via the tissues or via high endothelial venules in the lymph nodes.

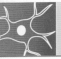

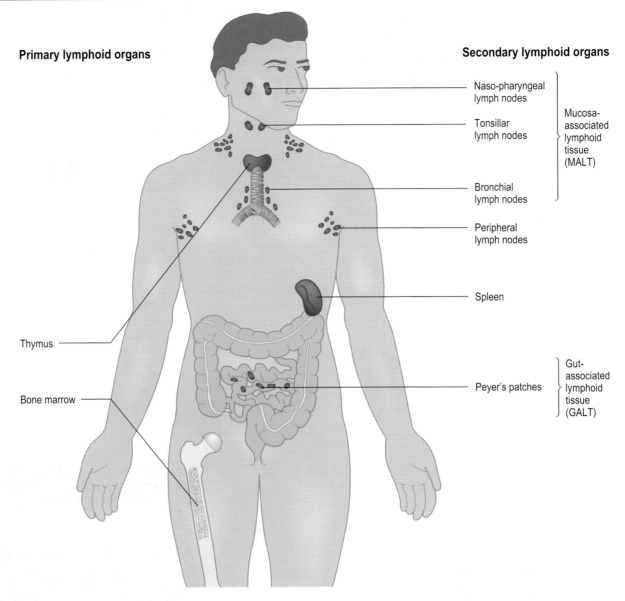

Fig. 1.4 Anatomy of primary and secondary lymphoid organs in humans.

microenvironment within the marrow and the influence of soluble mediators that act as **colony stimulation factors** are important determinants.

The thymus also constitutes something of an immunological 'black box', but a considerable amount is now known about the changes that take place within a pre-T lymphocyte as it matures in the thymus. The thymus develops from the third and fourth pharyngeal pouches in the sixth week of fetal life. Immature cells enter the cortex and receive the close attention of a mixture of thymic epithelial and other cells of myeloid origin, resulting in their development into immature T lymphocytes. The thymus is at its largest, in proportion to body mass, at birth and thereafter shows a relative decline in size. In some conditions

during adult life, the thymus may need surgical removal, for example because of a tumour, but this does not appear to compromise the normal functioning of the immune system.

Secondary lymphoid organs

The secondary lymphoid organs have three major functions. They are the residence for a variety of lymphoid cells (mainly T and B lymphocytes, dendritic cells); they are traps for antigen, the material against which immune responses are made; and they are the anatomical site in which immune responses are initiated.

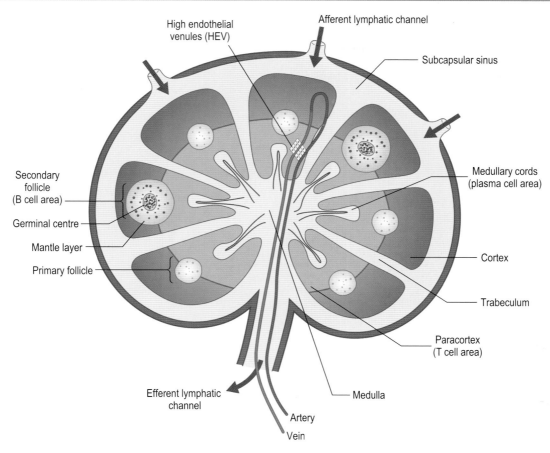

Fig. 1.5 **Structure of a lymph node.**
Lymph, containing lymphocytes, dendritic cells and soluble material (e.g. antigen) from the tissues, enters via the afferent lymphatic channels. Cells may also enter via the HEV structures directly from the blood. Cells leave via the efferent lymphatic channels. Note the T and B cell areas. The presence of secondary follicles with germinal centres indicates an ongoing immune response.

Lymph nodes

Lymphocytes and other migratory cells such as maturing dendritic cells enter the lymph nodes either through the lymphatics or from the blood (Fig. 1.5). The afferent lymphatics provide a route of entry into the subcapsular marginal sinus. From here, cells travel into the cortex and then the medulla of the node. The cortex of the lymph node contains follicles, which are organised aggregates of lymphoid cells. Primary follicles are characteristic of a resting state and suggest no recent immune activity. They are composed of B lymphocytes, macrophages and specialised dendritic cells with long cytoplasmic processes known as follicular dendritic cells. Secondary follicles arise following stimulation of a local immune response. The **germinal centre** of the follicle enlarges and B lymphocytes undergo proliferation and differentiation. The germinal centre is surrounded by a mantle of smaller, resting B lymphocytes. The **paracortical area** of the node is predominantly composed of T lymphocytes as well as the specialised **dendritic cells**, which are critical accessory cells in T lymphocyte responses. The medulla has characteristic **medullary cords** of lymphoid cells, which tend to become populated with plasma cells during immune reactions.

The speed of an individual lymphocyte's course through a lymph node will depend upon the state of activity of the node and whether the cell becomes involved in an immune response or not. Lymphocytes leave via the efferent lymphatics, ultimately passing into the thoracic duct and thence into the venous system. Lymphocytes may also enter lymph nodes via the blood. This is particularly true of naïve lymphocytes (i.e. those that have not yet become involved in an immune response). Naïve lymphocytes have a specific homing receptor for lymph nodes (called L-selectin) and its counter receptor is found on large cuboidal endothelial cells present on specialised structures called **high endothelial venules** (HEV). These are found in all lymph nodes, but their number can be regulated according to local requirements. Lymphocytes require 'homing' receptors on their surface to interact with HEVs, and such receptors are specific for different lymphocytes and different tissues. This implies a high degree of organisation within the lymphoid system, so that, for example, lymphocytes that protect against pathogens encountered in the gut will possess receptors specific for HEVs in GALT. GALT is composed of Peyer's patches and isolated lymphoid follicles within the gut submucosa. Peyer's patches are lymphoid aggregates with follicles, germinal centres and

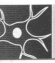

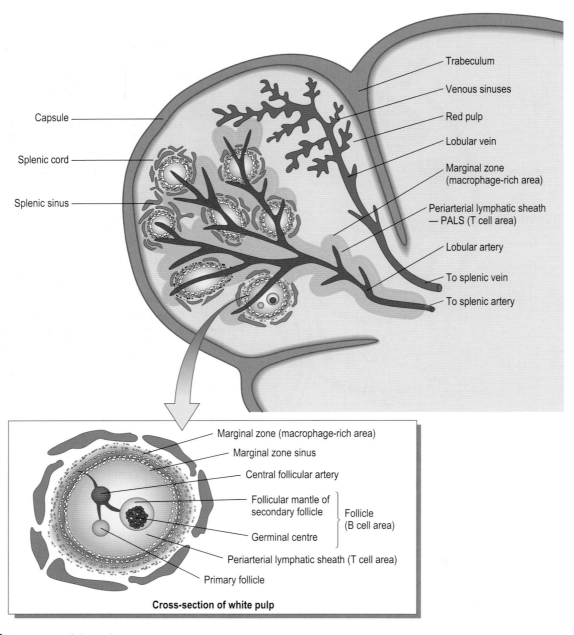

Fig. 1.6 **Structure of the spleen.**

a surrounding T cell area, but they differ from peripheral lymph nodes in lacking a capsule and afferent lymphatics. Anatomically they are closely associated with the intestinal lumen, being separated from it by a specialised epithelial dome composed of cells capable of sampling the milieu within the gut.

Spleen

If the lymph node is an antigen trap for the tissues, the spleen is an antigen trap for the blood. Its sponge-like qualities mean that the blood traffic of cells and proteins can be slowed down and inspected. The functions of the spleen represent a mixture between the haematological and the lymphoid activities. This is exemplified by its macroscopic appearance: a **white pulp** comprising lymphoid tissue and a **red pulp** comprising reticular tissue and sinuses bathed in blood (Fig. 1.6). The vasculature of the spleen forms a scaffold on which the white and red pulps are hung. Arteries entering the white pulp are surrounded by a sleeve of lymphocytes called the periarterial lymphatic sheath (PALS; predominantly a T lymphocyte zone). Lymphocytes enter the white pulp through venule walls, but the spleen does not have HEVs. Within the PALS, lymphoid follicles and germinal centres (B lymphocyte areas) similar to those seen in lymph nodes are found. In the red pulp, branches of the arteries transport blood into the splenic venous sinuses where its constituents interact with the marginal zone adjacent to the PALS. The marginal zone is rich in macrophages and its proximity to the T lymphocytes of the PALS allows close interaction between these cell types as the blood filters slowly through this area.

Functionally, the spleen is a combination of lymphoid organ, filter bed and reclamation site. The slow speed of circulation allows constant monitoring of the blood, particularly with regard to infectious agents and antigen–antibody complexes, which signify an active immune response. The red pulp is an important site for the removal of effete and defective red and white blood cells, which are cannibalised by resident macrophages. The resources, such as the iron in haemoglobin, are recycled, serving as a strong case for renaming this the 'green' pulp. For all this, the spleen is expendable, though its removal should not be undertaken lightly (Clinical Box 1.1).

SUMMARY BOX 1.2

Organs of the immune system

- Primary lymphoid organs (bone marrow and thymus) are sites of development and maturation of immune response cells.
- Secondary lymphoid organs — lymph nodes, spleen, mucosa-associated (MALT) and gut-associated (GALT) lymphoid tissue — organise the immune response.
- White blood cells become further specialised in secondary organs.
- Lymphocytes recirculate through blood, secondary lymphoid organs and lymphatics in a process of organised immune surveillance.

Further reading

Rich RR The human immune response and Lewis WE, Harriman GR Cells and tissues of the immune system. In: Rich RR, Fleisher TA, Shearer WT, Kotzin BL, Schroeder HW (eds) 2001 Clinical immunology, principles and practice, 2nd edn. Mosby: London

Vondenhoff MF, Kraal G, Mebius RE 2007 Lymphoid organogenesis in brief. Eur J Immunol 37 Suppl 1: S46–52

CLINICAL BOX 1.1

Defective immune function after removal of the spleen

The spleen may become diseased and require surgical removal for several conditions. Blunt trauma to the abdomen often leads to rupture of the splenic capsule and uncontrolled internal bleeding; the spleen may also become too voracious in its appetite for effete platelets, leading to low levels in the circulation and an increased tendency to bleeding. Splenectomy may, therefore, be necessary to save life, but it is not without risk, carrying a 40-fold increase in the incidence of severe microbial infection and a 17-fold increase in fatal sepsis. The infections encountered typically run a rapidly progressive course and involve encapsulated organisms such as *Streptococcus pneumoniae*. The importance of the spleen in protection against these bacteria probably results from a combination of its ability to slow and filter circulating blood and its capacity to act as a rapid response unit in generating specific antimicrobial antibodies. For these reasons, it is recommended that patients who have undergone splenectomy should receive prophylactic vaccinations against several organisms, including *S. pneumoniae, Neisseria meningitidis, Haemophilus influenzae* and influenza virus.

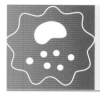
Innate immunity I: physical and humoral protection

Freedom from the burden of disease

The Latin *immunis*, meaning *free from burden*, has provided the English term immunity; it is often used in non-scientific contexts such as diplomatic immunity, crown immunity and so on. In biology, the burden is disease — caused by a variety of viruses, fungi, bacteria, protozoa, worms and toxins — and the physiological role of the immune system is to keep it at bay.

A broad definition of the immune system would be that it evolved to be able to identify **self**, and thus recognise **non-self**. The ability to make such a distinction is relatively primordial: sea anemones also have the capacity to recognise and react to non-self. The immune system in humans is often challenged by non-self, including pathogens such as those described above as well as organs transplanted from unrelated donors. Protection from these is afforded by a variety of cognitive and destructive processes, the understanding of which forms the basis of immunology.

Immunity from infection is the result of a complex process, as we shall see, but there are some general principles about immunity that we can deduce from our own everyday experience. For example, some features of protection from infection are obvious: if you have an open wound or burn, it is important to maintain cleanliness and protect the exposed tissues from becoming infected. Thus, loss of physical barriers lowers immunity. We also know that some infections can arise at any age and be dealt with by the immune system without necessarily needing antibiotics. On the other hand, we consider the newborn to be at greater overall risk of infection: they have less immunity. Other well-recognised truths relate to the infections of childhood. If you have chicken pox as a child, you are extremely unlikely to suffer the same illness again. However, having had chicken pox would not stop a child catching measles. We can conclude that we are born with some immunity and that the rest may be acquired during life; immune responses can be highly specific for a microbe: they may be learned and retained in an 'immunological memory'.

Types of immunity

Innate immunity

Immunity present at birth is termed innate. The innate immune system is the main, first-line defence against invading organisms. Its characteristics are that it is present for life, has no specificity and no memory. (An exception, to be discussed later, is the protective antibodies that babies acquire from their mothers.) Innate responses are most useful in protection against:

- pyogenic ('pus-forming') organisms, e.g. *Staphylococcus aureus*, *Haemophilus influenzae*
- fungi, e.g. *Candida albicans*
- multicellular parasites, e.g. worms such as *Ascaris*, the roundworm.

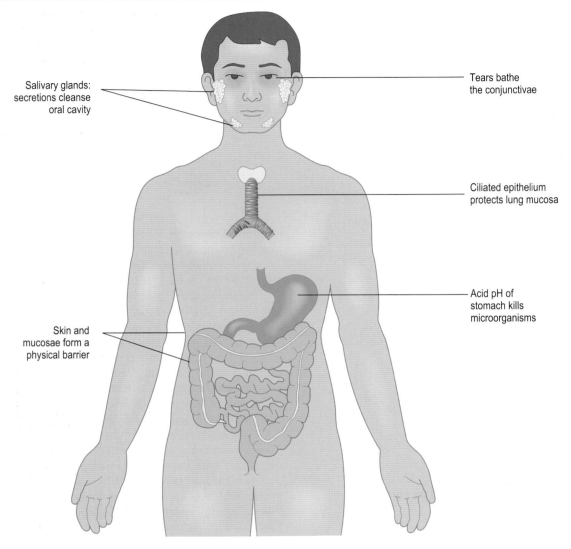

Fig. 2.1 Physicochemical barriers to infection which form the first line of innate defence against pathogens.
Secretions such as saliva and tears also contain antibacterial enzymes such as lysozyme.

Innate immunity has three components: physicochemical, humoral and cellular.

Physical barriers (Fig. 2.1) are the **skin** and **mucosae**, **secretions**, which continually wash and cleanse mucosal surfaces, and **cilia**, which help the removal of debris and foreign matter. Immunologically active factors present in mucosal secretions, in blood and in the cerebrospinal fluid (the *humors*) are termed humoral. The most important of these is **complement** and the **mannan-binding lectin**, as well as additional **opsonins** (an opsonin aids digestion of bacteria by neutrophils), such as **C-reactive protein**, and proteolytic **enzymes** (e.g. **lysozyme**). Cellular components are the **neutrophil**, the **eosinophil** and the **mast cell**, as well as the **NK cell**.

Acquired immunity

In contrast, some types of immune response are not present at birth but are gained as part of our development. The acquired or specific immune response is the antithesis of innate immunity. It is absent at birth, increases with age and has specificity and memory; hence it may also be termed **adaptive**.

Paralysis of one component of either of these two forms of immunity can have a profound effect on the host defence against infection.

SUMMARY BOX 2.1

Contrasting characteristics of innate and acquired immunity

Innate immunity

- Characteristics: non-specific, is present at birth and does not change in intensity with exposure.

- Components: mechanical barriers, secreted products (complement) and cells (granulocytes, dendritic cells, NK cells).

- Protects from: bacteria, fungi, worms.

SUMMARY BOX 2.1

Contrasting characteristics of innate and acquired immunity—cont'd

Acquired immunity

- Characteristics: specific responses, acquired from exposure and increases in intensity with exposure.

- Components: secreted products (antibodies) and cells (lymphocytes).

- Protects from: bacteria, including intracellular infection, viruses and protozoa.

Complement

Complement was described at the turn of the century during studies on the nature of immune reactions to bacteria in serum. Serum removed from animals that have been infected with a microorganism can subsequently agglutinate (clump together) and then lyse the same bacteria in a test tube (Fig. 2.2). Lysis, but not agglutination, is inhibited by pre-heating the serum at 56°C for 30 minutes. The lysing activity can be reconstituted using fresh serum from an animal not previously exposed to the bacteria. Therefore, a heat-labile factor without specificity for an organism is essential for its lysis.

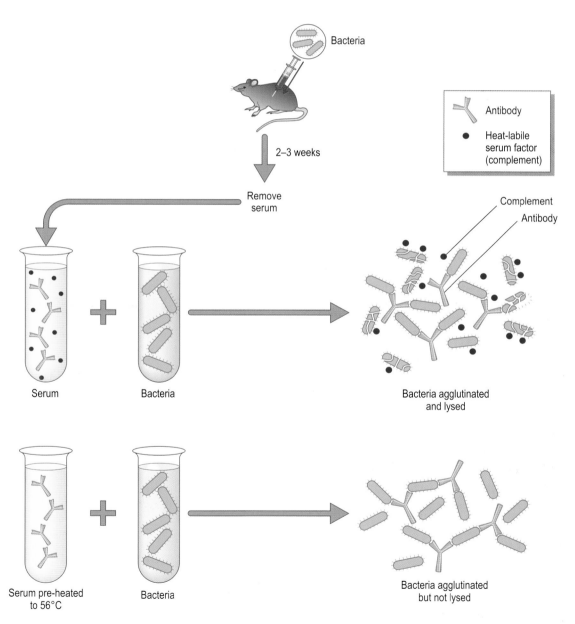

Fig. 2.2 Animals exposed to bacteria develop antibody, which specifically agglutinates ("binds together") the same organism. Lysis is achieved through the action of a heat-labile serum factor which *complements* the action of antibody.

Antibody

Antibody is a term we have all become used to. They are glycoproteins produced by lymphocytes following stimulation with a macromolecule (usually termed the antigen). An example of an antigen would be a protein coating the surface of a bacterium or virus. Antibody is a sophisticated glycoprotein that occurs in several different types with differing functions, but it is sufficient for the present to view it simplistically as a molecule with a shape like the letter 'Y'. The two smaller arms are identical to each other and each carries the ability to bind antigen; the trunk of the Y has specialised sites for interaction with complement proteins or specific receptors on cells. Granulocytes and mast cells, for example, bear receptors for antibody. Through interaction with complement and cells, antibody can provide the innate immune system with a specificity that, on its own, it does not possess. This serves as a reminder that the innate and acquired immune systems work best in concert.

These studies indicated the presence of two antibacterial agents in serum. One was fairly heat stable, inducible by the organism and capable of agglutinating but not killing it. This first factor was originally termed **antibody** (Science Box 2.1) and is specific for the target that induces it (the **antigen**), in this case a foreign organism. Since it is capable of specific reactions, antibody is part of the acquired/specific/adaptive immune system and will be discussed later. The second serum factor is heat labile and helps destruction of the organism by antibody. This factor was termed **complement**, now the name of a group of serum proteins that *complement* antibody in the destruction of organisms. It later became established that complement could, under many circumstances, be activated directly by pathogenic organisms without the need for antibody (therefore termed the alternative pathway), and is therefore a component of the innate immune system.

Complement is a protein cascade (cf. the kinin and clotting cascades) composed of more than 40 proteins including regulatory factors. The components are made in the liver, though some local production at sites of inflammation may be undertaken by macrophages. Complement has four pathways: the **alternative**, **classical** and **mannan-binding lectin** pathways, which are all capable of igniting the third pathway, known as the **common** or **membrane attack pathway**.

Complement proteins

The majority of complement proteins are soluble, although some are membrane bound. The soluble proteins circulate in an inactive state, and each must be activated sequentially for the reaction to proceed. Each activated molecule can catalyse

the conversion of several molecules of the next component in the sequence; this gives the cascade the key attribute of amplification. The overall serum concentration of complement proteins is 3–4 g/l (i.e. around 10% of serum proteins).

Several biological activities appear as a consequence of complement activation, the main ones being cell or bacterial **lysis**, the production of **pro-inflammatory mediators**, which amplify and perpetuate the process, and **solubilisation** of antigen–antibody complexes.

The confused and ever-changing terminology of the complement system was partly to blame for its past unpopularity with students and clinicians. In recent years the World Health Organization has proposed a standard nomenclature to obviate this (see Table 2.1). The precursor molecules, the fragments derived from enzymatic cleavage of the parent molecule, the inactivated component and the active state of isolated or integrated complement components are all clearly defined in the same way for every component of the pathways.

Complement activation

Activation of the complement system occurs through three distinct pathways, **alternative**, **classical and mannan-binding lectin**. These converge for the final common pathway, which provides most of the biological activity (Fig. 2.3). The alternative, classical and mannan-binding lectin pathways are composed of three distinct enzyme cascades that culminate in the cleavage of C3 and C5. Cleavage of C3 produces important biological consequences, while breakdown of C5 achieves the same and, in addition, provides the

Table 2.1 Terminology of the complement system

State of component	Nomenclature
Precursor molecules	Capital C followed by a number for the classical and common pathways, e.g. C1, C2 Capital letter followed by number for the alternative pathway, e.g. B1
Fragments	Small letter suffix, e.g. C4a, C2b ('a' fragments are smaller than 'b' fragments)
Inactivated components	Letter i prefix, e.g. iC3b
Active state	Bar over symbols, e.g. $\overline{C4b2b}$

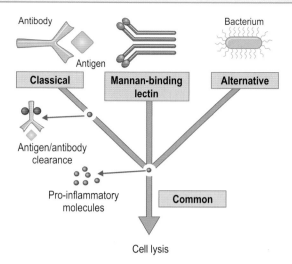

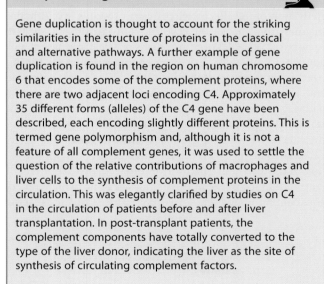

Fig. 2.3 Overview of complement activation pathways.
The final common pathway may be activated via the classical or alternative routes, which are initiated by antigen–antibody complexes and bacteria, respectively, or by mannan-binding lectin. Three main results of activation are clearance of complexes, release of biologically active mediators and direct cell lysis.

Complement genes

Gene duplication is thought to account for the striking similarities in the structure of proteins in the classical and alternative pathways. A further example of gene duplication is found in the region on human chromosome 6 that encodes some of the complement proteins, where there are two adjacent loci encoding C4. Approximately 35 different forms (alleles) of the C4 gene have been described, each encoding slightly different proteins. This is termed gene polymorphism and, although it is not a feature of all complement genes, it was used to settle the question of the relative contributions of macrophages and liver cells to the synthesis of complement proteins in the circulation. This was elegantly clarified by studies on C4 in the circulation of patients before and after liver transplantation. In post-transplant patients, the complement components have totally converted to the type of the liver donor, indicating the liver as the site of synthesis of circulating complement factors.

---

triggering stimulus to the final common pathway. The alternative, classical and mannan-binding lectin pathways bear striking resemblances, particularly in terms of protein structure (e.g. C2 and B, C1q and mannan-binding lectin), which is thought to arise from gene duplications occurring during the evolution of the cascade (Science Box 2.2). The pathways are, however, triggered by different substances and through different initiation mechanisms.

Complement

- Complement comprises a large number of serum proteins that are mainly made in the liver.
- Complement forms protein cascades, each activated component catalysing the activation of several molecules of the next component, causing amplification of the response.
- The consequences of complement activation are cell lysis, production of pro-inflammatory mediators and solubilisation of antigen–antibody complexes.
- There are four pathways.

Complement pathways

The three parallel initial pathways of complement each activate the final common pathway. In evolutionary terms, the alternative pathway is relatively primitive and a part of the innate immune system; the classical pathway, which is relatively recent, combines with antibody to initiate activation and is, therefore, an adjunct to the acquired immune system. The mannan-binding lectin pathway is probably somewhere in between — it interacts directly with pathogens and is therefore part of the innate immune system, but structurally it resembles early components of the classical pathway.

The classical pathway

The classical pathway is activated by an interaction between antigen and antibody, forming a so-called **immune complex**. Antibodies can bind to, or 'fix', complement only after reacting with their antigen. The formation of the complex provokes a conformational change in the antibody molecule that discloses a site for binding of the first complement component **C1**. C1 is a multimeric compound composed of six molecules termed **C1q**, and two each of **C1s** and **C1r**. C1q is an elongated protein with a rod-like stem composed of a triple helical structure and a globular head resembling a tulip (Fig. 2.4). It is the globular head that binds antibody. Six C1q molecules arrange themselves in a 'bunch' and the four C1r and C1s molecules attach in a calcium-dependent interaction. When antibody binds to two or more heads of C1q, C1r is cleaved to give an active molecule C1r, which cleaves C1s. C1s extends the activation process by cleaving the next complement component **C4** to C4b, which continues the reaction process, and C4a, which has other biological properties (see below).

Cleavage of C4 to C4b reveals an internal thioester bond, which is swiftly inactivated by binding water molecules unless it can form covalent bonds with cell surface proteins or carbohydrates. Should this happen, C4b becomes relatively stable and binds to **C2** in a magnesium-dependent reaction (Fig. 2.5). This illustrates one of the important forms of control over the complement cascade, namely that enzymatically active molecules are unstable and tend to degrade rapidly unless a solid surface, usually that of a target such as a bacterium, is available.

The C2 is itself then cleaved by C1s to form the complex C4b2b, known as the **classical pathway C3 convertase**. C3

is a similar molecule to C4, having an internal thioester bond. Two fragments derive from C3 cleavage. The smaller of these, C3a, has powerful biological properties; the larger, C3b, displays the labile binding site that allows the molecule to bind to membranes close to, but distinct from, C4b2b. The proximity of C3b to C4b2b leads to the generation of the last enzyme of the classical pathway, C4b2b3b (the **classical pathway C5 convertase**), which cleaves **C5**, a component of the membrane attack pathway.

In addition to antigen–antibody complexes, the activation of the classical pathway can be initiated by aggregated immunoglobulins and by non-immunological stimuli such as C-reactive protein.

The mannan-binding lectin pathway

This has only been uncovered relatively recently. The mannan-binding lectin, or MBL, closely resembles C1q in structure and is activated by binding to microbes. Like C1q, it forms a 'bunch of tulips' structure allowing two serine proteases to bind to the stalks (MBL-associated serine proteases 1 and 2, MASP-1 and -2). This activates the MASPs, which go on to activate C4, and the remainder of the classical pathway flows as described above.

The alternative pathway

Activation of the alternative pathway proceeds in a different manner from that of the classical pathway, since it appears to be based on a 'tickover' mechanism. The concept is analogous to an automatic car. If an engine is idling or 'ticking over', any movement of the throttle will accelerate the engine and cause the car to move. Similarly, in the alternative pathway, there is a continuous, slow reaction sequence that is insufficient to produce any measurable effect. Activators of the alternative pathway are substances that act on the throttle. Availability of C3b is the essential requirement for activation of the alternative pathway to proceed; this requirement is again fulfilled by the internal thioester bond, which undergoes continuous low-grade hydrolysis. Free C3b binds **factor**

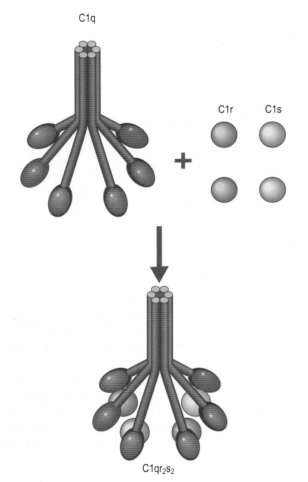

Fig. 2.4 'Tulip' structure of the C1q hexamer with dimers of C1r and C1s in place.
The globular heads of the C1q molecules bind antibody.

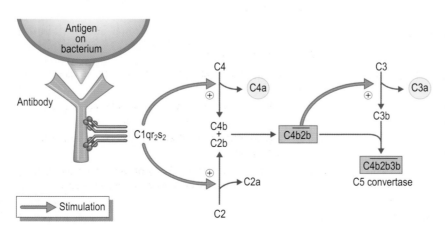

Fig. 2.5 Activation of the classical pathway.
Antigen–antibody complexes bind C1q. The C1qrs complex cleaves C4 and C2 to form the classical pathway C3 convertase C4b2b. Following C3 cleavage, the C5 convertase is formed. Biologically active fragments C4a and C3a are generated. C3b alone has other actions and may also 'drive' forward activation of the alternative pathway.

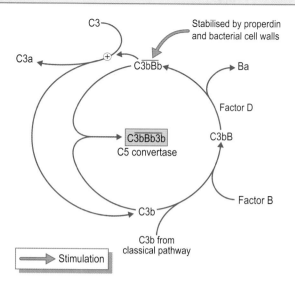

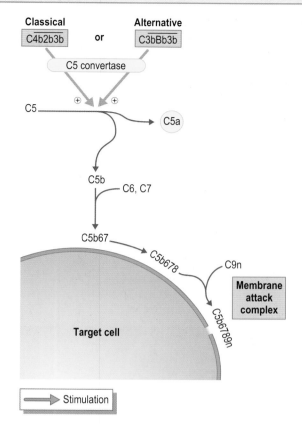

Fig. 2.6 **Alternative pathway activation.**
C3 'tick-over' generates C3b, C3bB and C3bBb, which in turn cleaves C3. The tick-over is accelerated if the active enzymes are stabilised on bacterial cell walls, or if more C3b is produced from the classical pathway. The alternative pathway C5 convertase C3bBb3b is generated.

B and the C3bB complex becomes the substrate of a circulating enzyme, **factor D**, which, by removing from C3bB the fragment Ba, generates C3bBb (Fig. 2.6). This complex, the **alternative pathway C3 convertase**, can cleave C3, detaching C3a from C3b, which can reinitiate the activation process.

How do the alternative pathway activators work? It is thought that bacteria provide a surface for C3b and C3bBb deposition and protection from the destructive action of circulating regulatory factors I and H, allowing the pressure on the throttle to increase. Further impetus is given by properdin, or **factor P**, which stabilises C3bBb and renders it more efficient. Positive feedback is provided here, since C3bBbP generates more C3b, which is capable of forming more enzyme. The complex C3bBb3b, analogous to C4b2b3b, is the **alternative pathway C5 convertase**, initiating the membrane attack pathway sequence.

The membrane attack pathway

This final common complement pathway (Fig. 2.7) generates one more biologically active component, C5a, but more importantly leads to the formation of the 'killer molecule' of the system. This is known as the **membrane attack complex (MAC)**, since it provokes membrane damage. The cleavage of C5 by the classical or alternative pathway convertases gives the smaller fragment C5a and the larger C5b split product, which continues the reaction sequence by binding to **C6** and inducing it to express a labile reactive site for **C7**. The C5b67 complex is highly lipophilic and binds to membranes, where it lies as a high-affinity receptor for **C8**. C8 has three chains, one of which inserts into the membrane, anchoring the C5b678 complex. C5b678 binds and polymer-

Fig. 2.7 **The final common pathway.**
The C5 convertases generate C5b and the pro-inflammatory C5a. C5b67 binds the target cell membrane and with addition of C8 and a C9 polymer the membrane attack complex forms.

ises **C9**, forming the MAC, the final component of the system. As many as 12 to 15 C9 molecules may cluster around one C5b678 complex, inserting into and traversing the membrane bilayer (Fig. 2.8). Holes are made in the membrane, and if a sufficient number are created death results through osmotic lysis.

SUMMARY BOX 2.3

Complement pathways

- Classical pathway is mainly activated by antigen–antibody complexes.

- Alternative pathway has a continual slow reaction that only produces effects if it is accelerated by the presence of a bacterial cell wall.

- The MBL pathway results in activation of the classical pathway.

- Each initial pathway produces a C5 convertase, which initiates the membrane attack pathway.

- The resulting membrane attack complex forms holes in cells causing lysis.

- Control is achieved by the lability of the components, by dilution and by specific regulatory proteins and receptors.

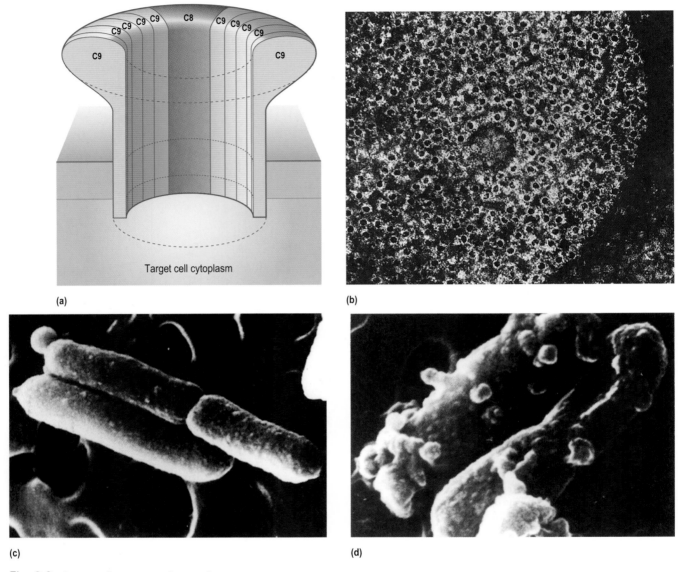

Fig. 2.8 **The membrane attack complex.**
(**a**) Schematic diagram. C5b678 is assembled and inserted into the membrane. Addition of multiple C9 molecules forms the MAC which punches holes in the membrane. (**b**) Electron micrograph of multiple MAC-induced holes in a red blood cell membrane. (**c**) Scanning electron micrograph of intact *Escherichia coli* bacterium and (**d**) after incubation with complement. Note dramatic expansion in size, caused by osmotic effects, and cytoplasmic blebbing (reproduced with permission from Upjohn Inc.).

Complement control mechanisms

Complement activation is kept in check by a variety of control mechanisms. The importance of such regulation is clear from the severity of the pathological states that result from congenital or acquired deficiencies of control proteins (see Ch. 19). We have already seen that lability of the active molecules is an inherent control mechanism, as is dilution into biological fluids. More specific regulation is provided by circulating or membrane-bound proteins. The classical pathway is controlled in its initial stage by **C1-inhibitor** (also known as C1 esterase), a protein in the blood that blocks the enzymatic function of activated C1 by combining with it in a virtually irreversible stoichiometric complex. In the circulation, **factor I** is an enzyme that degrades C3b while **factor H** binds C3b and accelerates the destructive action of factor I (Fig. 2.9). Factor I is also able to restrain activation of the classical pathway by destroying C4b. This destructive process is enhanced if C4b is complexed with a protein called **C4-binding protein** (C4bp). Two circulating proteins with a similar function are **protein S** and **SP-40,40**. Both are capable of binding the C5b67 complex to form an inactive moiety, preventing membrane insertion and formation of the MAC. Finally, a circulating enzyme, **carboxy-peptidase N**, cleaves the carboxy-terminal arginine from C3a, C4a and C5a and the resulting molecules (termed, for example, C5a-des arg) are inactivated.

Other regulatory proteins are membrane bound. A membrane attack complex inhibitory factor — also known as **CD59** or **protectin** — exemplifies membrane-bound control

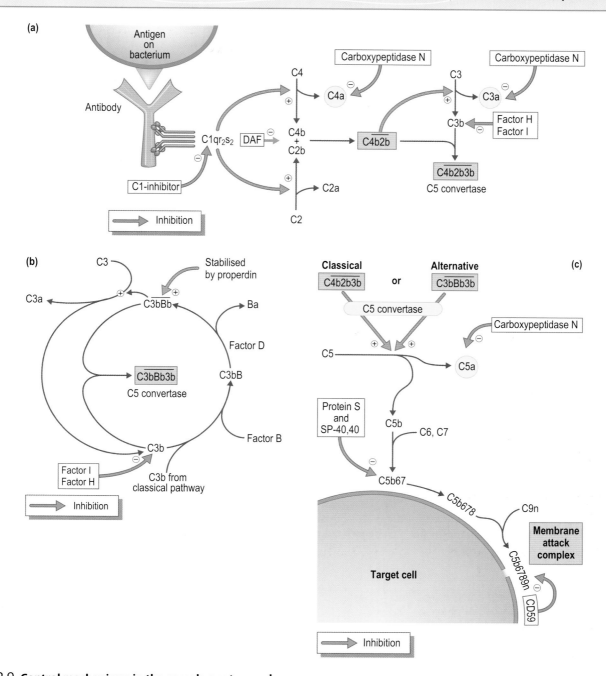

Fig. 2.9 Control mechanisms in the complement cascades.
(**a**) The classical pathway. (**b**) The alternative pathway. (**c**) The final common pathway. See text for details.

proteins. (CD is the abbreviation for **cluster of differentiation**, and CD numbers are widely used to identify surface molecules in the immune system. An outline of the CD system is given in Science Box 2.3: 'The CD classification', p. 20.) CD59 is designed to avoid bystander damage: the accidental insertion of MACs destined for a bacterium into the cell wall of a lymphocyte or other host cell. CD59, constitutively expressed on mammalian cells, interferes with the MAC insertion, thus preventing cell lysis. **Decay accelerating factor** (DAF), a transmembrane glycoprotein found on most blood cells, competes for C4b, thus inhibiting formation of the classical pathway C3 convertase.

Complement receptors

In addition to these membrane proteins, there are a group of receptors that have a more restricted distribution. The **complement receptors** (CR), CR-1 to CR-4, bind breakdown products of C3 predominantly and are found on cells of the immune system (see below). They have a variety of functions, but CR-1 is also involved in regulation of the classical pathway, binding C4b and enhancing the action of factor I in much the same way that C4bp does.

There are two main groups of complement receptors; CR-1 to CR-4 and receptors for the biologically active molecules

SCIENCE BOX 2.3

The CD classification explained

You can be forgiven for thinking that CD has only ever meant 'compact disk', but actually the immunologists got there first. The CD classification is ultimately the new way of defining a cell.

Lymphocytes, monocytes, dendritic cells, granulocytes and a host of other cells have surface receptors and molecules that are vital in a whole range of immunological functions: cell–cell signalling, cell activation, hormone–receptor signalling and many others. The surfaces of immune cells are literally covered with such proteins. Different cells with particular functions have distinct surface proteins, whilst other molecules will be common to several cell types. A major breakthrough in defining surface molecules came in the 1970s, with the discovery of monoclonal antibodies. In a nutshell, monoclonal antibodies are proteins tailor-made to bind to a specific target. They are usually raised by injecting the target protein into mice. Researchers in the 1970s and 1980s raised monoclonal antibodies by injecting mice with crude extracts made from various types of immune cell, to try and find cell and lineage-specific markers. Some of the monoclonal antibodies generated were able to bind to structures on the surfaces of the target cells. These could be used as tools to distinguish populations of lymphocytes with different functions, as well as identifying neutrophils and monocytes.

By the mid-1980s, however, so many monoclonal antibodies were being produced around the world in so many laboratories that confusion reigned: how did we know whether the surface molecule recognised by monoclonal antibody A produced in Atlanta was the same as that recognised by monoclonal antibody B produced in Baltimore? An international workshop was established. Monoclonal antibodies were exchanged by researchers and panels of experts sat to judge whether the antibodies recognised the same target protein. Because several different antibodies (a cluster) could recognise the same surface protein, and because surface proteins indicated the differentiation of a cell (e.g. granulocyte or lymphocyte), the monoclonal antibodies were assigned a number according to the **cluster of differentiation** to which they bound. A cluster of differentiation is, therefore, a surface molecule found on cells according to the cells' lineage and differentiation and identifiable by one or more monoclonal antibodies.

This means that cells can now be defined by the CDs they possess. For example, as you will see later on, a helper T cell could be defined as possessing the CD3 and CD4 markers, but not CD8 (i.e. 'CD3$^+$CD4$^+$CD8$^-$'). International Workshops to define new CDs are organised periodically. The most recent was the 8th, held in 2004, at which 100 new DC designations were confirmed; up to and including CD340 (http://hcdm.org). A list of commonly used CD numbers is given in Appendix 1.

C4a, C3a and C5a. The main properties of these are shown in Table 2.2 and will be considered in the next section and Chapter 3.

Biological activities generated by complement activation

Opsonisation

The Greek word *opson* means a relish or sauce, i.e. something to make food more 'attractive'. When applied to cells such as neutrophils, which engulf microorganisms, the concept of opsonisation is that opsonins coat bacteria and thus facilitate their removal. One of the major opsonins derives from complement. The ability to bind membranes is a feature of various complement fragments, but C3b accounts for most of the complement opsonic activity. Once organisms are coated with C3b, it is simple to see how the presence of CRs 1, 3 and 4 on neutrophils can result in more efficient engulfment.

Cell recruitment and activation

The low-molecular-weight fragments C4a, C3a and C5a are known as **anaphylatoxins**. This name derives from their putative role in a clinical syndrome **anaphylaxis** (see p. 143) in which they activate mast cells and basophils directly through specific receptors. C5a and, to a lesser extent, C3a are also **chemotactic**, a term used to describe the ability to attract cells, in this case neutrophils (see p. 28).

Cell lysis

Complete complement activation through either pathway occurring on cell surfaces leads to cell lysis. Typical targets could include bacteria and enveloped viruses, but host erythrocytes, platelets and lymphocytes may also become victims in certain pathological conditions.

Removal of immune complexes

Immune complexes of antibody and antigen are forming in the circulation continuously in small numbers, with periodic increases during infections or inflammatory episodes. These are potentially harmful, since they can become deposited in vessel walls or tissues and incite complement activation, with all the pro-inflammatory effects that that entails. Larger complexes, composed of a lattice of antibodies and antigens

Table 2.2 Complement receptors

Receptor	Ligands	Cell distribution	Function/comments	CD number
CR-1	C3b and C4b	Erythrocytes Granulocytes, monocytes	Clearance of immune complexes Enhances phagocytosis	CD35
CR-2	C3d, iC3b	B lymphocytes	B cell activation Receptor for Epstein–Barr virus	CD21
CR-3	iC3b, C3b	Monocytes, granulocytes	Cell adhesion	CD11b/CD18
CR-4	iC3b, C3b	Neutrophils, monocytes, dendritic cells	Enhances phagocytosis	CD11c/CD18
C3a/C4a receptor	C3a, C4a	Mast cells, basophils	Degranulation	Not known
C5a receptor	C5a, C5a-des arg	Mast cells, basophils Neutrophils Endothelial cells	Degranulation Chemotactic Increases vascular permeability	CD88

(Fig. 2.10), are more likely to become insoluble and fixed in the tissues. Complement has two key protective functions to prevent such damage: the ability to maintain immune complexes in solution and the ability to expedite their removal from the circulation. The covalent binding of C3b to antibody in a complex inhibits lattice formation and maintains solubility. In addition, C3b-coated complexes attach to erythrocyte CR-1, which acts to remove them from the circulation via the liver and spleen, where they are released and taken up by resident macrophages.

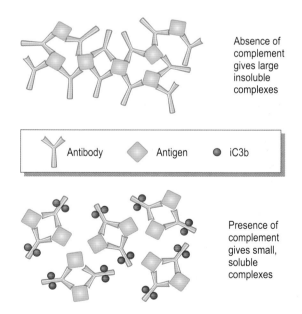

Absence of complement gives large insoluble complexes

Presence of complement gives small, soluble complexes

Fig. 2.10 Lattice formation and the role of complement in immune complex solubilisation.
Since antibodies are divalent (two antigen-binding arms), large antigen–antibody complexes form. C3b binds antibody and forms a complex that stoichiometrically inhibits other antibodies from binding. Soluble complexes can be transported to the spleen and liver for clearance by red blood cells bearing C3b receptors (CR-1).

SUMMARY BOX 2.4

Biological results of activation of the complement system

- Coating pathogens with complement proteins (opsonisation) to enhance phagocytosis.
- Cell recruitment, e.g. C5a attracts neutrophils.
- Cell activation, e.g. mast cells and basophils, directly by C3a, C4a and C5a.
- Cell lysis, e.g. completion of the complement cascade on the surface of a target cell.
- Removal of immune complexes to prevent a harmful build-up of pro-inflammatory molecules.

Other factors in humoral immunity

Other proteins may play a role in the innate immune response. One such is **C-reactive protein** (CRP), so named because of its property of binding to the C-polysaccharide of the pneumococcus. CRP is produced in the liver and binds direct to bacterial cell walls, activating complement through the classical pathway. One of the most striking features of CRP, however, is that its blood levels rise 10- to 100-fold within hours of the start of an infective or inflammatory process. Since it has a relatively short half-life, it has, therefore, become extremely useful in monitoring infective or inflammatory processes, and particularly their response to treatment. It is widely used to monitor responses to treatment in conditions such as rheumatoid arthritis. Recently it has been hailed as a marker of coronary artery disease, although its value as a risk factor remains unclear.

Fibronectin is a circulating protein capable of binding bacteria, particularly staphylococci and streptococci. Since it also binds macrophages and monocytes, it enhances clearance of these organisms. Fibronectin levels decline during infection and, like CRP, it is also used in disease monitoring, particularly in premature babies in whom the innate immune system is especially important.

Lysozyme is a bactericidal enzyme secreted in saliva, tears and other body fluids, as well as being present in neutrophil granules. It cleaves bacterial cell wall proteoglycans at a precise point, breaking the bonds between *N*-acetylglucosamine and *N*-acetylmuraminic acid.

Further reading

Endo Y, Takahashi M, Fujita T 2006 Lectin complement system and pattern recognition. Immunobiology 211: 283–293

Li K, Sacks SH, Zhou W 2007 The relative importance of local and systemic complement production in ischaemia, transplantation and other pathologies. Mol Immunol 44: 3866–3874

Mollnes TE, Jokiranta TS, Truedsson L, Nilsson B, Rodriguez de Cordoba S, Kirschfink M 2007 Complement analysis in the 21st century. Mol Immunol 44: 3838–3849

Zipfel PF, Mihlan M, Skerka C 2007 The alternative pathway of complement: a pattern recognition system. Adv Exp Med Biol 598: 80–92

Innate immunity II:
cellular mechanisms

Working alongside the soluble effector molecules of the innate immune system are a series of cells, which are present and functional at birth and constitute the innate cellular immune system. The granulocytes — neutrophils, eosinophils and basophils — are each present in the blood and have the capacity to migrate into the tissues. Migration of these cells into tissues is unidirectional and may be rapidly up-regulated as required. The mast cell is resident in the tissues, particularly at epithelial surfaces, and is characterised by the presence of abundant intracellular granules. A fifth circulating cell type involved in innate immunity, the NK cell, has a more specialised function in immune surveillance against viral infection and possibly against tumour cells, but in view of its similarities with the T lymphocyte, it will be described in a later chapter (p. 113).

Neutrophils, eosinophils and basophils are involved in different areas of the immune response. Neutrophils are adapted to the killing and removal of bacteria and fungi, while eosinophils have a predominant role in the control of infection with multicellular parasites, such as worms. Basophils and mast cells have a less well-defined physiological role in immunity, but are important in that they are involved in the pathogenesis (i.e. the mechanism of pathological tissue damage) of the clinical syndrome known as allergy, a common and debilitating immune-mediated disorder. Whilst the functional activity of granulocytes and mast cells varies with the cell type, all four of these different cells discharge some of their functions through the release of granules. As we have seen with the complement system, it is artificial to make strict divisions between the innate and acquired immune systems. Just like complement, granulocytes and mast cells can have their innate functions in the immune response modified and given more direction by specific antibody (see Ch. 2 and p. 29).

The sequence of events that leads from a granulocyte in the resting state to the completion of its role in an immune response includes signalling, activation, migration from the blood and effector function. Migration into tissues is not a random but rather a directed process. It involves adhesion between receptors on the granulocyte surface and their ligands on the membranes of endothelial cells, which provide the gateway to the tissues. Some of the adhesion molecules involved are also employed for migration by lymphoid cells.

In the present chapter the mechanisms through which granulocytes become activated, their adhesive and migratory properties and the toxic effector molecules that they generate will be discussed. In Chapter 8, it will be possible to see the way in which these responses dovetail with other elements of the immune system to provide protection from pathogens. In the case of the mast cell, the present section will outline the mechanisms and effects of cell activation, whilst its role in allergy will be discussed in Chapter 10.

Neutrophils

The neutrophil has a distinctive appearance, with its polymorphic nucleus and neutral staining granules. The multilobed nucleus is important for the cell to make rapid transit from the blood through tight gaps in the endothelium. The neutrophil is abundant in the circulation, present at a concentration of $2-7 \times 10^9$ per litre. The half-life in blood is

6 hours and in the tissues 1–2 days; the cells are replaced from the bone marrow, which can produce between 10^{11} (healthy state) and 10^{12} (during infection) new cells per day. In health, few neutrophils will be seen in the tissues.

Neutrophil granules

Neutrophils have two main types of granule: the first appear during their development in the bone marrow (primary or azurophilic granules) and the second group appears later (secondary or specific granules); secondary granules are three times more common in the cytoplasm. There are approaching 100 different molecules in the granules — a simplified list of the major granule contents, and the functions associated with them, are shown in Table 3.1.

Both primary and secondary granules may be released intracellularly or extracellularly following fusion with the plasma membrane. Granules are mobilised in response to several stimuli: the products of bacterial cell walls, complement proteins, the leukotriene group of lipid mediators and small bioactive peptides called cytokines. **N-formylated peptides** (for example, *N*-formyl-methionyl-leucylphenylalanine; FMLP) are bacterially derived and bind to receptors on the neutrophil surface. The ability of neutrophils to respond to bacterial proteins is clearly a major advantage for their innate responses. Activation products from **complement**, such as iC3b, also bind to specific surface membrane receptors. **Leukotrienes** (LT) are biologically active products of the lipooxygenase pathway of arachidonate metabolism and some, such as LTB_4, have potent stimulatory effects on neutrophils (see Science Box 3.1). Finally, natural chemical mediators such as the **chemokine** CXCL8 (also known as interleukin-8; IL-8) and the **cytokines** tumour necrosis

factor-α, (TNF-α) and granulocyte–monocyte colony stimulating factor (GM–CSF) have potent effects on neutrophils (for an introduction to these chemical mediators, see Science Boxes 3.2 and 3.3).

As might be expected, the major functions of granule contents are the killing and digestion of microorganisms. Within the primary/azurophilic granules are important anti-bacterial effector molecules, especially myeloperoxidase, which participates in a major microbicidal system (see p. 31). Cathepsin G and its related serprocidins, proteinase-3 and elastase, are deadly to a range of Gram-positive and Gram-negative organisms, as well as some *Candida* species. Cathepsins B, D and E are also present and bactericidal. Defensins are naturally occurring cysteine-rich antibacterial and antifungal polypeptides (29–35 amino acids). Three defensins (human neutrophil peptides 1–3; HNP1–3) make up 5% of all the protein in a neutrophil and act by insertion into pathogen membranes to disrupt ion fluxes. Bactericidal/permeability increasing protein (BPI) is toxic to Gram-negative bacteria.

The secondary granules contain preformed receptors and an assortment of proteins. Particularly notable are the cytochrome b_{558} and its associated proteins, which constitute a major bactericidal mechanism. The secondary granules also contain presynthesised receptors for some of the molecules capable of activating them (FMLP, complement). As secondary granules are released at a site on the neutrophil surface, therefore, the pole of the membrane that is involved shows an increase in specific receptors, enhancing the directional nature of the response. This may be particularly important in the process known as chemotaxis, the directed movement of cells (see p. 28). Collagenase and elastase break down fibrous structures in the extracellular matrix, facilitating progress of the neutrophil through the tissues.

Table 3.1 Contents and function of neutrophil granules

Function	Primary/azurophilic granules	Secondary/specific granules
Microbicidal	Myeloperoxidase (MPO) Cathepsin G Proteinase-3 Elastase Lysozyme Defensins Bactericidal/permeability increasing protein (BPI)	Cytochrome b_{558} and other respiratory burst components Lysozyme Lactoferrin
Migration		Collagenase CD11b/CD18 (CR-3) *N*-formyl-methionyl-leucylphenylalanine receptor (FMLP-R)

SCIENCE BOX 3.1

Arachidonic acid metabolites in inflammation

Following the activation of several different types of cell — especially the mast cell (see p. 32), but also macrophages, granulocytes and lymphocytes — lipids in the cell membrane are converted de novo into inflammatory mediators that have potent effects on the vasculature and on inflammatory cells such as the neutrophil. There are three different classes of such lipid mediators, all deriving from precursor membrane phospholipids and being converted by the action of the enzyme phospholipase A2 (see Fig. 3.1).

The first major lipid mediator to be described was **prostaglandin D$_2$** (PGD$_2$), derived from the cyclooxygenase pathway of arachidonic acid metabolism. This binds receptors on smooth muscle in the vascular endothelium, leading to vasodilatation. This increases blood supply and slows leukocytes passing through the tissues, allowing them to migrate from the blood. Other types of prostaglandin (e.g. PGE$_2$ and PGF$_2$, produced by macrophages) also have potent pro-inflammatory effects.

The second major group of mediators are termed the **leukotrienes** and are formed when arachidonic acid is converted through the lipooxygenase pathway. Mast cells synthesise LTB$_4$, LTC$_4$, LTD$_4$ and LTE$_4$, whilst the neutrophil synthesises LTB$_4$. These mediators also cause vasodilatation, as well as extravasation of fluid into the tissues.

The third lipid-derived mediator, **platelet-activating factor** (PAF), is produced by mast cells and also has the effect of relaxing vascular smooth muscle.

Perhaps one of the major driving forces behind the research in this field has been the knowledge that the lipid derivatives released as a result of these inflammatory reactions have a profound effect on smooth muscle in the lung, causing bronchial constriction. This is manifest as tightness of the chest and wheezing, symptoms of the chronic chest condition called **asthma**. In addition, these mediators are involved in pathways that lead to inflammation and pain sensation. The class of drugs known as **non-steroidal anti-inflammatory drugs (NSAIDs)**, such as

aspirin, which block cyclooxygenase, are thus important in the control of symptoms of diseases like arthritis. However, they have the side-effect of increasing stomach inflammation, which in severe cases leads to fatal haemorrhage. In recent years two different forms of cyclooxygenase have been identified, Cox-1 and Cox-2. Cox-2 inhibitors are a particularly attractive therapeutic option, since the Cox-2 pathway is selective for pain and inflammation, but spares gastric effects. It was thus an important breakthrough when the Cox-2 inhibiting drug Vioxx® appeared on the market. Unfortunately its safety profile was not as good as hoped, and several high profile lawsuits following fatal clot formation led to its withdrawal, serving to illustrate the complexity of this class of mediators.

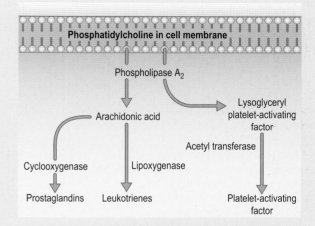

Fig. 3.1 **Biosynthetic pathways of lipid mediators, the leukotrienes, prostaglandins and platelet-activating factor.**

Neutrophil activation and migration

Neutrophils are activated by numerous stimuli: major molecules involved include the complement component C5a, LTB$_4$, FMLP and CXCL8. Each of these is likely to be released at sites of infection and inflammation. To make their contribution to the inflammatory process, neutrophils must migrate to the relevant site in the tissues. This requires some organisation: the affected organ must signal the focus of injury and the neutrophil must bind and adhere specifically to that tissue. This process of crossing into tissues is highly organised, has a similar basis for all immune cells, and has three basic steps: rolling, adhesion and trans-migration, which are achieved through the use of specialised **adhesion molecules**.

The interface between tissues and blood is formed by endothelial cells. Tissue signals are given out by endothelial

cells lining the post-capillary venules, where blood flow is at its slowest. Tissue damage, whether it is caused by infection or other injury, results in the release of mediators, such as histamine from mast cells (see p. 32), with profound effects on vessel walls. The resulting dilatation of vessels, with increased 'leakiness' and further reduction of the rate of blood flow facilitates neutrophil access to the site of tissue damage. Neutrophils have a tendency even in the resting state to adhere very lightly to the endothelium, in a process termed 'rolling'. This slows their movement right down, but is not sufficiently strong for them to stop. The neutrophils roll along the margin of the vessel, hence the term **margination**. The molecules responsible for rolling are the **selectins** (see below).

More specific mechanisms are now required for the neutrophil to halt and exit the bloodstream. Chemokines such as CXCL8 released from damaged tissues, bacterial cell-wall

SCIENCE BOX 3.2

Introducing cytokines

Cytokines can be defined as polypeptides (15–20 kDa molecular mass) released by a cell in order to change the function of the same or another cell. Cytokines are important chemical messengers in many contexts, and especially in the immune system. In immunological disease, cytokines have become both therapeutic agents and the *targets* of therapeutic agents in their own right (see pp. 317–322). There are several important features of cytokines:

- Each cytokine has many different effects on different cells: this property is called **pleiotropy**.

- A cytokine can have a direct effect on the cell that releases it: this is called an **autocrine** function and serves as a feedback mechanism.

- Cytokines can also have effects on cells immediately around them: this is a **paracrine** function.

- In addition, cytokines may act like hormones and have **endocrine** effects on cells and organs remote from the site of release.

- Cytokines often induce the release of other cytokines.

- One final property is that of **synergism**: cytokines may act in concert to achieve an effect greater than the summation of their individual actions.

The main cytokines you will encounter are the interferons (IFNs) and the interleukins (IL). The IFNs are limited to a few major types, and you will mainly encounter α, β and γ. In contrast, as of mid-2008 we are up to IL-35 and rising.

SCIENCE BOX 3.3

Introducing chemokines

Chemokines are a more recently recognised group of the type of immunological molecules that we have loosely termed 'natural chemical mediators' than are the cytokines. The defining feature of chemokines is that they function as chemotactic molecules — that is, they attract cells along a gradient of low to high chemical mediator. Thus chemokines have an important role in the trafficking of cells of the immune system. Chemokines have also gained notoriety from the fact that two members of their family of receptors, CXCR5 and CCR4, are co-receptors used by the human immunodeficiency virus to gain entry into target cells.

The nomenclature has suffered slightly from the fact that some molecules were identified as important immune mediators before the family of chemokines became a defined entity. Thus you may encounter some mediators (e.g. IL-8, which is CXCL8) being referred to by more than one name. There are now in excess of 50 chemokines. They are small (8–10 kD in size) and have a strikingly similar structure revolving around the configuration of cysteine residues at the amino terminus and giving rise to four families. Two cysteines

separated by any other amino acid residue is CXC; two cysteines next to each other is CC; one cysteine is C and two cysteines separated by any three amino acids are CX3C. The receptors are denoted by 'R', and are all distinctive G-coupled protein receptors with seven transmembrane spanning domains. There are more chemokines than receptors — it appears that the receptors can be shared.

Some chemokines are released by most nucleated cells in response to inflammation and have a role in chemotaxis, attracting immune cells to inflammatory foci (e.g. CXCL8); others are released in a programmed fashion by specialised cells in the immune system and have specific functions, especially in relation to development of secondary lymphoid organs (e.g. CXCL12). Like cytokines, however, chemokines are highly pleiotropic. Chemotactic chemokines appear to function in one of two ways. Either there is release of soluble chemokine and direct binding to the receptor, which leads to target cell changes; or the chemokine binds to components of the extracellular matrix, and forms a gradient or 'paper trail', along which attracted cells flow.

---

products such as FMLP, or cytokines such as TNF-α can have a direct effect on the endothelial cells, causing them to express stronger adhesion molecules, so that they become 'sticky' and the neutrophils adhere firmly. Stickiness results from the increased expression of a family of adhesion molecules on the endothelium (**ICAMs**; see below); at the same time, the counter-ligands for these are up-regulated on the rolling neutrophils (**LFA-1**; see below), again as a result of mediators such as CXCL1–3, 5, 6 and 8, as well as FMLP, C5a, which they are now beginning to encounter as they slow down near to the inflammatory focus. Similar stimuli up-

regulate the ligands and counter-ligands on the migrating cell and the vessel wall, so that adhesion is a concerted process. These adhesion molecules are found on all leukocytes and a variety of other cells. The interaction between complementary molecules on neutrophils and endothelial cells results in adhesion of the neutrophils and the opportunity for them to enter the tissue.

The whole process of margination, rolling and transmigration can be likened to a motorway with several lanes of traffic. If a driver wishes to be able to exit he must be in the slow lane to be ready for the slip-road, whilst the speed

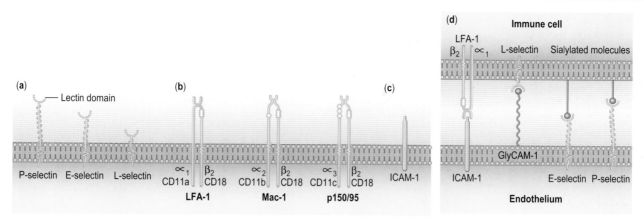

Fig. 3.2 **Adhesion molecules.**
(**a**) The selectins have N-terminal domains that are homologous to a variety of sugar-binding lectins. (**b**) The β_2 integrin family have similar structures with α and β chains that are non-covalently associated. (**c**) The ICAMs have a domain structure similar to immunoglobulin. (**d**) Interaction between these molecules (modified with permission from Springer 1990 Nature 346: 426–427).

Table 3.2 The selectins

CD	Selectin type	Cell type expressed on	Ligand and its site
CD62	P-selectin	Endothelium	Sialyl Lewis^X (CD15s) on neutrophils
CD62E	E-selectin	Endothelium; platelets	Sialyl Lewis^X (CD15s) on neutrophils
CD62L	L-selectin	Neutrophil	GlyCAM-1 on peripheral lymph node endothelium; MAdCAM-1 on mucosal endothelium

Note: Sialyl Lewis^X (CD15s) is a carbohydrate moiety on leukocytes, especially neutrophils; GlyCAM-1, glycoprotein cell adhesion molecule-1; MAdCAM-1, mucosal vascular addressin cell adhesion molecule-1.

of flow makes exiting from the fast lanes much more difficult.

Adhesion molecules

Broadly speaking, there are three main families of surface proteins whose prime role appears to be intercellular adhesion, and these are defined on the basis of shared structural features (Fig. 3.2): the **selectin** and **integrin** families and a third group, the **intercellular adhesion molecules** (ICAMs).

Selectins

Selectins were named because their N-terminal domain resembles various lectins (lectins are molecules with affinity for sugar moieties); the selectins have diverse roles in cell adhesion. Currently, there are three well-described selectins, P-selectin, E-selectin and L-selectin (Fig. 3.2a; Table 3.2). The

'P', 'E' and 'L' stand for platelet, endothelium and leukocyte, respectively, indicating the predominant cell type expressing each selectin. Despite its name, P-selectin is also found on activated endothelium. P-selectin and E-selectin bind a sialylated carbohydrate residue, which is constitutively expressed on circulating immune cells (called sialyl Lewis^X, CD15s); this interaction mediates the rolling. L-selectin is used for homing to lymph nodes — it is expressed on naïve lymphocytes and binds a glycoprotein cell adhesion molecule (GlyCAM-1) found on the high endothelial venules of lymph nodes. It can also bind a distinctive glycoprotein cell adhesion molecule found on mucosal endothelium, termed MAdCAM-1. GlyCAM-1 and MAdCAM-1 guide leukocytes to particular tissues and have thus been termed 'addressins'.

Integrins

The integrins are heterodimers; in other words the functional unit is composed of two different polypeptide molecules,

Table 3.3 The integrins

CD designation	Integrin	Cell type expressed on	Ligand and its site
CD11a/CD18	Leukocyte function associated antigen-1 (LFA-1)	Neutrophils; lymphocytes; monocytes	ICAM-1 and ICAM-2 on endothelium
CD11b/CD18	Macrophage-1 (Mac-1); complement receptor-3 (CR-3)	Neutrophils; monocytes; some lymphocytes	ICAM-1 on endothelium; iC3b following complement activation
CD11c/CD18	p150/95; complement receptor-4 (CR-4)	Tissue macrophages (to a lesser extent neutrophils and monocytes)	iC3b; C4b

in this case termed the α and β chains. They are responsible for stopping cells on the vessel wall, by interacting with ICAMs. There are two families of integrins, defined according to the structure of the β chain. The β_2 integrins are important in adhesion in all leukocytes including lymphocytes: these will be discussed here (Table 3.3). The β_1 integrins are a family of adhesion molecules of particular importance in T and B cell function: these will be discussed in a later section (see p. 85).

The β_2 integrins have a common β chain and three different α chains (Fig. 3.2b). Using the CD nomenclature, the common β_2 chain of 750 amino acid residues is CD18, the α chains (1100 residues) are CD11a, CD11b and CD11c. The heterodimer combination CD11a/CD18 is leukocyte function associated antigen-1 (LFA-1) and is found on lymphocytes, monocytes and neutrophils. CD11b/CD18, which is also complement receptor-3 (CR-3), is present mainly on granulocytes and monocytes. CD11c/CD18 is also termed complement receptor-4 (CR-4).

The main adhesion molecule amongst these, LFA-1, is present on most immune cells, including neutrophils, at a reasonably high level all of the time. However, unless the cell has received the correct signalling, the 'resting' form of LFA-1 is inactive, and has very low affinity for the ICAMs. The resting form of LFA-1 has to undergo a change of conformation so that it now becomes able to bind ICAM. This is termed functional up-regulation. It can be achieved by a variety of signals, which differ from cell to cell, but in the case of neutrophils the main signal is probably provided by CXCL8.

Intercellular adhesion molecules (ICAMs)

The ligands for the integrins are shown in Table 3.3. In the context of neutrophil adhesion, the most important interactions are between CD11b/CD18 and CD11c/CD18 with ICAMs 1 and 2, respectively, on the luminal surface of endothelial cells. ICAMs are single-chain molecules that form part of the so-called immunoglobulin superfamily. They have a structure comprising five immunoglobulin-like domains (Fig. 3.2c). ICAM-1, as well as its physiological role as the ligand for integrins, is also the receptor for rhinoviruses, which cause the common cold. ICAMs are expressed on resting endothelium, but are up-regulated by inflammatory mediators such as TNF-α.

It is worth noting that the CD11/CD18 interaction with ICAMs is not just used within the immune system for cell migration. These molecules provide such a good degree of adhesion that they are used during other forms of cell-to-cell contact, such as when antigen presenting cells interact with T cells (see p. 104).

Chemotaxis

Chemotaxis is defined as the directed movement of a cell along a gradient of increasing concentration of the attracting molecule (termed a chemoattractant). It is a property used by neutrophils when they migrate to the site in the tissues where the concentration of chemotactic factors is highest: in other words, the epicentre of the inflammatory process. The most potent chemotactic factors are the C5a complement component, FMLP, CXCL8 and LTB_4.

Neutrophils have a constant process of random movement akin to the Brownian motion of molecules in the gaseous phase. When a chemotactic factor binds at one pole of the cell, two processes take place: there is granule release, to up-regulate receptors for the chemotactic factors at that pole; and the neutrophil extends its membrane and cytoplasm into thin, foot-like processes known as pseudopodia (Fig. 3.4). After extending, the leading pseudopodium anchors itself and the remainder of the cytoplasm is drawn up. A new pseudopodium is extended and the process repeated; the motion can best be described as resembling that of a caterpillar. Pseudopodia are rich in microtubules, actin, myosin and actin-binding protein, which forms the actin into a lattice structure.

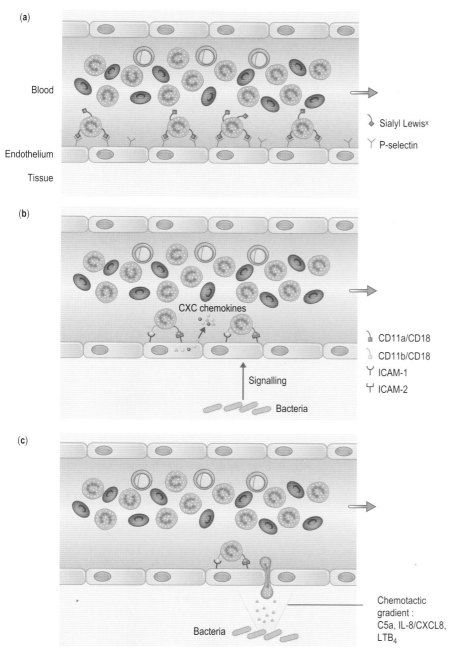

(a)

Blood

Endothelium

Tissue

γ Sialyl Lewis^x

Υ P-selectin

(b)

CXC chemokines

Signalling

Bacteria

$\blacksquare$ CD11a/CD18

$\circ$ CD11b/CD18

Υ ICAM-1

$\sqcup$ ICAM-2

(c)

Bacteria

Chemotactic gradient : C5a, IL-8/CXCL8, LTB$_4$

Fig. 3.3 **Neutrophil adhesion.**
(**a**) Margination and rolling of neutrophils, due to weak interactions between constitutively expressed molecules on these cells and endothelium.
(**b**) Activation of neutrophils and endothelium causes expression of integrins and ICAMs, and the neutrophil stops. (**c**) Permeation of the neutrophils through the endothelium (diapedesis).

Phagocytosis

The ability to ingest and kill microorganisms is a key component in host defence. Neutrophils have the capacity to ingest more than one bacterium or fungus at once in the process of phagocytosis, and this is equally applicable to other macromolecular structures. When large numbers of phagocytes are involved in an infective process, an abscess filled with pus (dead or dying neutrophils) may form.

Phagocytosis is comparatively ineffective in the absence of **opsonins**, the co-factors that coat microorganisms and enhance the ability of neutrophils to engulf them (opsonisation; Fig. 3.5). Receptors for the opsonins are

present on the neutrophil surface, forming a bridge between cell and organism. Typical high efficiency opsonins are the complement component C3b, C-reactive protein and antibody. The role of antibody, raised against a particular organism, is a good example of the specific immune system giving direction to the innate.

Phagocytosis is achieved using pseudopodia. These are extended to surround an organism or particle and eventually meet and fuse to form an enclosed vacuole termed a **phagosome**. The intracellular phagosome can now be fused with neutrophil granules, releasing their digestive and toxic contents to attack the phagosome contents (Fig. 3.6). Occasionally, granule contents may be discharged into the external

Basic and clinical immunology

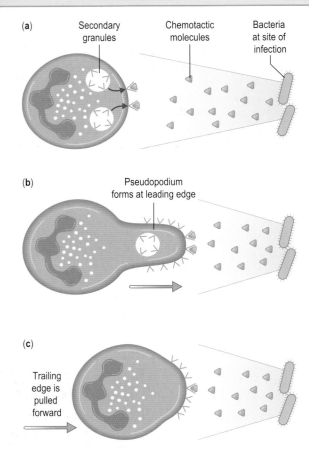

Fig. 3.4 **Neutrophil chemotaxis.**

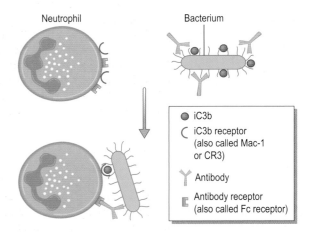

Fig. 3.5 **Opsonisation.**
Opsonins coat microorganisms and enhance the neutrophils' ability to engulf them.

milieu, for example if a particle is too large to engulf, leading to tissue damage; this process is termed 'reverse phagocytosis'. In fact, when this happens, the granule proteins and chromatin combine to form extracellular fibres that bind Gram-positive and Gram-negative bacteria. These **neutrophil extracellular traps** (**NETs**) appear to be a form of innate response that binds microorganisms, prevents them from

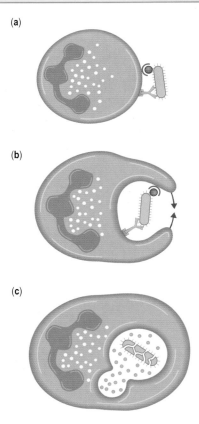

Fig. 3.6 **Phagocytosis.**
(**a**) Opsonised bacterium binds to neutrophil. (**b**) Pseudopodia extend around the bacterium. (**c**) Bacterium is engulfed inside a phagosome to which granules fuse and release their contents.

spreading, and ensures a high local concentration of antimicrobial agents to degrade virulence factors and kill bacteria.

Neutrophil killing

Killing bacteria and fungi is a critical, life-saving activity of neutrophils. In some disorders, killing by these cells is impaired and although the ability to phagocytose may remain intact, the individual suffers recurrent, often fatal infections (see Clinical Box 3.1). Killing is the end result of complex molecular and biochemical mechanisms. There are two major microbicidal routes: one is **oxygen dependent** and the other **oxygen independent**. The oxygen-independent mechanisms are those alluded to earlier; microbicidal enzymes such as lysozyme and the cathepsins. There are two oxygen-dependent mechanisms: the **respiratory burst** and the **hydrogen peroxide–myeloperoxidase–halide system**. The best known is the respiratory burst, so called because of its use of oxygen (see Science Box 3.4). The respiratory burst results from the interaction of several membrane-bound components in the secondary granules and the main toxic metabolites generated are:

- superoxide anion O_2^-
- hydrogen peroxide H_2O_2

CLINICAL BOX 3.1

When neutrophils fail us

Nothing has been more graphic in illustrating the critical role of normal neutrophil function in maintaining a physiological balance of immunity than the elucidation of genetic abnormalities in which one component of the neutrophil is missing or impaired. In all of these abnormalities, recurrent bacterial and fungal infections lead to failure to thrive, organ damage and premature death.

For example, several cases have been described of a condition in which the secondary granules are absent. The affected children suffer lung and skin infections, the main organisms involved being *Staphylococcus aureus* and *Candida albicans*. In a slightly more common abnormality, the respiratory burst fails, usually because of the absence of one of the required secondary granule membrane components. Again, pus-forming organisms and fungi cause frequent and prolonged infections of bone, skin and lungs. In another condition, the common β chain of the integrins is not synthesised. The resulting failure of leukocyte adhesion severely impairs immunity in the tissues, giving rise to repeated infections and premature death (**leukocyte adhesion deficiency syndrome; LAD**).

- singlet oxygen $^1O_2$
- hydroxyl radical $^\bullet OH$.

In the hydrogen peroxide–myeloperoxidase–halide system, H_2O_2 generated by the respiratory burst, myeloperoxidase from the primary granules and a halide such as Cl^- combine to give chlorine and hydroxyl ions, both of which are toxic to microorganisms.

SUMMARY BOX 3.1

Neutrophils

- The neutrophil is an essential component of the cellular innate immune system, involved in killing bacteria and fungi.
- A pool of neutrophils continuously rolls along the endothelial surface of blood vessels tethered by weak cell–cell interactions mediated by specific receptors.
- Following activation of both neutrophil and endothelium, specialised adhesion molecules halt neutrophil rolling and facilitate their entry into the tissues.
- Neutrophils move towards chemical attractants, and engulf microorganisms by phagocytosis.
- Killing is mediated by oxygen-dependent and oxygen-independent routes: the most important involves the generation of a respiratory burst.

SCIENCE BOX 3.4

Oxygen-dependent mechanisms to produce toxic metabolites

The respiratory burst
1. *Generation of superoxide anion*

   $O_2 + electron \rightarrow O_2^-$
   (It is not clear where the electron comes from: probably a $NADPH \rightarrow NADH + H^+$ reaction.)
2. *Generation of hydrogen peroxide*

   $HO_2 + O_2^- + H \xrightarrow{\text{superoxide dismutase}} O_2 + H_2O_2$
3. *Generation of singlet oxygen*

   $H_2O_2 + OCl^- \rightarrow {}^1O_2 + H_2O + Cl^-$
4. *Generation of hydroxyl radical*

   $O_2^- + H_2O_2 \rightarrow O_2 + OH^- + {}^\bullet OH$

The hydrogen peroxide–myeloperoxidase–halide microbicidal system
$H_2O_2^- + 2Cl^- + H^+ \xrightarrow{\text{myeloperoxidase}} H_2O_2 + Cl_2 + OH^-$

Eosinophils

The eosinophil comprises some 3–5% of all granulocytes in the circulation. This statistic hides the reality, however, since several hundred times more eosinophils are present in the tissues, where they collect preferentially at epithelial surfaces and may survive for several weeks. The distinctive staining of eosinophils is a result of the granule contents, mainly cationic (i.e. basic) proteins with affinity for acid aniline dyes such as eosin, and this remains the best method of identification. The main role of eosinophils in host defence is in protection against multicellular parasites such as worms (helminths), which is afforded by the release of toxic, cationic proteins. Outside the tropics, however, they are important for their contribution to allergic disease, particularly asthma.

Eosinophil granules

There are two main types of granule in the eosinophil: specific (95%) and primary (5%). The specific granules contain the cationic proteins, of which there are four main types. **Major basic protein** (MBP; so-called because it is the most abundant cationic protein), **eosinophil cationic protein** (ECP) and **eosinophil neurotoxin** are all potently and exquisitely toxic to helminths, while ECP also has some bactericidal properties. **Eosinophil peroxidase** is distinct from myeloperoxidase in neutrophils but catalyses a similar reaction generating toxic metabolites.

The primary granule enables swift release of LTC_4 and LTD_4. LTC_4 and another mediator, platelet activating factor (PAF), to produce changes in airway smooth muscle and vasculature, which are important in allergic reactions (see below).

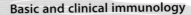

Eosinophil activation and migration

Like neutrophils, eosinophils are activated and recruited by a variety of mediators for which they have receptors. Specific receptors for C3b/C4b (CR-1), iC3b (CR-3), C5a and LTB$_4$ are present on the membrane. In addition, there is a pair of CC chemokines, termed **eotaxin-1** (CCL11) and **eotaxin-2** (CCL24) that are highly selective in eosinophil recruitment. Ligand binding to any of these receptors may activate the cell. Receptors are also present for the cytokines IL-3 and IL-5, which promote the development and differentiation of eosinophils, and for GM-CSF, which also acts on other cells as the name suggests (granulocyte monocyte colon stimulating factor). IL-5 is an essential and sufficient growth factor for eosinophils and may also be produced by them.

Eosinophils in host defence

The most important factors in neutrophil recruitment and activation are thus IL-5 (released by a subset of T lymphocytes termed T$_H$2) and the eotaxins. Although in vitro studies demonstrate that eosinophils are capable of phagocytosis and intracellular degranulation, in vivo they probably employ complement and antibody-guided local release of toxic cationic proteins onto the surface of helminths. There is increasing evidence that their defensive properties overlap with those of the acquired immune response. Eosinophils can synthesise and express on their surface CD4 and HLA-DR (see p. 88), which are associated with T lymphocyte responses. This evidence, taken with their longer life, compared with neutrophils, ability to secrete cytokines and maintain and perpetuate a state of cell activation, indicates that they are a markedly more sophisticated cell than the neutrophil.

SUMMARY BOX 3.2

Eosinophils

- The eosinophil contains several cationic proteins that are vital in host defence against helminthic parasites.
- At a more sophisticated level, eosinophil responses are under cytokine control and may involve interaction with lymphocytes.
- Eosinophils are a feature of the infiltrate in tissues involved in allergic responses, though their role remains unclear.

Mast cells and basophils

Mast cells and basophils share many features in common. The two main features of these cells are the histamine-containing granules and the possession of high-affinity receptors for IgE (contrasting with the low-affinity type on eosinophils). Basophils probably derive from a precursor cell in common with eosinophils; mast cells are thought to have a separate lineage, although controversy over the origins of these cells remains.

Mast cell and basophil granules

Mast cell and basophil mediators are categorised as pre-formed and as those synthesised de novo (Table 3.4; Figs 3.7 and 3.8). The best known is **histamine**, a low-molecular-mass amine (111 Da) with a blood half-life of less than 5 minutes and which constitutes 10% of the cell's weight (see Clinical Box 3.2). Injected into the skin, histamine induces the typical 'wheal and flare' or 'triple' response. Initially there is reddening (erythema) of the skin at the site as arterioles dilate and post-capillary venules contract. This is followed by increased vascular permeability, with leakage of plasma fluid into the tissues causing swelling (wheal). Finally, histamine acts directly on local axons to induce more widespread vascular changes distant from the injection site (flare).

Mast cell and basophil activation

Activation of mast cells and basophils by the antibody class IgE is an important feature of allergic disease that will be dealt with subsequently (Ch. 10). The anaphylatoxins C3a, C4a and C5a activate basophils and may activate lung mast cells, while FMLP probably acts on basophils alone.

CLINICAL BOX 3.2

Histamine

Histamine has two receptors. The H$_1$ receptor mediates the vascular and bronchial smooth muscle effects and is blocked by drugs such as mepyramine and terfenadine, which form the basis of many proprietary antihistamines used for allergic reactions such as hay fever. The H$_2$ receptor mediates gastric acid secretion and is blocked by the now famous drugs cimetidine and ranitidine, which have revolutionised treatment of gastric and duodenal ulceration.

The consequences of mast cell and basophil degranulation depend upon the site of release. In contact with the airways, histamine induces smooth muscle contraction, a process that underlies the airway obstruction seen in asthma. At other mucosal sites, there may be tear formation, nasal discharge (coryza), conjunctival redness, gritty eyes and itching. Widespread activation of mast cells and basophils with release of mediators into the circulation results in the state termed **anaphylaxis** — a syndrome of circulatory shock and collapse with low blood pressure and chest tightness leading to arrested breathing and death unless treated.

Table 3.4 Mast cell and basophil mediators

Mediators	Actions/comments
Pre-formed mediator	
Histamine	Vasodilatation Vascular permeability $\uparrow$ Smooth muscle contraction in airways
Protease enzymes	Mainly tryptic enzymes (cf. pancreatic trypsin) Digestion of basement membrane causes $\uparrow$ vascular permeability Digestion of connective tissue to $\uparrow$ cell migration Cleavage of C3 $\rightarrow$ C3a
Proteoglycans	Mainly heparin in mast cells Mainly chondroitin sulphate in basophils Responsible for distinctive blue staining Anticoagulant activity
Chemotactic factors	Eosinophil chemotactic factor of anaphylaxis Neutrophil chemotactic factor
Synthesised de novo	
Platelet activating factor (PAF)	Vasodilator
LTB_4, LTC_4, LTD_4	Eosinophil activators Neutrophil chemoattractants Platelet activators Vascular permeability $\uparrow$ Bronchoconstrictors
Prostaglandins (mainly PGD_2)	Vascular permeability $\uparrow$ Bronchoconstrictors Vasodilators

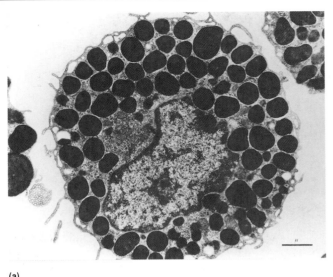

(a)

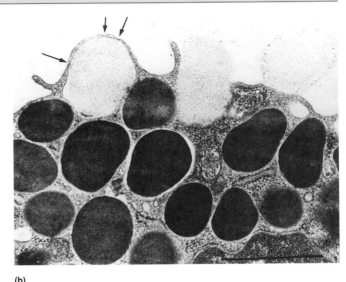

(b)

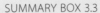

Fig. 3.7 **Granule release from mast cells.**

Electron micrographs of a normal mast cell (**a**) and a mast cell 20 seconds after activation (**b**). The release of granules (arrowed) results in a loss of electron density (reproduced with permission from Upjohn, Inc.).

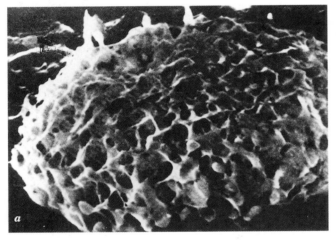

(a)

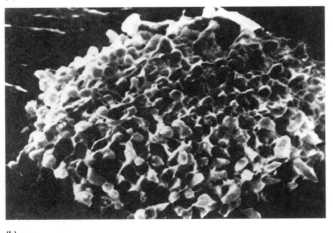

(b)

Fig 3.8 **Granule release from mast cells.**

Scanning electron micrograph of a resting (**a**) and a degranulating (**b**) mast cell (reproduced with permission from Upjohn, Inc.).

SUMMARY BOX 3.3

Mast cells and basophils

- ■ Mast cells and basophils are similar in structure and appear to serve similar roles in the tissues and blood, respectively.

- ■ Mast cell and basophil granule products, particularly histamine and the leukotrienes, have profound effects on blood vessels and bronchial smooth muscle.

- ■ The effect of release of mast cell and basophil granules differs according to the stimulus and site, producing anything from a localised wheal and flare to anaphylactic shock.

Further reading

Adamko DJ, Odemuyiwa SO, Vethanayagam D, Moqbel R 2005 The rise of the phoenix: the expanding role of the eosinophil in health and disease. Allergy 60: 13–22

Burg ND, Pillinger MH 2001 The neutrophil: function and regulation in innate and humoral immunity. Clinical Immunology 99: 7–17

Faurschou M, Borregaard N 2003 Neutrophil granules and secretory vesicles in inflammation. Microbes Infect 5: 1317–1327

Moser B, Willimann K 2004 Chemokines: role in inflammation and immune surveillance. Ann Rheum Dis 63: 84–89

Yang D, Liu ZH, Tewary P, Chen Q, de la Rosa G, Oppenheim JJ 2007 Defensin participation in innate and adaptive immunity. Curr Pharm Des 13: 3131–3139

Acquired immunity: antigen receptors

It is well known amongst mothers of young children that if a son or daughter catches chickenpox, then the chance of the child ever being troubled by the same virus again is minimal. The underlying explanation is that the immune system has 'learned' to 'recognise' what the chickenpox virus, herpes zoster, 'looks like'. This chapter and the next add flesh to that concept, in that they introduce the molecules in the immune system that are responsible for specific recognition of microbes: antibodies, T cell receptors and MHC molecules, whilst at the same time explaining how we can recognise such a vast array of different microbes.

These molecules are part of the acquired immune system. Before the development of an acquired immune response, the host immune system is in a state of ignorance and naïvety towards the provoking stimulus, which might be, for example, a virus or bacterium. During the first encounter between host and microbe, the immune system begins to 'identify' and 'learn' distinctive structural features of the microorganism. This enables the process of specific recognition. Effector responses (e.g. killing, neutralisation of toxins) can now be initiated, giving the host protection. At the same time, a memory bank of the most effective components of the immune response to that microbe can be laid down. Thus, in future responses to the same organism, host defences are already present or mobilised quickly, with a greater initial force. In the acquired immune response, then, we can see the cardinal features of **specificity**, **memory** and **variable intensity**.

In general, the innate and acquired immune responses do not become activated independently. They perform optimally when complementing each other. In particular, antibodies generated through acquired immunity are capable of directing components of the innate immune system (e.g. complement, neutrophils, mast cells) onto relevant targets.

Antigens and antibodies

Antigens

Antigens may be defined as structures which **gen**erate an **anti**-response by the immune system. If we take as an example of an antigen a core viral protein (Fig. 4.1), the immune system has three elements that are used in the binding and recognition of this antigen:

- antibodies
- T cell receptors
- MHC molecules.

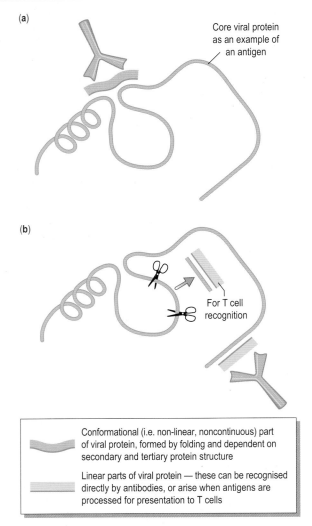

(a)

Core viral protein as an example of an antigen

(b)

For T cell recognition

Conformational (i.e. non-linear, noncontinuous) part of viral protein, formed by folding and dependent on secondary and tertiary protein structure

Linear parts of viral protein — these can be recognised directly by antibodies, or arise when antigens are processed for presentation to T cells

Fig. 4.1 Viral core protein as an example of an antigen. (**a**) Antibodies see 'shapes' derived from the conformational or linear parts of the antigen. (**b**) T cells and MHC molecules bind short peptides that are essentially linear in structure and can be derived from any part of a molecule. Antibodies can also bind linear epitopes.

Antibodies are generated by B lymphocytes and plasma cells. They are large glycoprotein structures with recognition sites for part of an intact antigen. The antibody–antigen interaction is shape dependent: imagine the antigen as the jelly and the antibody-binding site as the jelly mould. The shapes are sometimes termed conformations, and antibody binding is, therefore, conformation dependent. Antibodies can bind antigens that are free in solution, so-called soluble antigens. Alternatively, the antigen may be fixed on the surface of a cell or tissue. The part of the antigen with which the antibody interacts is termed an **epitope**. This region of the antigen determines which antibody will bind and may also be referred to as an **antigenic determinant**.

T cell receptors are the second type of receptor for antigen; they are found on T lymphocytes and, like antibodies, are large glycoproteins. However, there are some important differences between the two. T cell receptors interact not with whole intact antigens, but with a short segment of amino acids (termed the **peptide epitope**) derived from the intact antigen by proteolysis. A further difference is that the T cell receptor cannot interact with soluble peptide epitope directly; the epitope must be held and presented by other glycoprotein molecules. These 'other molecules' are the third element of the immune system that binds antigen: the **major histocompatibility complex** (**MHC**) **molecules**. MHC molecules hold the peptide antigen enclosed within a groove. What is recognised by the T cell receptor, therefore, is the combination of shapes formed by the peptide epitope and the walls of the groove in the MHC molecule (see Ch. 5).

Antigens, whether intact or short peptides, interact with these three types of receptor through non-covalent forces, such as hydrogen bonding, electrostatic attraction and van der Waals forces. The interaction is typically reversible, and obeys the laws of mass action. Taking antibody–antigen interactions as an example:

$$\text{antigen} + \text{antibody} \rightleftarrows \text{antigen} - \text{antibody complex}$$

There is a dynamic equilibrium between the dissociated antigen and antibody and the antigen–antibody complex (called an **immune complex**). The strength, or **affinity**, of the interaction can be defined as the concentration of antigens allowing half the antibodies to be complexed and half to remain in solution. This concentration is expressed in moles and is called the **dissociation constant** (K_d). The smaller the value of K_d, the higher the affinity. In general, of the three immune molecules designed to bind antigen, antibody has the highest affinity for antigen (estimated to be as high as 10^{-11} M for binding to natural antigens), with MHC molecules having a lower affinity for peptides (approximately 10^{-6} M) and the T cell receptor a lower affinity still for the peptide–MHC complex.

Because of their characteristic structure, with two 'arms', antibodies have at least two sites for binding antigen. In some cases, this number is even higher (e.g. one type of antibody, IgM, has five 'arms' and, therefore, 10 sites). Antibodies have a flexible hinge between the arms and, therefore, may be able to use more than one binding site in certain circumstances, for example when an antigen repeats itself as part of the coat of a bacterium. This increases the overall strength of binding, compared with when a single site is used. The overall strength of attachment is termed the **avidity**.

Antibodies

Antibodies are soluble glycoproteins that exhibit antigen-binding ability and belong to a group of large polypeptides termed the **immunoglobulins**. The term immunoglobulin derives from the facts that they have an immune function and they are identifiable in the fraction of serum proteins termed the globulins (see Science Box 4.1 and Fig. 4.2). The terms antibody and immunoglobulin are often used interchangeably.

Antibodies have a range of functions and uses, both biological and as clinical tools:

SCIENCE BOX 4.1

Separation of serum proteins by electrophoresis

Red and white blood cells circulate in a fluid enriched with many different proteins. This fluid is termed plasma. If blood is taken and allowed to clot, the fluid remaining after removal of the clot of cells and fibrin is termed **serum**. One of the earliest methods to be used for the separation and analysis of the different components of serum was **electrophoresis** (Fig. 4.2a). This can be carried out in a gel (e.g. agarose) or on a paper filter across which an electric field is applied. Proteins migrate within the field according to their charge. Once separated, the proteins can be stained in the gel or filter. Albumin is a major constituent of serum proteins and at pH 8.6 migrates fast as a negatively charged molecule towards the anode. Other proteins follow at

different speeds and form discrete zones, termed α and β. The Greek letters are often used as prefixes to name serum proteins found in these regions (e.g. β_2-microglobulin). The term globulin relates to the globular nature of many of the serum proteins.

Early studies indicated that most antibodies migrate cathodally, to a region termed γ, giving rise to the term gamma-globulins. As shown in Fig. 4.2b, the gamma-globulin region looks like a smear in contrast to the discrete band for albumin. This is because the γ region is composed of many forms of immunoglobulins (for example each one having a different antigen-binding site) so that each one differs slightly in its migration.

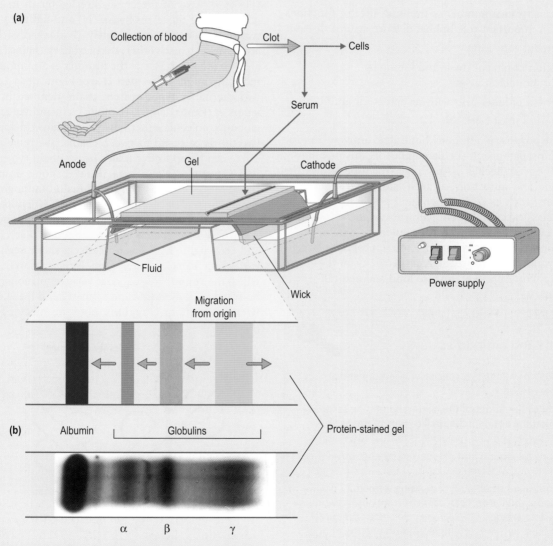

Fig. 4.2 **Separation of serum proteins by electrophoresis.**

1. In host defence:
   - targeting of infective organisms
   - recruitment of damaging host effector mechanisms such as complement
   - neutralisation of toxins
   - removal of foreign antigens from the circulation.

2. In clinical medicine:
   - specific anti-pathogen antibody levels used in diagnosis/monitoring infectious disease
   - pooled antibodies administered passively for host therapy/protection
   - antibodies used therapeutically to target cells or molecules (e.g. to eradicate tumours).

3. In laboratory science: antibodies are used in a vast range of diagnostic and research applications.

Antibodies activate a number of immune effector functions that have an important role in host defence against disease:

- complement activation
- stimulation of phagocytosis and killing by polymorphonuclear cells
- recruitment of killer cells with receptors for antibody
- activation of mast cells.

What is the purpose of antibody binding to antigen? In protection against pathogenic (i.e. damaging) organisms, binding of an antibody molecule to the intact microbe allows the recruitment and direction of host antibacterial effector mechanisms, such as complement and polymorphonuclear cells. The classical complement pathway cannot 'recognise' a foreign organism. Antibodies act as a guidance system, focusing effectors such as complement onto appropriate targets. In this way, antibodies provide target specificity for the innate immune system. Antibody can also bind and neutralise bacterial toxins.

SUMMARY BOX 4.1

Antigens and antibodies

- Acquired immunity has specificity, memory and a variable response.
- The molecular target of the acquired immune response is termed the antigen: the precise part of the antigen bound by an immune molecule is termed the epitope.
- Antigens are bound and recognised by antibodies, T cell receptors and MHC molecules.
- Antibodies are soluble glycoproteins termed immunoglobulins and can vary substantially in the range of possible antigen-binding sites. Because each molecule has at least two sites, multiple binding to large antigens is possible, increasing the avidity, or strength, of the attachment.
- Antibodies target foreign antigens, neutralise toxins and activate immune effectors: complement, mast cells, NK cells and phagocytes.

SUMMARY BOX 4.1

Antigens and antibodies—cont'd

- Antibodies are displayed on the surface of B cells or circulate as soluble proteins.
- Antibodies are used in clinical and research science as diagnostic tools.

Immunoglobulins

Structure

The typical immunoglobulin molecule has a molecular mass of 150–200 kDa and is made up of four polypeptide chains (Fig. 4.3). Two of the chains are lighter in mass than the others: hence the terms **heavy** (H) and **light** (L) chains. The two light chains (approximately 23 kDa) in each molecule are identical to each other; the two heavy chains (50–80 kDa) are also identical. Hence the formula of an immunoglobulin molecule might be written Heavy$_2$Light$_2$ or H_2L_2. There are two alternative types of light chain, denoted by the Greek letters κ (kappa) and λ (lambda). An individual immunoglobulin molecule either has two κ chains (in approximately two thirds of cases) or two λ chains (the remaining third). There can be up to five major heavy chain types, termed α, β, δ, ε, γ and μ (alpha, beta, delta, epsilon, gamma and mu; see below). Again, in each individual immunoglobulin molecule, the two heavy chains used will be identical.

When the structures of different antibody molecules are compared, several facts become apparent. Each heavy chain and each light chain has a relatively stable segment, which varies little between different molecules, as well as a zone in which the amino acid sequence varies enormously from antibody to antibody (see Science Box 4.2 and Fig. 4.4). The relatively constant, or **C regions**, hold the effector functions of

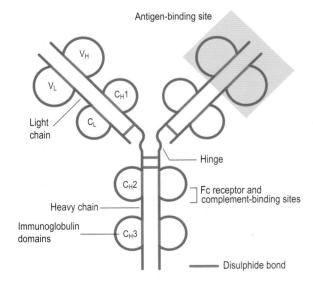

Fig. 4.3 **Typical structure of an immunoglobulin molecule.**

SCIENCE BOX 4.2

Variability and hypervariability in antibodies

Comparison of the amino acid sequences of different antibody molecules reveals that some areas frequently use the same or similar stretches of amino acids, with limited variability. In contrast, some areas demonstrate much greater variability, and at some points on the molecule a peak of variation in the choice of amino acids is seen. The variability can be plotted as histograms (called Wu and Kabat plots; Fig. 4.4). The regions of variability, of which there are three in each heavy and light chain, are termed **hypervariable** or **complementarity-determining regions** (**CDRs**; because they form the antigen binding site, which is a surface complementary to the three-dimensional surface of the antigen). Not surprisingly, this diversity is generated for a specific purpose: the CDRs come together after the folding of the immunoglobulin molecule into its tertiary structure and form the binding site for antigen (see Fig. 4.5). This explains the structural basis for the enormous variability available for recognition of a vast array of antigens by antibodies.

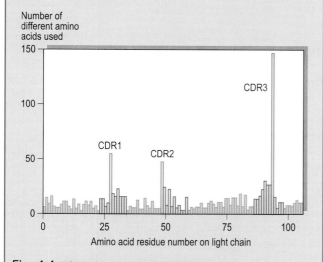

Fig. 4.4 **Diversity in antigen binding.**
This is dependent upon variation in the antibody structure and this diversity can be assessed by counting the number of different amino acids used at each position in a range of antibody molecules. This is called a Wu and Kabat plot and shows regions of the molecule where there is hypervariability between different antibodies (CDRs) (modified with permission from Kabat 1980 Journal of Immunology 125: 963).

interchain disulphide bond. The carbohydrate content of the glycoproteins varies between 2 and 12%. Within the heavy and light chains, there are intrachain disulphide bonds. These serve to bend segments back onto themselves, creating regions called **domains** within the heavy and light chains. This gives the immunoglobulin molecule a very distinctive structure. All immunoglobulin domains contain two layers of β-pleated sheet with three or four strands of anti-parallel polypeptide chain. When first discovered, the domain structure and its genetic basis were considered highly distinctive. Subsequently, many molecules in the immune system (MHC molecules, adhesion molecules, T cell receptors and cellular co-receptors) have been shown to share a similar domain structure, giving rise to the term **immunoglobulin super-gene family** to highlight this structural similarity.

In an immunoglobulin molecule the domains are named according to which chain (H or L) they are in, and numbered. Therefore, the light chain is referred to as having one V_L and one C_L domain (Fig. 4.5), while the heavy chain has a V_H and either three or four C_H domains (C_H1–4). The V_L and V_H domains combine to form the antigen-binding site. The C_H domains contain the major effector functions, such as the complement-binding site and the location for interaction with receptors on polymorphonuclear cells and mast cells. There is a **hinge region** in the middle of the molecule, which allows some freedom to the two arms bearing the antigen-binding sites. This flexibility enables antibody molecules to maximise the chances of binding two antigenic epitopes at one time.

The immunoglobulin molecule can be cleaved with different enzymatic treatments (Fig. 4.6). The enzyme papain cleaves at the hinge region, breaking the two interchain disulphide bonds between the heavy chains in the process, to produce three fragments. Two of the fragments are identical and retain antigen-binding ability. These are termed **Fab fragments** (for fragment antigen binding) and have a molecular mass of about 45 kDa. The other fragment is larger (55 kDa) and has no antigen-binding site but retains the effector functions (e.g. binding to cell surface receptors). This fragment is also crystallisable and is termed the **Fc fragment** (for fragment crystallisable: numerous cells express surface receptors for immunoglobulin molecules, and since these interact with this portion of the molecule, they are termed **Fc receptors**). Cleavage of the immunoglobulin molecule with pepsin leaves the heavy–heavy interchain disulphide bond intact. Therefore, the two Fab fragments are linked, into a **F(ab′)₂ fragment** with two antigen-binding sites, but no effector functions remaining.

As stated above, the part of the antibody molecule that holds the effector functions can be varied, for different roles. This is achieved through variation in the genes encoding the H chains. There are five different major types of H chain gene, giving rise to H chains denoted by a Greek letter: α, δ, ε, γ and μ, with the γ chains being further subdivided into γ₁, γ₂, γ₃ and γ₄ and the α chains into α₁ and α₂. When referring to the whole immunoglobulin molecule, **Ig** is used for short: the presence of the different heavy chains gives rise to the major **classes** of immunoglobulins: **IgA, IgD, IgE, IgG** and

the molecule, such as complement activation. The variable, or **V regions**, include the antigen-binding sites; the variability is critical for generating the potential to bind to more than 10^{11} different antigen structures. The genetic basis for this variability is discussed below (p. 46).

To form the full antibody molecule, the two heavy chains are linked together by two interchain disulphide bonds. Each heavy chain then has a light chain attached to it, again by an

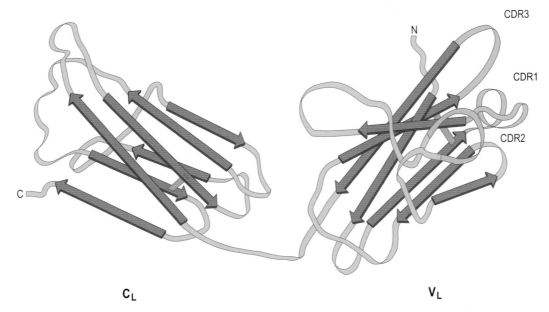

CDR3

N

CDR1

CDR2

C

C_L

V_L

Fig. 4.5 Immunoglobulin domains in a human light chain.
The V and C regions each fold independently. The brown arrows represent β-pleated sheets; the short purple bars are intrachain disulphide bonds; and the CDR1, CDR2 and CDR3 variable regions are coloured in light blue. The last group together form the antigen-binding site (adapted with permission from Edmundson et al 1975 Biochemistry 14: 3953–3961).

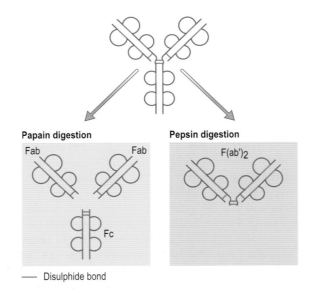

Papain digestion

Fab   Fab

Fc

Pepsin digestion

F(ab')$_2$

—— Disulphide bond

Fig. 4.6 Cleavage of antibody molecules to give Fab and Fc fragments.
Papain digestion produces two antigen-binding fragments (Fab) and one fragment that activates complement and binds to Fc receptors (Fc). Pepsin digestion produces a single F(ab')$_2$ fragment with two antigen-binding sites.

IgM. The IgG molecules can be further subdivided into the IgG1, IgG2, IgG3 and IgG4 subclasses and IgA into the IgA1 and IgA2 subclasses.

All of these immunoglobulin molecules have the same basic structure, of heavy and light chain constituents. Variations in the heavy chains, giving rise to the different classes and subclasses, confer distinctive functions, and these will now be examined in more detail.

Immunoglobulin classes and subclasses

Immunoglobulin G (IgG)

IgG is the most abundant immunoglobulin, having an average serum concentration of 10 g/l in an adult. The IgG molecule has three constant domains in the heavy chain (C_H1–3) (Table 4.1). IgG occurs as a monomer and can be subdivided into four subclasses. The variability between the four IgG subclasses is mainly located in the hinge regions and functional domains (Fig. 4.7). The IgG subclasses vary in their relative ability to perform some of the effector functions and also in their serum concentration (Table 4.2). IgG2 responses may be most important in combating capsulated bacteria. IgG1 and IgG3 are the main activators of the classical complement pathway. Binding of the complement component C1q to IgG in its native state is very weak; binding is greatly increased when the IgG is complexed to antigen. C1q interacts with the C_H2 domain.

There are three cellular receptors for the Fc portion of IgG, termed Fc$_\gamma$RI, II and III (Table 4.3). These are used to bind, recruit and activate cells such as polymorphs, mononuclear phagocytes and NK cells. The Fc$_\gamma$ receptors are also important in the active process of placental transfer of IgG from the mother to the fetus. This is an important feature of the late stages of pregnancy since it confers some specific protection on the newborn during the period when its own immune system is immature.

Immunoglobulin A (IgA)

IgA is the next most abundant immunoglobulin molecule. It is distinctive in two ways. First, it can occur not only as a monomer but also as a dimer, in which two IgA molecules

Table 4.1 Physical properties of immunoglobulins

	IgG	IgA	IgM	IgD	IgE
Usual structural form	Monomer	Monomer (circulating IgA) Dimer (secretory IgA)	Pentamer	Monomer	Monomer
Accessory chains		J chain polyimmunoglobulin receptor (secretory chain)	J chain		
Subclasses	IgG1, IgG2, IgG3, IgG4	IgA1, IgA2			
Heavy chain	γ	α	μ	δ	ε
Number of domains in heavy chain	3	3	4	3	4
Molecular mass (kDa)	150	160 (monomer), 385 (secretory)	950	180	190
Adult serum concentration (g/l)	6–12	1–4	0.5–2	0.04	0.003
Half-life (days)	23	6	5	3	2.5
Proportion found in circulation (%)	50	50	80	75	50

are joined by a short peptide (the **J chain**; Fig. 4.8). The second distinctive feature is that IgA is the major immunoglobulin secreted onto the external surfaces. It is an important aspect of host defence that mucosal surfaces, which are warm and moist, are protected from unwanted microbial growth, and this is achieved through the presence in secretions (e.g. saliva, bronchial fluid, gut secretions, tears, etc.) of **secretory IgA**. Although IgA is detected abundantly in serum (usually in the monomeric form), secretory IgA (dimeric) is found in saliva, lung fluids, gastrointestinal secretions, tears, breast milk and vaginal secretions. Secretion is achieved through the attachment of dimeric IgA to a molecule (termed the polyimmunoglobulin receptor, poly-IgR) synthesised by epithelial cells lining mucosal surfaces (Fig. 4.9). The IgA–poly-IgR complex is endocytosed, transported through the epithelial cell and secreted into the lumen. At this point the IgA–poly-IgR complex is cleaved, releasing IgA and a remnant of poly-IgR, termed the **secretory chain**, of approximately 70 kDa. The importance of this

process is highlighted in patients with selective IgA deficiency, in whom severe, intractable infections of the major mucosal surfaces (gastrointestinal, upper and lower respiratory tracts) are common (see p. 274). As the major secretory immunoglobulin, IgA has an important role in protection against bacterial, viral and protozoal infections of mucosae and can activate complement through the alternative pathway as well as having specific receptors (FcαR) on monocytes and neutrophils.

Immunoglobulin M (IgM)

IgM is highly distinctive, occurring primarily as a pentamer composed of five IgM monomers joined by the J chain (Fig. 4.8). Monomeric IgM molecules have the same basic structure as the other immunoglobulin molecules. IgM is the first immunoglobulin synthesised in an antibody response (the so-called primary response; see below, Fig. 4.10). As a pentamer it has multiple functional domains and is,

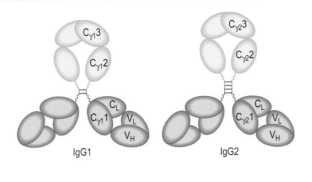

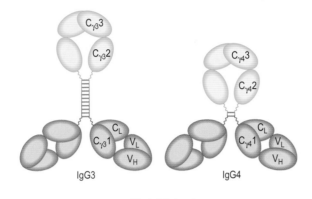

— Disulphide bond

Fig. 4.7 The four subclasses of human IgG.
IgG3 has a distinctive extended hinge region.

therefore, a potent activator of complement. In theory, it also has 10 potential antigen-binding sites. To utilise several of these at once, the IgM molecule can become flexed (resembling a crab) so that when reacting with repeating epitopes on a cell or bacterial surface several of the antigen-binding sites may be used. This is an important property: as the first antibody to be produced in response to an antigen challenge, many IgM antibodies do not have the high affinity of later, more refined antibody responses (see below). However, by utilising multiple binding sites, an enhancement of binding can be achieved at lower antibody affinity, a major advantage in the primary response.

Immunoglobulin D (IgD)

IgD is the least well characterised of the immunoglobulins from a functional viewpoint. Serum concentrations are extremely low, and it is unlikely that in this soluble form it has any major function as an immune effector. However, surface expression of IgD is evident at a relatively immature stage of the B cell cycle, and the signalling provided by this receptor on interaction with antigen in a lymphoid follicle is a critical part of B lymphocyte activation.

Immunoglobulin E (IgE)

IgE is the largest immunoglobulin monomer, having four CH domains. It is present in the serum of healthy individuals at extremely low levels. IgE levels rise in response to parasitic infections and in individuals who have allergy (see p. 138).

Table 4.2 Properties of IgG subclasses

		IgG1	IgG2	IgG3	IgG4
Proportion total IgG (%)		65	20	10	5
Activation of complement		++	+	+	−
Placental transfer		++	++	++	++
Binding to:					
	Fc$_\gamma$RI	++	−	++	+
	Fc$_\gamma$RII	++	−	++	−
	Fc$_\gamma$RIII	++	−	++	−
Major antibody responses:					
	e.g. tetanus	++	+	+	++
	e.g. bacterial polysaccharides	+	++	+	+

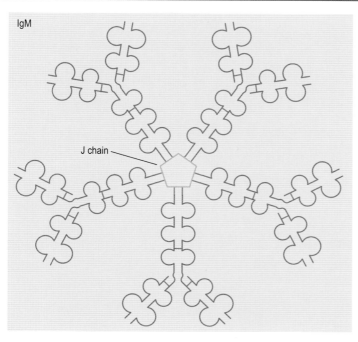

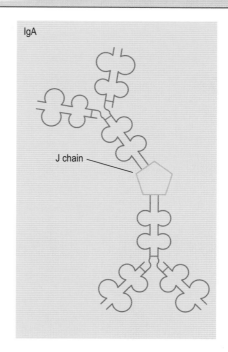

—— Disulphide bond

Fig. 4.8 **The structure of the IgM pentamer and the secretory IgA dimer.**
Both are stabilised by the J chain.

Table 4.3 Cell surface receptors for IgG

Receptor	Type	CD designation	Present on
Fc$_\gamma$RI	High affinity	CD64	Monocytes, macrophages (and activated neutrophils)
Fc$_\gamma$RII	Low affinity	CD32	Monocytes, neutrophils, eosinophils, B lymphocytes
Fc$_\gamma$RIII	Low affinity	CD16	Monocytes, neutrophils, NK cells

Allergic reactions and immune responses to parasites both involve activation of mast cells, which is the main effector function of IgE. Each mast cell bears 10^4–10^6 high-affinity surface IgE receptors (Fc$_\varepsilon$RI). Mast cells resident in the skin or mucosa will thus acquire surface IgE. If there is then an interaction between surface IgE and its specific antigen, mast cell activation is the result, with potent localised, and occasionally generalised, vascular effects. In physiological terms, the generation of these types of itchy, hypervascular responses is probably important in defence against parasitic infections such as intestinal worms. A low-affinity receptor, Fc$_\varepsilon$RII (CD23), is present on B lymphocytes and eosinophils. Interaction between Fc$_\varepsilon$RII on B lymphocytes is an important part of the regulation of IgE production.

Isotypes and allotypes

Isotypes are structural features of a particular immunoglobulin class or heavy or light chain type in a species. For example, the ε heavy chain has structural features peculiar to IgE molecules, which are present on all of the IgE molecules in the members of that species. Other parts of immunoglobulins have genetically determined differences between individuals. These are termed **allotypes**.

SUMMARY BOX 4.2

Immunoglobulins

- The basic molecule is composed of two light and two heavy chains connected by interchain disulphide bonds. Within the chains, distinctive motifs (domains) are formed by intrachain disulphide bonds.

- Many immunological molecules have similar domain structures: the immunoglobulin supergene family.

continued

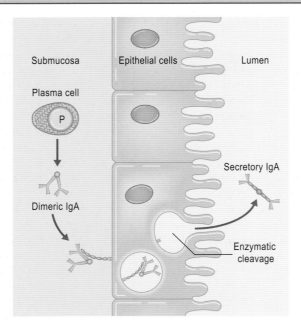

Fig. 4.9 **Dimeric IgA (two IgA monomers joined by the J chain) is secreted across the epithelial surfaces lining the mucosa.**
This is achieved using the poly-Ig receptor present on the surface of the epithelial cell.

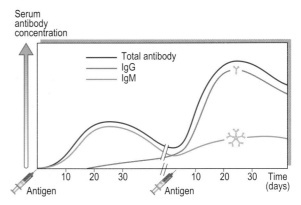

Fig. 4.10 **Primary and secondary antibody responses.**
Administration of an antigen at day 0 is followed by a primary antibody response, comprising predominantly IgM, at about 10–20 days. Rechallenge with the same antigen some weeks later causes a much more rapid rise in antibody levels and to a higher peak; this time the response is predominantly IgG (secondary response).

SUMMARY BOX 4.2

Immunoglobulins—cont'd

- Antibodies contain regions that are highly variable in their amino acid content in different molecules: these zones form the antigen-binding site.

- Antibodies also have relatively constant parts; on the heavy chain these hold different functional properties, such as the ability to activate complement.

- Different heavy chains give rise to different classes of immunoglobulin: IgA, IgD, IgE, IgG and IgM.

Immunoglobulin expression

B cell surface expression

A short extension of immunoglobulin molecules at the carboxy-terminus during synthesis enables insertion into the B lymphocyte surface membrane. Surface-expressed antibody has an important role in B lymphocyte activation and binding of antigen is an early event in the B lymphocyte cell cycle. In the case of mature B lymphocytes, interaction with surface IgG, IgA and IgD leads to internalisation of the antigen. Complex antigens may then be broken down (an event called **antigen processing**) and presented to T lymphocytes (see p. 94). Through this process, antigen-specific B lymphocytes can activate T lymphocytes, leading to a concerted immune response.

Primary and secondary antibody responses

When antigen not previously encountered is injected into an animal, and the antibody response measured, several observations can be made. The antibody response is detected 5–10 days after antigen challenge, rises over the next 10–20 days, and then declines to a low level without ever completely disappearing. If the same antigen is administered again several weeks later, the antibody response is **more rapid**, hits a **higher peak level**, and declines, but to a higher **baseline level** than previously seen (Fig. 4.10). These two responses, therefore, differ qualitatively and quantitatively, and are termed **primary** and **secondary**. If a different antigen is given at the second challenge, a primary response to that antigen is seen. The secondary response is, therefore, **antigen-specific**, and demonstrates **acquisition of memory** in the immune response. There is also a higher **intensity** to the secondary response. These are the 3 cardinal features of the adaptive immune response mentioned earlier — **specificity**, **memory** and **variable intensity**.

The qualitative differences between primary and secondary responses extend further than just the speed of appearance of antibody. The primary response is seen predominantly as antibody of the IgM class. IgG antibody specific for the same antigen begins to appear towards the end of the primary response. The secondary response, however, is predominantly IgG class antibody. There is another feature of the IgG in the secondary response: it has a higher affinity for antigen than antibody in the primary response. The genetic and cellular basis for switching from IgM to IgG class antibody is discussed below. The generation of high-affinity antibodies will also be discussed in greater depth, but in simplistic terms it can be viewed as the application of Darwinian evolutionary principles to B lymphocyte survival: those B cells with antibodies that have the highest affinity for an antigen in short supply compete most effectively and undergo positive selection.

Haptens

Some molecules are too small of themselves to generate an antibody response when administered to an animal. However, if coupled to a larger protein (a **carrier**), these small molecules may elicit production of antibodies that are able to bind the small molecule directly, in the absence of the carrier. Such molecules are termed **haptens**. The concept of haptens is especially important in unwanted immune responses, for example against drugs and toxins (see p. 296).

Clonality in antibody responses

Plasma cells — the end stage of B lymphocyte differentiation — produce and secrete immunoglobulin. More specifically, a single plasma cell produces a single antibody, with one heavy chain type, one light chain type and one conformation of antigen-binding region. This gives rise to the concept of a clone — a group of cells that is descended from the same common ancestor. A clone of plasma cells produces a **monoclonal antibody**, unvarying in its amino acid sequence. Most antibody responses to complex macromolecular antigens involve the targeting of multiple epitopes on the antigen. Each epitope may be targeted by more than a single antibody molecule. Thus, many different clones of plasma cells, and many different antibody types, are produced in a typical antibody response. Such a response is termed **polyclonal**. Antibody responses to a large macromolecular antigen are not evenly distributed throughout the antigen; some areas are targeted more frequently than others and are termed the **dominant epitopes**.

Monoclonal immunoglobulins are only identifiable in any quantity in two circumstances. The first is a clinical condition in which a tumour of plasma cell origin leads to the expansion of a single clone of cells, producing a single immunoglobulin molecule (a disease termed myeloma, see p. 300). The second is when such a tumour is fused with a B lymphocyte to give an immortalised, antibody-producing clone of B lymphocytes; such a manoeuvre is central to monoclonal antibody technology (see Science Box 4.3).

SCIENCE BOX 4.3

Generation of monoclonal and polyclonal antibodies

Monoclonal antibodies were 'invented' by George Köhler and César Milstein at Cambridge in 1975. Ironically, the two ended their article in *Nature* doubting whether their discovery was of any value in future science. In 1984, they were awarded the Nobel prize for what is unquestionably one of the single most important contributions to the biosciences. B lymphocytes are removed from the spleens of mice immunised with an antigen (Fig. 4.11). These B cells are then fused with a tumour cell line to provide a hybrid with the best of both worlds: specific antibody production and immortality. The hybridoma is grown, and antibody appearing in the culture fluid is tested to see whether it binds the antigen of interest. Since each hybridoma is derived from a single B lymphocyte, the immunoglobulin that it produces is monoclonal. Selected hybridoma cells can be grown in culture for many years and the monoclonal antibody purified in large quantities. Thus, an antibody can be raised to almost any antigen imaginable, providing the ultimate tool for many aspects of laboratory research and clinical science.

Antibodies raised in larger mammals (rabbits, guinea-pigs, sheep, donkeys, horses) can also be of great use. Here the antigen is administered and then the animal is bled some 2–3 weeks later. The serum obtained contains a high concentration of antibodies to the antigen of interest. These polyclonal antisera can also be applied widely in the laboratory. They were also used for one of the earliest attempts at manipulating immunity to the advantages of humans. Horse serum, obtained from animals injected with diphtheria toxin, was used successfully to combat the toxin-mediated effects of diphtheria infection in the early part of the twentieth century.

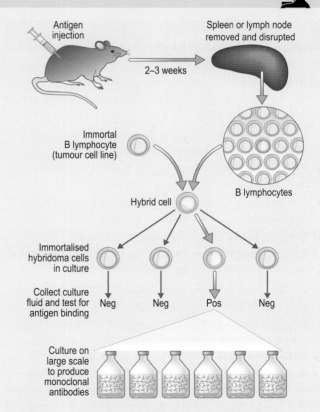

Fig. 4.11 **Production of monoclonal antibodies.**

SUMMARY BOX 4.3

Immunoglobulin expression

- Immunoglobulins on the surface of B lymphocytes bind antigen, which is then internalised, broken down and a portion is presented to T lymphocytes to activate their response to the antigen.

- Immunoglobulins can be characterised by their own ability to act as antigens: *isotypes* are epitopes that are present on all molecules of a class or chain type in a species; *allotypes* vary between individuals, *idiotypes* reflect variation in the antigen-binding sites of the immunoglobulin.

- Primary antibody responses are slow, mainly IgM and decline to low levels. Repeated exposure to the antigen at a later time elicits a more rapid response to a higher peak level that declines to a higher baseline level; this secondary response is predominantly IgG.

- Each plasma cell produces a single antibody; tumours formed from a single plasma cell will produce large quantities of this monoclonal antibody. A population of plasma cells will respond to different epitopes on macromolecular antigens giving rise to many clones of plasma cells and many antibody types: a polyclonal response.

Immunoglobulin genes

It is clear that the immunoglobulins are quite distinctive molecules. When examining the genes that encode these complex glycoproteins, we are looking for the explanation to some key characteristics.

- The immunoglobulin molecule has four chains; two identical heavy and two identical light chains.

- Each chain contains both highly variable *and* essentially constant regions.

- Antibody is IgM class in the primary response and IgG or other classes in the secondary response.

- Different heavy chains can be selected for an immunoglobulin molecule, hence modifying its effector function without altering antigen binding.

- During the generation of an antibody response, there is an increase in overall affinity for antigen.

- Potential binding capacity exceeds 10^{11} different antigen 'shapes', implying an equivalent number of different antibody molecules.

To summarise these points, it could be said that the genetic system for antibodies is required to generate enormous **diversity** for antigen binding at one end of the molecule and a limited choice of functional characteristics at the other. Two theories could easily explain such a model. One, favoured for many years because it did not require a rewriting of the genetics textbooks, stated that a separate gene existed for every different antibody molecule. In other words, there were

10^{11} different genes for 10^{11} different antigen-binding molecules. The other explanation was that a limited number of genes were available, but that they could combine randomly; such chance associations offered diversity. When the immunoglobulin genes were eventually identified, they were indeed limited in number, confirming the second hypothesis. However, the number was actually *too* limited to account for the enormous diversity achieved; additional mechanisms for the **generation of antibody diversity** were subsequently identified.

At a basic level, the organisation of genes for an immunoglobulin molecule can be viewed as follows. Each chain (heavy and light) is encoded by a gene complex. Within the complex are groups of genes (termed segments) that encode the variable regions (V genes), and genes that encode the constant regions (C genes) of each chain. Other genes are responsible for joining these two (J genes), or make an additional contribution to the generation of diversity (D genes). Up-to-date information on all gene types, structures and nomenclature for immunoglobulins and T cell receptors, as well as other resources, are available at http://imgt.cines.fr. The genes are known by the capital letters IG, followed by the name of the chain (for example κ and λ light chains are K and L), the name of the gene region (V, D, J, C) and a number (for example IGKV1 for immunoglobulin kappa variable chain gene number 1) (Fig. 4.12).

Light chain genes

The κ and λ light chain genes (named IGK and IGL, respectively) are on chromosomes 2 and 22, respectively, in humans (Fig. 4.13). The sequence of genes runs V to J to C, from the 5' to 3' end of the chromosome (there is no D segment for light chains). For the κ chain genes, there are some 40 functional IGKV gene segments, 5 IGKJ segments and one IGKC segment. In theory, then, there is the potential for $40 \times 5 \times 1 = 200$ different combinations of these gene segments to form 200 different κ light chains. The λ chain gene segments comprise some 30 IGLV and 5 IGLC gene segments, each C gene being accompanied by its own IGLJ gene. The potential diversity in the λ genes is, therefore, 30×5, or 150 different light chains.

Heavy chain genes

The human heavy chain genes, on chromosome 14, have a similar basic structure to the light chains, with two differ-

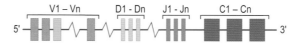

Fig. 4.12 Representation of the overall organisation of immunoglobulin genes.
The number of different genes in each gene segment is given by *n*.

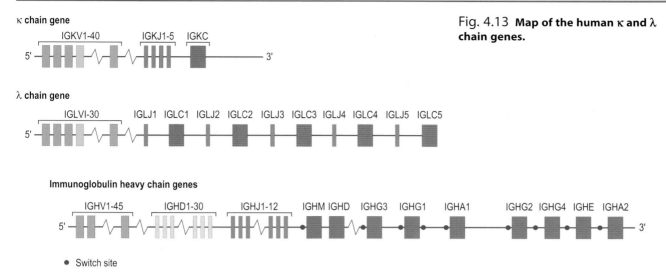

Fig. 4.13 **Map of the human κ and λ chain genes.**

Fig. 4.14 **Organisation of the human heavy chain genes.**

ences (Fig. 4.14). First, additional diversity is achieved by the presence of a small number of diversity (D) gene segments. Second, the different constant region gene segments encoding the heavy chain isotypes (IGHG1–4 for the IgG subclass heavy chains; IGHA1–2 for the IgA subclasses; IGHM, IGHD and IGHE for IgM, IgD and IgE heavy chain genes, respectively) are located together, downstream from the IGHV, IGHD and IGHJ segments, rather than on separate chromosomes.

IGHV gene segments fall into approximately seven families, each with numerous members, which are not always functional (some are pseudogenes), so that the total number of functional IGHV genes is estimated at 45. There are approximately 30 IGHD and 12 IGHJ gene segments. The maximum diversity achievable from this range of genes is, therefore $45 \times 30 \times 12 = 16\,200$. When combined with a κ light chain, for example, the total potential diversity of molecular structure in an immunoglobulin molecule is thus $200 \times 16\,200 = 3.24$ million. Since an alternative would be to combine with a λ chain, there is an additional potential diversity of $150 \times 16\,200 = 2.43$ million, making a potential combined range of 5.67 million potential molecules, although it is probably much less. This process of forming different antibody specificities through combining different genes randomly is termed **combinatorial diversity**, since it relies upon combinations of different genes.

Generation of immunoglobulin diversity

We have seen how, by careful manipulation of a large pool of genes encoding different parts of the immunoglobulin molecule, an enormous range of different immunoglobulin structures can be created (Fig. 4.15). However, there are two other manipulations that add to the diversity. First, there is a 'deliberate' imprecision in the joining together of IGHD and IGHJ, IGHV to the IGHD–IGHJ combination that forms, and also in the equivalent V–J segments as they join

for the light chain genes. Remembering that three nucleotides (a codon) in the gene are required per amino acid, loss or retention of whole codons when two genes join together determines whether an amino acid is present or not. Loss or addition of single nucleotides can lead to frame-shift mutations, altering the meaning of the whole of the genetic code after the join. This phenomenon is termed **junctional diversity** and is thought to increase the total potential diversity of immunoglobulin structure by a factor of 30 million. Combinatorial and junctional diversity tend to focus the changes introduced into the hypervariable regions (CDRs), which are mainly encoded from the joining regions of the genes. Thus, they create the potential for many different shapes in the parts of antibodies that bind antigen — a perfect system for coping with diversity in the microbial world.

In 1983, a further discovery identified the second additional mechanism by which antibody diversity is broadened. It was found that parts of the variable regions of different antibodies differed by a single amino acid residue, or their genes differed by a single nucleotide sequence, from the version of that gene encoded in the germline (i.e. non-rearranged DNA). This finding implied a single mutation. Subsequently, it was shown that such differences appeared *after* antigenic stimulation and, therefore, *after* the initial gene rearrangements occurring in that cell. This process has been termed **somatic hypermutation**. It may involve the substitution, deletion or addition of a single nucleotide, occurring after gene rearrangement. This occurs when the cell is undertaking the class switch between the primary and secondary responses. The process of somatic hypermutation introduces an additional diversity and is frequently focused in and around the CDRs. It is now known that somatic hypermutation is dependent upon the activity of an enzyme, **activation induced cytidine deaminase.** Genetic defects in this enzyme result in a failure of B cells to generate diversity through this process, resulting in poor production of high affinity antibodies and a rare immune deficiency state called Hyper IgM syndrome type 2.

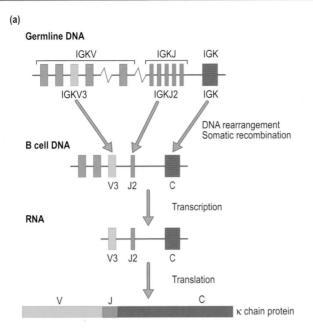

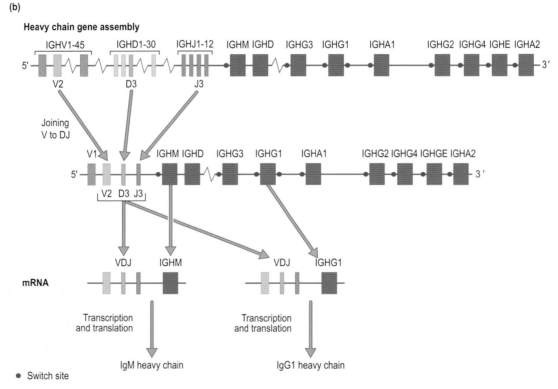

Fig. 4.15 The overall scheme of gene rearrangements to achieve a final immunoglobulin chain.
(**a**) For an immunoglobulin light chain. (**b**) For a heavy chain, with or without class switching.

The mechanisms for the generation of antibody diversity are summarised in Table 4.4.

Class switching

In the process of assembling the different gene segments necessary to make an immunoglobulin molecule composed of two light and two heavy chains, random combinations of the different component genes produce an enormous potential diversity. At this point in the development of B lymphocytes, the cells are able to express the rearranged immunoglobulin on the cell surface. Invariably, at this stage, the surface immunoglobulin (sIg) is a monomer of the IgM class. As we shall see in a later chapter (Ch. 6), the rearrangement of immunoglobulin genes into sIgM is a very early

Table 4.4 Contribution of the different mechanisms of generation of diversity for immunoglobulin molecules and TCRs

Mechanism	Immunoglobulin		TCRαβ		TCRγδ	
	Heavy chain	**Light chain**	α	β	γ	δ
Number of variable (V) segments	45	30–40	50	50	8	10
Number of diversity (D) segments	30	0	0	2	0	2
D segments read in all three reading frames	Rare	—	—	Frequent	—	Frequent
Joining (J) segments	12	4–5	50	13	2	3
Combinatorial diversity	$3–5 \times 10^6$		~2500		80	
Somatic hypermutation	3×10^6					
Total potential repertoire including allowance for functional diversity	$10^{11}–10^{12}$		$= 10^{16}$		$= 10^{18}$	

Adapted with permission from Davis & Bjorkman 1993 Nature 334: 395.

event in the B cell life cycle and is independent of any encounter with antigen. When sIgM binds specific antigen, the B cell may become activated. One of the results of such activation is the transformation into a B cell with surface IgG, IgA or IgE, as an alternative for IgM. This process of class switching must be carried out without the B cell changing its antigen specificity: it would be no good the B cell being activated for expressing anti-X and becoming a cell capable of an anti-Y response. What has been achieved by the process of class switching, however, is to modulate the functional capabilities of the antibody produced, according to whether IgG, IgA, IgE or IgM is chosen. This is termed **class switch recombination**. It is thought that activation induced cytidine deaminase is responsible for this process. Here we see the genetic and molecular basis for the qualitative change in the antibody repertoire seen when a primary response (mainly IgM) becomes a secondary one (mainly IgG).

Affinity maturation

One final major difference between antibodies produced in the primary and those produced in the secondary response

is their affinity. IgM antibodies produced in the primary response to an antigen tend to be of relatively low affinity and may rely upon the additional avidity afforded by their pentameric structure to bind antigen efficiently. However, the IgG and other class antibodies produced in the secondary response tend to be of much higher affinity. This change in the characteristic of antibody binding to antigen is termed **affinity maturation**. It is assumed that the process is something of a Darwinian evolutionary change. It is probable that in the lymph node during an antigen challenge, many different IgM-expressing B cells are present, binding antigen with relatively low affinity. They receive positive differentiation signals and undergo class switching. It is at this stage that the process of somatic hypermutation also takes place. The product of these manipulations is a range of antibodies with single affinity, available for selection. Only those B cells receiving the necessary signals to continue their expansion (signals provided by lymph node T cells in the main) will proliferate. In the presence of a limited supply of antigen, the law of the 'immunological jungle' will apply, and only the highest affinity antibodies, which compete most effectively, will receive the next selection signal. We will see the cellular basis of this part of B cell maturation in a later chapter (see p. 81).

Genetic basis for immunoglobulin gene rearrangement and class switching

We have talked blithely of combinatorial processes, class switching and hypermutation; but what are the genetic processes that underlie these? The heavy chain genes on one chromosome are assembled first, with an IGHD and IGHJ segment combining, before an IGHV segment is added. If a successful VDJ gene is produced through this rearrangement, it is likely that the other chromosome is inhibited in some way from undergoing the same process (allelic exclusion). The constant heavy chain is then added to the rearranged IGH VDJ segment. Invariably, the IGHM is selected, and it is worth noting that the appearance in the cytoplasm of this protein product (i.e. the IgM heavy chain) is one of the earliest indications that a cell is of the B lymphocyte lineage. Next, the light chain gene V and J segments are rearranged and combined with the constant region gene. In humans, the IGK gene is selected first, and only if the rearrangement is unsuccessful on both strands of chromosome 2 is the IGL gene then sought (the majority of κ chain gene rearrangements must be successful, since the κ:λ ratio of antibodies in the periphery is 2:1). At this point, sufficient genetic material to produce an immunoglobulin molecule has been constructed. When class switching takes place, the IgM heavy chain must be replaced by selection of the IGHG, IGHA or IGHE gene. This is achieved by the use of switch regions, 5′ to the IGH genes. The only IGH gene not to have a switch region is the IGHD gene: this may explain why few mature B cells express sIgD, and why very little

immunoglobulin of the IgD class is made. The precise mechanism by which switch regions allow the new CH gene to be transcribed is not known, although it may involve loops and excisions, or straight deletions, as proposed in the models of VDJ recombination (see Science Box 4.4 and Fig. 4.16).

SUMMARY BOX 4.4

Immunoglobulin genes and antibody diversity

- Antibody diversity is achieved through a variety of genetic mechanisms, the changes tending to focus on the hypervariable regions.

- Combinatorial diversity is the random recombination of some of a large pool of gene segments for the light and heavy chains.

- Junctional diversity is the random imprecision in the joining of the segments caused by loss or retention of codons or nucleotides, which results in frame-shifts.

- Somatic hypermutation is the occurrence of a single mutational change after the initial gene rearrangements, probably during class switching.

- In class switching in B cells, the early expression of IgM gives way to the mature, activated expression of other classes of immunoglobulin. B cells with the highest affinity will be stimulated to proliferate further — affinity maturation.

SCIENCE BOX 4.4

Immunoglobulin gene recombination: twists and palindromes

Immunoglobulin gene rearrangements have always been an interesting area of study for molecular geneticists. One early question was how differing gene segments were successfully selected and combined. Careful analysis of the nucleotides flanking each V, D and J gene segment revealed an interesting set of repetitive sequences (Fig. 4.16). Downstream from each V gene segment, for example, is a sequence of seven particular nucleotides (a heptamer), followed by a random set of nucleotides (invariably 12 or 23 in number) and then a further nine defined nucleotides (a nonamer). At the approach to each gene segment (i.e. upstream) is a similar set, but this time running in the sequence nonamer → random 12 or 23 nucleotides → heptamer. Particularly intriguing was the fact that the two heptamers and nonamers were palindromic (remember a palindrome reads the same forwards and backwards: 'madam', for example). In DNA terms, this means that when read in opposite directions the heptamers and nonamers are complementary with each other. In other words, if the gene region were doubled back onto itself, for example by formation of a loop, the heptamers and nonamers could form

a region of double-stranded DNA. This is made easier since the heptamer and nonamer sequences are separated by random sequences of fixed length, 12 or 23 bases, which correspond to one or two complete turns of a DNA helix. There is one final 'twist' in the story, however. Analysis of the sequences reveals that for two gene segments to join, the heptamer and nonamer must be separated by a 12-mer on one side and a 23-mer on the other. This is termed the 12–23 rule. Several enzymes have been identified that catalyse this process, forming what is termed the **V(D)J recombinase**. Within this are two **recombination-activation genes (*RAG-1* and *RAG-2*)**, which are critical to this process in developing B lymphocytes and the similar process that takes place in developing T lymphocytes. Mice in which the *RAG* genes are knocked out cannot rearrange immunoglobulin genes or T cell receptors and are profoundly immune deficient. Careful studies on the flanking sequences of immunoglobulin gene segments indicate that the 12–23 rule is important because it dictates that VH cannot joint JH directly, because such a recombination would involve two 23-mers. This ensures the addition of the DH region in-between.

Immunoglobulin gene recombination: twists and palindromes—cont'd

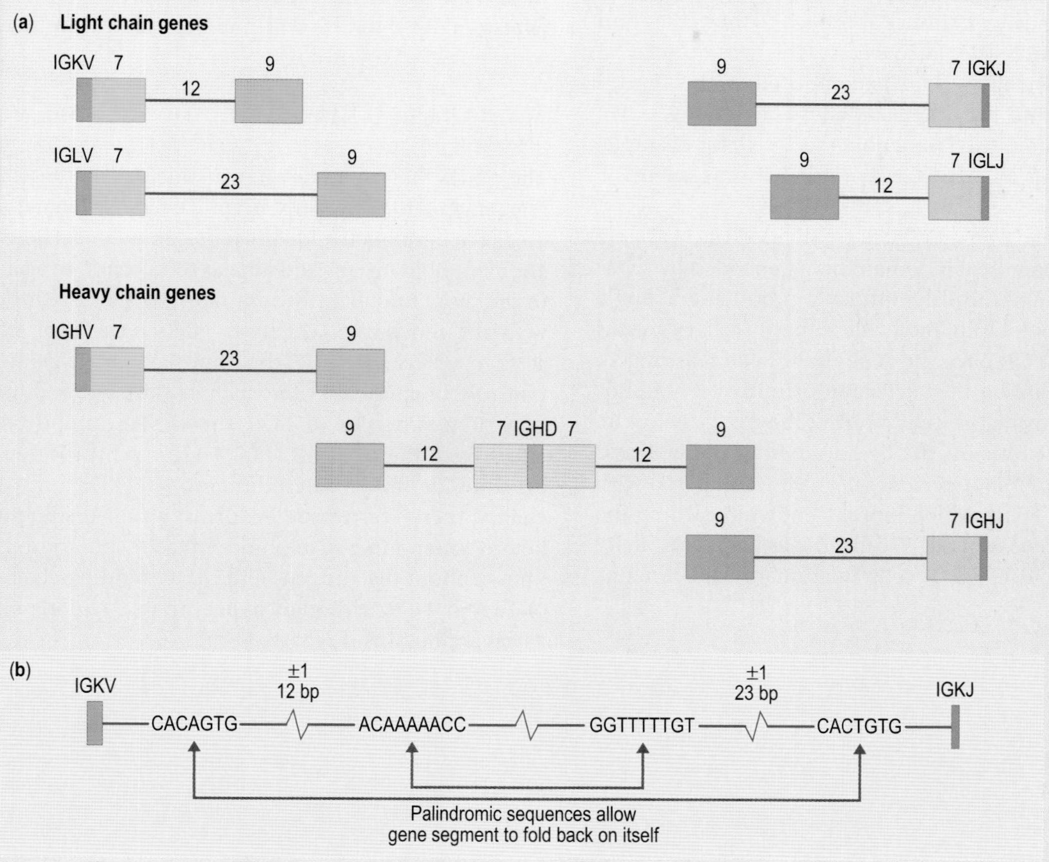

(a)   Light chain genes

IGKV   7 — 12 — 9   9 — 23 — 7 IGKJ

IGLV   7 — 23 — 9   9 — 12 — 7 IGLJ

Heavy chain genes

IGHV   7 — 23 — 9

9 — 12 — 7 IGHD 7 — 12 — 9

9 — 23 — 7 IGHJ

(b)

IGKV —CACAGTG— ±1 12 bp —ACAAAAACC— —GGTTTTTGT— ±1 23 bp —CACTGTG— IGKJ

Palindromic sequences allow
gene segment to fold back on itself

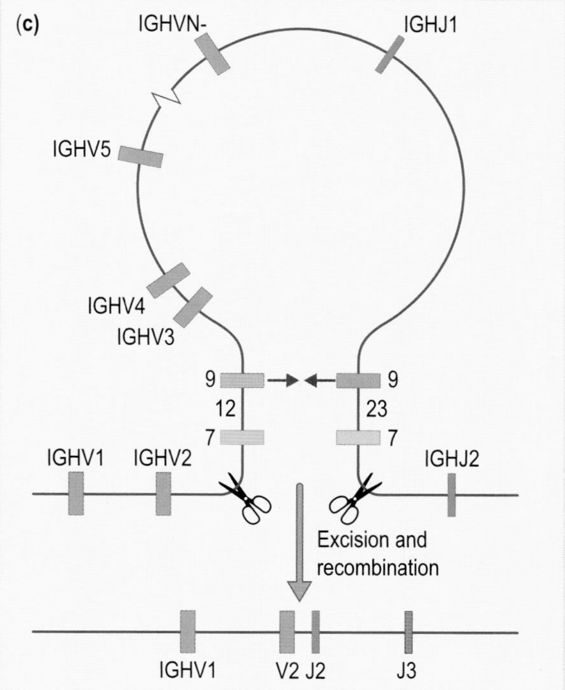

(c)

IGHVN-   IGHJ1

IGHV5

IGHV4
IGHV3

9 — 12 — 7   9 — 23 — 7

IGHV1   IGHV2   IGHJ2

Excision and
recombination

IGHV1   V2 J2   J3

**Fig. 4.16 Mechanisms of gene rearrangements
for immunoglobulin segment genes.**
(**a**) Heptamer and nonamer consensus sequences
flanking the VJ and VDJ joining sites, showing the
12–23 rule. Note that V–J joining in the heavy chain
is forbidden and that the D segment insertion
between V and J is obligatory. (**b**) Examples of the
palindromic heptamer and nonamer sequences
flanking the κ light chain segments. (**c**) Probable
mechanism of rearrangement of genes within
different segments on a chromatid to bring two
genes together. Here V2 and J2 are brought
together by the formation and excision of a loop of
redundant DNA.

T cell receptors for antigen

In broad terms, the genomic organisation of T cell receptor (TCR) genes is similar to that of immunoglobulin genes, with each cell type using a similar approach to the generation of receptor diversity. The TCR exists as a heterodimer, of which there are two types. One is composed of an α and β chain (αβ TCR), and the other of γ and δ chains (γδ TCR). The TCR type is often used to denote the T cell: for example, a T cell expressing an αβ TCR is referred to as an αβ T cell.

The chains of each type of TCR are divided into variable and constant domains, each domain being encoded by separate gene pools. Like the B lymphocyte producing a single clone of immunoglobulin molecules, the T cell expresses only one form of TCR once the genes have been rearranged. The γδ TCR appears on the surface of primitive T lymphocytes in the thymus before cells bearing the αβ TCR can be seen. The αβ TCR remains the best studied in humans and is present on over 90% of peripheral T cells (compared with 1–10% for the γδ TCR). Much more is known regarding the antigen responsiveness of αβ T cells; the antigen specificity and functional role of γδ T cells in humans still remains unclear.

Structure and function of the αβ T cell receptor

The αβ TCR is a disulphide-bonded heterodimer comprising an α chain (43–49 kDa) and a β chain (38–44 kDa) (Fig. 4.17). The variable and constant domains follow the nomenclature of the immunoglobulin molecules V_α, V_β, C_α and C_β. The structure of the domains in the TCRs is analogous to that of the immunoglobulin domains, and they form part of the immunoglobulin supergene family. As for antibodies, it appears that TCRs have hypervariable regions in the variable domains, forming CDRs 1–3. Remembering that the func-

tion of the TCRs is to recognise and bind the shape formed by the peptide embedded within an MHC molecule groove, it is now known that CDRs 1 and 2 interact with the two α-helices of the α1 and α2 domains of the MHC molecule, as these run along the sides of the antigen-binding groove, whilst CDR3 interacts with the peptide within the groove.

Structure and function of the γδ T cell receptor

The γδ TCRs are somewhat distinctive in that their gene rearrangement is an early thymic event. As stated above, γδ T cells in humans are equally represented in peripheral blood and lymphoid organs and appear to function in a similar way to the more numerically dominant αβ T cells. This contrasts with the mouse, in which γδ TCRs have been extensively studied, where it appears that they have a particularly important role in epithelial sites, such as skin, gut and lungs.

Structurally, the γδ TCR shows some important differences from the αβ TCR (Fig. 4.17b). Whilst it does exist as a disulphide-linked heterodimer of γ (50 kDa) and δ (40 kDa) chains, there are two other forms: a non-disulphide-linked heterodimer and a disulphide-linked γγ homodimer. Less is known about the antigen- and MHC-binding characteristics of the γδ TCR, although hypervariable regions within the variable domains do exist.

The T cell receptor genes

The repertoire of T cell antigen receptors is required to have a similar depth of diversity as that for antibodies. For the α, β, γ and δ chains, the genes are divided into two separate groups, one encoding the variable domains using multiple gene segments, the other for the constant domains. As for immunoglobulin genes, TCR genes must undergo rearrangements from the germline before they are transcribed and translated.

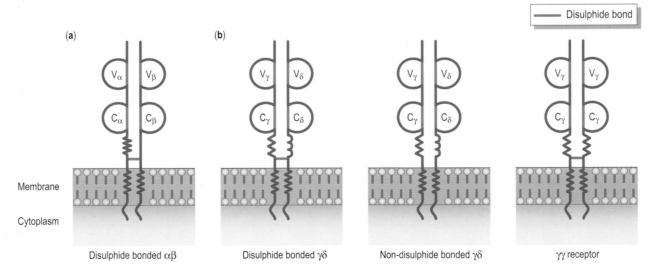

Fig. 4.17 **The structure of the T cell receptor.**
(**a**) The αβ TCR. (**b**) The different types of γδ TCR.

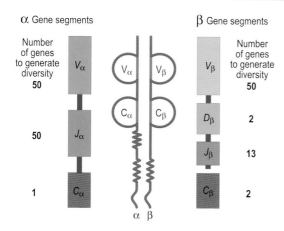

Fig. 4.18 Numbers of different gene segments used to generate αβ TCR diversity.

Genes for the α and β chains

Analogous to the heavy and light chain gene segments of immunoglobulin molecules, the gene encoding the α chain is formed by the recombination of segments from different gene groups, in this case TRAV (of which there are ~50 functional genes), TRAJ (~50) and a single TRAC gene segment (Fig. 4.18). The potential diversity achievable for the α chain is, therefore, 2500.

The β chain genes comprise the following different functional segments: TRBV (~50), TRBD (2), TRBJ (13) and TRBC (2), giving 2600 possible forms.

Overall, the diversity achievable from a set of α and β chain genes rearranging and producing two polypeptide chains is 2500 × 2600 = 6.5 million.

There are some important differences in the genes and in the genetic processes that give rise to the assembled TCR product compared with immunoglobulin genes. First, the TRAC and TRBC genes do not encode segments typical of secreted proteins, indicating that secretion of TCRs is not an important functional characteristic. Second, there is no somatic hypermutation in the genes encoding a complete αβ TCR. This is an important difference from immunoglobulins since, as we shall see, it would be dangerous to allow a T lymphocyte, once selected for its antigen receptor and allowed into the periphery in a mature form, to alter subsequently its receptor configuration.

Genes for the γ and δ chains

The human γ chain gene locus contains three gene segment pools: TRGV (10 genes), TRGJ (6) and TRGC (2). The diversity achievable is, therefore, relatively limited, to 10 × 6 × 2 = 120 different rearranged genes. The δ chain genes are located within the middle of the α chain gene locus, and are arranged in four pools of TRDV (3 genes), TRDD (3), TRDJ (4) and TRDC (1). The diversity produced is 3 × 3 × 4 × 1 = 36 possible rearrangements; combined with the γ chain genes the total diversity in the receptor is 120 × 36 = 4320.

Generation of T cell receptor diversity

The mechanism for bringing different gene components of the TCRs together in order to construct a rearranged TCR gene is virtually the same as that used for the immunoglobulin genes, and nonamer and heptamer sequences as well as the 12 and 23 nucleotide sequences (the '12–23' rule; see Science Box 4.4).

Apart from the presence of randomly associating gene segments and the possibility of V–D–D–J and V–J combinations as well as V–D–J, TCR diversity is derived from other mechanisms. In particular, imprecise joining, as for the immunoglobulin gene segments, is common, and the resultant new nucleotide sequences and frame-shift mutations contribute considerably to diversity (see Table 4.4). The extent of the total diversity is difficult to estimate, but it is thought to be many orders of magnitude in excess of that indicated in the number of individual gene segments in each of the V, D, J and C pools (see Table 4.4).

SUMMARY BOX 4.5

T cell receptors for antigen

- TCRs have a basic molecule composed of two chains; these may be α/β (90%) or γ/δ. Within the chains are the distinctive motifs which make these molecules members of the immunoglobulin supergene family.

- Like antibodies, TCRs have distinctive regions that are highly variable between different molecules; these regions interact with antigen.

- TCRs vary in structure through: selection from a large pool of gene segments for individual receptor chains; and random imprecision in the joining together of the selected variable, diversity and joining genes.

- TCRs do not mutate somatically after gene rearrangement.

- The function of the TCR is to recognise and bind the complex of a specific antigen with a self MHC molecule, which is formed when the antigenic peptide becomes embedded within the MHC groove.

Further reading

Jardetzky T 1997 Not just another Fab: the crystal structure of a TcR-MHC-peptide complex. Structure 5: 159–163

Krogsgaard M, Davis MM 2005 How T cells 'see' antigen. Nat Immunol 6(3): 239–245

Lefranc MP 2004 IMGT-ontology and IMGT databases, tools and web resources for immunogenetics and immunoinformatics. Mol Immunol 40: 647–660

Maizels N 2005 Immunoglobulin gene diversification. Annu Rev Genet 39: 23–46

Papavasiliou FN, Schatz DG 2002 Somatic hypermutation of immunoglobulin genes: merging mechanisms for genetic diversity. Cell 109 Suppl: S35–44

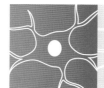

The human leukocyte antigens

This chapter is centred around a collection of genes, termed the **major histocompatibility complex (MHC)**, that in humans represents about 0.1% of the whole genome, is sited on the short arm of chromosome 6, and plays a critical role in immune function. In particular, the MHC contains a group of genes that code for proteins expressed on the surface of a variety of cell types. In humans, these are known as the **human leukocyte antigens**, or HLA system. So, use of the term MHC refers to this collection of genes in general, while the term HLA refers only to the human MHC. **HLA/MHC molecules** are involved in **antigen recognition by T lymphocytes**. The T lymphocyte receptor only recognises antigen that is presented as a short peptide embedded within a physical groove created by a HLA molecule.

Several other features of the MHC make it interesting for clinicians and biologists. First, it has been known for many years that differences in HLA molecules between individuals are responsible for tissue and organ graft rejection (hence the name histo- (*tissue*) compatibility; see Science Box 5.1). Second, genetic studies have revealed that possession of certain HLA genes is linked to greater susceptibility to particular diseases, such as multiple sclerosis, type 1 diabetes and ankylosing spondylitis (see Science Box 5.2). Finally, it has been demonstrated that differences in the ability of mouse strains to respond to particular antigens can be mapped to genes in the MHC, implying that at the level of antigen-specificity, these genes control the immune response. Armed with the knowledge that HLA molecules present antigen, we must now set about accounting for these original observations.

The major histocompatibility complex

The immune response

In 1974, two scientists, Zinkernagel and Doherty, published a series of classic experiments that can be considered as the turning points in our understanding of the physiological role of MHC genes in the immune response (Fig. 5.2), for which they received the 1996 Nobel Prize in Medicine. The studies demonstrated that in strain A mice infected with lymphocytic choriomeningitis virus (LCMV), cytotoxic T lymphocytes appeared that were capable of killing LCMV-infected cells. However, LCMV-infected target cells obtained from strain B, which differed from strain A at certain genetic loci in the MHC, were not susceptible to killing by cytotoxic T lymphocytes from strain A. LCMV-infected target cells obtained from strains other than A were susceptible to killing by cytotoxic T cells from strain A, as long as they shared identical genes at these key MHC loci.

It appeared from these studies that recognition of a viral antigen by cytotoxic T cells required the presence on the target cell of molecules encoded by the MHC. More than this, the MHC molecules had to be the same as those present in the animal from which the cytotoxic T cells were obtained. This principle was termed the **law of MHC restriction**: antigen-specific cytotoxic T cell responses are *restricted* to kill only those target cells that bear the correct MHC molecule. Antiviral responses were convenient for these early studies, but, subsequently, the universality of this principle was established for all forms of T lymphocyte response to antigen. Once the law of MHC restriction was established, researchers set about interpreting it. Clearly, it implies that a T lymphocyte is compelled to recognise a specific antigen

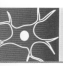

SCIENCE BOX 5.1

MHC genes and organ transplantation

Some of the proteins encoded by genes in the MHC are at the heart of organ graft rejection. Attempts to transplant tissue from one animal to another have been made for over 200 years, with limited success. Early studies on animals revealed that transplanted organs, for example kidneys, did not survive because of a destructive process termed 'rejection', taking place within 1 or 2 weeks of implantation. By the middle part of the twentieth century, surgical techniques had advanced sufficiently for human organ transplantation to be considered viable, and this became a major driving force in the study of rejection. The use of inbreeding in mice to achieve pure strains with complete genetic identity — syngeneity — between individuals demonstrated that skin grafts between such animals were not rejected, while grafts between animals of two genetically different inbred strains were. By careful cross-breeding between different inbred strains, the genes most important in conferring skin graft compatibility between individual mice were soon identified. In mice, the gene complex involved is on chromosome 17, and because of its determinant role in whether tissues are compatible, it was termed the major histocompatibility complex (Table 5.1; Fig. 5.1).

Identification of the human MHC took a little longer for the obvious reason that inbred strains are not readily available. Clues to its existence came from the results of a series of kidney transplants performed in Boston in the early 1950s. Those performed between unrelated individuals were uniformly unsuccessful, but the survival of one of these patients for 6 months encouraged further operations to be undertaken, this time between identical twins. The unqualified success of these grafts was confirmation of the existence of genes determining tissue types in humans, and this was soon followed by the identification of the human MHC. Very much like the ABO blood group system, it was established that the molecules actually involved in determining the 'foreignness' of a graft were present as proteins on the surface of white blood cells, hence the name human leukocyte antigens.

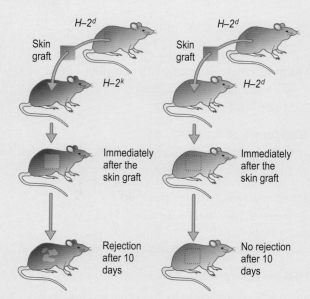

Fig. 5.1 Influence of MHC genes on skin grafting. A graft from a mouse possessing the *d* gene at the *H–2* locus is rejected after 10 days by a mouse possessing the *k* gene at this locus. The *H–2* locus in mice is the MHC region, equivalent of the HLA genes in humans.

Table 5.1 Terminology and definitions

Term	Definition
Major histocompatibility complex (MHC)	Large collection of genes that includes those responsible for determining rejection of transplanted tissue by the immune system; versions of the MHC are possessed by all mammals, and by animals as low as coelenterates (e.g. sea anemones)
Human leukocyte antigens (HLA)	Term for human MHC gene products involved in antigen presentation to T lymphocytes
Haplotype	A collection of genes (i.e. a section of chromosome) inherited as a whole group
Gene polymorphism	The availability in the gene pool of the population of many different allelic forms of a gene at a particular locus
Linkage disequilibrium	Alleles appearing *together* on the same haplotype more frequently than their single gene frequencies suggest; this implies that meiotic recombination is non-random

MHC and disease susceptibility

The association between the inheritance of particular genes in the MHC and a higher risk of developing certain diseases was first clearly demonstrated in 1973, when Brewerton showed that over 90% of patients with ankylosing spondylitis, an inflammatory disease of the spine, had *B27* as one of their HLA types. Possible explanations for such associations are discussed in a later chapter (see p. 127), but they serve to underline that this group of genes was known for its relationship with disease and graft rejection before a physiological function could be assigned to it.

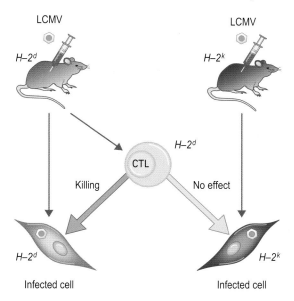

Fig. 5.2 MHC restriction of immune responses.
The experiments that led to a Nobel Prize in Medicine. Mice infected with the lymphocytic choriomeningitis virus (LCMV) produced cytotoxic T lymphocytes (CTL) capable of killing LCMV-infected target cells from the same animal. Cells infected with LCMV but possessing different genes at the *H–2* locus to those of the mouse providing the CTL cells are not susceptible to killing. These studies indicated that CTLs need to recognise both LCMV *and* a self MHC molecule.

(e.g. a virus) *and* MHC molecules simultaneously. It is the molecular basis of this recognition that forms the major subject of this chapter.

Structure of the HLA

The human MHC, or HLA, comprises three major classes (I, II and III) of genes involved in the immune response (Fig. 5.3). In addition, there are several genes that lie in the HLA region but do not fall into any of the three major categories. These include the genes for 21-hydroxylase (an enzyme important in steroid metabolism), tumour necrosis

factor-α, and heat-shock protein 70 (one of a family of proteins produced by cells in response to heat and other injuries). An extended map of the HLA region can be found at http://www.sanger.ac.uk/HGP/Chr6/XMHC/.

Genes in the HLA are designated using capital italic letters. The protein molecules produced by them are designated with capital roman letters and the Greek letters α and β describe the polypeptide chains.

Class I region

The 'classical' (also called class Ia) class I HLA genes are found furthest from the centromere and are designated by capital letters, *HLA-A*, *HLA-B* and *HLA-C*. They are 'classical' in the sense that they present peptide antigens to T cells — such responses are the main topic in this chapter. These class I genes encode the class I α chains (the *H–2* region is the mouse equivalent). The class I β chain that combines with an α chain to form the class I HLA molecule is an invariant molecule (i.e. the same β chain is used for all α chains) called **β₂-microglobulin**, the gene for which is on chromosome 15. Once α and β chains are assembled, the class I molecule has the role of presenting peptide antigens to T lymphocytes.

Unlike the β chain, the genes encoding the α chains vary. In some cases, the number of different alleles is considerable, a phenomenon termed **gene polymorphism**. The result of such gene polymorphism is that there is enormous potential for individuals to differ in the *HLA* genes they possess, and hence the HLA molecules they express. We identify these differences by **HLA typing**. As an example, there are nearly 200 allelic versions of the *HLA-A* genes.

In the same region of the genome are some 'non-classical' HLA class I genes, known as class Ib. They are less polymorphic, have a more restricted expression on specialised cell types, and present a restricted type of peptide or none at all. The main genes here are *HLA-E*, *F* and *G*, and some of the encoded molecules have an important interaction with natural killer cells. In addition, in the region between class I and class III lies a set of genes that give rise to proteins with a similar overall structure to class I molecules, but that differ in key respects — notably they do not bind peptide antigen to present it to T lymphocytes. These are MHC class I-related (MIC, or class Ic) genes, *A* and *B*. These are also highly polymorphic gene regions, with over 70 MICA and MICB alleles. The MIC genes are expressed mainly on epithelial surfaces and participate in an interaction with lymphocytes that signals cellular stress.

Class II region

The class II genes have three major subregions, *DP*, *DQ* and *DR* (there are two equivalent regions in the mouse, *I–A* and *I–E*) (see Fig. 5.3). In these subregions are genes encoding molecules that, like those in the class I region, present peptide antigen to T lymphocytes. Other molecules encoded here aid this process: *HLA-DM* and *-DO*, *TAP* genes; and *PSMB* genes.

Two distinct polypeptide chains, termed the α and β chains, combine to form the class II HLA molecules -DR,

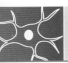

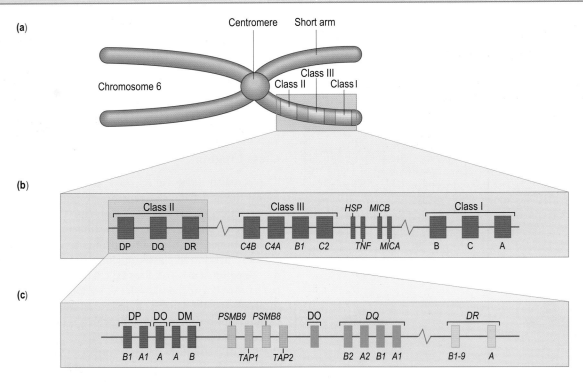

Fig. 5.3 **The three classes of genes in the human MHC.**

(**a**) Site on short arm of chromosome 6 where the HLA region is. (**b**) The major subregions (classes I, II and III) and genes within each. (**c**) Detailed map of class II region showing the major genes. TAP, transporter associated with processing; HSP, heat-shock protein; TNF, tumour necrosis factor; MICA and MICB, MHC class I-related A and B molecules; PSMB, proteasome subunit beta.

-DQ and -DP, that present antigen to T lymphocytes. Like the class I molecule, the HLA class II molecule is termed a **heterodimer** because it is made up of two different chains. The *DR* subregion contains only a single α chain gene (*DRA*), and, therefore, all HLA-DR molecules have the same α chain. There is more than one *DRB* gene locus (see http://www.sanger.ac.uk/HGP/Chr6/XMHC/II_list.shtml), but the best known is *DRB1*, encoding a distinct β chain, which can combine with the single invariant α chain to form the DR molecule DRαβ1. The number of other DRB genes expressed in an individual depends upon the **haplotype** inherited (a haplotype is a group of genes inherited as a unit).

At each locus of the functional DRB genes, there is the potential for different alleles (i.e. different forms of the same gene). While *DRA* has no allelic forms, and hence as stated the α chain is invariant, the *DRB* genes are highly variable and so, like the class I region, this area is highly **polymorphic**: the *DRB1* locus has over 60 different alleles. Since only the *DRB* genes are polymorphic, it is these that determine the particular HLA-DR type.

The *DQ* region contains two pairs of genes for the α and β chains. *DQA1* and *DQB1* are the better characterised and encode the DQ α and β chains that combine to form the DQ molecule, which is expressed on cell surfaces. Both DQ α and β chains are polymorphic (i.e. have numerous possible alleles at the locus) though the DQ β chain bears the majority of the polymorphism.

In the DP region, *DPA1* and *DPB1* encode the DP α and β chains that form the expressed DP molecule. The DP α

chain displays low levels of polymorphism, whereas the DP β chain is highly polymorphic.

Finally, there are related gene regions, *DM* and *DO*. The product of the *DMA* and *DMB* genes is an αβ heterodimer that, unlike the heterodimers produced by genes in the *DP*, *DQ* and *DR* subregions, is very rarely expressed on the cell surface, if at all. HLA-DM αβ molecules play a critical role in loading peptide into the other, 'more conventional' class II HLA molecules (see p. 96). HLA-DO has a role in regulating the antigen loading process.

There are other gene groups of importance in the class II region, of which we shall hear more when the mechanism through which antigenic peptides are loaded onto HLA molecules is discussed in greater depth (see p. 94). *PSMB8* and *9* genes code for **p**roteasome subunit, **b**eta type, 8 and 9. These are proteins contained within a large, multimolecular enzyme complex called the **proteasome**, which can actually be visualised at the electron microscopic level (see p. 98). The role of the PSMBs is in the cleavage of proteins into smaller peptides for binding to class I HLA molecules. *TAP-1* and *TAP-2* genes (for transportation associated with processing) each encode one half of a peptide transporter responsible for transporting peptides of the required length into the class I synthesis compartment for loading.

Class III region

Between the class I and II regions is the class III region, which contains several genes coding for complement components, which we encountered in Chapter 2.

Structure of the HLA gene region

- MHC genes (HLA in humans) encode for proteins involved in the immune response.

- There are three classes of genes: I, II and III.

- Class I and II genes encode for proteins that physically present peptide antigens to T lymphocytes, whilst class III genes encode complement proteins.

- Each of us possesses a discrete number of different class I and II genes.

- Gene polymorphism in the class I and II regions ensures that at a population level there are many different versions of class I and II genes.

Inheritance of the MHC

Two complementary chromosome strands, one maternal and one paternal, are inherited, each strand providing an MHC haplotype, i.e. a string of MHC genes linked together on the same chromosome. For example, in the class I region, an individual might have inherited the *A1* and *B7* genes on a single maternally derived chromosome. The paternal genes at these loci might be *A28* and *B14*. When the genes of maternal and paternal haplotype are transcribed and translated into their protein products, *both* maternally and paternally derived allelic forms are expressed as cell surface proteins, a feature known as **co-dominance**. In our example, A1, A28, B7 and B14 class I molecules are expressed (Fig. 5.4).

Haplotypes encoding class II HLA molecules are inherited in a similar fashion. The major difference is that haplotypes in this region do not necessarily contain a full complement of the *DRB* loci. However, all haplotypes contain the *DRB1* locus, which is the location of the best studied HLA-DR genes.

Although genes in the MHC follow a Mendelian inheritance pattern, two additional features of this complex serve to set it apart in terms of genetics. One of these is the degree of gene polymorphism and the other is linkage disequilibrium between different loci. **Linkage disequilibrium** describes the fact that certain alleles are found together on the same haplotype with greater frequency than should occur if recombination during meiosis was random. For example, genes for HLA-B8 and HLA-DR3 are found in a Caucasian population with frequencies of 9% and 12%, respectively. Therefore, the expected frequency of a haplotype containing *HLA-B8* and *DR3* is 0.09 × 0.12, giving 0.0108, or approximately 1%; this haplotype is actually found in over 7% of Caucasians. Linkage disequilibrium results in the inheritance of large portions of the MHC that are intact and have not undergone recombination. It gives rise, therefore, to what are termed **extended haplotypes**; long segments of chromosome that incorporate genes from all three MHC classes and are passed on undisturbed from generation to generation.

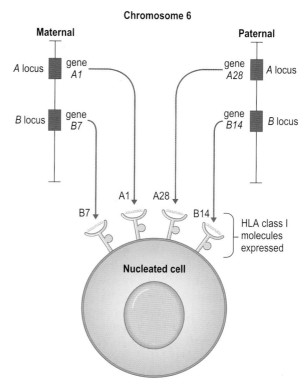

Fig. 5.4 Inheritance of HLA genes and expression of the gene products, demonstrating co-dominance.
This typical nucleated cell expresses gene products from both maternal and paternal chromosomes. Thus the HLA class I type of the individual from whom this cell comes is A1, 28; B7, 14.

Studying the MHC: HLA typing

As we shall see in later sections on autoimmune disease (Ch. 13) and transplantation (Ch. 11), examining the **HLA type** of an individual has become a part of mainstream clinical practice. HLA typing is now carried out almost entirely at the DNA sequencing level. The challenge is to have a technique to tell the difference between different genes in this highly polymorphic region. The favoured approach is to amplify the DNA of a particular locus using the polymerase chain reaction (PCR) using a technique in which there is only successful DNA amplification when the genomic DNA sequence matches that of the primer used. By using a range of primers for different alleles, particular alleles, corresponding to the HLA type, can be identified.

Tissue distribution of HLA molecules

Important differences exist in the tissue and cell distribution of HLA molecules. These are governed by cell lineage and state of maturation/activation (Table 5.2). Broadly speaking, class I HLA molecules are expressed everywhere and class II molecules at specialised sites of active immune response, such as the lymph node. More precisely, whilst **class I**

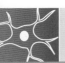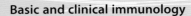

Table 5.2 Cells constitutively expressing HLA molecules

Class I	Class II
Virtually all nucleated cells	Dendritic cells
	Macrophages and monocytes
	B lymphocytes

molecules are expressed on the surface of virtually all cells except for mature erythrocytes and trophoblast cells, **class II molecules** are only expressed as a matter of routine (so-called constitutive expression) on the surface of a small number of cell types, including macrophages, monocytes, dendritic cells and B lymphocytes (but not plasma cells). These are all cells with the ability to carry out a process termed **antigen presentation** (see p. 95).

Under the influence of cytokines released during inflammation (e.g. interferons-α and γ, tumour necrosis factor) a whole range of cells that typically only express class I may be induced to express class II MHC molecules and also to up-regulate the number of surface MHC class I molecules. This ability to up-regulate MHC expression is important in the eradication of intracellular viral infections.

SUMMARY BOX 5.2

Genes in the HLA

- Each of us expresses on the cell surface both maternally and paternally derived HLA molecules; the genes are inherited in large 'chunks' called haplotypes.

- Class I HLA molecules are almost ubiquitously expressed on the surface of nucleated cells.

- Class II HLA molecule expression is highly restricted to cells that present antigens to T lymphocytes.

Structure of HLA molecules

The class I molecules, HLA-A, HLA-B and HLA-C, are formed from polymorphic heavy-chain glycoproteins (44 kDa) that bind non-covalently to the β chain, β_2-microglobulin (12 kDa). The class II molecules, HLA-DP, HLA-DQ and HLA-DR, are formed from two glycoproteins, an α chain (34 kDa) and a β chain (29 kDa) (Fig. 5.5).

Three-dimensional structure of HLA molecules

In 1987 the first crystal structure of class I MHC protein was obtained for HLA-A2 and much is now known about the

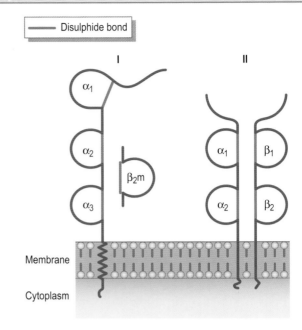

Fig. 5.5 Schematic illustration of the structure of class I and class II molecules.
In class I molecules, the heavy or α chain carries three distinct extracellular regions, or domains, formed by disulphide bonding, while the lighter β_2-microglobulin is a much smaller one-domain structure. The α and β chains are not covalently linked. The α chain is anchored into the cell membrane. The class II molecule is formed from two similar polypeptide chains (α and β). These are non-covalently linked and both are membrane anchored. Each chain has two domains formed by disulphide bridging. Because the class II HLA molecule is made from two different chains it is often referred to as a heterodimer. The domains present in both class I and II molecules can be subdivided into two 'immunoglobulin-like' domains and two 'peptide-binding' domains. For class I MHC molecules, the heavy chain inserts into the cell membrane and contains both peptide-binding domains (α_1 and α_2) and one immunoglobulin domain (α_3). Class II molecules have a symmetrical arrangement in which the two polypeptides each insert into the membrane and each supply one peptide-binding (α_1 and β_1) and one immunoglobulin domain (α_2 and β_2).

structure–function relationships in this molecule. Perhaps the most comprehensible view to have is to take the position of an approaching T cell about to interact with the HLA class I molecule and the peptide antigen it is holding for presentation. The T cell receptor encounters a deep-grooved binding site, 2.5 nm long, 1 nm wide and 1 nm deep, closed at either end and occupied by an antigenic peptide of around 9 amino acid residues in length. The groove is fashioned by two α-helices which make up the sides, on top of a floor comprising eight anti-parallel β-pleated sheets (Fig. 5.6). The α-helices and floor contain holes ('pockets') that can accommodate side chains poking out from the different amino acids in the bound peptide. When HLA-A2 was crystallised, this binding site actually contained tightly bound electron-dense material; this was the bound peptide. On the basis of these observations, it is now possible to visualise T cell rec-

(a)

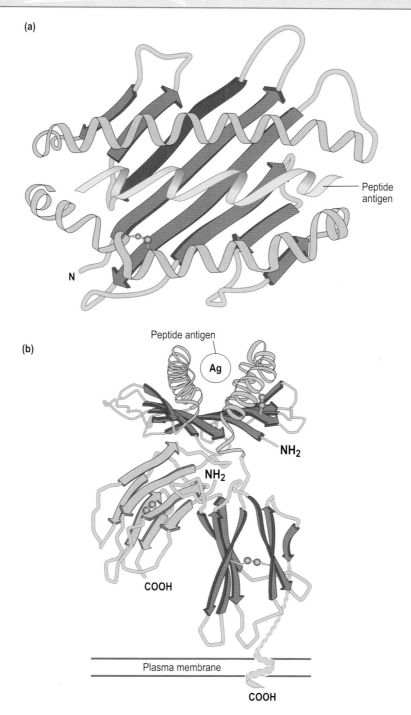

Peptide antigen

N

(b)

Peptide antigen

Ag

NH₂

NH₂

COOH

Plasma membrane

COOH

Fig. 5.6 Structure of the HLA class I molecule.
(**a**) As seen by an approaching T cell receptor, the class I molecule has a deep groove, the antigen-binding site, occupied by a short antigenic peptide. The groove is constructed from two α-helices on either side and has a floor made from β-pleated sheets.
(**b**) Lateral view of the molecule with a peptide in the antigen-binding groove (modified with permission from Bjorkman et al 1987 Nature 329: 506–512).

ognition as a T cell receptor clinging to both α-helical sides of the HLA groove and also embracing the peptide lying within it.

Comparisons between the crystallographic structures of HLA class I molecules such as A2 and A68 show that, with minor perturbations, the polypeptide backbones are extremely similar. The differences between them relate almost entirely to the nature of the amino acids that occupy positions lining the floor and sides of the groove. The side chains of amino acids at these positions influence the composition of the pockets mentioned above. This means that even an apparently small number of differences between two HLA

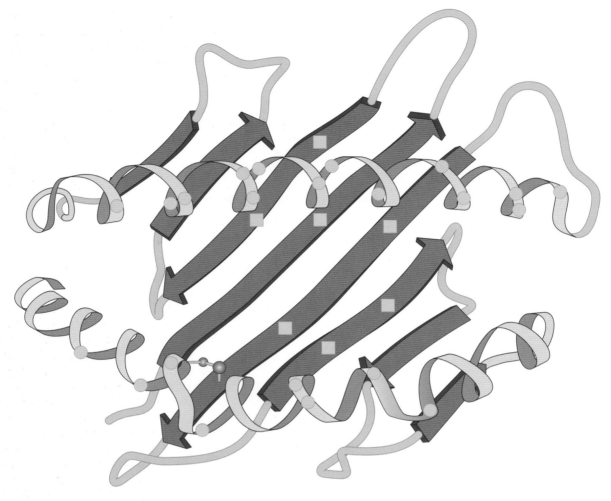

Fig. 5.7 Examples of sites at which amino acids tend to vary in HLA class I molecules (i.e. polymorphic residues).
Polymorphic residues shown as circles in the α-helices and as squares in the β-pleated sheets. Note how polymorphism affects all parts of the peptide antigen binding site (modified with permission from Bjorkman et al 1987 Nature 329: 506–512).

molecules can have a profound effect on the peptides they can bind (Fig. 5.7).

This is a critically important point, as it gives a physiological explanation for polymorphism (see p. 58) in HLA molecules. Each HLA molecule has a limited repertoire of antigenic peptides that can bind into its groove. At an individual level, we each express several different class I molecules (by having multiple loci A, B, C, etc., and co-dominance). This increases the range of different antigenic peptides an individual can present to T lymphocytes. In the context of presenting peptides from infectious agents to T cells, it is not difficult to see that these features are of benefit to the individual. Similarly, at the population level, there are many polymorphisms (i.e. slightly altered versions) of HLA molecules, which further increases the potential range and diversity of peptides that can be bound across the human race. Again, in the context of presenting peptides from infectious agents to T cells, it is not difficult to see that this polymorphism is of benefit to the species.

The crystallographic structure of a class II molecule, HLA-DR1, was solved in 1993. It has a remarkably similar appearance to that of class I (Fig. 5.8), with some key differences. First, the peptide binding groove is larger and is not closed at either end, allowing the peptide to protrude. This feature is consistent with the finding that class II binding peptides are roughly double the length of those binding class I molecules (see below).

Interaction of the HLA molecule and peptide

The function of HLA molecules is to bind short peptide fragments of whole antigens. The antigens are degraded inside cells and the peptides, bound to HLA, are presented on the cell surface in order to interact with the receptors of T cells. As a general rule of thumb, the source of the peptide dictates whether it is presented in association with class I or class II molecules. Under physiological conditions, peptides derived from proteins synthesised endogenously, within the cell presenting the antigen, are presented bound to class I HLA molecules. Note that this can include peptides from virus proteins — during a viral infection, viral proteins are synthe-

complex. The nature of the T lymphocyte recognition is dictated by another law of MHC restriction: only T cells bearing a surface glycoprotein molecule (termed CD4) that binds to a fixed, non-varying point on the class II β chain, are able to interact with class II-presented peptides. Conversely, only T cells bearing a surface glycoprotein (CD8) that binds to the α chain of the class I molecule are able to recognise peptide presented by class I HLA molecules. With very few exceptions, mature T lymphocytes express either CD4 or CD8, but not both. It seems probable that one of the main functions of these CD4 and CD8 'accessory' molecules is to stabilise the interaction of the T cell receptor and the HLA molecule–peptide complex, which is typically of quite low affinity.

Peptide binding to class I HLA molecules

Since the crystallisation of HLA-A2, and the intriguing view of a tightly bound peptide in the groove, extensive studies on the characteristics of this binding have been carried out. One approach has been to use acid dissociation to disrupt the class I molecule and free the bound peptides. From a class I MHC molecule, the eluted peptides are typically nine amino acid residues long and composed from endogenous proteins (Table 5.3). They fit tightly into the groove using non-covalent forces such as hydrogen bonding, van der Waals and electrostatic forces. Side chains from the peptide squeeze into pockets in the groove. The pockets are numbered 1 to 9, according to the length of the peptide, and for HLA class I molecules, the major anchoring pockets are P2 and P9 (Table 5.3; Fig. 5.9a). For a given HLA molecule, therefore, the amino acids at positions 2 and 9 are usually constant. The intervening peptides provide some auxiliary binding but show more variability. The characteristic sequence of a peptide for a particular HLA molecule is termed the **motif**.

It appears that the peptide itself may occasionally be required to bend to fit into the class I groove, which is closed at both ends. As we shall see later (p. 69) this may force the middle region of the peptide to bulge out of the groove towards the approaching T cell receptor. It is this middle, 'bulging' part of the peptide that the T cell receptor interacts with.

The binding of peptide to class I molecules is tighter than to class II molecules and can be considered irreversible. This irreversibility correlates with the trap-like geometry of the peptide-binding groove. The kinetics of MHC molecule–peptide interactions can be represented by the dissociation constant, a measurement of the ratio between the rate at which molecules associate and dissociate. This has a value of between 10^{-5} and 10^{-6} M^{-1}, interpreted as indicating a slow association and a very slow dissociation. This dissociation constant is five orders of magnitude higher than interactions between antibody and antigens (i.e. antigen and antibody associate faster and dissociate slower). The half-life of the MHC–peptide complex on the cell surface is some 30 hours.

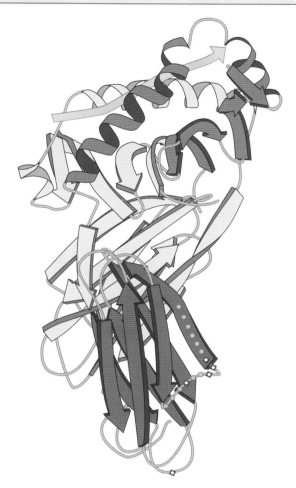

Fig. 5.8 Structure of HLA class II.
Three-dimensional structure of the class II αβ heterodimer, showing the orientation of the peptide binding groove (modified with permission from Brown et al Nature 364: 33–39).

sised endogenously using the host cell's 'machinery'. Hence, viral peptides may also be presented through this **endogenous pathway**, bound to class I HLA molecules. In contrast, peptides derived from outside the cell (exogenous antigens) are taken into the cell, processed using proteolytic enzymes (see Ch. 7) and presented after binding into the groove of class II HLA molecules. Antigens presented through this so-called **exogenous pathway** will include a variety of molecules from the external milieu: plasma proteins, for example. However, it should be noted that during infection or injury, the nature of the exogenous antigens will change. This is an opportunity for 'foreign' antigens, such as those derived from bacteria, to be processed and presented by HLA class II molecules to T lymphocytes. The uptake and presentation of foreign antigens to T cells is a pivotal event in the initiation of immune responses (see p. 95).

The role of the HLA molecule is the presentation of the peptide antigen fragment in its groove to a responding T lymphocyte. The T lymphocyte, as we shall discuss later, bears a receptor that recognises the HLA molecule–peptide

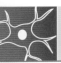

Table 5.3 Examples of self peptides eluted from the class I molecule HLA-B27

	Peptide									Source
	P2							P9		
	↓							↓		
R	R	I	K	E	I	V	K	K		Heat-shock protein 89β
R	R	V	K	E	V	V	K	K		Heat-shock protein 89β
G	R	I	D	K	P	I	L	K		Ribosomal protein
R	R	S	K	E	I	T	V	R		ATP-dependent RNA helicase
F	R	Y	N	G	L	I	H	R		60S ribosomal protein
R	R	Y	Q	K	S	T	E	L		Histone H3.3
R	R	W	L	P	A	G	D	A		Elongation factor 2

Marked with arrows are the amino acids that fit into the P2 and P9 pockets of HLA-B27. Each letter denotes an amino acid (e.g. R = arginine, see Appendix 4).

Peptide binding to class II HLA molecules

Peptide binding to class II HLA molecules runs along similar principles. The major differences are that the peptide is longer; and that the groove is open at each end, encouraging peptides to 'hang out' at either end. This promotes a looser fit for peptides in the HLA class II molecule groove.

The pathway leading to the generation of class II-binding peptides is designed to present fragments from the external milieu (e.g. from bacteria), but when a cell that expresses class II HLA molecules is 'at rest', it will present a range of peptides from plasma membrane-associated proteins. These proteins are internalised into the endosomal and lysosomal compartments, where class II HLA molecules are loaded — if a bacterium is internalised at the same time, peptide fragments from this pathogen will also be presented (Table 5.4).

On average, the peptides found in class II HLA molecule grooves are between 13 and 18 amino acid residues long (although the range is from as few as 10 to over 30). The pockets for interaction between peptide and the HLA class II groove are also numbered P1 to P9. The major pockets are P1, P4, P6 and P9 (Fig. 5.9b). Again, different HLA molecules have different structural features in these pockets because of polymorphism, and this dictates the type of amino acid side chain that will be preferred. Again, therefore, HLA class II molecules can be characterised by a **peptide-binding motif**. Apart from length, there are other important differences between class I- and II-associated peptides (Table 5.5). Class II peptides display 'promiscuity': in other words,

the same peptide may bind to several different types of class II molecules.

HLA polymorphism

With such a clear vision of the peptide-binding site, it is now possible to visualise the regions of the molecule that are characterised by the extensive polymorphism associated with the MHC. Polymorphism is the phenomenon whereby numerous different alleles — **allotypes** — can occur at a single locus. Gene polymorphism in the HLA region is the most extensive yet described. In evolutionary terms, polymorphism has arisen by gene duplication and point mutation to provide a mechanism for increasing the variety of peptides that can be presented to T lymphocytes. The higher the number of different HLA genes possessed by an individual, the wider the range of peptides that can be bound and the broader the ability of T cells to respond. In addition, because MHC genes are co-dominant, heterozygotes will have an advantage over homozygotes by being able to construct a wider range of chain combinations. The groove of a single HLA molecule can accommodate a variety of different peptide antigens, but it cannot bind all peptides against which it would be beneficial to mount an immune response.

Each person is capable of mounting strong responses to some organisms and weaker responses to others. Viewed in

Table 5.4 Examples of self peptides eluted from the class II molecule HLA-DR4 (B1*0401)

				P1 →			P4 →			P6 →			P9 →						Source
D	T	Q	F	V	R	F	D	S	D	A	S	Q	R	M	E	P	R		HLA-A2
D	T	Q	F	V	R	F	D	S	D	A	S	P	R	G	E				HLA-Cw9
G	S	L	F	Y	N	I	T	T	N	K	Y	K	A	F	L	D	K		VLA-4
P	E	D	F	Y	Q	F	K	M	K	C	Y	F						Q	HLA-DQβ
S																			

Marked with arrows are the amino acids that fit into the P1, P4, P6 and P9 pockets that are important for HLA-DR4 (B1*0401). Each letter denotes an amino acid (e.g. R = arginine, see Appendix 4).

(a)

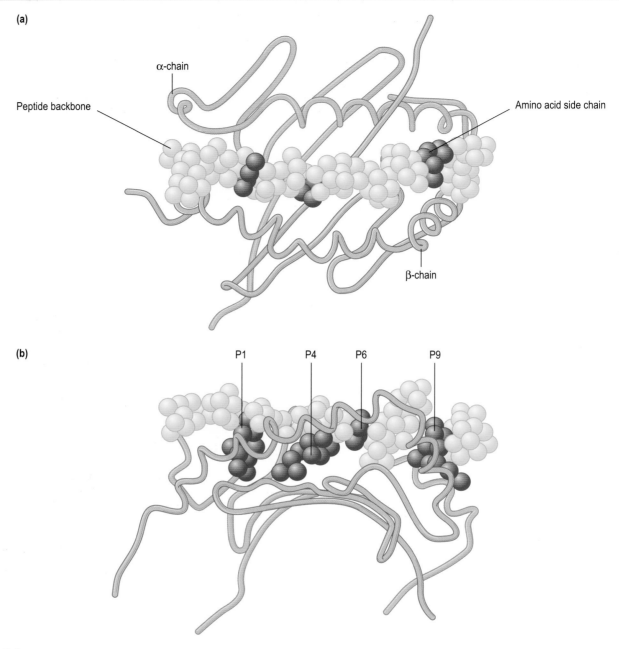

(b)

Fig. 5.9 Schematic representation of peptide binding to HLA class II molecule (a) as viewed from above by the approaching T cell and (b) lateral view. Panel (b) represents a cross-section through the peptide-binding region, showing pockets that receive side chains from the antigenic peptide. The main anchor residues for HLA class II molecules are P1, P4, P6 and P9. Side chains in the middle of the peptides project upwards towards the T cell receptor.

evolutionary terms, polymorphism decreases the chance of a population being annihilated by a microorganism against which not all individuals are capable of mounting an effective immune response. Within a species, therefore, the greater the MHC polymorphism, the greater the collective immunity (see Science Box 5.3). Polymorphism of HLA genes has two important consequences for the individual: unrelated individuals have a diverse susceptibility to disease and, as we

shall see later (p. 153), also promptly reject organ transplants between each other.

The variable regions responsible for HLA polymorphism generally lie along the α-helices that form the margins of the groove and the β-pleated sheets where the pockets are (see Fig. 5.7). Polymorphism, at these sites, serves to dictate the type of peptide fragment that binds and thus dictate the nature of presentation to the T cell receptor.

Table 5.5 Comparison of major features of class I and class II MHC molecules

	Class I molecules	Class II molecules
Genetic organisation	Polymorphic α chain genes in MHC (on chromosome 6 in humans) Monomorphic β chain gene (on chromosome 15 in humans)	Polymorphic α and β chain genes in MHC (on chromosome 6 in humans)
Molecular structure	Non-covalently associated αβ dimer	Non-covalently associated αβ dimer
Binding groove	Two α-helices flanking a floor of β-pleated sheets	Two α-helices flanking a floor of β-pleated sheets
Peptide size	Average 9 (range 8–10) amino acid residues	Average 15 (range 10–34) amino acid residues
Peptide source	Endogenous proteins (including virus-infected cells)	Exogenous and endogenous proteins derived from endosomal compartments situated near plasma membrane
Cellular site of peptide binding	Early: during assembly of class I molecule Peptide required for correct folding of dimer	Late: in a specialised endosome Invariant chain (but not peptide) required for folding of dimer
Affinity for peptide	High	Moderate
Role	Presentation of endogenous peptides to the TCR of T lymphocytes bearing the accessory molecule CD8	Presentation of exogenous peptides to the TCR of T lymphocytes bearing the accessory molecule CD4
Tissue distribution	Almost all nucleated cells	Dendritic cells, cells of monocyte lineage, B lymphocytes, activated T lymphocytes

SCIENCE BOX 5.3

HLA haplotypes — too much of a good thing?

Selective pressures during the course of evolution may have been the major factor in the survival of certain HLA gene combinations in a haplotype. Inherited together, a collection of class I, II and III genes could offer the optimum protection against a particular infection, providing a positive selection pressure. In contrast, studies since the late 1970s have shown that possession of certain HLA haplotypes is disadvantageous. For example, the extended haplotype of *HLA-A*0101*, *HLA-B*0801*, *HLA-DRB1*0301* and complement *C4AQ0* alleles present together on a single chromosome is found much more frequently than could occur by chance in patients with a range of diseases that go under the umbrella of 'inflammatory' (e.g. vasculitis) or 'autoimmune' (e.g. the autoimmune form of diabetes) conditions. It has been proposed that these particular gene combinations, which are common in Caucasians, enhanced survival from a viral or bacterial epidemic afflicting northern Europe millennia ago. Those who survived mounted an appropriately vigorous immune response to the infection. It is further speculated that this tendency to aggressive hyper-responsiveness may leave such individuals prone to developing inappropriate immune responses, giving a greater tendency towards chronic inflammatory conditions and responses to self antigens.

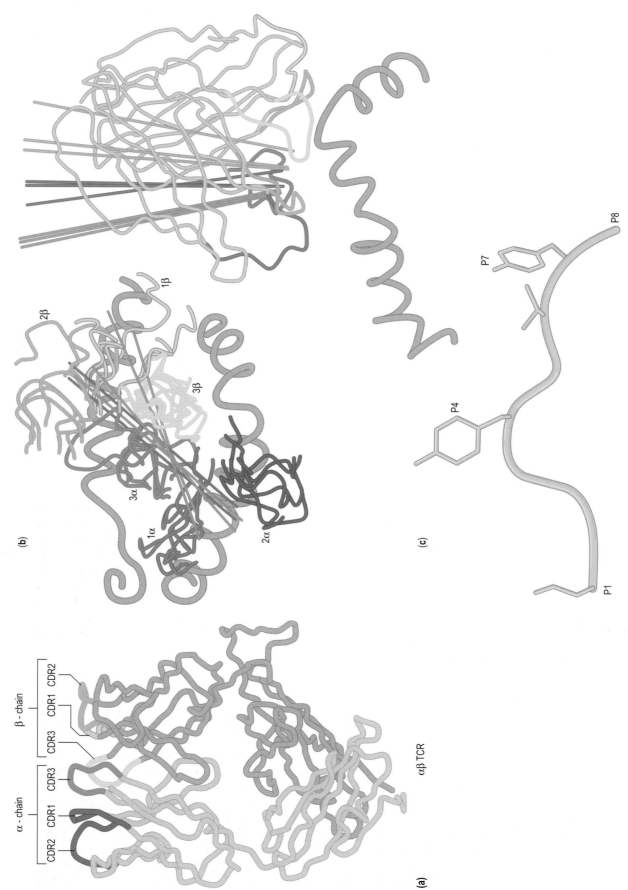

Fig. 5.10 **Crystal structures of peptide–HLA–TCR complexes reveal how TCR binds.**
(**a**) The TCR has 6 major regions involved in antigen recognition. These are the CDR1–3 regions for the α and β chains. (**b**) The TCR binds at an angle (the direction of which is shown by the straight lines) such that the CDR1 and CDR2 regions of the α chain (1α and 2α regions as shown), and the CDR1 and CDR2 regions of the β chain (1β and 2β) of the TCR bind to either of the α-helices of the HLA molecule. The CDR3 region of α and β chains of the TCR (3α and 3β) are the only parts to interact with the peptide. (**c**) For its part, the peptide may 'bulge' upwards out of the groove to make contact with the CDR3 regions. Adapted with permission from Rudolph MG, Wilson IA. The specificity of TCR/pMHC interaction. Current Opinion in Immunology 14: 52–65, 2002.

Table 5.6 Examples of the nomenclature for HLA alleles

General formula for nomenclature			
Locus	Type (i.e. allele)	Variant	
HLA-X*	00	00	
Allele given by new nomenclature			**Frequently used shorthand**
Class I			
HLA-A*0101			HLA-A1
HLA-B*0801			HLA-B8
Class II			
HLA-DRB1*0101			HLA-DR1
HLA-DRB1*0401			HLA-DR4
HLA-DRB1*0301			HLA-DR3

How the T cell receptor and peptide–HLA complex engage

The discussion about HLA structure, and the binding of peptide, has one important element missing — what is the nature of the interaction with the T cell receptor? How does it engage the peptide–HLA complex. One could have several possible hypotheses. Does the TCR make contact along the length of the peptide-binding groove, contacting most of the peptide and each α-helix? Or, does the TCR bind at 90° to the direction of the peptide, and interact with very little of peptide or MHC? For several years the answer to these questions was held back by an inability to obtain a crystal of the tri-molecular complex of peptide–HLA–TCR. In recent years technical advances in making crystals of this complex have enabled a clear view to be obtained. And the answer to the question? As shown in Figure 5.10, it is now apparent that the TCR straddles the peptide-binding groove of HLA at an angle of perhaps 45°. TCR binding at this angle means that two of the hypervariable regions (the CDR1 and CDR2 regions of the α chain) bind one α-helix whilst two other hypervariable regions (the CDR1 and CDR2 regions of the β chain) bind the other α-helix of the HLA molecule. The CDR3 regions of α and β chains of the TCR are the only parts to interact with the peptide. For its part, the peptide may 'bulge' upwards out of the groove to make contact with the CDR3 regions. This topography of TCR across HLA actually has important implications. It means that a single TCR could potentially bind to different peptides in the HLA molecule groove as long as the region in the centre of the groove contains the same or similar amino acids. Essentially, one TCR can recognise more than one peptide. As we shall see, this could have important implications for the development of autoimmune disease.

Nomenclature

A major revision of the nomenclature of factors in the HLA system has been in progress since 1989. It has been devised in order to assimilate new alleles and gene sequences as easily as possible as they are discovered. The nomenclature is gradually catching on, and makes the naming and identification of HLA molecules much more precise than ever before. Originally, when HLA typing for class I and class II alleles was based on recognition of differences using antibodies, types were assigned according to the antibodies with which an individual's cells reacted. This typing method is

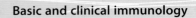
relatively imprecise, as the antibodies may bind epitopes common to more than one molecule. Therefore, molecules shown to be identical by this technique (called serology) may differ at the amino acid sequence level.

In the new nomenclature — as previously — an allele is first identified by the letter or letters that designate that locus (e.g. *HLA-A*, *DR*, *DP*). For class I alleles, this is followed by an asterisk and then a two-digit number (e.g. 01, 02, 03, etc.) defining the HLA type. Where possible, for class I and II alleles, this two-digit number is the same as that of the antibody-defined equivalent. A further two digits (01, 02, 03, etc.) define the variants of that type (Table 5.6). For class II, the letters defining the locus are followed by *A* or *B* (corresponding to genes coding for α or β chains), a number defining the locus if more than one exists (e.g. *DRB1, 3, 4, 5, DRB1* being the main one) and an asterisk followed by the types (01, 02, 03, etc.) and their variants (01, 02, 03, etc.) defined in an identical fashion to class I. The new system thus allows for novel variants at a locus to be identified at the genetic level and then identified using the next number in sequence. A selected list of HLA types is given in Appendix 3.

SUMMARY BOX 5.3

HLA molecule: structure and function

- HLA crystal structures reveal a class of molecules designed to project from the cell surface, presenting a small peptide antigen to T cells.

- Class I HLA molecules present relatively short peptides (9 amino acids) typically derived from endogenously produced proteins (including viruses that may infect cells).

- Class II HLA molecules present slightly longer peptides (typically about 15 amino acids) usually derived from exogenous material (e.g. a bacterium).

- The sequence of the peptide presented is heavily influenced by the HLA type of the molecule.

- The T cell receptor 'straddles' the peptide–HLA complex in a diagonal fashion, interacting with the two α-helices of the HLA molecules and the central core of the embedded peptide.

Further reading

Larsen CE, Alper CA 2004 The genetics of HLA-associated disease. Curr Opin Immunol 16: 660–667

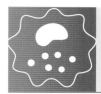

Cellular immune responses I: dendritic cells, macrophages and B lymphocytes

In this chapter we begin to encounter the main cell types involved in the events that lead to an adaptive immune response. The discussion of cell-mediated immune responses is complex when encountered for the first time. Description of the individual cell types and their functions in isolation is artificial. It is a bit like listening to an orchestra by hearing all of the different sections — woodwind, brass, strings, percussion — on their own one after another. None of it appears to harmonise or relate, and the common themes are lost. Bear in mind, then, that in this chapter and the next we are 'hearing' the dendritic cells, macrophages, B lymphocytes, T lymphocytes and natural killer cells on their own. In Chapter 8 we will be hearing the full symphony, as these cells combine to regulate one of the most vital but complex systems in mammalian physiology.

Some general principles may help your reading. Phylogenetically and ontogenetically (i.e. in terms of development of the species and development of the individual), macrophages, dendritic cells and natural killer cells are the more 'primitive' cells, followed by the B, then the T lymphocytes. **Dendritic cells** and **macrophages** are key components of the **innate immune system** and have none of the cognitive capacities (memory, specificity, amplification) of the acquired immune system on their own. However, they have highly specialised systems to enable them to 'sense' pathogens, a key event that starts the process towards the adaptive immune response against the same pathogen. Dendritic cells, in par-

ticular, are highly specialised for pathogen sensing, and are the most powerful cells for converting naïve into activated T lymphocytes. Dendritic cells, as we shall see, form a bridge between the innate and adaptive immune systems, since they are the vehicles for **presentation of antigens** to T lymphocytes leading to the activation of adaptive immunity. The **B lymphocyte** has specificity in the form of a surface receptor (immunoglobulin) capable of direct binding to antigens of any size in solution or in solid form. The B lymphocyte may differentiate further into a **plasma cell**, which resides in the tissues and secretes antibodies into the circulation. The T lymphocyte, in contrast, does not 'see' soluble antigen. As we have learned in our discussions of the function of the MHC system, the receptor on T lymphocytes requires simultaneous interaction with both MHC molecules and antigen in the form of a bound peptide. The gulf between the need of a T cell to respond to short peptides that come from large, complex antigens is bridged by cells specialised in **antigen presentation** (this is a particular feature of dendritic cells) so that antigens become 'visible' to the T cell.

Cytokines

We have already briefly discussed cytokines, in Chapter 3, as the small, soluble peptides used extensively by the immune system to communicate and influence cell growth, differentiation and function. The importance of their role is graphically illustrated by some of the rarest immune defects, which we will encounter later (see Ch. 19). In one of the syndromes described, the molecule responsible for activation of T lymphocytes, interleukin-2 (IL-2), is absent, resulting in a fatal immune deficiency disease. In another, one of the chains of a cytokine receptor is missing, and, again, a severe, fatal (if untreated) immune deficiency disorder follows.

The discussion of cytokines in teaching texts is difficult and frequently results in a sterile list of cells and functions. For this reason, and the fact that cytokines alone are nothing without the cells that release them and the cells that they affect, only a few general principles will be illustrated at this stage. Individual cytokines will be discussed as and when they are relevant. In Appendix 2 a list of cytokines and

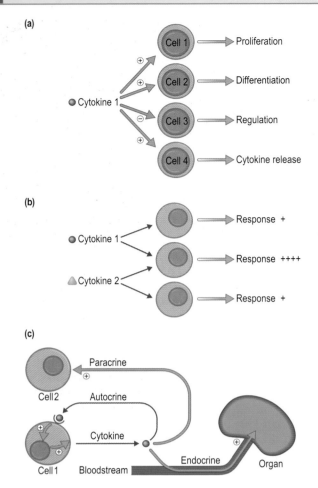

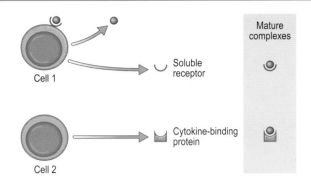

Fig. 6.2 **Molecules regulating cytokine functions.**

Fig. 6.1 **Important general properties of cytokines.**
(a) Pleiotropy. (b) Synergism. (c) Autocrine, paracrine and endocrine effects.

functions is provided for reference purposes. The important features of cytokines — **pleiotropy**, **autocrine function**, **paracrine function**, **endocrine effects** and **synergism** — are illustrated in Figure 6.1.

Cytokines require specific cell surface receptors through which to mediate their range of actions on different cells. Frequently, the action of a cytokine on a cell will include the up-regulation of surface expression of its receptor, as well as enhanced release of the molecule itself. Receptors have been broadly categorised into class I (includes interferon receptors) and class II (cytokines such as IL-2, IL-4) according to family resemblances, and there is also a TNF receptor family and a distinctive set of receptors for chemokines. Receptors may be released as soluble forms and can be detected in the circulation. This could be a form of regulation, and there are also soluble binding proteins for some cytokines, that neutralise their effects (Fig. 6.2).

Dendritic cells

A famous dendritic cell (DC) expert was once asked, in the early days of their discovery, how he would define a DC. He answered that there was no definition — 'They can be what-

ever you want them to be'. His comment reflects the enormous plasticity of these cells, characterised by a wide range of functions and morphologies. Several years on, we have a much firmer idea of their identity and role, but this remains a highly active area of research.

A current definition would be a cell that has (i) dendritic morphology (Fig. 6.3), (ii) machinery for sensing pathogens, and (iii) the ability to process and present antigens to CD4 and CD8 T lymphocytes, coupled with (iv) the ability to activate these T cells from a naïve state and (v) to dictate the T cell's future function and differentiation. Quite powerful cells then!

Dendritic cells exist as several subtypes, with common origins (Fig. 6.4). The major ones are the **myeloid DC (mDC)**, the **plasmacytoid DC (pDC)** and a variety of specialised DCs, which resemble mDCs, found in tissues (for example the **Langerhans cell** in the skin, p. 240). It is possible to recognise DCs and their different forms from the molecules they express, and some of the key ones are shown in Table 6.1. Using these markers it has been possible to track DCs and study their migration patterns. It is apparent that mDCs and pDCs are present in the blood, but at very low levels (<0.5% of lymphocyte/monocyte cells), where they exist in immature form. These **immature DCs** are also abundantly present in the tissues.

Pathogen sensing by dendritic cells

Pathogen sensing is the first major function of DCs. It is achieved through expression of a limited array of specialised molecules. These are called **pattern recognition receptors (PRRs)** and they are capable of binding to structures common to pathogens. For example, there is a PRR capable of binding to lipopolysaccharide, a molecular pattern found in the cell walls of many Gram-negative bacteria. Another binds flagellin, also found on many bacteria. Yet others bind double-stranded and single-stranded RNA from viruses. The key finding here is that the immune system has devised a means of identifying most types of invading microorganisms by their **common molecular patterns** — these are called **pathogen associated molecular patterns (PAMPs)**. Another important point is that this system requires only a handful of different PRRs, giving an important economy of scale. These receptors have been strongly

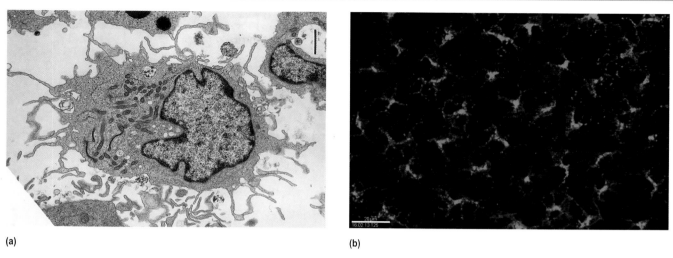

(a)

(b)

Fig. 6.3 **Images of dendritic cells.** (a) Electron micrograph of dendritic cell showing dendrites (from Patterson S et al 1999 Immunology Letters 66 111–116, with permission). (b) Dendritic cells in situ. Picture (b) shows skin of a mouse stained for dendritic cells in situ, showing the large number in normal skin and the ability of each cell to 'cover' large tracts of tissue (courtesy of Dr Jessica Strid and Professor Adrian Hayday).

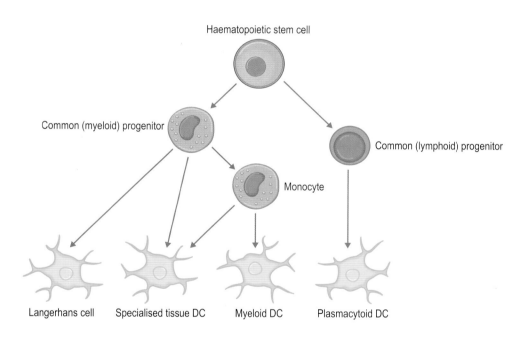

Fig. 6.4 **The origins of different blood and tissue dendritic cell types.**

conserved throughout evolution, and the name given to many of them (**Toll-like receptor**; **TLR**) is derived from their resemblance to Toll, a molecule first identified in the fruit fly, *Drosophila melanogaster*. Using the PRR-PAMP system, an mDC cannot necessarily tell the difference between staphylococcus and streptococcus, but it senses that each is equally potentially dangerous. The sensing of this danger is the first step in initiating an adaptive immune response against the pathogen.

A list of some of the main PRRs is shown in Table 6.2, along with the DC subsets that express them and the PAMP that activates them. A further important point can be made in the light of this list. The mDC and pDC subsets differ in

terms of which PRRs they express. In fact, it looks like, broadly speaking, the pDC is more specialised for antivirus responses and the mDC for antibacterial responses (Fig. 6.5). This concept is backed up by some of the specialised functions of these cells (see below).

The consequences of DC activation

The binding of a PAMP to a PRR activates the DC. This results in one of the most amazing phenomena in cell biology. As an immature DC becomes activated it changes its shape, gene and molecular profile and function within a matter of

Table 6.1 Markers for dendritic cell subsets

Marker	Myeloid DC		Plasmacytoid DC	
	Immature	Mature	Immature	Mature
1. DC subset markers				
CD1c	+	++	−	−
CD123 (IL-3 receptor)	−	−	+	++
2. DC molecules important for their function				
Molecules involved in co-stimulation of T cells (CD80, CD86)	+	+++	+	+++
HLA class I for antigen presentation to CD8 T cells	+	+++	+	+++
HLA class II for antigen presentation to CD4 T cells	+	+++	+	+++

Table 6.2 Pattern recognition receptors expressed by dendritic cells

Pattern recognition receptor (PRR)	Pathogen associated molecular pattern (PAMP)	PAMP present on:	PRR present on:
TLR2	Peptidoglycan	Gram-positive bacteria	mDC
TLR3	Double-stranded RNA	viruses	mDC
TLR4	Lipopolysaccharide	Gram-negative bacteria	mDC
TLR5	Flagellin	bacteria	mDC
TLR7	Single-stranded RNA	viruses	pDC
TLR9	Double-stranded DNA	viruses	pDC

hours to take on its mature form. In the case of the immature mDC its function is to sample the environment, searching for pathogens. This is achieved in the tissues through its long dendrites, which vastly increase its reach. In addition, the mDC is enormously pinocytotic — in other words it is constantly drinking material from its surroundings. Once activated, the mDC takes on its mature form, during which there are several key changes, as shown in Table 6.3.

Changes in immature pDCs, which are small rounded cells, are equally dramatic. Once activated, pDCs enlarge and take on a true dendritic shape. They up-regulate molecules required for T cell activation and secrete enormous quantities of interferon-α, which has potent antiviral and pro-inflammatory effects (see Science Box 6.1, and Ch. 8).

The net result of these changes is that the mature DC is ready to activate naïve T cells in the lymph node. The mature DC is the most powerful cell for activating T cells from a naïve into an effector state, and in vivo is probably the only cell that does this (Fig. 6.6). The mature DC provides three major signals:

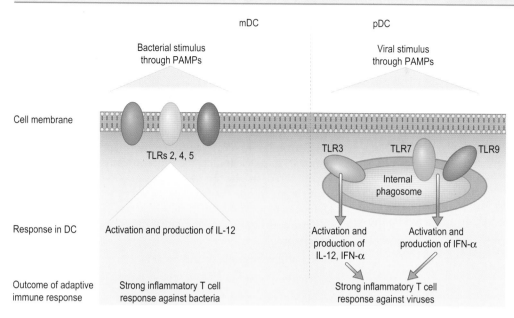

Fig. 6.5 **Activation of myeloid and plasmacytoid dendritic cells.** Myeloid DCs appear predominantly equipped for activation by bacteria through TLRs 2, 4 and 5 on the cell membrane. Both mDCs and pDCs share internal TLR3, which is sensitive to dsRNA from viruses inside the cell. pDCs have further internal sensors for viruses in the form of TLRs 7 and 9.

Table 6.3 Changes in myeloid DCs during maturation

Immature mDC	Mature mDC
Highly pinocytotic	Ceases pinocytosis
Low level expression of molecules required for T cell activation	Up-regulates CD80, CD86 and HLA molecules
Low level expression of machinery required to process and present microbial antigens	Begins to process microbial antigens (break down into small peptides) in readiness to present them to T cells (using HLA molecules)
Generally localised and sedentary	Begins active migration to local lymph node
Minimal secretion of cytokines	Active secretion of cytokines in readiness to stimulate T cells; in particular IL-12

- **Signal 1** = presentation of peptide antigen from a pathogen, bound to surface MHC molecules.
- **Signal 2** = co-stimulation, typically through CD80 and CD86.
- **Signal 3** = cytokines, notably IL-12 from mature mDCs.

In Chapter 7 we will discuss the consequences of these three signals for the T cell that receives them.

The picture emerges that, in their immature state, DCs are waiting and ready for activation by pathogens. Activation of DCs will involve internalisation of the pathogen, either by

SCIENCE BOX 6.1

The interferons

Interferons were first noticed as part of the innate immune system as natural antiviral agents. Overall, there are two types of interferon: I and II. The type I interferons have antiviral activity and are found in two main forms, α and β (the type II interferon, interferon-γ, is discussed later). IFN-α may be produced by most cells, but especially the plasmacytoid dendritic cell which makes 100–1000 times more. IFN-β is derived mainly from stromal cells such as fibroblasts; both act through the type I IFN receptor. These cytokines can act on all cell types in the body in a paracrine protective effect to inhibit virus growth through inhibition of replication of viral RNA and DNA. In addition, these IFNs potentiate the activity of natural killer cells and myeloid dendritic cells, as well as enhancing MHC class I molecule expression on a range of cell types. In the context of an intracellular infection (e.g. by a virus) increased expression of class I MHC molecules renders a cell more susceptible to killing by cytotoxic T cells (see p. 108). Class II MHC molecule expression is increased on dendritic cells and macrophages, enhancing antigen presentation. All in all, these functions greatly enhance the ability of the host defence systems to eradicate viruses, and recombinant IFNs have been used with some considerable success in patients who are chronic carriers of viruses, such as the hepatitis viruses.

pinocytosis/phagocytosis or in the case of viruses, through actual infection. Once activated, DCs migrate and change their function towards a DC ready to activate T cells of the adaptive immune system. Migration to the lymph node is usually via the lymphatics and involves up-regulation of the lymph node homing chemokine, CCR7. During migration, DCs are breaking down pathogen proteins into 'bite-size' chunks ready for presentation to naïve T cells, which are waiting to encounter pathogens in the nearest lymph node.

Monocytes and macrophages

Cells of the monocyte/macrophage lineage are frequently referred to as mononuclear phagocytes (MNPs). These cells are highly sophisticated phagocytes, with complex and refined properties over and above cells such as neutrophils. Monocytes are in the blood (10–15% of the non-granulocyte population) and macrophages in the tissues (see Fig. 6.7). Importantly, monocytes spend only a matter of days in the circulation before seeding the tissues, where they differentiate to form macrophages and dendritic cells. This is especially likely to happen during episodes of inflammation.

Blood monocytes can be divided into two subsets: those expressing CD14 (like TLR4, a component of the receptor for lipopolysaccharide) and those expressing CD14 and

CD16 (the Fc$_\gamma$RIII). Both subsets seem to have the potential to differentiate into mDC-like cells in vitro (by culturing them with IL-4 and GM-CSF) and into macrophages, although some studies support the view that the CD14$^+$ CD16$^+$ monocyte subset is the main mDC precursor.

The role of tissue macrophages can be generally defined as being involved in tissue homeostasis. These cells clear cellular debris, particularly after inflammation. In the lung, **alveolar macrophages** are more specialised towards removal and clearance of microorganisms and debris encountered in the air. Macrophages in the **gut lamina propria** are more specialised towards bactericidal activity. **Osteoclasts** are multinucleate giant cells that resorb bone. Other important end general properties of cells of the MNP system are:

- the ability to process and present antigens to T cells
- release of soluble factors (cytokines)
- killing, especially of engulfed organisms.

In addition to CD14 and CD16, the following markers are often found on cells of the MNP system:

- **CD35** complement receptor 1 (CR-1) for C3b
- **CD11b/CD18** leukocyte function-associated antigen 1 (LFA-1)
- **CD4** (but at a considerably lower surface concentration than on CD4 T cells)
- **CD64** Fc$_\gamma$RI
- **MHC class II** molecules.

Monocytes and macrophages during inflammation

Following an inflammatory stimulus at a tissue site, monocytes up-regulate their migration into tissues and differentiation to macrophages. Under strong pro-inflammatory conditions (e.g. the presence of LPS acting through TLRs, or interferons) macrophages take on a pro-inflammatory and microbicidal phenotype. The microbicidal components are very similar to those found in neutrophils (see p. 30). There is also increased induction of antigen presentation machinery (see p. 94) and, like DCs, of co-stimulatory and HLA

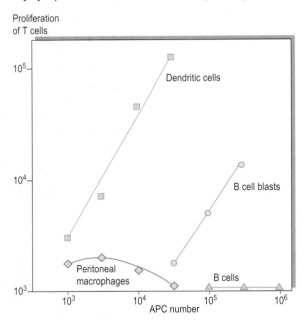

Fig. 6.6 The ability of different APCs to activate naïve T cells showing the overriding potency of DCs.
In this experiment the incubation consisted of 3 million naïve T cells, antigen and varying numbers of APCs; proliferation of T cells is measured by the incorporation of [^{3}H] thymidine, see page 101 (with permission from Inaba and Steinman 1984 Journal of Experimental Medicine 160: 1717).

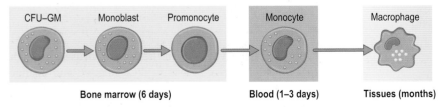

Fig. 6.7 The life cycle of the monocyte.
CFU-GM is a colony forming unit (i.e. stem cell pool) for granulocytes and monocytes.

molecules (see Table 6.3). Inflammatory macrophages also secrete a range of cytokines, including TNF-α (see Science Box 6.2), IL-1 and IFN-γ. Thus macrophages are capable of many of the bactericidal activities of neutrophils and have comparable phagocytic, chemotactic, opsonic and cytotoxic activities, but also appear to be particularly important in the ingestion and killing of **intracellular microorganisms**, such as *Mycobacterium tuberculosis*. Tissue macrophages involved in such chronic inflammatory foci may undergo terminal differentiation into **multinucleated giant cells**, typically found at the site of the **granulomata** characteristic of tuberculosis and other conditions.

B lymphocytes

Source and site

In humans, B lymphocytes develop initially in the fetal liver and transfer to the bone marrow around the 12–16th weeks of fetal life. From then the marrow is the only site of B lymphocyte generation. Rearrangement of immunoglobulin genes (see Ch. 4) takes place early during B lymphocyte development with the result that each B cell has a unique receptor for antigen (i.e. antibody). Two major changes then take place during further B cell differentiation, which is driven by a combination of antigen and T lymphocyte help. First, somatic mutations in the rearranged immunoglobulin genes lead to subtle changes in the antigen binding ability of the antibody they produce (see p. 47), giving rise to a coterie of selected B cells that produce high affinity antibodies. Second, there is a change in the heavy chain constant region used by the antibody, refining its effector functions (see p. 48). B lymphocytes reside in lymph nodes, mucosa-associated lymphoid tissue (MALT) and the spleen and in these structures they are found in the middle of germinal centres in lymphoid follicles. B cells traffic through the blood, where they constitute 5–15% of lymphocytes. B lymphocytes

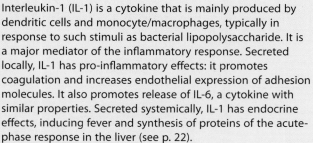

SUMMARY BOX 6.1

Cytokines, dendritic cells and monocyte/macrophages

- Cytokines are small soluble peptides used by the immune system to communicate and to influence cellular function.

- Dendritic cells are present in the blood and lymph nodes, and characterised by their distinctive morphology, ability to sense pathogens, and activate naïve T lymphocytes.

- Monocyte/macrophages have an important role in innate immune defence, exploiting their characteristic properties of phagocytosis, killing and secretion.

SCIENCE BOX 6.2

Interleukin-1 and tumour necrosis factor

Interleukin-1 (IL-1) is a cytokine that is mainly produced by dendritic cells and monocyte/macrophages, typically in response to such stimuli as bacterial lipopolysaccharide. It is a major mediator of the inflammatory response. Secreted locally, IL-1 has pro-inflammatory effects: it promotes coagulation and increases endothelial expression of adhesion molecules. It also promotes release of IL-6, a cytokine with similar properties. Secreted systemically, IL-1 has endocrine effects, inducing fever and synthesis of proteins of the acute-phase response in the liver (see p. 22).

TNF is a principal mediator in the host inflammatory response, to Gram-negative bacteria in particular, and also plays a role in many aspects of immune pathology. Like IL-1, with which it shares many similarities, the main cell types secreting TNF are monocyte/macrophages, dendritic cells and T cells. There are two structurally and functionally similar forms of TNF: α and β (the latter also known as lymphotoxin). The name derives from early experimental work that demonstrated the existence of a soluble factor capable of lysing a range of tumour cell types. T cells and natural killer cells, when activated, may also secrete TNF. Local release of TNF has many effects, including killing of target cells, up-regulation of adhesion molecules to enhance cell migration;

activation of neutrophils and macrophages to kill microbes; stimulation of release of other cytokines (e.g. IL-1, IL-6 and more TNF); increased expression of MHC class I molecules to enhance presentation of peptides in intracellular (e.g. virus) infections; and induction of expression of class II MHC molecules (this action requires the presence of other cytokines, such as interferon-γ) to enhance presentation of pathogen peptides. It can be seen that this range of activities is important in the immune response to bacteria and viruses.

Systemic release of TNF has the same fever-inducing and acute-phase response properties as IL-1. In addition, systemic TNF contributes to a clinical syndrome similar to shock: low blood pressure, reduced heart muscle contractility and intravascular thrombosis. These are features of the shock associated with Gram-negative bacterial sepsis, malarial and meningococcal infections, in all of which TNF is thought to have a major role.

Finally, it should be noted that TNF release may play a critical role in some inflammatory conditions, and the advent of monoclonal antibodies that neutralise its effects has revolutionised the treatment of diseases such as rheumatoid arthritis (see p. 182).

may undergo end-stage differentiation into **plasma cells**. These are non-circulating cells found predominantly in the bone marrow, lymph node medulla and gut and whose role is the production and secretion of antibody. Plasma cells are identified by their distinctive appearance (eccentric nucleus with a 'clock face') and by their cytoplasmic contents: immunoglobulin heavy and light chains.

Surface molecules on B lymphocytes

B lymphocytes are indistinguishable from T lymphocytes by light or electron microscopy. They are best identified by surface protein structures, several of which have important functions, the most obvious being the **B cell receptor (BCR)**, which is composed of a membrane bound, or **surface immu-** noglobulin molecule (**sIg**) (Table 6.4). Through this the B cell displays its receptor for antigen.

B lymphocyte functions

B lymphocytes are a component of the **acquired** immune response. The major roles of B lymphocytes are:

1. To ensure antibody production against appropriate target antigens, with the help of T cells.
2. To present antigen to T lymphocytes and provide signals for T lymphocyte activation.

It is difficult to dissociate these two functions: a B cell presents antigen to a T cell and receives a positive signal for antibody production in return, whilst the T cell receives a

Table 6.4 B lymphocyte surface molecules and their function

Marker	Function	Comments
B cell receptor composed of a surface immunoglobulin molecule	Binding to specific antigen	Specific for B cells
CD79α and CD79β, also called Igα and Igβ	Transduce activation signals after antigen binding	Specific for B cells
CD19 and CD21	Promote transduction of activation signals after antigen binding	Both are specific for B cells. CD21 is the CR-2 complement receptor which binds C3d-tagged antigens to enhance signalling
CD20	Unclear; capable of signal transduction	Specific for B cells; CD20 is the target of Rituximab, a monoclonal antibody used to deplete B cells for therapeutic purposes (see p. 308)
CD22	Promotes adhesion to interacting cells to enhance signalling	Specific for B cells
CD23	Regulation of IgE production	Low affinity receptor for IgE (Fcε RII), present on numerous cell types
CD40	Essential co-receptor for T cell dependent antibody responses	The ligand for CD40 (CD40L or CD154) is expressed on T cells; CD40L defects give rise to severe antibody deficiency (see p. 272)
MHC class II	Constitutively expressed by B cells at high levels for antigen presentation to T cells	Expressed on other antigen presenting cell types (see p. 74)
CD80 and CD86	Co-stimulation of T cells	Expressed on other cells with antigen presenting capacity such as DCs (see Table 6.1)

further stimulus to maintain its activated state. This is the so-called **cognate interaction** between T and B lymphocytes, which will be dealt with in a later section (see p. 107).

B lymphocyte life cycle

In humans, B cell development takes place in three phases: initially within the bone marrow; in other sites (e.g. lymph nodes) after export from the marrow; and then within the lymph node germinal centres as responder B cells are selected. The nomenclature is carefully chosen to represent these phases:

- **pre-B cells** (bone marrow) do not have fully rearranged antigen receptors

- **immature B cells** (bone marrow) are not ready to respond to antigen

- **virgin B cells** (lymph node, spleen) have fully rearranged immunoglobulin genes but have not encountered antigen

- **mature B cells** (lymph node, spleen) have encountered antigen and possess antigen specificity

- **memory B cells** maintain memory of the encounter with antigen and reside in the lymphoid system.

In the first phase of B cell development, progenitor cells (pro-B cells) migrate from the periosteal region to the centre of the bone marrow (Fig. 6.8), acquiring markers of maturation and differentiation and rearranging immunoglobulin genes. This process goes on throughout life and in the adult rodent gives rise to some 20 million cells per day. It is estimated that, during this transition, a single progenitor beginning the journey undergoes six mitotic cycles, giving rise to 64 progeny in 3–4 days. Maturation is supported by marrow stromal cells, with secretion of IL-7 a key signal (see Science Box 6.3). The first recognisable stage of B cell development

(the pre-B cell) is the appearance of cytoplasmic heavy chain of the IgM class. This μ heavy chain associates with a surrogate light chain and CD79α and CD79β to form a pre-BCR. Of the pre-B cells generated in this process, 75% are killed before they leave the marrow. The basis for this selection is not clear: both *positive* (i.e. active selection of a cell for its attributes) and *negative* (i.e. removal of a cell with undesirable attributes) selection processes are involved. One factor known to lead to negative selection is the generation of immunoglobulin gene rearrangements that do not lead to productive expression of heavy and light chains: these cells are deleted.

In the second phase of B cell development, virgin B cells leave the marrow to join the peripheral B cell pool. The blood phase may last as little as 1 hour, before the virgin B cells migrate to the spleen and lymph nodes, at this stage expressing surface IgM and IgD. Again, a minority of these virgin B cells survive. Negative selection of 'autoreactive' B cells (i.e. those with dangerous sIg capable of recognising self antigens) takes place in this period. For those B cells remaining in the pool, the length of their life span is a matter of weeks or months, bearing in mind that the pool is being replenished daily. While the majority of the peripheral B cell pool comprises virgin B cells, some members of the pool are memory cells, involved in the process of recirculation.

All of the B cell development described so far is antigen independent (Fig. 6.9). At this stage the B cell typically expresses sIg composed of μ and δ heavy chains (i.e. IgM and IgD). The B cell is ready to encounter specific antigen, and this usually takes place in the lymph node or spleen. Given the correct signals during this meeting, B cell proliferation and diversity generation take place. At this point, diversity generation is restricted to somatic hypermutation; there is no further rearrangement of genes contributing to the variable segments (see p. 47). Alternative heavy chain genes are now selected, in the process of class switching (see p. 48). A single B cell may select any one of the major classes or

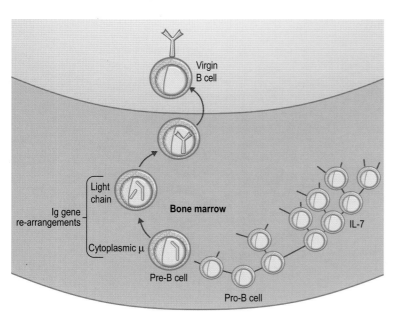

Fig. 6.8 The first phase of B cell development.
Pro-B cells are generated in the bone marrow and undergo several rapid rounds of mitosis under the influence of IL-7. They become recognisable as pre-B cells once cytoplasmic μ chains appear following *VDJ* gene rearrangements. At the point of export from the marrow into the stable peripheral B cell pool the uniquely arranged immunoglobulin is expressed on the cell surface.

...n. At this point various different ...panded in number in response to ... different clones recognise different ... antigen, or the same epitope. The ...sponse will require selection of the B ...st affinity for antigen. This selection will result naturally from competition for antigen. Those B cells best able to bind and internalise antigen will be able to present the antigen to T cells and receive in return the positive signal for expansion. This is the lymph node version of 'survival of the fittest' (Fig. 6.10) and results in the affinity maturation of antibody responses (see p. 49).

SCIENCE BOX 6.3

Colony-stimulating factors

Numerous cytokines have been identified whose most potent activity is the stimulation of growth and differentiation of bone marrow progenitor cells. Some of the colony-stimulating factors (CSFs) are restricted in their target cell, whilst others are quite broad in their range of actions. IL-3, released by CD4 T helper cells, has effects on the growth of cells of most lineages and especially on plasmacytoid dendritic cells (Table 6.1). IL-7, released by bone marrow stromal cells, has effects on the development of B cells within the marrow and on T cell activation — it is also a cytokine that opposes the natural tendencies of cells towards cell death (apoptosis) during periods when they are not receiving activation signals.

Some of the most interesting molecules within this grouping are granulocyte-monocyte-CSF (GM-CSF),

granulocyte CSF (G-CSF) and monocyte-macrophage CSF (M-CSF). G-CSF and GM-CSF have already found their way into the clinic, being used extensively in patients whose white blood cells have been ablated temporarily as part of another treatment (e.g. anti-leukaemic cytotoxic chemotherapy). GM-CSF is made by CD4 T cells, monocyte/macrophages and endothelium. It acts to promote growth of bone marrow cells already committed to the granulocyte and monocyte lineage; it may also activate mature forms of these cells. G-CSF is released by similar cell types but acts preferentially on cells committed to the granulocyte phenotype. M-CSF is made by monocyte/macrophages and endothelial cells and is primarily produced within the bone marrow to promote development of these cell types.

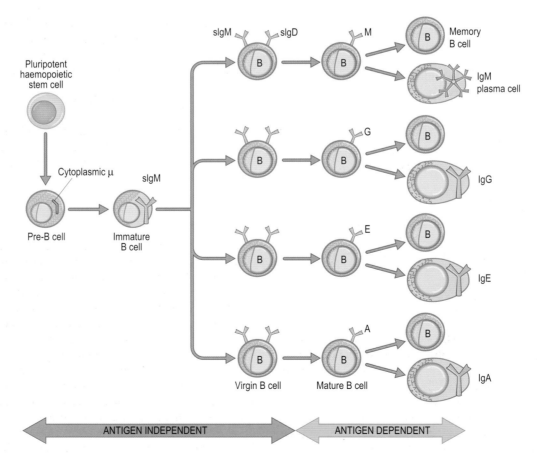

Fig. 6.9 The life cycle of the B cell in relation to antigen.
Note how much B cell development is antigen independent.

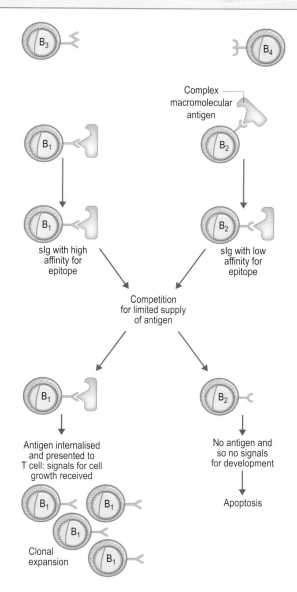

Fig. 6.10 Selection of B cells with highest affinity for an antigen.
A complex macromolecular antigen arriving in the lymph node causes expansion of a small number of B cell clones (oligoclonal expansion). Some (e.g. B_1 and B_2) bind the same epitope on the antigen, others (e.g. B_3 and B_4) do not bind antigen and die. In the presence of a limited supply of antigen, the highest affinity sIg (on B_1) is able to compete successfully against lower affinity sIg (B_2) for its epitope. B_1 internalises antigen and presents it to a T cell, which provides the necessary growth signals for clonal expansion of B_1.

The pool of effector B cells (memory B cells and plasma cells) is constantly being replenished. Cells not receiving appropriate signals within the lymph node germinal centre are lost. Some of the B cells in the peripheral pool are recirculating memory cells, already committed to a specific immune response through a previous encounter with antigen. Memory B cells are more easily primed and can give a swift, specific, high-affinity, class-switched secondary response. If such a response is not needed over a long period (several years), these cells also may die.

Molecular and genetic events in B cell development

During development in the bone marrow, pre-B lymphocytes arise following immunoglobulin gene rearrangements in B lymphocyte precursors (*D–J* segments first, then a *V–DJ* recombination; see p. 47). Pre-B lymphocytes can be identified by the presence of cytoplasmic μ chains but no light chains are found. In the next phase, light chain *V–J* recombinations occur. These genetic recombinations give rise to a unique immunoglobulin gene sequence and, hence, a unique antibody structure. This provides the basis for the **antibody specificity** of a given B lymphocyte, which, interestingly, arises long before that cell ever encounters the antigen with which it is capable of binding. Only *one* antigen-binding specificity of immunoglobulin is produced per B lymphocyte, composed of the variable regions of light and heavy chains. The structure of these regions will be maintained without change for the rest of the life cycle of the B lymphocyte (apart from a degree of somatic mutation; see p. 47) while the constant region of the heavy chain, which determines the class (G, A, M, D or E) of antibody, will be changed. The immature B lymphocyte has sIg of the IgM class. This is accompanied by IgD expression, particularly in lymph node germinal centres. Surface IgD is important in the receipt and transduction of activation signals and signifies a virgin B lymphocyte (i.e. one which has not encountered its specific antigen). Surface IgD is lost from the cell after antigenic stimulation. Once activated by encounter with specific antigen under the appropriate conditions during a primary immune response, the B lymphocyte matures and is now restricted to display only one isotype of surface immunoglobulin (e.g. a particular G subclass, A subclass, M, D or E) (see Fig. 6.9).

B lymphocytes at this stage have two main differentiation pathways. They can become memory B lymphocytes, ready for further rounds of activation and differentiation should the specific antigen be encountered again. Alternatively, they can end-differentiate into a mature plasma cell (Fig. 6.11).

Plasma cells

Plasma cells have lost all surface immunoglobulin but remain committed to production and *secretion* of a *single* antibody specificity with a *single* light and heavy chain type.

Immunoglobulin production and secretion by plasma cells give rise to the soluble IgG, IgA, IgM, IgE (and rarely IgD) molecules found in the circulation and to the IgA secreted across the mucosa. These circulating antibodies are an important component of maintaining host defence against pathogens. If the levels fall, for example from ~10 g/l of IgG in a healthy adult to <0.5 g/l, there is a dramatically increased risk of infection. If a plasma cell is committed to the production of neutralising antibody to a pathogen (e.g. poliovirus), immunity is retained in an ever-ready state for as long as that plasma cell continues to secrete antibody. Prolonged or repeated stimulation of antibody production (e.g. by immunisation boosters) will enhance the process of B cell

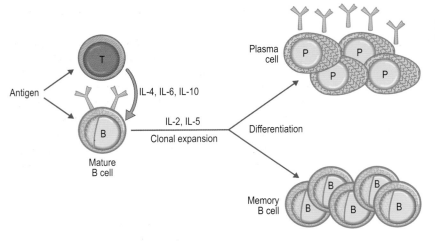

Fig. 6.11 Differentiation of mature B cells into plasma cells or memory B cells. See text for detail.

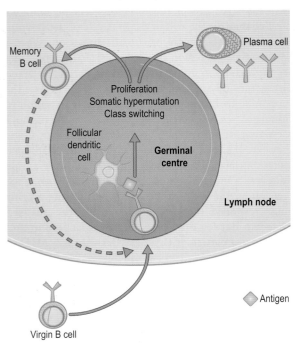

Fig. 6.12 B cell activation in lymph nodes.
Virgin B cells from the stable peripheral pool enter lymph node germinal centres. Here, antigen is presented on the processes of follicular dendritic cells. B cells holding sIg recognising the antigen are stimulated into mitosis, during which sIg is lost and there is somatic hypermutation and class switching. B cells with the highest affinity for antigen after this phase are selected as memory B cells or plasma cells, as required. Memory B cells may join the stable peripheral B cell pool.

differentiation, more plasma cells will appear, protective antibody levels will be maintained and immunity will be maintained and augmented.

B lymphocyte activation

B cell activation takes place in the lymph nodes (Fig. 6.12). In secondary follicles, activated B cells form the germinal centre, a process that is dependent on antigenic stimulation.

Very few secondary follicles are found in congenitally athymic mice, indicating that their formation is also largely T cell dependent. Secondary follicles consist of a mantle, or corona, of packed resting small B cells (sIgM$^+$ and sIgD$^+$) of the peripheral pool. In the centre of a secondary follicle is the germinal centre, a collection of activated B (mainly) and T lymphocytes. Here, B cell activation and maturation process takes place.

Follicular dendritic cells (FDCs) make up about 1% of the cells in these follicles, and have a key role in B cell activation. First, they are able to present antigen on their surface, mainly in the form of immune complexes (formed by binding of antigen, antibody and complement) directly to B cells. Second, they can retain antigen in this form for long periods of time, presumably while the B cells with the 'best fit' for antigen are selected (reminiscent of the story of Cinderella and her lost slipper). Third, they provide additional signals to activate B cells, including B cell activating factor of the TNF family (BAFF), IL-15 and adhesion molecules such as ICAM-1. This is a pattern of activation of lymphocytes that we will also encounter for T cells — the combination of presentation of antigen with additional membrane-derived and soluble molecular signals.

By this process, B cells with sIg complementary to the antigen presented by FDCs undergo proliferation, and the germinal centre begins to develop. These blasts, termed centroblasts, lose sIg and are typically localised at one pole of the follicle (Fig. 6.13). Centroblasts begin to generate progeny (termed centrocytes) that now express sIg and migrate towards the outer zone of the follicle. During the generation of centroblasts and centrocytes, somatic hypermutation (see p. 47) and class switching, leading to selection of heavy chains, takes place.

At this stage, further survival of the B cell depends on how successful the BCR is in binding to the antigen currently being presented in that germinal centre. If binding is strong, there are three separate pathways of maturation. First, the centrocyte interacts with a CD4 helper T cell (see p. 107) through the cell surface molecule CD40, leading to the generation of memory B cells. The ligand for CD40 (CD40 ligand; CD40L or CD154) (see Clinical Box 6.1) is expressed on T cells almost exclusively, and its expression is tightly

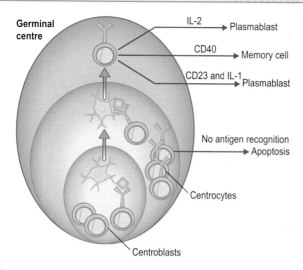

Fig. 6.13 B cell development within the germinal centre. B cells recognising specific antigen are stimulated into an oligoclonal expansion (centroblast stage). These expanded cells migrate further into the germinal centre. There are several possible outcomes of the centrocyte stage. If affinity for antigen is lost after somatic hypermutation, there is no positive signalling and the cells cannot be rescued from apoptosis. Centrocytes remaining highly specific for the antigen may be influenced in three different ways. Interaction with T lymphocytes expressing CD40L stimulates CD40-expressing centrocytes to become memory cells. Either IL-2 or a combination of CD23 and IL-1 influence centrocytes towards the plasmablast and then plasma cell stage.

CLINICAL BOX 6.1

X-linked hyper IgM syndrome: the importance of CD40–CD40L

The identification of the CD40–CD40L interaction in rescuing antigen-specific B cells from apoptosis has elucidated the pathogenesis of a disease characterised by deficiency of antibody production. This immune deficiency is termed X-linked hyper IgM syndrome, since it is found only in males, who typically have high levels of IgM antibodies but no mature B lymphocytes producing the other immunoglobulin classes. The IgM produced tends to be ineffective in protection against bacterial infections, and boys affected with the disease are at risk of serious infections unless treated. It was known for some years that the B cells themselves are not particularly abnormal and could be stimulated effectively using T cells from unaffected donors. It was then demonstrated that the genetic basis for this syndrome is the presence of mutations in the *CD40L* gene, which is present on the X-chromosome. In the absence of a CD40L–CD40 interaction, some developing B cells are not rescued from apoptosis, whilst some remain viable but do not receive the correct maturation signals. These latter B cells may escape cell death, but in the absence of T cell help remain only as producers of IgM, hence the high levels of this antibody class seen in this condition.

---

controlled, being inducible by T cell activation within 2–8 hours but being lost again from the surface after 24 hours. The second manoeuvre that saves centrocytes from apoptosis is exposure to soluble CD23 (a surface protein found on B cells and FDCs) and IL-1α, inducing differentiation into plasmablasts (i.e. pre-plasma cells). This is followed by migration into the lymph node medullary cords and then out to the gut lamina propria, bone marrow and spleen, which are the main resident sites for plasma cells, the end-stage differentiated B cells. A third mechanism of rescue from apoptosis can be provided by IL-2, which also induces the production of plasmablasts.

The role of T cells in B cell activation

Immature B lymphocytes may become activated with or without the help of T cells (so called thymus-dependent and thymus-independent pathways, respectively) (Fig. 6.14). This should remind you of the classic experiment described on page 3, when the thymus was removed from mice. They lost the ability for T cell responses and, surprisingly, also to some

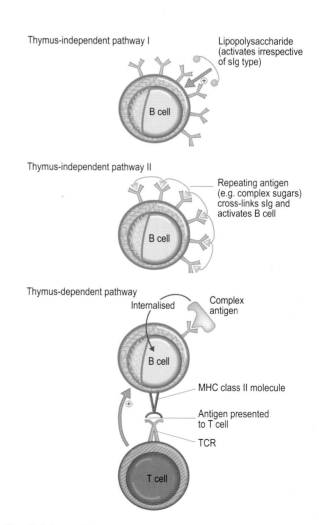

Fig. 6.14 T cell dependent and independent pathways of B cell activation.

extent for B lymphocyte responses, indicating the dependence of B cells on the T lymphocyte.

The dominant pathway of B cell activation in vivo involves T cell help. Thymus-independent B cell activation can result from the effects of certain bacterial products, such as cell wall lipopolysaccharides, which have the capacity to activate *all* B lymphocytes directly (so-called **polyclonal activation**). Activation here is not related to the antigen specificity of the B cells and generally gives rise to an IgM response with little memory generation or affinity maturation.

The thymus-dependent pathway is clearly the most important in that it generates high-affinity, class-switched, specific antibodies. It is this process that has been described in the previous sections: B lymphocytes use their sIg as a receptor for antigen, which is internalised. Inside the B cell, a combination of enzymes and physical effects such as low pH degrade the antigen (**antigen processing**, see p. 95), and a small peptide fragment of the whole antigen becomes attached to a class II MHC molecule and is exported to the surface (**antigen presentation**, see p. 96). The B lymphocyte is here acting as an APC. T lymphocytes with a T cell receptor able to recognise the peptide-MHC class II complexes are activated (the B lymphocyte acting as T lymphocyte activator) and, in turn, the T cell activates the B lymphocyte. This elaborate system ensures that (1) only B lymphocytes and T lymphocytes specific for the same antigen are given the activation signal and (2) only antigens against which the immune system is fully committed (i.e. have both T and B lymphocyte recognition for) invoke an immune response. The latter is a protection against developing anti-self reactions. Do not forget that B lymphocytes are designed to produce millions of different specificities, some of which may cross-react with self. This potentially dangerous complication is the price paid for diversity.

Signals in B lymphocyte activation

The B cell receptor complex (composed of sIg and the CD79α/β) provides the major signal in B cell activation and transmits the message that there has been productive interaction with an antigen. The signal is transduced via the cytoplasmic portions of the CD79 molecules, which contain immunoreceptor tyrosine-based activation motifs (ITAMs). We will encounter exactly the same process for T cell activation (see p. 106). An intracellular activation cascade is initiated, triggering tyrosine kinase activation and calcium signalling, ultimately leading to changes in gene expression profiles.

For subsequent development of T cell dependent activation pathways, additional signals from the T cell are required. These include B cell accessory molecules that interact with their ligands on the T cell, such as CD40 and CD80/CD86, as well as the provision of cytokine signals. (Again, we will see exactly the same pattern for T cell activation — the requirement for additional molecular interactions at the cell surface and soluble factors in the form of cytokines.) Several T lymphocyte-derived interleukins are important in B

lymphocyte activation, growth, clonal expansion and class switching. **IL-4** is the main B lymphocyte activator (see Fig. 6.9). It also stimulates B lymphocyte growth. **IL-5** and, to some degree, **IL-2** promote clonal expansion. **IL-6** is a B lymphocyte growth factor that also enhances the switch to IgG production. What influences production of different Ig isotypes is not fully characterised. Control by cytokines undoubtedly exists, but also local factors have a role (e.g. IgA production by mucosal B lymphocytes).

The outcome of B lymphocyte activation

The important results of B lymphocyte activation are **clonal expansion** with the generation of memory B lymphocytes and plasma cells. When a B lymphocyte is activated by antigen, the first response is IgM production, beginning after 5–10 days, followed 2–3 days later by the appearance of IgG in the serum. This constitutes the primary response. When there is a re-challenge with the same antigen, memory cells are already primed and present. Activation of primed cells is quicker and leads to the secondary response. This has several different characteristics: it is quicker (3–5 days), IgG is produced early and it is produced in much greater quantities (see p. 44).

Physiological importance of B lymphocyte responses

The role of B lymphocytes in host protection is exemplified by rare genetic diseases, such as X-linked agammaglobulinaemia (see p. 273). Children born with the syndrome have no circulating B lymphocytes, although pre-B lymphocytes can be identified in the bone marrow. No B lymphocytes means no antibodies, and patients suffer from repeated life-threatening infections.

In medical practice, we have found ways of manipulating B lymphocytes, especially in **vaccination/immunisation**. In these processes, a harmless, inactivated form of a pathogen is used to stimulate the primary antibody response, so that when the real pathogen is met, there is pre-existing immunity and the secondary response can be invoked to boost the level of immunity very quickly (see Ch. 23).

Class and subclass switching, and the production of IgE

Class switching involves the selection during B cell development of different *IGH* genes. To what extent this takes place as a spontaneous event and to what extent it is driven remains a moot point in immunological circles. Certain facts relating to the results of in vitro culture studies are pertinent. In particular, the control of IgE production has been quite well studied, for the obvious reason that it may be relevant to the development of allergy (see Ch. 10). For example, co-culture of B cells with a polyclonal activator alone typically results in IgM production in the culture fluid. Addition of IL-4 induces switching to IgE production. In contrast, addition of

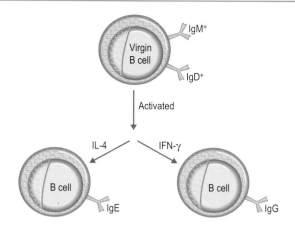

Fig. 6.15 **The control of IgE production by cytokines.** See text for details.

IFN-γ induces production of IgG class antibodies, and no IgE (Fig. 6.15).

The other factors that clearly must have an effect on class switching are the nature of the antigen, since some antibody responses are skewed to certain isotypes (see Table 4.2), as well as the site of production, since antibodies produced in mucosally associated lymphoid tissue tend to be of the IgA class. It seems likely that the T cells at these sites have an influence: B lymphocytes from other sites co-cultured with mucosally derived T cells can be switched to IgA production.

SUMMARY BOX 6.2

B lymphocytes

■ B lymphocytes mature from bone marrow precursors and express surface immunoglobulin molecules unique to each cell.

■ B cells are selected for expansion and differentiation by T cells, with the generation of plasma cells to produce circulating protective antibodies, and memory B cells.

■ A complex interaction of T and B cells, with the important influence of cytokines, takes place in lymph nodes to achieve B cell activation.

■ In this unique position of presenting internalised antigens to T cells, the B cell is also an important source of antigen-presenting function, with consequent T cell activation.

Adhesion molecules in lymphocyte functions

The integrins and selectins are important in T and B cell functions and serve the same purpose as they do for granulocytes, namely directed adherence to endothelium and migration into the tissues (the molecular basis for these has already been discussed). LFA-1 (one of the β_2 integrins) is expressed on virtually all mature resting and activated peripheral T and B cells. LFA-1 is particularly important in migration of lymphocytes into the tissues. In addition, the ligand for LFA-1, ICAM-1, is frequently expressed on other immune cells, as well as on the endothelium. Therefore, when lymphocytes make contact with other lymphocytes or APCs, LFA-1/ICAM-1 adhesion can enhance the interaction and the passage of cell–cell signals. L-selectin is also expressed on the majority of T and B lymphocytes and is present at its highest levels on naïve forms of these cells — this ensures that naïve cells are attracted to lymph nodes, where they may be required for an immune response. The chemokine receptor, CCR7 (main ligands CCL19 and CCL21), is also a surface molecule that is important in lymph node homing. For example, subsets of T cells destined to become lymph node-resident memory cells after activation (often termed 'central memory cells') will acquire CCR7.

Another group of integrins are termed the β_1 integrins, and these share expression of a common β chain, CD29. The β_1 integrins are also called the **very late activation** (VLA) molecules. VLA-4, VLA-5 and VLA-6, are particularly strongly expressed by resting T cells and are highly up-regulated on activation. VLA-4 mediates binding of lymphocytes to endothelium at sites of inflammation, where its ligand, VCAM-1, is typically up-regulated.

Further reading

Kawai T, Akira S 2006 Innate immune recognition of viral infection. Nat Immunol 7: 131–137

Ollila J, Vihinen M 2005 B cells. Int J Biochem Cell Biol 37: 518–523

O'Neill LA 2004 TLRs: Professor Mechnikov, sit on your hat. Trends Immunol 25: 687–693

Reis e Sousa C 2006 Dendritic cells in a mature age. Nat Rev Immunol 6: 476–483

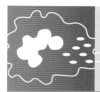

Cellular immune responses II: T lymphocytes, antigen presentation and natural killer cells

In the previous chapter we began to appreciate that a key component of the immune response is the ability of DCs to sense pathogens. This information must be passed on to the adaptive arm of the immune response, in order for the recognition and removal of pathogens to be organised. In the adaptive immune response, recognition and removal is controlled by T lymphocytes. T lymphocytes may be involved in pathogen removal directly (for example by killing) or indirectly (for example by recruiting B cells to make specific antibody). T lymphocytes are the immunological equivalent of the 'sweeper' in soccer, or the quarterback in American football. They make the plays. In this section we will cover the final components of the cellular and molecular processes that are required for an adaptive immune response.

T lymphocytes

T lymphocyte source and subsets

Key studies in the 1950s indicated that lymphocytes were the cells responsible for two measurable immune responses: antibody production and graft rejection. Surgical removal of the thymus effectively abolished the ability of a host to reject a tissue graft, and the lymphocytes assumed to derive from the thymus were named T lymphocytes. These cells play a pivotal role in the adaptive immune response. If, for any reason, T lymphocytes are absent or reduced in number or function (for example as a result of genetic abnormality, immunosuppressive therapy, or infectious agents), the host is at greatly increased risk of a range of infections.

Understanding the complexities of T lymphocyte function is vital for a clear understanding of their role in protective immunity and in disease. Major diseases of interest are those resulting from T cell deficiency (Ch. 19), or those arising when the fine tuning of T cell responses is impaired, which can lead to a range of inflammatory disorders, including hypersensitivity (i.e. allergy, Ch. 10) and autoimmune disease (such as rheumatoid arthritis, type 1 diabetes and multiple sclerosis, Chs 12, 13 & 18).

The T lymphocyte life cycle

Like B cells, T cells are generated from precursors in the bone marrow. In the case of T cells, they then migrate to the thymus. Here, like B cells in the bone marrow, rearrangement of the genes they will use to generate a receptor for antigen takes place. Like B cells, T cells then leave to populate the lymph nodes, in a **naïve**, immature state having been selected for certain key properties, mainly (i) the functional rearrangement and expression of their surface receptors for antigen and (ii) a reduced or absent tendency to recognise self antigens (and thus avoid autoimmunity). Naïve or immature T cells become activated for the first time in the lymph node by antigens presented to them as short peptides bound to MHC molecules on the surface of antigen presenting cells. Of all APCs, only the DC is capable of activating naïve T cells. The activation process involves much more than just the presentation of antigen. A series of co-ordinated signals are used, some involving the interaction of molecules on the DC and T cell surface, others involving secretion of cytokines by DCs. The outcome is **T cell activation** and then **functional polarisation**. Functional polarisation means that the T cell takes on a particular set of tasks that promote the adaptive immune response (e.g. organising B cell responses). These are often also called **effector** or **regulatory** functions, depending on their nature. An overview of the T cell life cycle is shown in Figure 7.1.

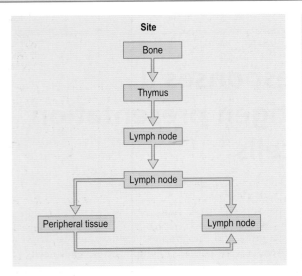

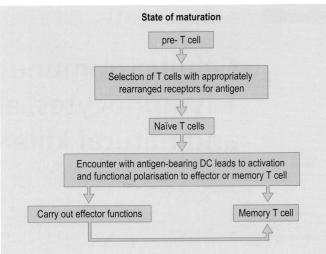

Fig. 7.1 **Schematic overview of the life cycle of the T lymphocyte.**

Table 7.1 Identification of T cells and major subsets by surface molecules

T cell population	Marker	Typical percentages in blood	Additional information
T lymphocytes	T cell receptor CD3	100% of T cells (70% of lymphocytes)	All T cells are thymus-derived
Helper T lymphocytes (T_H)	CD4	66% of T cells	Interact with antigen presented by MHC class II molecules
Cytotoxic T lymphocytes (CTLs)	CD8	33% of T cells	Interact with antigen presented by MHC class I molecules

Identification of T lymphocytes by surface molecules and by function

Like the B cell (see p. 78), the T cell is defined by the surface expression of a receptor for antigen. It is composed of T cell receptor α and β chains (which bind antigen and are the equivalent of sIg) and a collection of molecules that transduce activation signals, called the CD3 complex. A proportion (typically 5% in humans) of T cells use TCRs composed of γ and δ chains. The genetic basis for the generation of α and β or γ and δ chains (rearrangement of genes coding for variable and constant chains of these molecules) has been described already (Ch. 4). Cells expressing the different receptor chains are typically referred to as $\alpha\beta$ or $\gamma\delta$ T cells.

There are two major subsets of T cells to be found in the blood and lymph nodes, defined by the expression of two accessory molecules, CD4 and CD8. Some two thirds of $\alpha\beta$ T cells express the surface glycoprotein CD4 (CD4 T cells). Some years ago it was shown that the mature form of these cells was capable of promoting immune responses such as antibody production by B cells, and they were therefore termed **T helper** (T_H) cells. The remaining third of $\alpha\beta$ T cells do not express CD4, but express a related glycoprotein, CD8. T cells expressing CD8 (usually called CD8 T cells) are typically associated with the killing of target cells, and therefore the term **cytotoxic** T lymphocytes (**CTLs**) is often used (Table 7.1). The majority of $\gamma\delta$ T cells express CD8 or neither of these accessory molecules. Cells can be recognised and measured in the blood using these different surface proteins as markers of **T cell subsets**, using immunofluorescence and flow cytometry (see Science Box 7.1 and Fig. 7.2).

It is worth stressing at this point that the most precise nomenclature to use for T cells when describing them are the terms $\alpha\beta$ or $\gamma\delta$ and CD4 or CD8. Functional terms such as T_H and CTL should really only be used when referring to cells or populations for which these functions have been clearly defined. The CD4 and CD8 accessory molecules perform very precise functions. **CD4 binds to MHC class II molecules** on antigen presenting cells during antigen presentation, stabilising the interaction and providing additional signalling. **CD8 binds to MHC class I molecules** on antigen presenting cells or target cells, also adding stability and signalling strength. Thus, the narrowest definition of a CD4 T

Measuring T cells in the blood

It has become an absolute mainstay of the management of patients with a variety of disorders to count the numbers of different T cell subsets in the blood. Nowhere has this been more graphically illustrated than in the management of patients with HIV infection, in which CD4 T cells are progressively lost and their quantification is an important prognostic tool (see p. 287). However, this approach has now extended to numerous clinical settings, and especially those in which immune deficiency is suspected (see p. 267) or a patient is being treated with monoclonal antibodies designed to deplete a particular subset of cells (see p. 311). The approach is also widely used in research.

Cell subset quantification exploits three items: (i) the existence of a subset-specific cell surface molecule (e.g. CD4 for T cells); (ii) a monoclonal antibody specific for the molecule; and (iii) chemicals called fluorochromes that fluoresce at a particular wavelength when exposed to an excitatory light source. The fluorochromes most frequently used are fluorescein, phycoerythrin and allophycocyanin, which fluoresce green, orange and red, respectively, when exposed to an ultraviolet light source. A suspension of cells from the patient is incubated with monoclonal antibodies that have been tagged with the fluorochrome of choice. The labelled cells then need to be exposed to a laser, viewed and counted. This is done in a technique called flow cytometry, a technique for the study of cells in flow.

The basic skeleton of a flow cytometer is shown in Figure 7.2a. Cells are identified first by the way they scatter light in a forward direction (dependent upon cell size) and at 90° (dependent upon granules in the cytoplasm) since this is distinctive for lymphocytes, monocytes and neutrophils (Fig. 7.2b). Then the machine analyses whether a particular cell has been bound by the monoclonal antibody used. In clinical practice four different fluorochromes will be used simultaneously, so that the machine identifies a lymphocyte and asks: Are you a T cell (using monoclonal anti-CD3 antibody)? Are you a helper T cell (anti-CD4) or a cytotoxic T cell (anti-CD8)? Other questions can be added — Are you expressing homing receptors for the skin (using monoclonal anti-cutaneous leukocyte antigen)? In research practice, the machinery used is sufficiently sophisticated to add three more dimensions to the analysis. First, antibodies can be directed *inside* the cell, for example to see what kind of cytokines are being secreted and thus examine functional polarisation (see p. 104). Second, up to 18 different coloured fluorochromes can be used at once, to add fine specificity. Finally, cell subsets of interest can be transiently exposed to a magnetic field, allowing them to be 'pulled' into a collection tube for further analysis.

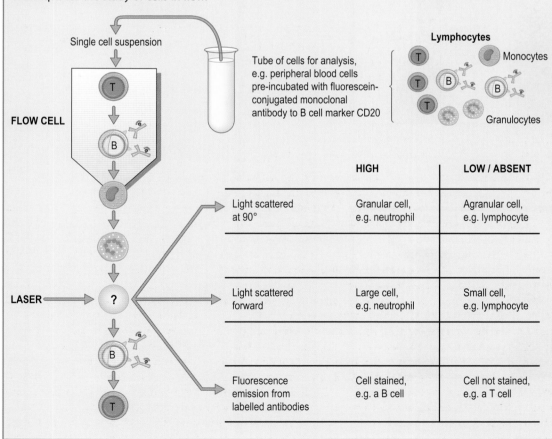

Fig. 7.2 Flow cytometry. (**a**) Principle of flow cytometry. The detection of different cellular subsets on the basis of physical characteristics (size, granularity) and binding of fluorochrome-tagged monoclonal antibodies.

Single cell suspension

Tube of cells for analysis, e.g. peripheral blood cells pre-incubated with fluorescein-conjugated monoclonal antibody to B cell marker CD20

FLOW CELL

LASER

Lymphocytes — Monocytes — Granulocytes

	HIGH	LOW / ABSENT
Light scattered at 90°	Granular cell, e.g. neutrophil	Agranular cell, e.g. lymphocyte
Light scattered forward	Large cell, e.g. neutrophil	Small cell, e.g. lymphocyte
Fluorescence emission from labelled antibodies	Cell stained, e.g. a B cell	Cell not stained, e.g. a T cell

(continued)

SCIENCE BOX 7.1

Measuring T cells in the blood—cont'd

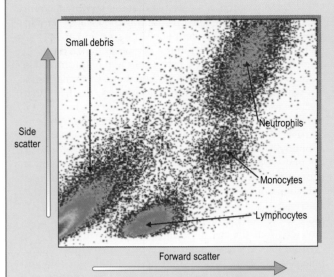

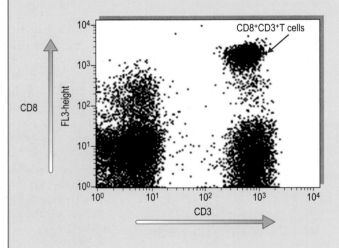

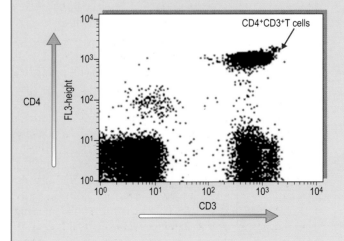

Fig. 7.2 **Flow cytometry—cont'd**

(**b**) Flow cytometry in action. In the upper panel, a blood sample has undergone red blood cell lysis and then been analysed for the physical characteristics of forward and side scatter of light. Each 'dot' represents a single cell analysed in this way. This reveals cells with relatively low forward scatter (small) and low side scatter (few granules) that are the lymphocytes (T, B, NK cells). Cells that are slightly bigger and more granular are the monocytes, and cells that are considerably bigger and highly granular are the neutrophils. In the lower panels, only the lymphocyte population is shown. Monoclonal antibodies (tagged with different coloured fluorescence molecules) against CD3 (identifies T cells), CD4 (identifies helper T cells) and CD8 (identifies cytotoxic T cells) have been used to identify these specific subsets. In the scatter plots shown, each dot is a cell, analysed to see whether it expresses the indicated markers. Cells that are CD8$^+$ CD3$^+$ T cells are shown as a cluster in the middle panel, and CD4$^+$ CD3$^+$ T cells in the lower panel.

cell is that it receives signals through antigen presentation by MHC class II molecules, and of CD8 T cells that they received signals through MHC class I molecules.

Development of T cells: thymic education

A view of the adaptive immune system emerges from Chapter 4 that T and B lymphocytes have the capability to react against a vast array of antigens, through the rearrangement of sets of genes to provide antigen receptor diversity. The clear consequence of this process is the ability to respond not just to viruses and bacteria, but also to self proteins. We have discussed how the DC, through its ability to guide responses only when danger signals are present, could provide 'stop' and 'go' advice when initiating an immune response, and thus help to prevent reactions against self. But this level of control can only operate when the T cells present require strong signals, acting in series, in order to be activated. What would happen if T cells were allowed to generate TCRs that bound with such high affinity to self peptides that they did not require DCs to become activated? Clearly, the result would be uncontrollable autoimmunity! The thymus is the key organ in the immune system for ensuring that this state of affairs does not arise, and, as discussed below, it does so by deletion of T cells with high affinity for self.

The bone-marrow-derived precursor cells that enter the thymus (Fig. 7.3) are not identifiable as T cells. They do not have a T cell receptor rearranged and bear none of the surface molecules typical of T cells. The precursor T cells mature within the thymus, where they are termed **thymocytes**. The process of thymic education for a cell emerging successfully into the periphery takes about 3 weeks. The length of time spent in the thymus by a cell not destined for selection (true of approximately 99% of thymocytes) is about 3.5 days. Any description of the events that take place during the development of thymocytes before release into the periphery must take account of this, and the following facts about a mature T cell:

- in mature T cells, TCR genes are rearranged and the TCR dimer expressed, along with CD3 and one accessory molecule, either CD4 or CD8
- CD4 T cell responses require presentation of peptide antigens by *self* MHC class II molecules
- CD8 T cell responses require presentation of peptide antigens by *self* MHC class I molecules.

In other words, in the thymus, T cells acquire the 'tools of their trade' (receptors and accessory molecules) and the ability to use them within the laws of MHC restriction described earlier. This process is often referred to as **thymic education**.

Other facts which must be accounted for in the explanation of thymic development are:

- there is extensive thymocyte death, and only 1% of precursor cells entering the thymus leave as mature T cells
- despite the enormously broad repertoire of possible TCR configurations, in health relatively few mature

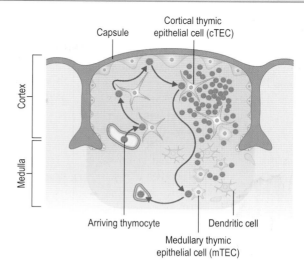

Fig. 7.3 Life cycle of the developing thymocyte.
The thymocyte arrives via the blood from the bone marrow, migrates to the cortex, expands and then follows a series of interactions with epithelial cells in the cortex and medulla, as well as with dendritic cells before leaving the thymus as a naïve T cell.

peripheral T cells are able to make responses to self antigens.

An explanation for these observations is that having acquired the tools of the trade, thymocytes undergo a selection process that has three basic elements. The first is to discard all TCRs that are incapable of interacting with self MHC molecules. As we observed in Chapter 5, quite a large amount of the TCR interaction with peptide-MHC is with the MHC itself. If a TCR cannot interact with self MHC, it is useless and is discarded. The second element is to discard all TCRs with dangerously high affinity for self MHC. As discussed above, this is highly undesirable and is termed **negative selection**. The third element is to select TCRs that are between these two extremes — i.e. have an operationally useful affinity for self MHC that is not too high as to be dangerous and not too low as to be useless. This is termed **positive selection**.

An overview of T cell development in the thymus

The arriving thymocyte (Fig. 7.3) migrates to the cortex of the thymus and undergoes a twenty-fold expansion. At this stage, there is no T cell receptor. Neither is there any CD4 or CD8 expression, hence this is termed the **double-negative**, or **DN** stage (Fig. 7.4). The first point at which a developing DN thymocyte takes on something approaching the form of a T cell is when the TCRβ chain genes are rearranged (see p. 53) and the protein expressed on the surface. At this stage of development, the surface expressed TCRβ chain pairs with an invariant pre-TCR α chain that assists signalling through the CD3 complex. Should the thymocyte fail at this stage (the first checkpoint) then it will die. Assuming there is productive expression of a TCRβ chain the DN cells progress to express both CD4 and CD8 (**double positive**, or **DP** stage) and rearrange the TCRα chain genes and now express a productive TCRαβ dimer. This represents the second checkpoint. The DP cells now lose either CD4 or CD8 and become **single positive** for one or the other (**SP4 or SP8**). If cells are separated from an active thymus, stained for CD4 and CD8 and analysed by flow cytometry (as described in Science Box 7.1) the different stages of DN, DP and SP are clearly seen (Fig. 7.5).

At this point, the developing T cells are ready for the careful selection process discussed above, which centres around the ability of the TCR to interact with self MHC molecules. It is now clear that the majority of TCRs generated at the SP stage fail, within a 3–4 day window, to make productive interactions with self MHC and thus these cells (probably 90–95% of thymocytes) do not receive any survival signals. This is known as '**death by neglect**' and is mainly confined to the **thymic cortex** and mediated by **cortical thymic epithelial cells** (**cTECs**).

At the next stage, SP cells migrate towards the thymic medulla, where they mainly interact with medullary TECs (mTECs). mTECs have a unique set of properties. In particular, they express proteins that would not, under normal circumstances, be found anywhere other than in specialised peripheral organs. For example, mTECs express insulin, trypsin, complement (see Table 7.2). It is said that this promiscuous, or ectopic gene expression of tissue-specific antigens (TSAs) 'mirrors the peripheral self'. The expression of such proteins would normally be regulated by tissue-specific transcription factors. However, mTECs possess transcription factors that allow them to express this wide variety of gene products. One such transcription factor is the AIRE gene (for autoimmune regulator). A genetically determined failure to express AIRE in humans, and knockout of the gene in mice, gives rise to a syndrome in which there are multiple manifestations of self reactivity by T cells (see p. 201). This tells us that the function of mTECs is to display peripheral self antigens to enable the deletion of any SP T cells possessing TCRs capable of very strong binding to self. Any TCRs showing strong avidity (strength of binding) for these self

antigens when presented by MHC molecules are actively deleted. This is a further example of **negative selection** and is used to remove from the repertoire any T cells with **high avidity** for self antigens.

The end result of the 3 weeks that a thymocyte might spend developing in the thymus is as follows:

1. To survive there must be productive rearrangement and expression of TCRαβ chains.

2. To survive further, the TCR must be capable of moderate affinity interaction with self MHC.

3. To undergo final selection for export into the periphery, the TCR affinity for self antigens must not be too high.

Should all of these criteria be fulfilled, the T cell is chosen for survival by a process termed **positive** selection and exported to the periphery, where, as a naïve T cell it resides in the lymphatic system, recirculating between lymph nodes and the blood. In this state, it is ready for the first encounter with antigen presented by activated DCs.

CD4 T lymphocyte functions

As the pivotal cell in immune responses, one would expect the T cell to influence most aspects of immunity, and this is not far short of the truth. Much of the functional 'outreach' is done through the secretion of cytokines, although direct cell–cell interaction with DCs is key in 'licensing' these cells for other functions, and direct interaction with B cells is important in the maturation of antibody responses — in both cases the pairing of CD40 and CD40 ligand (CD154) is particularly powerful in these respects. Major functions of T cells are as follows:

● Activation of DCs during antigen presentation.

● Recruitment and activation of specialised cytotoxic CD8 T cells in antiviral responses.

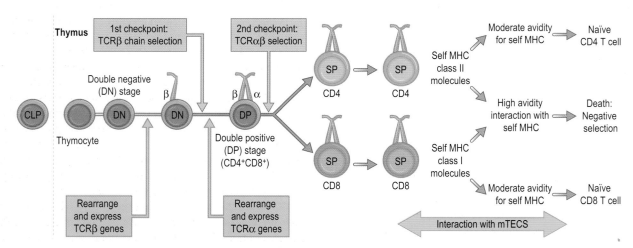

Fig. 7.4 Development of the thymocyte.
Thymocytes at the double negative stage (DN; i.e. negative for CD4 and CD8) rearrange the β chain of the TCR, acquire both CD4 and CD8 (double positive or DP stage) and then α TCR chains, before losing CD4 or CD8 to become single positive (SP). Inability of the newly formed TCR to interact with self MHC leads to 'death by neglect' and the SP cells then migrate to the thymic medulla for selection on the basis of moderate avidity for self MHC ("positive selection").

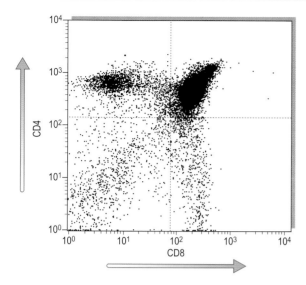

Fig. 7.5 Flow cytometry.
Plot (see Fig. 7.2b) of developing thymocyte populations, showing cells that are single CD4 and CD8 positive (SP4 and SP8) as well as cells that are double positive (DP) and double negative (DN) (courtesy of Deena Gibbons and Bruno Silva-Santos in Adrian Hayday's laboratory, King's College, London).

Table 7.2 Examples of ectopic expression of peripheral self antigens by thymic medullary epithelial cells

Peripheral proteins	Peripheral tissue represented
α-fetoprotein	Liver
Serum amyloid P	Liver
Trypsin	Pancreas
Insulin	Islets of Langerhans
Glutamic acid decarboxylase	Islets of Langerhans
Somatostatin	Islets of Langerhans
Crystallin	Eye
Retinal S antigen	Eye
Thyroglobulin	Thyroid

- Signalling for B cell expansion, inducing them to produce antibody and mature into plasma cells or memory cells.
- Secretion of cytokines responsible for growth and differentiation of a range of cell types, especially other T cells, macrophages and eosinophils.
- Regulation of immune reactions.

It can be seen from this list that few cells in the immune system remain untouched by the influence of T cells.

Molecules involved in T lymphocyte function

In addition to the TCR, which interacts with specific antigen, there are numerous cell-surface molecules critically involved in T lymphocyte functions. Some of the molecules (e.g. the CD3 complex) are an absolute requirement for T cell function. Others have a role in stabilising cell–cell interactions; and yet others provide important additional activation signals; frequently these so-called **accessory molecules** provide adhesion between communicating cells *plus* a signal for T cell activation. As stated earlier, some accessory molecules (e.g. CD4, CD8) are permanently expressed and denote a **functional subset** of T lymphocytes. Other accessory molecules are up- and down-regulated according to need (e.g. CD28, required for T cell activation, see p. 106) and yet others change as the T cell differentiates.

In clinical laboratory practice, monoclonal antibodies able to identify the different T cell-associated molecules can be used to subdivide the total T cell population into what are broadly termed **T cell subsets** (see Science Box 7.1). This is of importance in the diagnosis and management of a range of inflammatory diseases, most notably infection with the human immunodeficiency virus (HIV). In this disorder, CD4-expressing T cells are selectively depleted (see Ch. 20), at a rate which correlates with the progression of the disease. Once a critically low level of CD4 cells is reached, patients are immune deficient and at high risk of developing infections — hence the importance of measuring numbers of CD4 T cells in managing patients.

The CD3 complex: signal transducer for the T cell receptor

Analogous to the B cell receptor complex (see Ch. 6), a group of molecules (collectively termed the CD3 complex) has been identified that closely associates with the TCR and functions to transduce signals that follow from interaction with peptide-MHC molecules, to initiate the process of T cell activation. TCR-mediated activation follows the same general principles as for B cells — the antigen receptor itself has no intrinsic signalling property; it recruits additional molecules of the CD3 complex that have immunoreceptor tyrosine-based activation motifs (ITAMs); this leads to activation of an intracellular activation cascade, triggering tyrosine kinase activation and calcium signalling and ultimately leading to changes in gene expression profiles (see p. 106).

The CD3 complex is composed of five different transmembrane protein chains, denoted by Greek letters: γ (25–28 kDa), δ (20 kDa), ε (25 kDa), ζ (zeta, 16 kDa) and η (eta, 22 kDa). One ε chain associates non-covalently with a δ chain and this complex lies adjacent to the α chain of the TCR. An ε–γ complex associates with the β chain, and nearby lies a disulphide-linked ζ–ζ homodimer (90% of T cells) or ζ–η heterodimer (10%) (Fig. 7.6).

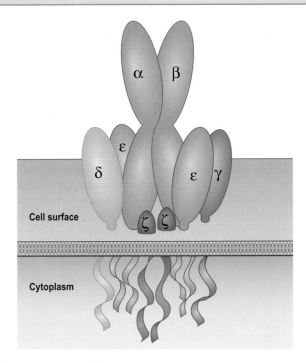

Fig. 7.6 Schematic representation of the TCR and CD3.
CD3 chains transduce activation signals emanating from the TCR interaction with presented antigen.

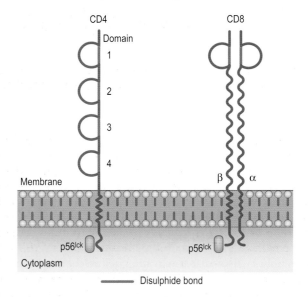

Fig. 7.7 Schematic representation of CD4 and CD8 accessory molecules.
Note immunoglobulin-like domain structure and the associated protein tyrosine kinase, p56^{Lck}.

CD4 and CD8, accessory molecules in T cell function

CD4 and CD8 are the major accessory molecules in T cell function. CD4 is typically present on about two thirds of mature peripheral blood and lymphoid T cells, and CD8 on the remaining one third.

CD4 is a transmembrane glycoprotein of 55 kDa expressed as a monomer and a member of the immunoglobulin

supergene family. As such it has four immunoglobulin-like domains (Fig. 7.7). CD4 has a dual role in T cell activation: it provides some adhesive forces between interacting cells by binding to the β_2 domain of class II MHC molecules on the APC, and it also provides an accessory activation signal through a lymphocyte-specific protein tyrosine kinase, called Lck (or p56^{lck}) (Fig. 7.8). One other important fact about CD4 will become apparent: it is the cellular receptor for human immunodeficiency virus, HIV (see p. 288).

The CD8 molecule differs from CD4 in being a disulphide-linked dimer, each chain (32–34 kDa) having a single immunoglobulin-like domain (Fig. 7.7). The CD8 molecule is similar in function to CD4. As a cell-adhesion molecule it binds to the α_3 domain of the class I MHC molecule, stabilising T cell interactions with APCs or target cells, whilst its cytoplasmic domain becomes phosphorylated (Fig. 7.8).

SUMMARY BOX 7.1

T lymphocyte characteristics

- T lymphocytes arise in the thymus and carry an antigen-specific receptor, the TCR.
- Other key surface molecules acquired in the thymus are CD3 (signal transduction) and accessory molecules (e.g. CD4, CD8).
- CD4 occurs on the surface of two thirds of T cells; it interacts with class II MHC molecules on cells presenting antigen and increases the affinity of binding. CD4 T cells are termed T helper (T$_H$) cells.
- CD8 interacts with class I MHC molecules on cells, stabilising T cell interactions with cells presenting antigen. Effector CD8 T cells (CTLs) kill target cells.

T cell activation: antigen processing and peptide presentation

When B cells are incubated in vitro with antigen to which their surface immunoglobulin can bind then the whole intact antigen is internalised; this provides an important signal for B cell activation. In contrast, when T cells are incubated with whole intact antigen, there is no TCR recognition event. As stated previously, TCRs do not 'see' native intact antigens. For TCR recognition, the native antigen must be 'presented' in the form of short peptides bound to MHC molecules. The short peptides are derived from the whole, intact antigen by 'processing'. Therefore, a discussion of **antigen processing and presentation** is required to understand T cell activation. Antigen processing is different for CD4 and CD8 T cells, broadly reflecting the different sources of antigenic targets (external antigens, e.g. from microbes for CD4 T cells; internal antigens, e.g. from intracellular viruses, for CD8 T cells). In the experiments required to show antigen processing and presentation, the T cell response is used as the read-out; a T cell response means that the correct peptide ends up bound in the correct MHC molecule groove. The T cell response

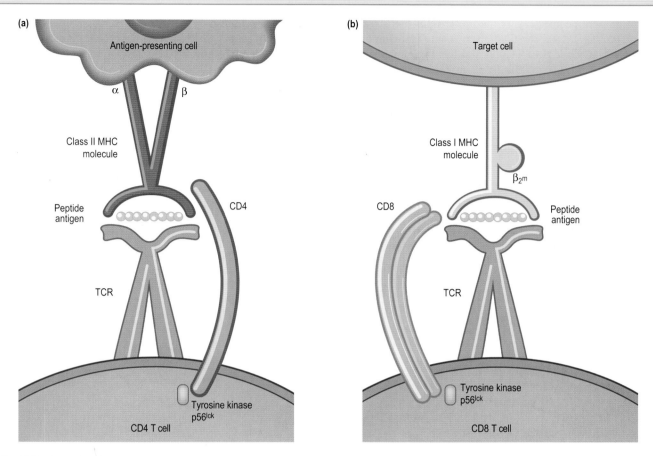

Fig. 7.8 The role of CD4 and CD8.
Schematic representation of the interaction between TCR and antigenic peptide presented by class II MHC molecules. CD4 stabilises this configuration by binding the class II MHC molecule. (**b**) CD8 has a similar role, but in the interaction with antigen presented by a class I MHC molecule.

can be measured in a variety of different ways (see Science Box 7.3).

Antigen processing and presentation to CD4 T cells

It has been established for many years that when cultured on their own, CD4 T cells cannot respond to antigen. Antigen must be *presented* by a cell bearing the same class II MHC type as that expressed in the thymus in which the T cell developed. Antigen processing is a specialised, active function of cells and is almost exclusively carried out by specialised APCs, namely dendritic cells, B cells and monocyte/macrophages. The requirements of APCs are to be able to **internalise antigen**; activate **proteolytic enzymes** for degradation into peptides; and carry out **peptide loading** into MHC molecules ready for surface presentation to CD4 T cells.

The process begins with the acquisition of antigens from outside, and it is therefore often termed the **exogenous pathway** of antigen presentation. The mechanism of antigen internalisation varies according to the APC (Fig. 7.9). Dendritic cells are highly pinocytotic (i.e. 'drink' from their surroundings) and also express specialised surface receptors

that can bind particular types of antigen. Two of the best examples are the mannose receptor and DC-SIGN (for dendritic cell-specific ICAM-grabbing non-integrin), which bind microbes. Antigen is internalised by B cells through surface immunoglobulin, and is thus highly specific for a particular target. Whatever the route of uptake, antigen from the external milieu arrives in compartments termed **late endosomes**, because of their proximity to the cell surface. Endosomes may then migrate towards the cell interior and fuse with lysosomes. Both endosomes and lysosomes contain proteolytic enzymes and are able to lower their pH, a combination of events that leads to antigen degradation.

At the same time in APCs, as part of a continuous process, class II MHC molecules are being generated from gene transcription and translation and assembled in the endoplasmic reticulum (ER). This process is up-regulated when APCs are activated, as is likely when DCs encounter pathogens through their PRRs (see Ch. 6), providing an increase in MHC class II molecule availability and expression. Newly-synthesised class II MHC molecules travel via the Golgi apparatus to come into contact with the late endosomes. The antigen-binding groove of the MHC class II molecule is protected throughout this journey through the cytoplasm from accepting peptide antigens by the presence of the **invariant chain (Ii)** (Fig. 7.10). The Ii chain thus acts as a **chaperone** for new MHC class II molecules and has three major functions in antigen presentation; it promotes assembly of new MHC class II α–β heterodimers; it targets newly synthesised

class II MHC molecules into the endosomal pathway, guiding them to the site at which antigenic peptide binds; and most importantly it *protects the peptide-binding groove* until the class II MHC molecule has arrived at the appropriate site for peptide loading. The protection of the class II binding groove is achieved by a part of the Ii chain called the **CLIP region** (class II-associated invariant chain peptide), which occupies the MHC groove and prevents any other self peptide from binding, ensuring that the desired, internalised peptides are loaded preferentially. There is still controversy over some of the locations of subsequent events, but a major proportion of antigenic peptide loading into MHC class II molecules takes place in a group of vesicles in a late endosomal compartment termed **MIIC** (for MHC class II compartment). Here, the Ii chain is released and new peptides from exogenous antigens (typically 12–25 amino acid residues long) are inserted into the MHC molecule groove. This reaction is catalysed by molecules that resemble conventional HLA class II molecules (but do not bind peptide) called HLA-DM. In B cells an additional set of similar molecules (HLA-DO) assist in peptide loading.

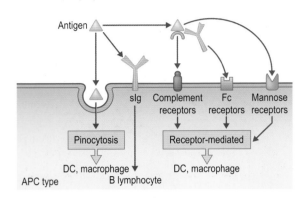

Fig. 7.9 **Differing mechanisms for antigen internalisation for different antigen presenting cell types.**

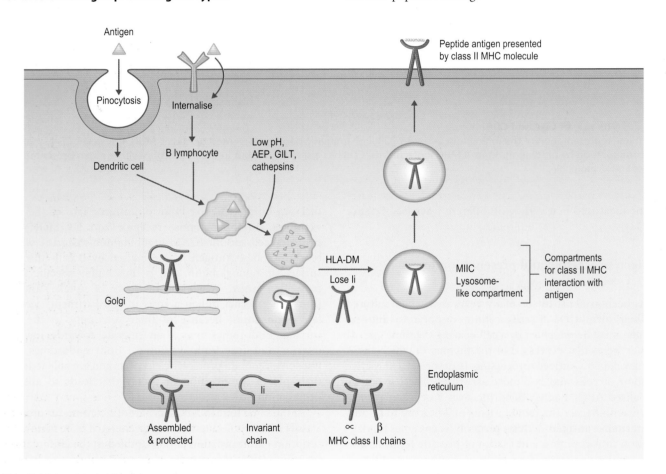

Fig. 7.10 **Processing and presentation of exogenous antigen via the MHC class II (exogenous) pathway and assembly of class II MHC molecules with antigenic peptide.**
MHC class II molecules are assembled in the endoplasmic reticulum and the peptide-binding groove is protected by the presence of the invariant chain. After modification in the Golgi apparatus, MHC class II molecules migrate to the late endosomal compartments (e.g. MIIC) where they meet antigen that has been internalised and processed by proteolytic enzymes (e.g. AEP, GILT, cathepsins) and low pH in late endosomes. The invariant chain is removed and antigenic peptide added to the binding groove, in a process catalysed by the HLA-DM molecule. The MHC–peptide complex now migrates to the cell surface.

The mechanism through which complex protein antigens are degraded is not yet fully determined. It is known to involve proteolytic enzymes. Two important enzymes with **specific cleavage** patterns are **GILT** (for gamma-inducible lysosomal thiol reductase), which cleaves disulphide bonds, and **AEP** (for asparaginyl endopeptidase), which cleaves after asparagine (N) residues. These enzymes are critical for the unfolding of complex folded antigens, which 'relax' after disulphide bond cleavage or removal of N. The **cathepsins** are a group of enzymes with broad specificity that cleave at both ends of proteins. In combination with acid pH, these enzymes reduce complex proteins to peptides, which then load onto the waiting MHC class II molecule.

Antigen presentation to CD8 T cells

Antigenic peptides are presented to CD8 T cells through what is termed the **endogenous pathway**, since the peptide fragments come from endogenously synthesised cellular proteins (which would include microbe-derived peptides in the case of an intracellular infection, e.g. with a virus) (Fig. 7.11). Antigen peptide loading takes place at the site of assembly of class I MHC heavy chains with β_2-microglobulin (β_2-m), in the ER. The assembly of a peptide-loaded MHC class I molecule depends upon all 3 components (heavy chain, β_2-m and peptide of 8–10 amino acids) being available. Analogous to the Ii chain in class II MHC molecule assembly, a molecule termed **calnexin** acts as the molecular chaperone for class I MHC molecules. Calnexin is an ER resident protein that ensures that assembled class I MHC molecules associate with peptide in the correct compartment (in this case peptides derived from the cytoplasm and moved into the ER), and also that any assembled class I molecules with empty peptide-binding grooves are not allowed to leave. **Calreticulin**, another chaperone molecule, ensures that the α heavy chain and β_2-m are stable until antigenic peptide is loaded.

How do the peptides arrive in the ER and how are they formed and selected for loading? Working backwards, from the site of peptide binding to HLA, the first question to address is how the peptides arrive in the MHC class I molecule assembly compartment. This is achieved with two ATP-dependent molecules termed TAP-1 and TAP-2 (for transporter associated with processing; note that their genes lie in the class II MHC region, see p. 58). The TAP transporters act as funnels into the ER and also have a selection capability to choose peptides of the correct size (8–10 residues), as well as of an appropriate sequence for class I binding. TAP transporters are kept in close proximity to the waiting class I molecule by a molecule called **tapasin**. Tapasin also enhances the overall stability of these intermolecular interactions, and has a peptide-editing role. Together the above named proteins come to form what is termed the **peptide loading complex** for MHC class I, which has an overall stoichiometry of 4 MHC class I heavy and light chains; 4 calreticulin, 4 tapasin and 1 of each TAP molecule (Table 7.3).

The supply of appropriate peptides into TAP requires a proteolytic machinery. The major known pathway for cata-

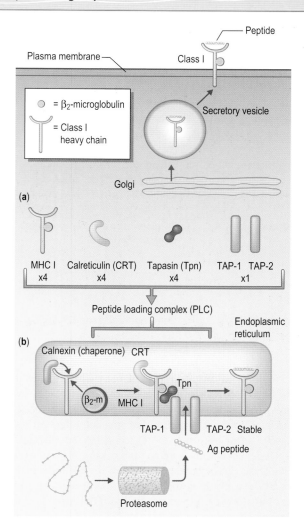

Fig. 7.11 Processing and presentation of endogenous antigen, via the MHC class I (endogenous) pathway. Cytoplasmic proteins derived from the cytoplasm are cleaved into peptides by the action of enzymes in the large proteasome complex. The peptide is transported into the site of class I molecule assembly by specific transporter molecules (TAP-1 and TAP-2). Peptide, α chain and β_2-microglobulin (β_2m) combine and are protected and loaded using the peptide loading complex (PLC). The stable, peptide-loaded complex is then guided out of the endoplasmic reticulum by the chaperone proteins via the secretory vesicle, to the cell surface.

lytic turnover of any cytoplasmic protein is a large complex of proteases with multicatalytic capabilities, termed the **proteasome**. The proteasome is large enough to be visible by electron microscopy and has a cylindrical shape like a cotton reel (Fig. 7.12) composed of 4 rings of 7 cylinders each, with a hollow core. It is the cell's recycling machinery, taking proteins that have been tagged by a process termed ubiquitination as being surplus to requirement or mis-folded. A subset of the catalytic complex can be formed that contains two components, PSMB8 and PSMB9 (see p. 58) and is called the immunoproteasome, typically only found in dendritic cells (note that PSMB molecules are also encoded in the class II

Table 7.3 Components involved in loading MHC class I with antigenic peptide

Molecule	Function
Calnexin	Chaperone for protecting empty groove
Calreticulin	Chaperone for maintaining stability in absence of peptide loading
Tapasin	Brings empty class I molecule close to loading site
TAP-1 and TAP-2	Transportation into ER and editing of cytoplasmic peptides
Proteasome	Generation of peptides for loading

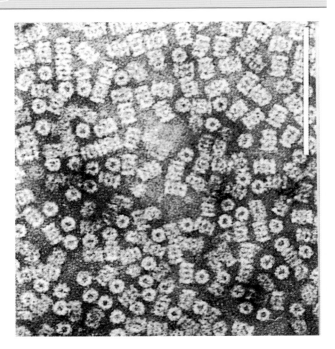

Fig. 7.12 The proteasome.
Electron micrograph of a proteasome: the large proteolytic complex responsible for catalytic breakdown of cytoplasmic proteins. Note the cotton reel shape. Proteasomes cleave endogenous peptides for antigen presentation (reproduced with permission from Peters 1994 Trends in Biochemical Sciences 19: 377–382).

MHC region, indicating a mechanism by which genes in one region of the MHC can influence those in another).

One final component of antigen presentation to CD8 T cells relates to viral proteins that are actually synthesised inside the ER: how do these become loaded through the proteasome–TAP route? Current thinking is that proteins such as these can be transported from the ER into the cytoplasm by **retrograde translocation** (i.e. protein movement in the opposite direction to normal) and that this is achieved through an ER-associated degradation (ERAD) system. Thus, there should be no escape for viruses from being tracked by the immune system, although, unsurprisingly, viruses have devised many systems for avoiding the immune system, including interference with viral antigen processing (see Science Box 7.2).

How are viral antigens taken in by DCs presented to CD8 T cells?

Now that the essential mechanisms of antigen presentation to CD4 and CD8 T cells have been discussed, there is an important issue to consider. Take the following scenario. A virus infects epithelial cells in the respiratory tract. As part of the viral replication process to generate new infective virions, some virus proteins will undergo processing and presentation through the endogenous pathway in the epithelial cells and be loaded into class I MHC molecules for surface display. There will be activation of DCs, which will internalise viruses and transport them to the local lymph node. Some days later, when the cellular immune response to this virus has been generated, CD8 cytotoxic T cells (CTLs) will arrive in the respiratory tract and kill the virus-infected cells — this is a major means of host protection. The CTL response that achieves this will be directed against epithelial cells displaying virus peptide-MHC class I complexes

on the cell surface. The CTL response will have been generated in the regional lymph node, through the combined efforts of DCs bearing viral antigens and CD4 T$_H$1 cells, to activate the naïve CD8 T cell. And here is the conundrum — the DC arrives in the lymph node bearing viral proteins that it has acquired by *internalisation into endosomes*, yet the viral antigens must be located in the *endogenous pathway of antigen presentation* in order to be loaded into MHC class I molecules to activate the CTL response.

The answer to the conundrum is a process termed **cross presentation**. This is mainly a property of DCs. Once viral proteins are acquired from the external milieu and internalised into endosomal compartments for antigen presentation, they must then undergo **retrograde translocation** into the cytoplasm under the influence of a protein conducting channel called **Sec61**. This allows DCs to process, present and display in the lymph node the same virus peptide–MHC complex that the CD8 CTL will encounter in the respiratory tract (Fig. 7.13). See Science Boxes 7.3–7.6.

Molecules involved in T cell activation — on the outside

The key cells and molecules involved in T cell activation have all now been encountered. Picture an immune response to a virus not encountered before. DCs arriving from the tissues into the lymph node laden with viral antigens are

---

SCIENCE BOX 7.2

How viruses, bacteria and parasites avoid immune surveillance

It should come as no surprise that successful microorganisms have evolved mechanisms for avoiding the innate and adaptive immune response. The selective pressure on viruses, bacteria and parasites exerted by the immune surveillance systems in their host will naturally give rise to successfully resistant variants, which thus acquire a selection advantage. The terms that have been coined for these processes are 'subversion' of the immune system and 'anti-immunology'. In some cases they undoubtedly contribute to chronicity and pathogenicity. Since there is a myriad examples of such avoidance strategies, only a few will be considered here for illustrative purposes.

Simple examples are obvious ways of 'hiding' from the immune system and include the surface expression on viruses and bacteria of structures that interfere with immune recognition. For example, *Streptococcus pneumoniae* and *Neisseria meningitidis* have developed complex capsular carbohydrates that prevent access of antibodies and complement to the bacterium. Viruses appear especially adept at generating their own versions of immune modulators (e.g. chemokines, cytokines, interferons, complement inhibitory proteins). An example is the Kaposi sarcoma-associated herpes virus (KSHV), the aetiological

agent in this rare tumour of lymphatic vessel endothelium. The genome of KSHV contains several viral homologues of human immune modulator genes, including 3 chemokines and IL-6. These genes, presumably 'pirated' from human cells, must be useful in survival and propagation of the virus. In addition, viruses, and especially RNA viruses, have high mutational frequencies that constantly generate mutants. If the mutations are located in important target antigens for the immune system (e.g. in a CTL epitope) and do not interfere with viral fitness, then mutants can develop that are highly resistant to killing. Whilst that is a fairly random and subtle means of avoiding immune recognition, many viruses have developed mechanisms for inhibiting antigen presentation, and it is clear that at almost every step of the endogenous pathway there is a repressing viral strategy. As one example, herpes simplex virus-1 encodes ICP47, a cytosolic protein that binds to TAP-1/2 dimers to prevent peptide binding and entry into the ER lumen, thus restricting presentation of viral peptides to CTLs. Uncovering these and other mechanisms of 'immunoevasion' is a high priority area of research, since it might reveal novel approaches for anti-viral therapies.

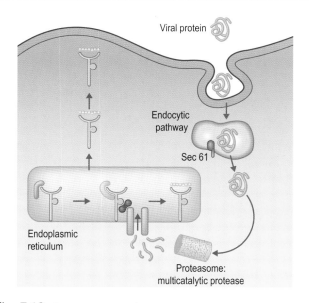

Viral protein

Endocytic pathway

Sec 61

Endoplasmic reticulum

Proteasome: multicatalytic protease

Fig. 7.13 Cross presentation.
Antigens internalised by dendritic cells into endosomes are translocated into the class I endogenous pathway by retrograde transport into the cytoplasm using proteins such as Sec61.

required to process these and present viral peptide epitopes bound to MHC molecules on the cell surface. The next step is a little like the story of Cinderella — the DC has to find a naïve T cell bearing a TCR that fits the peptide–MHC complex with sufficient snugness to induce activation. This is achieved in the lymph node, where naïve T cells reside.

Much of what we now know about this process has been revealed by intravital microscopy — actually viewing DCs and T cells in a live lymph node. It appears that the arriving DCs bearing antigens are surrounded by swarms of randomly migrating naïve T cells. It is estimated that each DC can contact 5000 T cells per hour. If the naïve T cell gets no signal from a DC, it moves on. The lymph node up-regulates adhesion molecules on high endothelial venule structures (see p. 7) to draw in more naïve T cells from the blood, increasing the pool of potentially useful TCR repertoires. This results in the swelling and tenderness of lymph nodes often noticed during an infection. At some point, there will be the 'Cinderella moment', when an appropriate TCR–pMHC interaction occurs. The T cell stops migrating and becomes more tightly adherent to the DC surface. This interaction between peptide–MHC and TCR, which is transduced by the CD3 complex, is termed **signal 1** in the process of T cell activation.

Of itself, signal 1 is insufficient to drive a naïve T cell into full activation. **Signal 2** is required, and is provided by the interaction of a group of complementary molecules in a process termed **co-stimulation**. On the DC side, the co-stimulatory molecules are CD80 and CD86. You may remember that these are present at low levels on immature DCs, but are massively up-regulated when the DC is activated, for example by a pathogen (see p. 74). CD80 and CD86 bind to CD28 on the T cell. This leads to a sequence of intracellular events (see below) initiated by the CD28 cytoplasmic domain, which binds a phosphoinositide 3-kinase to initiate an activation cascade, leading to transcription and translation of the IL-2 and IL-2 receptor genes (see Science Box 7.7).

The reliance on signal 1 and signal 2 to achieve full T cell activation has a number of important implications, the main one being that of acting as a **fail-safe mechanism** to avoid unwanted activation of the adaptive immune system (which could, for example, lead to autoimmunity). The requirement for signals 1 and 2 means that only highly activated DCs have the necessary power to activate a naïve T cell. This, in turn, means that the adaptive immune system relies very heavily upon whether the innate immune system is activated or not. For this to happen the DC must receive appropriate activation signals from a pathogen. This phenomenon has been termed by some the **danger hypothesis**. Without the element

---

SCIENCE BOX 7.3

Activating T cells and measuring responses in the laboratory I: separation and testing of lymphocytes for proliferative responses

To examine whether an individual has a T cell response to an antigen, it is conventional to carry out a proliferation assay (Fig. 7.14). First, the lymphocytes must be separated from the whole blood. This is done by exploiting the difference in density between lymphocytes and monocytes, on the one hand, and erythrocytes and granulocytes, on the other. Blood is layered onto a solution of fixed density and then centrifuged. Under these conditions, the denser cells pellet at the bottom of the tube, and the lighter lymphocytes, monocytes and DCs remain above the density medium. This population of cells is termed the 'peripheral blood mononuclear cell' or PBMC preparation. Selected populations can be further purified using monoclonal antibodies (e.g. anti-CD4, anti-CD8) coated with magnetic beads. The proliferation assay (Fig. 7.14b) requires responding T cells and antigen-presenting cells (e.g. monocytes, DCs) all of which are contained in the PBMC prep, to be incubated with the antigen for approximately 3–6 days. A radioactive source of the DNA base thymidine is then added and incorporated into the new DNA of dividing cells. The radioactive nuclei of the cells are collected onto a filter and the radioactive emission counted. This provides a measurement of the T cell proliferative response to antigen.

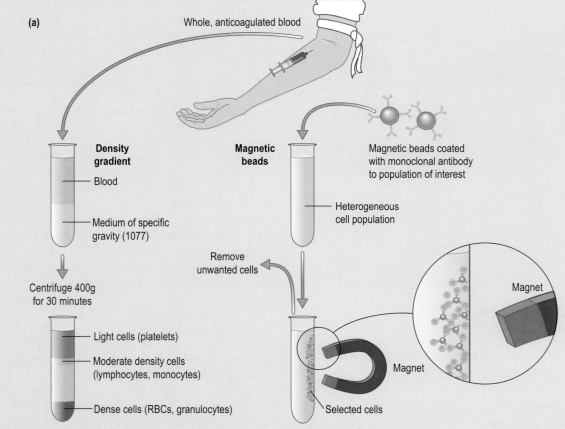

Fig. 7.14 **Purification of leukocyte populations and measuring T cell proliferation.**
(a) Separation of blood leukocytes using a density gradient. Purification may also be achieved using specific monoclonal antibodies tagged to magnetic beads.

SCIENCE BOX 7.3

Activating T cells and measuring responses in the laboratory I: separation and testing of lymphocytes for proliferative responses—cont'd

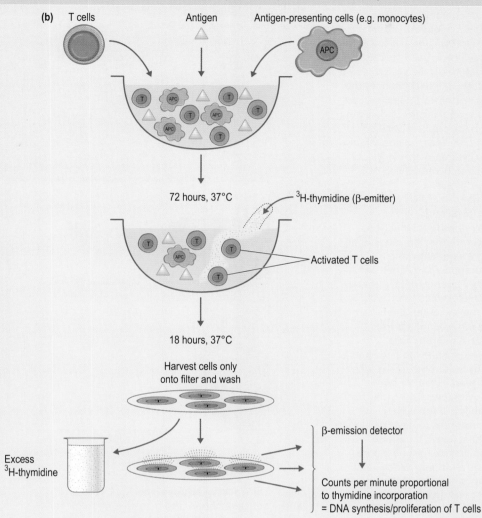

Fig. 7.14 **Purification of leukocyte populations and measuring T cell proliferation—cont'd** (**b**) Proliferation assay to measure T cell response to specific antigen.

SCIENCE BOX 7.4

Activating T cells and measuring responses in the laboratory II: polyclonal stimuli

Sometimes it is desirable to be able to activate T cells 'artificially' in the laboratory and measure the response. This is carried out not just for research purposes, but can also be an important diagnostic test in patients with a suspected immune deficiency (see p. 267). Broadly speaking, the stimuli used for activation fall into two camps. The first method of activation is to aim to stimulate most or all T cells using a **polyclonal activator**, or **mitogen**. Examples are the lectin phytohaemagglutinin (PHA), which cross-links surface glycoproteins on T cells; or monoclonal anti-CD3, which acts to cross-link the TCR complex. These stimuli force most T cells to proliferate and make effector cytokines. Phorbol myristate acetate (PMA; activates protein kinase C; see p. 106) along with a calcium ionophore is a very strong stimulus for inducing T cells to produce cytokines and reveal their

functional polarisation. **Superantigens** (e.g. staphylococcal enterotoxin B) are microbial compounds that bind simultaneously to domains on particular families of V_β chains of the TCR on the T cell surface, and to the β chain of the class II MHC molecule on the APC, and in doing so they activate and expand all T cells bearing this V_β. These polyclonal activators give an overview of how well the T cells in an individual subject can respond. Sometimes, however, it is important to be able to examine immunity to a specific stimulus, for example a pathogen. For this, a more physiological stimulus in the form of whole antigen from the microbe or a specific peptide epitope is added to cultures containing T cells and APCs. Under these conditions, the responses of antigen-specific T cells can be measured.

SCIENCE BOX 7.5

Activating T cells and measuring responses in the laboratory III: cytokines and tetramers

Measuring the T cell response is carried out in different ways, depending upon the information required. One of the simplest means of detecting a T cell response is to see whether the stimulus induces the cell cycle and leads to proliferation (see Science Box 7.1). More detailed information is often required, however, in the form of what cytokines the responder cells make. This enables responses to be classified as T_H1, T_H2, T_H17, or Treg. There are several means of detecting cytokine responses. The cytokine made can be measured in different assay formats, including ELISA. The cytokine can also be detected inside the cell by flow cytometry (see p. 89), or cytokine-specific mRNA transcripts can be quantified by polymerase chain reaction.

A new means of quantifying antigen-specific T cells has been developed in recent years. It involves using recombinant DNA technology to synthesise soluble HLA molecules, each of which is loaded with the peptide epitope of interest. These HLA molecules are assembled into complexes of four peptide–HLA components (termed an **HLA tetramer**) using a flexible hinge arrangement. Although a single soluble peptide–HLA molecule would not have sufficient affinity for a single TCR, the use of tetramers increases the overall avidity of the interaction (it is like hanging on to a rock face with both hands and feet compared with trying to grab the mountain with one hand!). The HLA tetramer is coupled to a fluorochrome (see p. 89) such that individual T cells able to bind to the specific epitope can be identified by flow cytometry (Fig. 7.15). This approach has revolutionised the ability to use widely available technology to measure responses to, say, Epstein–Barr virus (EBV, the cause of glandular fever). It has also revealed some surprises. During an acute virus infection, as many as 5–10% of CD8 T cells in the peripheral blood can be shown to be reactive to EBV epitopes, showing the massive expansion in CTLs that is required to control the infection.

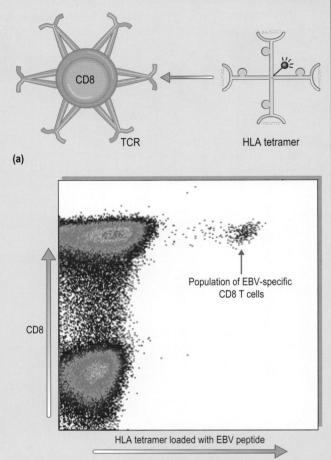

Fig. 7.15 **Tracking antigen-specific T cells.**
(**a**) The principle of HLA tetramer staining to identify antigen-specific T cells. The HLA tetramer is a reagent composed of 4 identical HLA molecules each loaded with the same peptide. The tetramer is able to bind to the surface of T cells bearing TCRs that bind to that peptide–HLA complex. The tetramer is labelled with a fluorescent molecule and thus able to indicate the T cells that are stained positive. (**b**) Staining and flow cytometry analysis of CD8 T cells using an HLA class I tetramer loaded with a peptide from the Epstein–Barr virus (EBV). Flow cytometry shows a cloud of cells that are termed 'tetramer positive' and represent CD8 T cells specific for this peptide from EBV. Identifying these cells allows laboratories to track and quantify the antiviral response.

of danger provided by a DC PRR interacting with a pathogen PAMP, there will be insufficient signalling to activate a naïve T cell.

Finally, there is a **signal 3** provided by DCs in the form of cytokines that polarise the T cell response (see Table 7.4). The nature of the DC stimulus dictates the quality of signal 3. The **T_H1-polarising cytokine IL-12** is critical at this stage for driving a CD4 T cell response dominated by IFN-γ (Fig. 7.18). Conditions which favour a T_H2 response are a lesser amount of IL-12 and the presence of **IL-4** (see Science Box 7.8). The newly described T_H17 pathway requires the combination of **IL-23**, **IL-6** and **TGF-β**. A Treg response is promoted by the presence of **TGF-β** and **IL-10**. IL-10 is produced by immature DCs. This would appear to represent

Activating T cells and measuring responses in the laboratory IV: measuring cytotoxicity

Cytotoxicity assays are useful research tools for examining specific lysis by CTLs and also killing by natural killer cells. The assay is based upon incubating together the effector cells and target cells and measuring damage to the targets. In the assessment of CTL activity, the appropriate MHC-matched target cell (e.g. a virus-infected cell from the same donor) must be used. Whether performing an assay of cytotoxicity mediated by CTLs or by natural killer cells the appropriate target cells are labelled by incubation with a solution of radioactive sodium chromate (^{51}Cr) or other types of indicator molecules that diffuse easily across the membranes of intact target cells and become retained within the cell cytoplasm as long as the cell is alive. The targets and effectors are then incubated together for 4–5 hours (Fig. 7.16). If target cells are damaged by the effectors, ^{51}Cr is released from the cytoplasm into the culture fluid. Levels of radioactivity in the culture fluid are, therefore, proportional to the degree of target cell lysis.

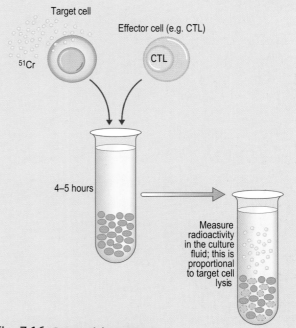

Fig. 7.16 **Cytotoxicity assays.**
See the box text for details.

Interleukin-2

IL-2, originally known as T cell growth factor, is the major cytokine responsible for T lymphocyte activation and proliferation. Its importance in T cell physiology cannot be stressed enough. A major feature of this 15 kDa polypeptide is the autocrine loop through which it operates: receipt of an appropriate activation signal by a T cell results in massive up-regulation of production of both the cytokine and its receptors, so that IL-2 can feed back activating signals through its receptor. Similarly, local release of IL-2 can lead to activation of nearby T cells in a paracrine fashion. IL-2 also has important growth-promoting functions in relation to B lymphocyte development. IL-2 is part of a family of interleukins (other members are IL-4, IL-7, IL-9, IL-15 and IL-21) that share a common receptor component (the γ chain). The receptor for IL-2 has three chains: α, β and γ (Fig. 7.17). The minimal receptor configuration for signal transduction is the IL-2Rβγ heterodimer, which binds its ligand with an intermediate affinity (K_d 10^{-9} M), whilst the combination of α, β and the common γ chain results in high-affinity (K_d 10^{-11} M) binding. The γ chain also appears to be critical for internalisation of the receptor–ligand complex. The IL-2Rα (CD25) also distinguishes cells with Treg activity, and Tregs are dependent upon IL-2 for their differentiation and function. IL-2 has been used therapeutically to activate the immune system in an attempt to eradicate tumours (especially renal cell cancer and malignant melanoma) and chronic viruses. The IL-2 pathway is the target of drugs designed to dampen down the immune system, either by interfering in the signalling (e.g. ciclosporin, tacrolimus) or using monoclonal antibodies against CD25 (daclizumab) (see p. 308).

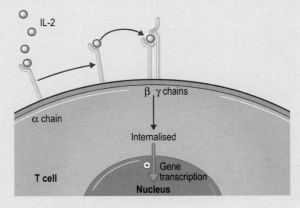

Fig. 7.17 **Receptors for IL-2.**
The T cell growth factor IL-2 binds the IL-2 α chain, which acts as a trap. Transfer of IL-2 to the βγ dimer of the receptor allows internalisation leading to cell proliferation.

Table 7.4 Identification of T cell subsets by function

T cell population	Main marker	Main ('signature') cytokines produced	Functions	Major role in physiological immune response
T helper 1 (T_H1) cells	CD4	IFN-γ, IL-2, TNF-α	Pro-inflammatory	Organise killing of bacteria, fungi and viruses; activate macrophages to kill intracellular bacteria; instruct CTL responses
T helper 2 (T_H2) cells	CD4	IL-4, IL-5, IL-13	Pro-inflammatory	Organise killing of parasites by recruiting eosinophils; promote antibody responses
T helper 17 (T_H17) cells	CD4	IL-17	Pro-inflammatory	Not yet fully defined; capable of recruiting cells and damaging targets
Regulatory T cells (Treg)	CD4	IL-10, TGF-β	Regulatory	Regulation of inflammation

---

SCIENCE BOX 7.8

Interleukin-4

IL-4 is a 20 kDa polypeptide released predominantly by T_H2 cells, which has important effects in relation to T and especially B cell function. It provides a potent stimulus for B cell switching to production of IgE antibody. As such it is important from a clinical viewpoint in relation to parasitic infections and allergy, in both of which IgE-mediated responses play an important role. IL-4 is an important promoting growth factor for the T_H2 subset of lymphocytes and is an equally important inhibitory cytokine in the growth and differentiation of T_H1 cells.

SUMMARY BOX 7.2

T cell selection and activation

- Only 1% of potential T cells entering the thymus will be selected for the periphery: selection is based on affinity for self MHC molecules. The optimum characteristic is moderate affinity for a peptide presented by self MHC molecules. Cells with high or low affinity for self fail to develop, and undergo apoptosis.

- CD4 T cells are activated by peptides that are derived from exogenous proteins, which are internalised and processed in APCs and presented bound to MHC class II molecule on the surface of the APC.

- CD8 T cells are activated by endogenously derived peptides presented by class I molecules.

- There are two distinct pathways of antigen processing for presentation.

- Chaperone molecules — invariant chain for class II and calnexin for class I — protect the peptide-binding groove of the MHC molecule until peptide antigen can bind.

- Cross-presentation is required for viral proteins internalised by DCs to find their way into the class I MHC presentation pathway.

---

another dimension of the fail-safe mechanism of control exercised by DCs. If there is antigen presentation by an immature DC that makes IL-10 (i.e. in the absence of PRR-PAMP interactions) then the T cell response is directed down a 'default' pathway of Tregs. This may be an important mechanism for generating Tregs to control autoimmunity. Each of these subsets of CD4 T cells maintain their programmed function through the expression of individual **transcription factors** (i.e. proteins that bind DNA regulatory elements) (see Fig. 7.18).

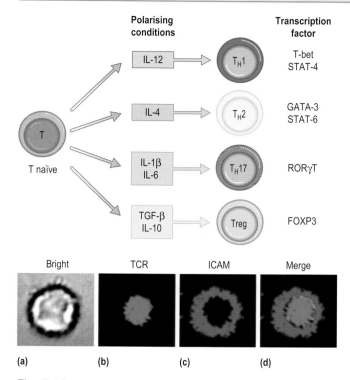

Polarising conditions		Transcription factor	Effector cytokines
IL-12	T$_H$1	T-bet STAT-4	TGF-β IL-10
IL-4	T$_H$2	GATA-3 STAT-6	IL-4, 5, 13
IL-1β IL-6	T$_H$17	RORγT	IL-17
TGF-β IL-10	Treg	FOXP3	TGF-β IL-10

T naïve

Fig. 7.18 Pathways for development of naïve T cells to mature effector T cells after encounter with antigen presented by dendritic cells. Depending upon the signal provided by DCs, in the form of secreted cytokines, the T cell develops into a particular type of effector with a specific set of transcription factors controlling its gene profile, and a specific set of effector cytokines, which represent the 'signature' for that cell type.

Bright   TCR   ICAM   Merge

(a)   (b)   (c)   (d)

Fig. 7.19 The immunological synapse.
The separate components of the synapse have been stained with different coloured antibodies after the cell in (**a**) has been activated. Staining for TCR (**b**) shows the central supramolecular complex, cSMAC and staining for the adhesion molecule ICAM (**c**) shows a 'doughnut' that represents the peripheral or pSMAC. The merged image is shown in (**d**). Reproduced with permission from Kaspar D, et al; Science 310: 1191–1193, 2005.

Molecules involved in T cell activation — on the membrane

We have described the pairing of individual surface molecules and their ligands between the DC and the T cell. However, this is only part of the membrane activity that takes place during T cell activation. Multiple sets of molecules and their respective ligands interact at the membrane interface between the two cells. The aim of this process is presumed to be to enhance the strength of the signal between the two cells and maintain contact for the amount of time required to complete the activation process. It also provides a polarising effect so that secretion of cytokines and chemokines between the cells is focused on the relevant area.

The interchange is highly organised into two zones, at what has been termed the **immunological synapse** (Fig. 7.19). The inner part of the synapse is termed the **central supramolecular complex** or **cSMAC** and is composed of TCRs pairing with peptide–MHC, CD28–CD80 pairing and expression of protein kinase C-θ. Around 100–150 TCRs will be present in the cSMAC, which forms a bull's eye surrounded by the peripheral SMAC (**pSMAC**) composed of adhesion molecules, especially LFA-1 and ICAM-1. There are slight differences in the configurations of the cSMAC and pSMAC in different APCs. Whilst B cells have what

resembles the true bull's eye configuration, for the DC it may appear more as a loose collection of microclusters, each containing about 100 TCRs. The earliest sign of TCR clustering, to form nanoclusters that migrate into the cSMAC zone, starts within approximately 30 seconds of cell contact, and the immunological synapse is fully formed within 5 minutes.

Molecules involved in T cell activation — on the inside

Binding of antigen to the lymphocyte receptor, accompanied by co-signals supplied through other surface receptors, is the common mechanism by which both B and T lymphocytes are activated. For each, activity at the membrane must be translated ultimately into nuclear events designed to equip the cell to make an appropriate response (e.g. proliferation, cytokine release). The two main themes overlying the intracellular processes of lymphocyte activation are signal **transduction** and **amplification**. These lead to the generation of **transcription factors** and **DNA-binding proteins**, which initiate the processes of gene transcription and translation. Knowledge regarding pathways of lymphocyte activation is beginning to be translated into the generation of drugs that might interfere in these intracellular events giving rise to powerful immunosuppressive drugs, which are so important for successful clinical organ transplantation programmes and treating inflammatory diseases (see Chs 11 and 22).

At its simplest, the intracellular events involve:

1. Early generation of enzymes capable of protein tyrosine phosphorylation (e.g. protein tyrosine kinases, PTK).

2. Early activation of the phosphatidylinositol membrane pathway, which leads to generation of high levels of intracellular calcium.

3. Recruitment of adaptor proteins, which act as signal relays.

4. Cascading of signals through molecular pathways.

5. Activation of nuclear transcriptional events.

These are the signal transduction events (Fig. 7.20). Additional amplification of the signals is required because the

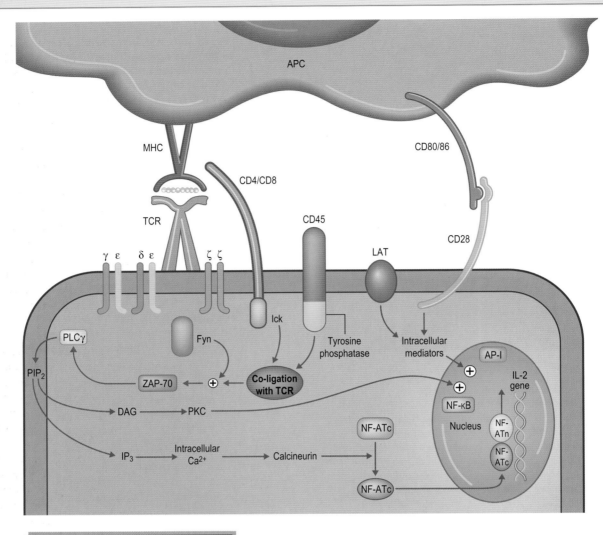

NF-ATc	Nuclear transcription factor (cytoplasm)
NF-ATn	Nuclear transcription factor (nucleus)
PTK	Protein tyrosine kinase
PLCγ	Phospholipase Cγ
PIP$_2$	Phosphatidylinositol (4,5) diphosphate
IP$_3$	Inositol (1,4,5) triphosphate
DAG	Diacylglycerol
PKC	Protein kinase C
ZAP-70	Tyrosine kinase
Fyn, Ick	Src family kinases
LAT	Linker for activated T cells

Fig. 7.20 **Activation of T lymphocytes.**

T cell activation follows interaction between the TCR and the MHC–peptide antigen complex, stabilised by CD4 or CD8 and accompanied by appropriate co-signals supplied by CD45 and CD28. The TCR signal is transduced through the CD3 complex. Early intracellular events that follow include activation of protein tyrosine kinases such as Fyn associated with the TCR, p56lck associated with CD4/CD8 and a tyrosine phosphatase associated with CD45. Subsequent events are the activation of other tyrosine kinases (ZAP-70), the phosphatidylinositol pathway, a rise in intracellular Ca^{2+} and the relocation of nuclear transcription factor NF-ATc (c, cytoplasmic; n, nuclear) to activate the IL-2 gene. The co-signal provided by CD28 to up-regulate the IL-2 gene has a similar mechanism of mediation, and the important transcription factor NF-κB is up-regulated via the PKC pathway.

number of surface antigen receptors actually being signalled through in a responding T or B cell is known to be quite small (e.g. as few as several hundred molecules per cell). Without these additional signals, it is unlikely that the lymphocyte could generate a sufficient head of steam to become activated. Since enzymes are generated in the signal transduction events, there will necessarily be an element of amplification of the signal. However, important amplification is also supplied through enzyme activities in the accessory molecules of T and B cells, notably CD4/CD8 in T cells, and the CD19–CD21–CD81 complex, CD20, CD22 and CD40 molecules in B cells. CD45 appears to supply critical amounts of tyrosine phosphatase activity to both cell types.

Neither the BCR complex (sIg plus CD79α and CD79β) nor the TCR complex (TCR plus CD3) have intrinsic PTK activity. Taking T cell activation as the example, it is known that CD3 complexes contain numerous distinctive repeating immunoreceptor tyrosine-based activation motifs (ITAMs) that become phosphorylated by Src family kinases (Fyn, Lck). This generates binding sites for ZAP-70, which becomes activated. The downstream events after this include generation of intracellular second messengers (e.g. calcium and protein kinase C). Recently it has become clear that an additional set of events involves adaptors (e.g. LAT; linker for activated T cells) that recruit other signalling molecules together into multimolecular complexes that relay signals further downstream.

The cascade of kinase activities draws nearer to the nucleus. One pathway activates **calcineurin**, a calcium-dependent protein phosphatase, which dephosphorylates a nuclear transcription factor present in the cytoplasm, **NF-ATc** (for nuclear factor of activated T cells$_{cytoplasm}$), which is thus enabled to translocate from the cytoplasm to the nucleus and there to initiate transcription of the IL-2 gene in concert with a similar nuclear transcription factor (**NF-ATn**). Further signalling events are provided by ligation of CD28 by CD80/86 co-stimulatory molecules on the DC surface, and this is especially important for IL-2 production. Other transcription factors that regulate genes important in lymphocyte activation are also promoted at this stage, including NF-κB and AP-1.

The sequelae of T cell activation: T lymphocyte-mediated immune responses

As already alluded to, once they have been activated in the lymph node against a particular pathogen or antigen, T cells develop a range of different activities (help, killing), allowing populations or subsets of T cells to be defined in terms of their functional polarisation. These functions are reflected closely by the types of cytokines secreted by T cells in a particular subset. The existence of these **functional subsets** gives rise to an additional type of nomenclature, particularly for CD4 T cells, as shown in Table 7.4.

The major areas in which T cells help the functions of other cells are in relation to DCs, macrophages, B cells, other

helper T cells and cytotoxic T cells. Within recent years, it has become recognised that T helper lymphocytes are not a homogeneous group of cells but can be divided into different subgroups. The subgroups are identifiable by the panel of cytokines they secrete and, thus, the *type* of help they provide. These cytokine profiles subdivide CD4 T cells into **T helper 1** and **T helper 2** subsets, or **T$_H$1** and **T$_H$2**. This subdivision is based on cytokine profiles alone; there are no surface markers or CD numbers that distinguish these two cellular subsets. Not every CD4 T cell falls neatly into these two categories: some cells may have a mixed cytokine secretion pattern. The cytokines released by the different T helper subsets are shown in Table 7.4 and the cytokines IL-4, IL-5, IL-6 and IL-10 are described in Science Boxes 7.8 to 7.14. The T$_H$ subsets arise from a common precursor, and the cytokine influence at a critical point of development determines whether a T$_H$1 (IL-12 providing the major maturation signal) or T$_H$2 (IL-4 the main signal) cell is produced.

The **T$_H$17** subset of T cells is newly described and derives its name from the secretion of IL-17. The role of T$_H$17 cells in the immune response is not yet entirely clear. They are capable of secreting numerous pro-inflammatory cytokines (e.g. IL-6, IL-8) and growth factors (GM-CSF). Studies in mice suggest that these cells are critically involved in the inflammation associated with the murine versions of diseases such as multiple sclerosis and rheumatoid arthritis, and it will be important to establish whether this is also true in man.

The mechanism through which T cells provide help to B lymphocytes is illustrated in Figure 7.21. The important point to remember here, as mentioned on page 84, is that the B cell will internalise specific antigen through sIg and process it through the exogenous pathway for presentation by class II MHC molecules. Only CD4 T cells that recognise peptides from this antigen will thus be able to interact with the B cell and provide help — this maintains the antigen

SCIENCE BOX 7.9

Interleukin-5

This 40 kDa cytokine is released by T$_H$2 lymphocytes and also by activated mast cells. The major actions of IL-5 are to promote B cell growth and immunoglobulin production; stimulate the growth and differentiation of eosinophils; and also to activate mature eosinophils to kill parasitic worms. The activities induced by IL-5 are, therefore, a key part of the antiparasitic response and the allergic immune response. It can be envisaged that during a typical response, IgE (promoted by the T$_H$2 cytokine IL-4) activates mast cells. These in turn recruit, promote the expansion of and activate eosinophils, through release of eosinophil chemotactic factors and IL-5. The T$_H$2 influence remains as IL-5 is also released by these T cells, strengthening the eosinophil-dominated response. Eosinophils are important in antiparasitic responses; their involvement in allergic responses is an important factor in the tissue damage caused in conditions such as asthma.

SCIENCE BOX 7.10

Interleukin-6

IL-6 is a cytokine of 26 kDa secreted mainly by T cells and APCs such a macrophages and DCs. The major stimulus for its secretion is IL-1, with which it shares many actions in common, but TNF-α also induces IL-6 release. IL-6 has a major role in the acute-phase response to inflammatory episodes. It induces the liver to synthesise plasma proteins that are involved in acute-phase reactions, such as clotting and complement factors and C-reactive protein. IL-6 also has potent effects on B cell differentiation, growth and immunoglobulin class switching. IL-6 is also an important cytokine in driving the differentiation of T$_H$17 cells.

SCIENCE BOX 7.11

Interleukin-10

IL-10, an 18 kDa peptide, is predominantly thought of as an immunosuppressive cytokine. It is produced by CD4 T cells (Tregs, Tr1 and also T$_H$2 cells) as well as macrophages, DCs (particularly immature DCs) and some B cells. Its inhibitory activity is mainly a result of effects on APCs, inhibiting their production of pro-inflammatory cytokines (e.g. TNF-α and IL-1) and down-regulating expression of MHC and co-stimulatory molecules. In contrast, the effect of IL-10 on B cells is stimulatory.

SCIENCE BOX 7.12

Interferon-γ

Interferon-γ is a homodimer composed of subunits of approximately 25 kDa. It is released by CD4 T lymphocytes (T$_H$1), CD8 T lymphocytes, as well as by activated natural killer cells. The interferons are known for their antiviral activity, and IFN-γ is no exception. In addition to these innate antiviral effects (similar to the type I interferons, see p. 75), IFN-γ has distinct immunological roles. First, IFN-γ is a potent activator of macrophages, inducing an increase in metabolic, phagocytic and killing activity (see p. 77). This role is an essential part of the response induced by T$_H$1-like lymphocytes. Second, IFN-γ has the ability to increase MHC class I molecule expression on a range of cell types and induce expression of class II MHC molecules on other cells, either alone or in concert with other cytokines (e.g. TNF). This may be an important component of antiviral protection, since it up-regulates presentation of viral targets by infected cells. Third, as a T$_H$1-cytokine, IFN-γ has profound effects on T cell development (favouring the development of T$_H$1 cells) and B cell differentiation (biasing the production of immunoglobulin in favour of IgG and away from IgE).

SCIENCE BOX 7.13

Transforming growth factor-β1

TGF-β1 is a member of a family of cytokines with many different actions, mainly in the realm of controlling proliferation, differentiation and function of cells. When TGF-β1 is released in a focused manner by immune cells during an immune response it has potent effects on immune function, and is predominantly viewed as an immunosuppressive cytokine. Tregs produce TGF-β as do macrophages and DCs, resulting in reduced proliferation of T and B cells, reduced cytokine release and inhibition of APC function.

SCIENCE BOX 7.14

Interleukin-12

IL-12 is a key cytokine produced by activated, mature DCs and has the profound effect of inducing naïve CD4 T cells to differentiate into T$_H$1 effector cells. The balance of IL-12 and IL-4 during naïve CD4 T cell activation thus determines whether these cells become T$_H$1 or T$_H$2. IL-12 thus promotes CD4 T cell production of the pro-inflammatory cytokines IFN-γ and TNF-α and also activates NK cells.

specificity of both the T and B cell response. This help is complemented by the cell–cell contact between co-signalling molecules (CD80/86 with CD28, CD40 with CD40L, adhesion molecules). The net result of this predominantly T$_H$2-type action is (1) the activation and expansion of B cells and (2) their differentiation along different pathways of antibody production. In addition, the memory T cell will receive an activation signal as a result of this interaction with the B cell.

This type of reciprocated interaction is also seen with other T cell–APC interactions. Thus T$_H$1 cells are able to activate macrophages to kill microorganisms that they have internalised and presented. CD4 T cells also influence DCs during antigen presentation. One example is the CD40–CD40L interaction, which is important in 'licensing' DCs for activation of other cells, especially naïve CD8 T cells to generate CTLs.

Cytotoxic T lymphocytes

Cytolytic, or cytotoxic, T lymphocytes (often abbreviated to CTL) are important in defence against virally infected cells, in rejection of foreign tissue grafts and possibly also in immune responses to certain tumour types. CTLs are capable of killing targets expressing a specific antigen. They are found predominantly amongst the CD8 population of T cells. We have already discussed the pathway for antigen presentation to CD8 T cells: peptide antigen is derived from internally synthesised proteins (the endogenous pathway of antigen

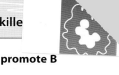

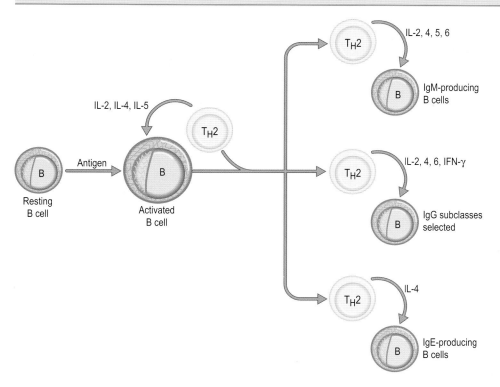

Fig. 7.21 **T$_H$2 cells promote B cell functions.**

presentation) and presented bound to MHC class I molecules. Target peptides for CTLs are fragments of virus, or tumour antigens.

CD8 T cells, remember, interact with antigen through presentation of peptides in the groove of class I MHC molecules. The induction of a CTL response is dependent upon CD4 T lymphocytes to provide help, in the form of activation stimuli and DC licensing. The life cycle of a CTL up to the point of killing is as follows. CD8 T lymphocytes with the potential to become CTLs exit the thymus expressing their specific TCR but cannot lyse target cells at this stage. In the periphery, when a cytotoxic response is required, the pre-CTLs are activated by the combined effect of CD4 T lymphocytes and DCs. The CD4 and CD8 T cells need to cluster on the same DC in order for sufficient activation stimuli to be generated (Fig. 7.22). This also ensures that the CD8 T cell is activated against a target for which there is a CD4 T cell response. Since naïve CD4$^+$ T cells are only activated by DCs when 'danger' signals are present, this is another process for ensuring that CTL generation is restricted to important targets such as viruses, rather than self antigens. The main cytokine signal is IL-2, but IFN-γ is also a stimulator of CTLs.

Following activation, the CTL must prepare the machinery required to lyse target cells. This falls into three categories: **cytotoxic granule** proteins, **toxic cytokines** and **death-inducing surface molecules**. Cytotoxic granule proteins are present in lysosomal structures proximal to the membrane. Upon activation of the CTL by a target bearing appropriate peptide-MHC, there is polarisation of granule release organised by the cell cytoskeleton onto the target cell surface. One type of cytotoxic granule protein is called **perforin**, which forms membrane pores (Fig. 7.22b) and is very

reminiscent of the membrane attack complex of complement C5–9 (see p. 17). At the same time, CTL granules containing **granzymes** are released. The perforin pores aid the arrival of granzymes into the cytoplasm where they activate a cytoplasmic protein caspase-3. This triggers a cascade that leads to **programmed cell death** also termed **apoptosis**. The second killing mechanism is cytokine release directed onto the target cell surface. IFN-γ and, notably, TNF-α are capable of inducing cell damage. Remember that IFN-γ, as the name implies, also has direct antiviral activity, which may be of local importance when a viral-infected cell is lysed and virions released. TNF-α is also toxic to a range of cell types, especially when released locally on the surface of a target cell. The third mechanism of inducing cell death relies upon the surface expression of death-inducing molecules by the CTL, and engagement of the appropriate ligand on the target cell surface (ligand expression may be induced by cytokines or as a consequence of viral infection). Examples include a molecule called **Fas ligand** (FasL), which binds Fas on target cells. Fas contains an intracellular 'death' domain, which leads to apoptosis via caspase activation.

Regulatory T cells

As discussed, the generation of B and T cells provides a potentially vast array of rearranged antigen receptors. Although there are severe selection processes to remove lymphocytes with 'dangerous' avidity for self, there remains a possibility that these do actually arise. These receptors for self proteins give rise to the potential for 'autoreactivity': reactivity to self. Lymphocytes with an antigen receptor that could indeed be self-destructive ('*horror autoxicus*' as Ehrlich put it) must either be weeded out or tightly controlled.

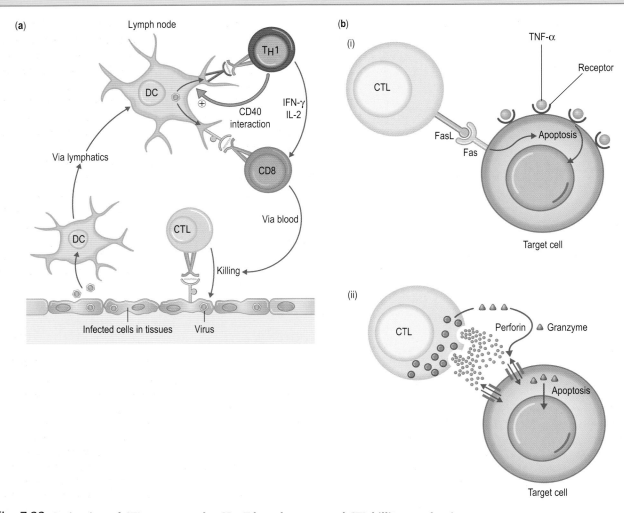

Fig. 7.22 Activation of CTL responses by CD4 T lymphocytes and CTL killing mechanisms.
(**a**) Virus particles excreted from a virally infected cell are endocytosed by DCs and brought to the lymph node for presentation to T_H1 cells. These provide activation signals for the DC through CD40–CD40-L interaction. This 'licenses' the DC to activate the CTL, along with additional cytokine signals from the T_H1 cell. Note that the DC has presented virus proteins through both exogenous (class II MHC, to the T_H1 cell) and endogenous (class I MHC, to the CTL via cross-presentation) pathways. (**b**) The CTLs with TCR specificity for viral peptides presented by class I MHC molecules on the DC will seek the same peptide MHC complexes on target cells in the infected tissues. CTLs can then kill target cells by (i) inducing suicide (apoptosis) through cytokine release, cell–cell contact using Fas–Fas ligand, or (ii) kill by forming pores in the target cell and secreting toxic proteins such as granzyme. The cell–cell interactions in CTL killing ensure no bystander cells are killed.

The immune system is thus empowered with (1) potentially lethal effector mechanisms and (2) the capacity to develop a sufficient array of receptors to be capable of self-recognition. Yet there is no self-destruction in the vast majority of people! When it does occur, and **autoimmune disease** results, the consequences may be life threatening (it is estimated that 5% of the population have an autoimmune disease during their life). Clearly, the *potential* for response to self is balanced for the most part by an *inability* to respond to self. This state is one of **immunological self tolerance**; the controlled inability to respond to self. It can be likened to living within a community and having a next-door neighbour with a penchant for playing loud heavy metal music every now and then. Rather than make a fuss, which would endanger our relationship with the neighbour, and perhaps on a larger scale damage the community, many of us would tolerate the noise. We have the capacity to respond, but we choose not to.

The immune system has the capacity for self-recognition, but for the most part avoids it. How is control exercised over individual T and B lymphocytes that may have unwanted specificities for self?

The mechanisms of immunological tolerance (Science Box 7.15), how they may be broken and what are the consequences are discussed in Chapter 9. Amongst these mechanisms, it has become apparent that there are subsets of CD4 T cells that are powerful mediators of immune tolerance. These have been given the generic term **Treg** (for regulatory T cells). At present, there is controversy over just how many types of Tregs there are, and how they are generated, but some general principles can be outlined.

First, there are Tregs generated in the thymus. These are thought to be important in regulation of autoreactive T cells, since removal of the thymus from neonatal mice at day 3 leads to the development of autoimmune disease such as autoimmune gastritis. The subset of cells within the thymus that has Treg activity is currently best identified by the surface expression of CD25 (the IL-2 receptor α chain). These cells also express Foxp3, a transcription factor that is important for their function, and they lack CD127 (the IL-7 receptor). These **CD4$^+$, CD25$^+$, CD127^{lo}, Foxp3$^+$ Tregs** may also be generated post-thymically in the peripheral immune system and work predominantly through **cell-to-cell contact** to regulate effector T cells, whilst also secreting IL-10 and TGF-β, known to be immune suppressive cytokines. Another potential mechanism of action of Tregs is surface expression of **CTLA-4** (for cytotoxic T cell antigen-4, or CD152). CTLA-4 is expressed on CD4 T cells and binds to CD80/86 co-stimulatory molecules with a higher affinity than CD28, delivering an inhibitory signal to the T cell and thus regulating immune responses (Fig. 7.24). Mice deficient in CTLA-4 have uncontrolled T cell activation and autoimmunity. In humans, approximately 5–10% of T cells in the blood may

have these markers, but they are not foolproof for identifying Tregs — CD25, CTLA-4 and Foxp3 can also be expressed on recently activated effector cells. Another Treg type produces copious amounts of IL-10 and has been termed the **Tr1** subset. Tr1 cells mediate immune suppression through the action of IL-10. Yet another Treg type is thought to work predominantly through **TGF-β** secretion. An important principle of these cell types is that they require recognition of specific antigen through the TCR to become activated, but once activated they can regulate any surrounding cells, including those specific for the same antigen as well as others in the vicinity (so-called '**bystander suppression**'; Fig. 7.25). If the regulated cell is on the same APC and is responding to the same or a related antigen this is called '**linked suppression**'. Interest in Treg biology is burgeoning, not just because these are key cells in the immune response, but also because of the potential therapeutic avenues they open (see Clinical Box 7.1).

SCIENCE BOX 7.15

The discovery of immunological tolerance

The discovery of the existence of immunological tolerance is credited to Burnet and Medawar, who were awarded the Nobel Prize in 1960 for their contribution. Medawar had become interested in graft rejection during treatment of severe burns in airmen during World War II: skin grafts from distant sites on the same patient usually took, but foreign grafts did not. The key study of Medawar and Burnet was based around the phenomenon of rejection of allogenic (i.e. non-self) skin grafts by mice, which they noted to be associated with heavy lymphocytic infiltration. Injection of allogenic bone marrow cells into the mice at the neonatal

stage did not impair general immunity, but when the mice became more mature, they now failed to reject skin grafts from the marrow donors (Fig. 7.23). They had acquired immunological tolerance to the antigens in the skin graft against which the lymphocytic response was raised. The same manoeuvre of bone marrow injection applied to adult mice had no tolerising effect. The importance of the work lay in the demonstration that tolerance to foreign antigens could be achieved, even though the route of neonatal injection was unlikely to become of use in human organ transplantation.

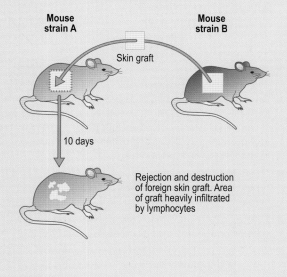

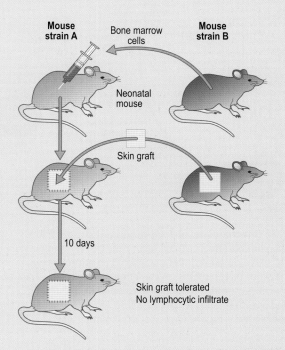

Fig. 7.23 **Induction of immunological tolerance to foreign skin grafts by injection of bone marrow cells into neonates.**

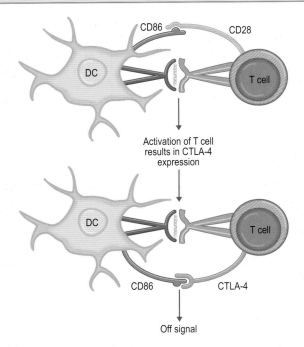

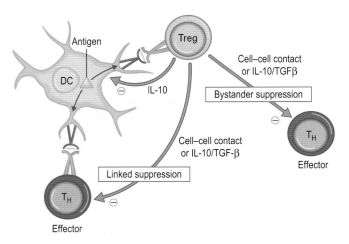

Fig. 7.24 Role of co-stimulatory molecules and their ligands in T cell activation and termination of the activation signal.
The T cell is activated through interaction of its TCR with the presented antigen and the co-stimulation of the CD80/86–CD28 interaction. During activation, CTLA-4 is induced and its ability to bind to CD80/86 with higher affinity represents an 'off' signal for the T cell.

Fig. 7.25 Mechanisms of Treg-mediated suppression.
Tregs can inhibit effector T cell responses by direct effects on the APC (IL-10 down-regulates MHC and co-stimulatory molecules) or direct effects on the effector T cells, which can be in the vicinity, perhaps responding to unrelated antigens (bystander suppression) or on the same APC responding to the same or related antigens (linked suppression).

CLINICAL BOX 7.1

Taking Tregs into the clinic

From a clinical viewpoint, there are several reasons to be excited at the current intense study of Treg biology. First, it may offer insights into how diseases that have an autoimmune component arise. An example is the rare genetic disease IPEX (for Immune dysregulation, polyendocrinopathy, enteropathy, X-linked syndrome). Children born with this have a defective *Foxp3* gene and develop severe inflammatory processes leading to gut and skin disease within the first year of life. Most notably, they also develop the autoimmune disease type 1 diabetes in which the insulin producing cells in the pancreas are destroyed by autoreactive T cells (see Ch. 13). The disease is thought to arise as a result of unchecked autoreactive T cells, due to the absence of thymus-derived, islet-reactive Tregs. This extreme example is indicative of the fact that, in general, autoimmune diseases may be the result, in part, of an underlying deficiency in Treg function. A second reason for interest in Tregs is therapeutic. Can the natural power of Tregs be harnessed in the form of therapies for autoimmune disease or to counter graft rejection in clinical transplantation? Many say yes, and there are already clinical trials planned that will use 'designer Tregs', generated ex vivo and then infused back into the patient.

SUMMARY BOX 7.3

Lymphocyte activation and sequelae

■ Lymphocyte activation requires at least two signals: antigen plus a co-signal. For T cells, CD4, CD8, CD45, adhesion molecules and co-stimulatory molecules such as CD28 provide the co-signals. For B cells, CD22, CD40, CD19, CD20 and CD45 have the same role.

■ To be effective, the signal must be transduced and amplified within the lymphocyte by a series of reactions.

■ Once in the periphery, T cells are the pivotal cells in immune responses. Through cell–cell contact and the secretion of a range of powerful cytokines, they activate and promote the growth of other T cells, B cells, monocytes and granulocytes.

■ The CD4 T helper cell subset is divided into T_H1 and T_H2 types, with different functions, according to the cytokines they secrete.

■ Cytotoxic T cells (CTLs) kill target cells expressing a specific antigen by inducing cell lysis or apoptosis.

■ The potential danger of autoreactive lymphocytes giving rise to autoimmune disease is avoided: this lack of response to self is termed tolerance, and several mechanisms of tolerance induction exist.

Natural killer cells

Natural killer (NK) cells are the third members (after B and T lymphocytes) of the cell populations of bone-marrow-derived lymphocytes. They are present in the blood and form about 10% of peripheral blood lymphoid cells. The name is derived from two features. Unlike B and T lymphocytes, NK cells are able to mediate their effector function (i.e. *killing* of target cells) *spontaneously* in the absence of previous known sensitisation to that target. Hence the terms '*killer*' and '*natural*'. Also unlike B and T lymphocytes, NK cells achieve this with a very limited repertoire of germ-line-encoded receptors that do not undergo somatic recombination. The lack of requirement for sensitisation and the absence of gene rearrangement to derive receptors for target cells mean that NK cells are part of the innate immune system. For identification purposes, the main surface molecules associated with NK cells are CD16 (see below) and CD56 (note, NK cells are CD3- and TCR-negative).

The role of NK cells is to kill 'abnormal' host cells, typically cells that are virus infected, or tumour cells. Killing is achieved in similar ways to CTLs, namely by the exocytosis of lytic proteins such as perforin and granzymes, and by the expression of FasL. NK cells also secrete copious amounts of IFN-γ and TNF-α, through which they can mediate cytotoxic effects (e.g. by inducing up-regulation of MHC molecules on target cells) and also activate other components of the innate (e.g. DCs) and adaptive immune system (e.g. T cells) (Fig. 7.26). The interaction between NK cells and the adaptive immune system is two-directional, in that NK cell function can be influenced by B and T cells. The best example of this is NK cell expression of CD16, the low affinity receptor for IgG (FcRγIIIA). Through this, NK cells can kill IgG-coated target cells in a process termed antibody-dependent cellular cytotoxicity (ADCC). The majority of NK cells are bone marrow derived.

NK cell activation

Much has been learned about this process in recent years, although it remains a complex area of immunological science. NK cells integrate the signal from a potential target cell through a series of receptor–ligand pairings. These pairings provide activating and inhibitory signals, and it is the overall balance of these that determines the outcome for the NK cell.

1. Inhibitory receptors

The discovery of these led to the coining of the 'missing self' hypothesis. NK cells use inhibitory receptors on their surface to survey targets for the presence of MHC class I molecules. If the molecules are present, inhibition of activation is the result. The inhibitory receptors are termed killer cell immunoglobulin-like receptors (KIRs). KIR gene loci have arisen relatively recently in evolutionary terms through multiple gene duplications, and are highly polymorphic between individuals and different receptors may be present on different NK subsets. Examples of inhibitory receptors and their ligands are shown in Table 7.5.

2. Activating receptors

Most activating receptors are expressed by all NK cells. A small number of examples of these are shown in Table 7.6.

As for T cells, NK cell activation requires initial contact, adhesion and polarisation. It is not known which of the inhibitory or activating receptors, if any, is the first to initiate target cell contact. Once contact is made, adhesion is

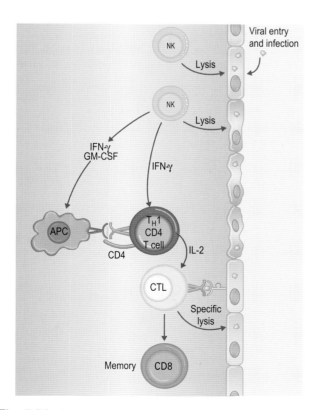

Fig. 7.26 **The role of NK cells in the immune response.**

Table 7.5 Examples of NK cell inhibitory receptors

Receptor on NK cells	Ligand
KIR2DL1	HLA-C molecules
KIR3DL1	HLA-B molecules
KIRDL2	HLA-A molecules
NKG2A	HLA-E

Table 7.6 Examples of NK cell activating receptors

Receptor on NK cells	Ligand
CD16 (low affinity receptor for IgG)	IgG
NKG2D	MHC class I chain related gene A (MICA)
KIR2DS1	HLA-C

important and is predominantly mediated by LFA-1 : ICAM-1 interactions. These events polarise the NK cell onto its target and direct the release of granules and cytokines. One of the important targets of NK cell activating receptors, MICA, is induced under conditions of cellular 'stress', such as might arise during infection or neoplastic transformation.

In practice, in vivo, how does the process of NK killing occur? As discussed (see Science Box 7.2), many viruses have developed immunoevasion strategies that avoid presentation of viral proteins to CTLs by interfering with the MHC class I presentation pathway. This renders infected cells susceptible to killing by NK cells, which detect the reduced levels of MHC class I molecules (hence, 'missing self'). Likewise, tumours that escape immune surveillance by CTLs through the outgrowth of daughter cells that have low MHC expression, then become NK cell targets. The relatively recent development of NK cell receptor diversity implies a strong evolutionary driving force, probably related to viral immunoevasion strategies. KIR–HLA interactions are thus vital to antiviral immunity, and this is confirmed by the numerous associations between KIR and HLA genotype combinations and susceptibility to chronic infection with viruses, notably the human immunodeficiency virus (see Ch. 20).

SUMMARY BOX 7.4

Natural killer cells

- Natural killer (NK) cells are a small population of cells that resemble lymphocytes morphologically but form a separate lineage from T and B cells.
- NK cells kill tumour cells and virally infected cells without the need for prior sensitisation.
- NK cells secrete cytokines (mainly IFN-γ), which promote a cellular immune response, activating phagocytic cells and recruiting T cells.
- NK cells are activated by the cytokines IFN-γ, IL-2 and IL-12, and have two mechanisms of killing targets. In one, target cells are bound by IgG antibody, for which the NK cell has a receptor. In the second, cell–cell contact with the target is required, during which the balance of activating and inhibitory receptor signalling determines the outcome.

Further reading

Chien YH, Konigshofer Y 2007 Antigen recognition by gammadelta T cells. Immunol Rev 215: 46–58

Corthay A 2006 A three-cell model for activation of naïve T helper cells. Scand J Immunol 64: 93–96

Hill JA, Benoist C, Mathis D 2007 Treg cells: guardians for life. Nat Immunol 8: 124–125

Hogquist KA, Baldwin TA, Jameson SC 2005 Central tolerance: learning self-control in the thymus. Nat Rev Immunol 5: 772–782

O'Connor GM, Hart OM, Gardiner CM 2006 Putting the natural killer cell in its place. Immunology 117: 1–10

Steinman L 2007 A brief history of T(H)17, the first major revision in the T(H)1/T(H)2 hypothesis of T cell-mediated tissue damage. Nat Med 13: 139–145

Watts C 2001 Antigen processing in the endocytic compartment. Curr Opin Immunol 13: 26–31

Williams A, Peh CA, Elliott T 2002 The cell biology of MHC class I antigen presentation. Tissue Antigens 59: 3–17

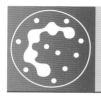

The immune response to microbes: an overview

The analogy between the players in the immune system and those in an orchestra has already been drawn in an earlier chapter. The orchestra is best appreciated, and the music best understood, when all of the instruments play and are heard together. It is likewise with the components of the immune system. Learning that IL-8/CXCL8 attracts neutrophils, for example, or that LFA-1 interacts with ICAM-1, does not give a full idea of how a pyogenic bacterium is identified and killed.

In this section, the balance of such excessive reductionism is redressed. The immune system is viewed acting in concert, from the moment of entry of a microbe, through to its eradication and the creation of a bank of memory cells equipped for any future encounter. The overview is necessarily general, but each figure panel is accompanied by cross-referencing, so that greater detail can be found if required.

Primary viral infection

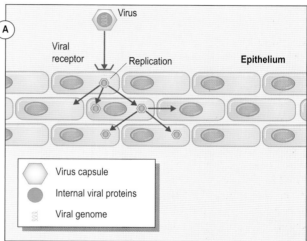

Virus infects epithelial cells and replicates amongst them.

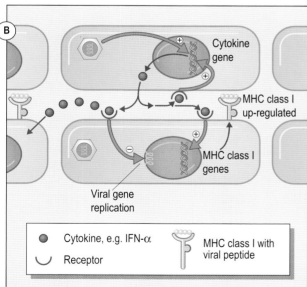

Effect of intracellular viral infection is the activation of cytokine and cytokine-receptor genes, especially the Type I interferons (e.g. IFN-α). Secretion of IFN-α involves autocrine feedback loop. Local effects of IFN-α are inhibition of viral gene replication, and up-regulation of MHC class I molecules. Viral peptides will appear in the MHC class I peptide-binding groove. (See *IFN-α*, p. 75.)

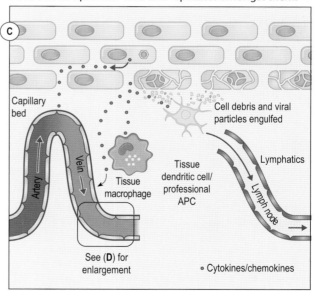

Viral infection results in cell death and viral replication. Virus components (e.g. single-stranded RNA) activate dendritic cells and locally released cytokines and chemokines amplify the activation of macrophages and antigen-presenting cells (APCs). These engulf and present viral proteins as well as cellular debris. Professional APCs (e.g. tissue dendritic cells such as Langerhans cells in the skin) transport antigen to local lymph nodes via lymphatics. (See *Macrophages*, p. 76; *Dendritic cells*, p. 72; *Antigen presentation*, p. 94.)

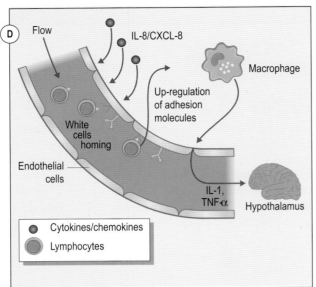

Cytokines and chemokines up-regulate endothelial cell expression of adhesion molecules such as ICAM-1. Chemokines (e.g. IL-8/CXCL 8) begin to attract cells through the endothelium towards the site of infection. Some locally released cytokines from cells such as macrophages and T cells (e.g. IL-1, TNF-α) enter bloodstream and have systemic effects of fever and arthralgia/myalgia. (See *Cell adhesion molecules*, p. 27; *IL-1*, p. 77; *TNF-α*, p. 72; *Chemokines*, p. 26.)

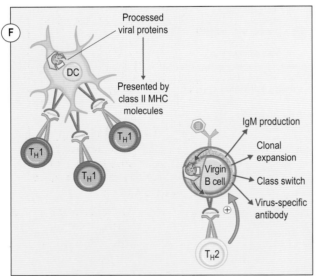

Dendritic cells and other APCs are surrounded in the lymph node germinal centre by T cells, where presentation of viral peptides takes place. T cells possessing TCRs complementary to the class II MHC molecule/viral peptide complex are activated and become T$_H$ cells. Virgin B cells, acquiring viral particles through attachment to surface IgM or IgD, process and present viral peptides to T$_H$2 cells, and in turn receive positive growth and differentiation signals. IgM antiviral antibody is produced as a result (primary antibody response) whilst some B cells differentiate and class switch, leading later to production of high affinity antiviral IgG (secondary antibody response). (See *Antigen presentation*, p. 94; *B cell activation*, p. 79.)

T$_H$1 cells recruit and activate virus-specific cytotoxic T lymphocytes (CTLs, see *CTL activation*, p. 110). The CTLs recognize virus peptides cross-presented by DCs (see Cross-presentation, p. 98). The same viral epitopes will be presented on the surface of infected target cells (see panel K).

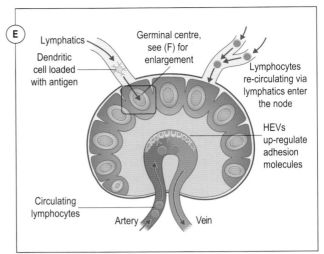

Dendritic cell enters local lymph nodes, and moves to germinal centre. Local inflammation leads to up-regulation of adhesion molecules on high endothelial venules of lymph node, and lymphocytes enter directly from the blood. Circulating lymphocytes in the lymphatics also enter. Many lymphocytes become trapped in the local inflamed node, and the consequent swelling, along with local hyperaemia, leads to the symptom of swollen painful/tender lymph nodes.
(See *Lymphocyte circulation*, p. 5.)

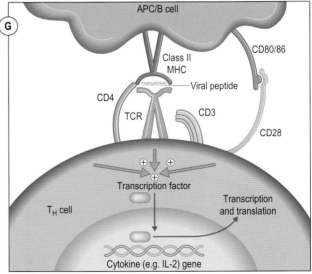

A viral peptide is presented by class II MHC molecules to a complementary TCR on a T$_H$ cell. The interaction is stabilised by CD4/class II MHC and CD80/86 binding to CD28, which also provides co-stimulatory signals to the T$_H$ cell. (See *T cell activation* and *co-stimulation*, p. 106.)

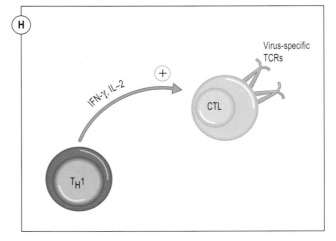

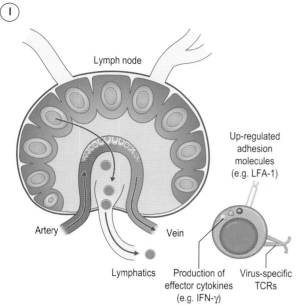

Up-regulated adhesion molecules (e.g. LFA-1)

Lymph node

Artery

Vein

Lymphatics

Production of effector cytokines (e.g. IFN-γ)

Virus-specific TCRs

T_H and CTLs leave the lymph node via the draining lymphatics towards other lymph nodes, and ultimately enter the blood. At this stage their key attributes are: (**1**) virus-specific TCRs; (**2**) up-regulated adhesion molecules, to allow migration into the inflamed tissues; and (**3**) up-regulated cytokine production.

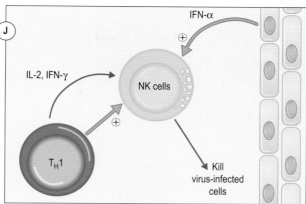

IFN-α

IL-2, IFN-γ

NK cells

T_H1

Kill virus-infected cells

NK cells may be recruited at two points at least during the virus infection. They may have an early, innate antiviral role following activation by epithelium-derived cytokines. Alternatively, at a later stage they are activated by T_H1 cells specific for the virus. (See *NK cells*, p. 113.)

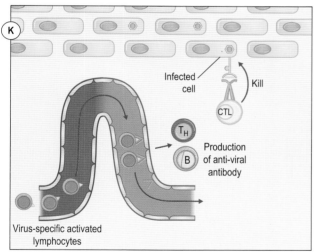

Infected cell

Kill

CTL

T_H

B

Production of anti-viral antibody

Virus-specific activated lymphocytes

Activated cytotoxic T cells kill virally infected cells. Local T_H1 and T_H2 cells now organise the local antiviral immune response. (See *Cytotoxic reaction*, p. 110.)

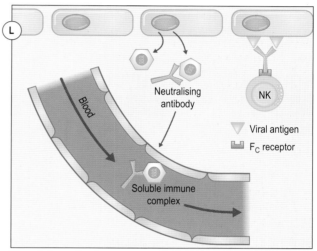

Blood

Neutralising antibody

NK

▽ Viral antigen

▭ F_C receptor

Soluble immune complex

Virus-infected cells secrete and express viral proteins. These may be neutralised or removed by antibody in the form of immune complexes, which are cleared, or antibody may be used to guide Fc receptor-expressing NK cells.

After resolution of the infection, virus-specific memory T and B cells reside long term in lymph nodes, spleen and bone marrow. Plasma cells ensure long-term circulation of protective, virus-neutralising antibody.

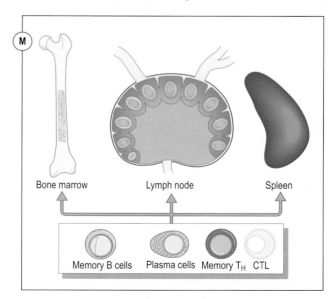

Bone marrow

Lymph node

Spleen

Memory B cells   Plasma cells   Memory T_H CTL

Primary bacterial infection

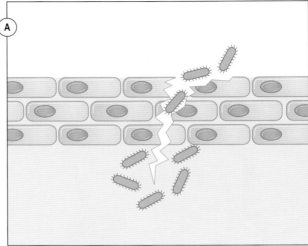

Break in epithelial surface allows bacterial entry and proliferation.

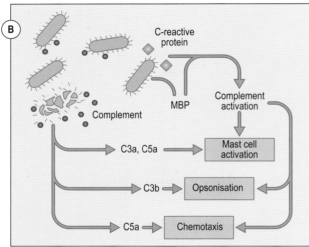

Surface lipopolysaccharide may activate the alternative complement pathway or mannan-binding lectin pathway leading to bacterial lysis. Other complement activators operating at this stage include C-reactive protein, which binds bacterial coat polysaccharides. (See *Complement*, p. 13; *Opsonisation*, p. 20; *Chemotaxis*, p. 20.)

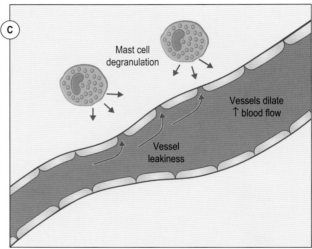

Mast cell degranulation enhances blood flow. The increased blood flow and local oedema are perceived as itchiness and irritation in the inflamed area. (See *Mast cell*, p. 32.)

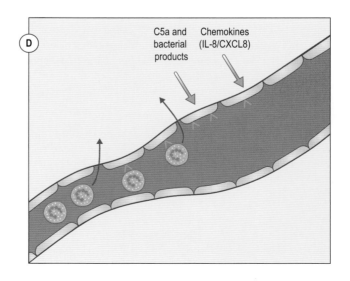

Rolling, marginating neutrophils adhere to the vein wall as locally released chemokines and bacterial-derived molecules (e.g. endotoxin) activate both the endothelium and the neutrophils, resulting in adhesion between the two. (See *Neutrophil adhesion*, p. 27.)

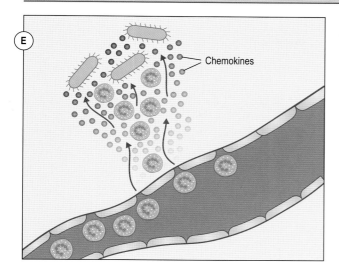

Chemokines

Bacterial products (e.g. f-MLP), complement fragments (C5a) and chemokines (IL-8/CXCL8) attract neutrophils to the site (chemotaxis).

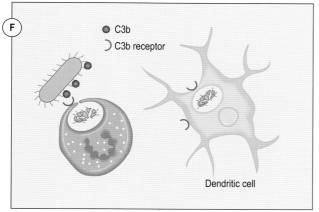

Opsonised bacteria are rapidly engulfed and killed by neutrophils. Dendritic cells (DC) engulf and internalise bacteria, are activated via pattern recognition receptors (e.g. Toll-like receptors) and migrate via the lymphatics.

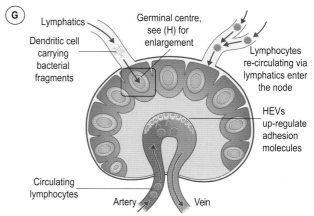

Bacterial antigens are processed and presented in local lymph nodes.

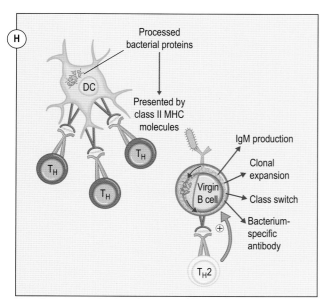

T_H cells are recruited and activated by professional APCs in the lymph node, and by B cells, promoting the production of bacteria-specific antibodies. Naïve T cells become differentiated towards T_H1 and T_H2, according to the dendritic cell signals. Initially, IgM class antibody is produced, followed by clonal expansion and switching to other classes, e.g. IgG or IgA for mucosal pathogens. (See *B-cell activation*, p. 79–80.)

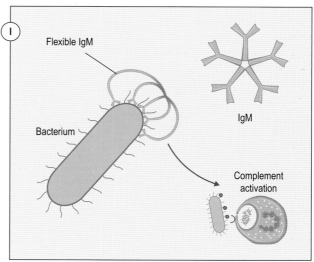

Early antibacterial antibody production is of the IgM class. This relatively low affinity interaction is enhanced by the five adhesion sites on IgM, leading to higher efficiency of binding. IgM is a very potent complement activator and opsonin. Opsonised bacteria are engulfed by phagocytes and lysed by complement. (See *IgM*, p. 41.)

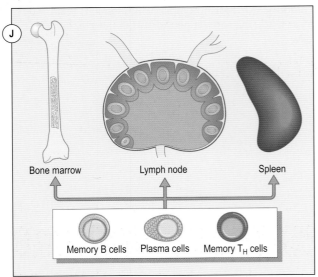

Following the resolution of the bacterial infection, protective mechanisms for future encounters are put in place by the laying down of memory cells and production of antibody.

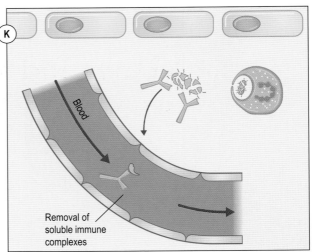

In the resolution of an infection, bacterial debris is removed by local neutrophils, or by antibody as soluble immune complexes.

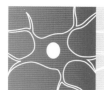

Tolerance and mechanisms of autoimmunity

Previous chapters have illustrated that the immune system is a complex orchestra comprising diverse cells and molecules. The tune it plays depends on the integration of many signals, but the overriding goal is eradication of microbes and parasites and the restoration of homeostasis. The immune system is a potentially powerful destructive agent — witness the rapid damage to, and rejection of, transplanted organs when tissue barriers are crossed. For the most part, the immune system focuses its activities on the outside, and we remain healthy. Given its complexity and power, though, we should not be surprised when occasionally the beast is unchained, unleashing itself in unhelpful directions and giving rise to such conditions as allergy and autoimmune disease. These occurrences are perhaps the price that must be paid for protection.

This chapter concentrates on one of these scenarios, the development of autoimmune disease. To understand autoimmunity, we must first understand tolerance — the process by which a fully armed immune system is prevented from self-destruction.

Immunological tolerance

How do we define tolerance? Tolerance can be defined as controlled unresponsiveness. I like the example of the irritating person that occasionally sits next to you during lectures. He or she may be chewing gum, humming, using their mobile telephone, snoring — whatever it is, they are annoying and distracting you. You have a very sharp pencil in your hand, and it crosses your mind to jab this into their flesh, gain their attention and tell them to behave! You could do it so easily — but you refrain; because you are a tolerant person. Likewise, immunological tolerance is the controlled inability to respond to self, despite having the capability to do so.

Immunological tolerance is many layered. We have already learned most of the general principles that confer immunological tolerance, and Figure 9.1 integrates these into a model that can then be used to understand autoimmunity. Here it is applied to T cells (there are similar mechanisms for B cells, and of course B cell responses are often, generally speaking, controlled by T cells). The broad distinction is into central and peripheral tolerance.

In the thymus, where central tolerance is achieved (as detailed on p. 91), there is deletion of T cells with the potential to react against self at too high an affinity. Some 95–99% of potential T cells entering the thymus fail to come out the other side — this is a major tolerance mechanism. In some circumstances these cells are killed, in others they survive but are rendered anergic (unresponsive). The critical difference here is that the anergic cells with potential for self-reactivity remain available, and could, if activated, participate in autoimmune responses at a later stage. Deletion and anergy represent the major forms of central tolerance induction. What happens if a self peptide is not available in the thymus? Indifference or ignorance describes a situation in which a T cell fails to encounter a peptide presented by MHC for which its TCR could have a correct fit. It may be that the antigen is not represented in the thymus, or that it is present at insufficient levels. This is a potentially dangerous scenario, however, since these T cells could acquire sufficient survival signals (e.g. through interaction with other, similar ligands) to exit into the periphery. In the periphery they are now available for subsequent activation, perhaps even by the self peptide that was not present in the thymus.

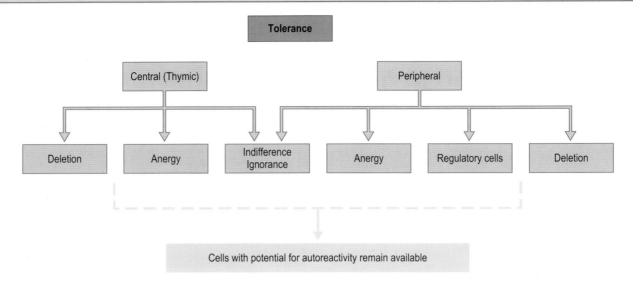

Fig. 9.1 **Mechanisms of T cell tolerance.**

Central tolerance is thus a broad screening programme to remove T cells with high affinity for self peptides represented in the thymus. Its major *modus operandi* is deletion. It is by no means complete, and therefore requires a complementary system to be active in the periphery.

In the periphery (i.e. tissues and lymph nodes), similar mechanisms of tolerance may apply. When peripheral T cells encounter exceptionally high peripheral antigen levels, this may lead to a process termed activation induced cell death (AICD) and consequent deletion. An example would be very common soluble proteins such as haemoglobin or serum albumin, which are constantly acquired and presented by APCs. Under other circumstances anergy may arise. This is thought to arise particularly when peptide-MHC as signal 1 is available to the T cell, but not the co-stimulatory signal 2. An example would be when a common self antigen is taken up by a resting, non-activated dendritic cell. In the absence of any danger signal, co-stimulatory molecules are not up-regulated by the DC. A final mechanism of peripheral tolerance is that self antigens may simply not be presented in the periphery as a mechanism of attaining and maintaining tolerance through ignorance. This can be achieved in several ways. One obvious mechanism is to limit the expression of MHC molecules, thus limiting antigen presentation. In particular, class II MHC molecules are normally present only on a restricted cohort of cells (antigen presenting cells). Another possible way to achieve ignorance to a self antigen is to restrict its expression to the intracellular compartment, or to a particular tissue, so that it is unavailable for presentation. Finally, should any of these mechanisms fail, there are the 'immunological police' available in the form of regulatory T cells (Treg). These take different forms, as shown in Table 9.1. Some of these are naturally available to keep autoreactivity in check (e.g. CD4+CD25+ Treg). Others are induced under particular conditions of antigen administration (e.g. Tr1, T$_H$3). The activation of Tregs is antigen specific. They express TCRs and require activation through the TCR in order to regulate. Once activated, Tregs can regulate the cells around

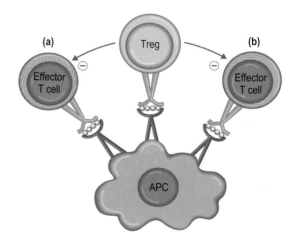

Fig. 9.2 **Treg suppression.**
The Treg is interacting with peptide-MHC presented by an APC. The Treg is able to suppress the activation of an effector cell recognising the same peptide (**a**) and an effector cell recognising a different peptide presented by the same APC (**b**).

them. These cells could be recognising the same antigen on an APC, or a different one (so-called bystander regulation; Fig. 9.2).

Autoimmunity

Now that we have a definition of tolerance, autoimmunity can be defined in a very straightforward way — as the loss of immunological tolerance to self. Autoimmunity is common. Indeed, all of us have the capacity and potential to mount autoimmune responses. The two main reasons for this are illustrated in Table 9.2. First, not all T cells are deleted in the thymus, and so some T cells remain available. Second, as discussed in Chapter 4, T cell receptors show enormous plas-

Table 9.1 Main types of regulatory T cell

Regulatory T cell (Treg)	Type of T cell	Actions	Mechanism of action	Other features
CD4$^+$CD25$^+$ T cells	CD4$^+$, TCR$^+$	Inhibits T cell responses (proliferation and cytokine production)	Not known, but needs cell-to-cell contact	Arise naturally; mainly thymus-derived; high expression of Foxp3, a transcription factor important in Treg function and low expression of CD127 (IL-7 receptor)
Tr1	CD4$^+$, TCR$^+$	Inhibits T cell responses (proliferation and cytokine production)	Production of IL-10	Arise naturally or may be induced (e.g. by repeated antigen injection)
T$_H$3	CD4$^+$, TCR$^+$	Inhibits T cell responses (proliferation and cytokine production)	Production of transforming growth factor-β	Induced by oral administration of antigen

Table 9.2 Spectrum of autoimmune responses

Level of response	Characteristics
Autoimmune potential	Ubiquitous; reflects T and B cell receptor diversity; healthy response
Physiological autoimmunity	Non-pathogenic; may include Tregs
Pathological autoimmunity	Results in autoimmune disease; common (5%); result of complex interactions of genetic and environmental factors

ticity for the peptide–MHC complexes with which they can interact. One TCR can interact with many more than one peptide. So, under normal circumstances, there are T cells available that can recognise self antigens. Some of these may even be regulatory T cells (i.e. physiological autoimmunity). However, should these T cells become activated as effector cells and cause tissue damage, then autoimmune disease will be the result. Autoimmune disease is relatively common, affecting up to 5% of individuals at some time during their life. This spectrum, from autoimmune potential, through physiological autoimmunity to pathological auto-reactions, holds the key to our understanding of the role of the immune system in many different diseases (Table 9.3).

Autoimmunity is frequently categorised according to the nature of the target tissues. Some autoimmunity is directed against particular cells in an organ: examples include the insulin-producing β cells of the islets of Langerhans in the pancreas, and the thyroxine-secreting cells in the thyroid. In these diseases, the autoimmune reactions are directed against one or more specific cytoplasmic constituents, plasma-membrane structures or secreted products of a particular cell. This is termed organ-specific autoimmunity. In contrast, non-organ-specific autoimmunity is directed against structures common to many tissues and found throughout the body: for example nuclear components, mitochondrial proteins or constituents of muscle. Examples of organ-specific and non-organ-specific autoimmune diseases are given in Table 9.3. Some disorders fall in the grey area between the two designations. In primary biliary cirrhosis, for example, although the liver is the organ predominantly affected by autoimmune attack, the target of the autoantibodies is a ubiquitous mitochondrial enzyme pyruvate dehydrogenase, and the disease itself often involves manifestations of non-organ-specific diseases, such as the rheumatic condition Sjögren's syndrome.

In organ-specific autoimmune diseases, target cells are frequently damaged irreparably, resulting in loss of endocrine secretions, such as insulin in type 1 diabetes, thyroxine in autoimmune thyroiditis, and adrenocorticosteroid hormones in Addison's disease due to autoimmune adrenocortical insufficiency. In non-organ-specific autoimmune diseases, inflammation and damage may be widespread, often involving the articular joints (rheumatoid arthritis) or small blood vessels (vasculitis) leading to damage to vital organs such as the eyes and kidney.

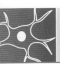

Table 9.3 The spectrum of autoimmune diseases, from organ-specific to non-organ-specific and the autoantigens typically targeted

Disease	Main autoantigens targeted
Organ specific	
Myasthenia gravis	Acetylcholine receptor
Graves' disease	Thyroid-stimulating hormone receptor
Hashimoto's thyroiditis	Thyroid peroxidase; thyroglobulin
Type 1 diabetes	Islet cell cytoplasmic targets; insulin; glutamic acid decarboxylase, IA-2, zinc transporter 8
Pernicious anaemia	H^+K^+ ATPase (gastric proton pump); intrinsic factor
Addison's disease	21α-hydroxylase
Pemphigus vulgaris	Desmoglein 3
Vitiligo	Tyrosinase
Autoimmune hepatitis	Cytochrome P4502D6
Autoimmune haemolytic anaemia	Various red blood cell surface targets
Overlap between organ- and non-organ-specific diseases	
Primary biliary cirrhosis	Pyruvate dehydrogenase complex in mitochondria
Goodpasture's syndrome	Collagen Type IV
Non-organ-specific diseases	
Rheumatoid arthritis	IgG
Systemic lupus erythematosus	Double-stranded DNA; Sm (small nuclear ribonucleoproteins); SS-A (Ro; a 60 kDa ribonucleoprotein); SS-B (La; a 47 kDa ribonucleoprotein); histones
Sjögren's syndrome	SS-A, SS-B
Systemic sclerosis	DNA topoisomerase I
Mixed connective tissue disease	Ribonucleoproteins

Tolerance and autoimmunity

- Immunological tolerance is the controlled inability to respond to self, despite the capacity to do so.
- Tolerance in the immune system is maintained by numerous control mechanisms.
- Breakdown of tolerance leads to autoimmunity, which may lead to autoimmune disease.
- Autoimmune disease can affect specific cells (organ-specific) or be diffuse (non-organ-specific).

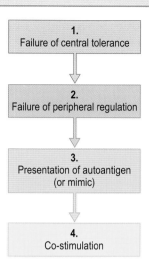

Fig. 9.3 **The four checkpoints in the development of autoimmune disease.**

Breakdown of tolerance: mechanisms of autoimmunity

The fact that there are several different mechanisms through which immunological tolerance can operate leads to an obvious conclusion: several different pathological processes could break tolerance and lead to autoimmunity. It has been argued that the multilayered nature of self-tolerance is a failsafe mechanism: all or several control mechanisms must be breached before disease results. This approach would explain several important principles regarding autoimmune disease: (1) it is usually multifactorial, requiring inheritance of at least one gene polymorphism and exposure to one or more environmental factors; (2) it often progresses much more slowly than immune reactions to pathogenic organisms, suggesting that control mechanisms may continue to work up to a point; and (3) it has a tendency to remit and relapse, indicating that control mechanisms may recover and temporarily restore tolerance.

In this section, we will highlight several events that could unlock one of the failsafe mechanisms of tolerance. We will use the template generated in Figure 9.1 to 'hang' these different pathogenic scenarios on.

The key event in developing an autoimmune disease is the activation of an effector CD4 T cell that recognises a self peptide. There are four checkpoints that must be overcome to result in this. These are shown in Figure 9.3; there must be a failure of central tolerance, failure of peripheral regulation, presentation of the autoantigen and co-stimulation.

Checkpoint 1 — Failure of central tolerance

As discussed, central tolerance is incomplete, and therefore in each of us it results in the release of T cells into the periphery that have the capacity to recognise self peptides. Situations that further compromise central tolerance (such as a failure to express a self protein) would be expected to favour the development of autoimmunity. Recently a very graphic example of this has been discovered. There is a group of

patients who develop multiple autoimmune disorders (Autoimmune Polyglandular Syndrome Type 1; APS Type 1; see Ch. 13). The disease is inherited in an autosomal dominant fashion, and when the gene responsible was identified, it was discovered to encode a nuclear protein that regulates the transcription of other genes in the thymus. Curiously, the gene, termed *AIRE* (for autoimmune regulator), seems particularly powerful at up-regulating the thymic expression of a host of autoantigen genes (e.g. the insulin gene, insulin being an important autoantigen in type 1 diabetes). Thus it would appear that in health the AIRE protein acts as a transcription factor promoting the expression of autoantigen genes in the thymus and enabling deletion of any potentially autoreactive T cells (see p. 92). In patients with a defective *AIRE* gene this cannot happen; the result is incomplete tolerance to a range of autoantigens and multiple organ-specific auto-immune disease.

AIRE gene defects are a rare cause of autoimmunity, but they illustrate the fact that any event that disturbs central tolerance could promote autoimmune disease.

Checkpoint 2 — Failure of peripheral regulation

This is perhaps the easiest concept to grasp, and is based on a similar concept to that of 'fewer policemen (Tregs) equals more criminals (autoreactive T_H cells)'. One of the critical Treg populations (CD4+CD25+) requires expression of a transcription factor, Foxp3, for its regulatory actions. Foxp3 appears to function by suppressing the activation of genes required for effector T cell function. There is a human condition in which the Foxp3 gene is defective (IPEX: immune dysregulation, polyendocrinopathy, enteropathy, X-linked syndrome (see Clinical Box 7.1)). Although very rare, a few patients with this syndrome have been studied. They have

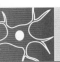

defective Tregs and develop a range of conditions, including organ-specific autoimmune disease.

The example of IPEX is a very rare, but robust and educational, example of how Treg defects can lead to autoimmune disease. Other examples of Treg defects are less obvious, the best being the fact that autoimmune disease is associated with polymorphisms in the gene that encodes CTLA-4, which we encountered earlier (see p. 111), as a molecule that switches off activated T cells. Mice in which the CTLA-4 gene is completely inactivated develop a severe, uncontrolled T cell activation and proliferation, with manifestations of autoimmunity. In humans, a particular CTLA-4 polymorphism is associated with an increased risk of developing autoimmune thyroid disease and type 1 diabetes (see p. 190), although precisely how this leads to reduced T cell regulation and autoimmunity is not known.

In summary, it is beginning to appear likely that at the important checkpoint of T cell regulation, patients with susceptibility to autoimmune disease are unable to apply the brakes on the immune system.

Checkpoint 3 — Presentation of an autoantigen (or its mimic)

It is obvious by now that for an autoimmune disease to develop, there must be presentation of autoantigens to CD4 T cells by professional APCs. This most likely happens in one of two ways.

First, it is possible that some form of tissue damage or injury leads to release of hidden self antigens. These will be taken up, processed and presented by tissue-resident dendritic cells, transported to the local lymph node and presented to T cells. This scenario is particularly likely if the tissue damage is originally caused by a virus or bacterial infection, which will stimulate the innate immune system and DC activation.

The second possibility is mimicry. This is also a simple concept, in which an antigen or epitope in the pathogen looks like a self antigen or epitope. In the process of making an entirely appropriate immune response against the pathogen, T or B cells are generated that also have the capacity to recognise self. It is called mimicry, rather than identity, because the amino acid sequences of the cross-reacting antigens or epitopes need not be identical — they must simply 'look' the same to an approaching TCR or antibody molecule.

In theoretical terms, there should be many opportunities for mimicry (examples are given in Table 9.4). There are only 20 amino acids with which to construct each epitope. For a T cell epitope, there may be as few as three required amino acids for binding to MHC and two for interaction with the TCR. Indeed, there are now several published examples of T cells obtained from patients with autoimmune disease that can be activated by both a self peptide from the relevant autoantigen and by a mimicking peptide from a human pathogen (Fig. 9.4). However, the evidence for the role of molecular mimicry in the majority of organ-specific autoimmune diseases is still being weighed in the balance at present. One of the problems is the fact that autoimmune diseases usually take many years from the initiation of the autoimmune process to the clinical disease. Associations with viruses and bacteria that were present at the beginning are, therefore, difficult to find; hence molecular mimicry is often termed the 'hit-and-run' theory of autoimmunity.

Checkpoint 4 — Co-stimulation

We have already learned that for a T cell to become activated, it requires two signals, peptide–MHC and co-stimulation from an APC. It is the same for an autoreactive T cell, and this is perhaps the most important checkpoint in the devel-

Table 9.4 Examples of viral or bacterial and autoantigen sequences that have been shown to exhibit immunological cross-reactivity in the context of autoimmunity

Disease	Autoantigen	Microbial antigen
Autoimmune cardiomyopathy in post-streptococcal rheumatic fever	Cardiac myosin	Streptococcal M protein
Chagas' disease with associated cardiomyopathy	Cardiac myosin	*Trypanosoma cruzi* B13 antigen
Autoimmune hepatitis Type 2	Cytochrome P4502D6	Hepatitis C virus E1 protein
Autoimmune gastritis	H^+K^+ ATPase (gastric proton pump)	*Helicobacter pylori* acetate kinase
Primary biliary cirrhosis	Pyruvate dehydrogenase complex-E2	Pyruvate dehydrogenase complex-E2 from bacteria

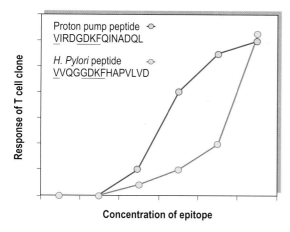

Fig. 9.4 Molecular mimicry as a mechanism of autoimmunity.
This graph shows T cell cross-reactivity in autoimmune gastritis. A single T cell has been obtained and grown from the gastric mucosa of a patient with autoimmune gastritis. The autoantigen in this disease is the proton pump (H⁺K⁺ ATPase). *Helicobacter pylori*, a gastric pathogen, has been implicated as causing inflammation in this disease. Here we see that the T cell responds to increasing amounts of both the proton pump peptide and the *H. pylori* peptide. They are mimics of each other, and share some identical amino acids (underlined). (Data adapted from Amedei A et al. Molecular mimicry between *Helicobacter pylori* antigens and H⁺, K⁺-adenosine triphosphatase in human gastric autoimmunity. J Exp Med 2003 20(198): 1147–1156.)

opment of autoimmune disease. Even if there is failure of central and peripheral tolerance, and an autoantigen is available for presentation, there must be an activated APC in order for the autoreactive T cell to be activated in turn. Therefore, in considering models of autoimmunity, those that include the capacity for APC activation are worthy of serious attention.

The most likely situation in which an APC is activated is infection. Two models of autoimmunity that include an infectious agent are molecular mimicry and bystander activation. Molecular mimicry, as we have seen above, thus provides the answer to two of the checkpoints, presentation of an autoantigen (or its mimic) and co-stimulation through infection. Bystander activation is also an appealing scenario (Fig. 9.5). Here, there is an active infection leading to cell and tissue damage and release of autoantigens. These are taken up, along with pathogen-related material, by tissue-resident DCs. These become activated by the pathogen-related receptors and migrate to the local lymph node. Here there is activation of effector T cells directed against the pathogen and the potential for similar immunity to be driven against self antigens; the DC is unable to distinguish one from another and will present both. The activation of autoreactive T cells will only be prevented if there has been effective central tolerance (no T cells with affinity for the self peptide) or if there is effective regulation. Relative defects at either of these checkpoints will favour autoimmunity.

We have discussed the fact that evidence for molecular mimicry remains elusive in human autoimmune disease. What about bystander activation? The only evidence that can be brought to bear is that from situations in which there may be a general increase in co-stimulatory signals. Co-stimulation is provided by both molecular interactions (e.g. CD80/86 and CD28) and by pro-inflammatory cytokines. There are several situations in which such cytokines are given therapeutically. For example, many patients who fail to clear hepatitis C virus have been given IFN-α as an antiviral agent. This has powerful effects on bystander activation as it mimics some of the effect of activated DCs. Many patients treated in this way have developed autoimmune thyroid disease, and there are also case reports of development of autoimmune type 1 diabetes.

We can now add this knowledge regarding the checkpoints onto the framework of immunological tolerance in Figure 9.1. The result (Fig. 9.6) is the assembly of a model of autoimmune disease in which each checkpoint must in some way be 'leaky'. For most of us, not all of them are leaky at the same time, and we resist autoimmune disease. For others, especially those with genetic backgrounds that have an adverse effect on the function of checkpoints, the risk is much higher.

The role of HLA in autoimmunity

One of the unsolved mysteries of autoimmunity is the role of HLA molecules. For most diseases, inheritance of particular HLA molecules is by far the strongest genetic influence on the disease (Table 9.5), but how this works remains unclear. Since the sole function of HLA molecules is antigen presentation, we can assume that the effect on disease is related to the effect on peptide–MHC–TCR interactions. Somehow we have to factor HLA into our model of autoimmunity.

First, let us analyse the nature of the association. One of the best studied diseases in this regard is type 1 diabetes, an autoimmune disease affecting 1 in every 300 people in the UK. The HLA association in diabetes is focused on particular HLA-DQ molecules, the major risk being conferred by HLA-DQ8 and HLA-DQ2 (see Table 9.5) whilst HLA-DQ6 is protective (i.e. it is found very rarely in a diabetic patient). In between these extremes are HLA-DQ molecules with moderate risk and those with a neutral effect. Analysis of the differences between these HLA molecules should indicate whether there is a structural basis for susceptibility and protection. From this type of analysis it has been established that the risk relates mainly to the structure of the antigen binding groove. In precise terms, a charged amino acid such as aspartate at position 57 on the HLA-DQβ chain is low risk, and a non-charged amino acid at this position (e.g. alanine, serine) confers high risk.

It is now well established that the HLA-DQβ57 position has a strong influence over the shape of the peptide binding

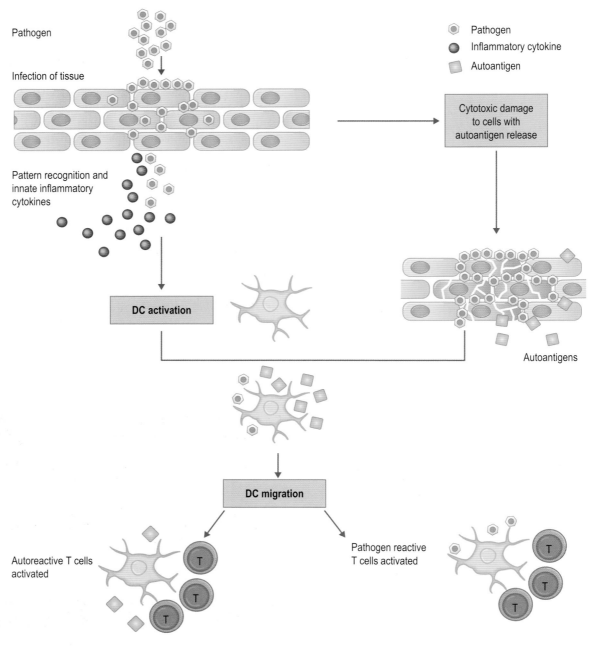

Fig. 9.5 **Bystander activation of autoreactive T cells.**
See explanation in text for details. Note that autoreactive T cells are activated only if they are available (i.e. failed central tolerance) and are not regulated (i.e. failed peripheral regulation).

groove at this point. HLA-DQβ57Asp gives rise to a closed groove whilst HLA-DQβ57Ala or Ser is more 'relaxed'. These differences have a major impact on the types of peptides that will bind (see Fig. 9.7).

So, how could this affect autoimmunity? Several options can be considered; in each case diabetes and HLA-DQ will again be used as the examples:

1. HLA-DQβ57Ala or Ser molecules favour presentation of an important epitope involved in the development of the disease. This could be an islet autoantigen epitope, or perhaps a mimicry epitope from a virus. Presentation of this epitope initiates CD4 T cell activation and the autoimmune cascade. In contrast, HLA-DQβ57 Asp molecules fail to present the critical epitope.

2. HLA-DQβ57Ala or Ser molecules are poor at presentation of critical islet autoantigen epitopes in the thymus, thus failing to delete potential islet autoreactive T cells. In contrast HLA-DQβ57 Asp molecules are very good at thymic deletion.

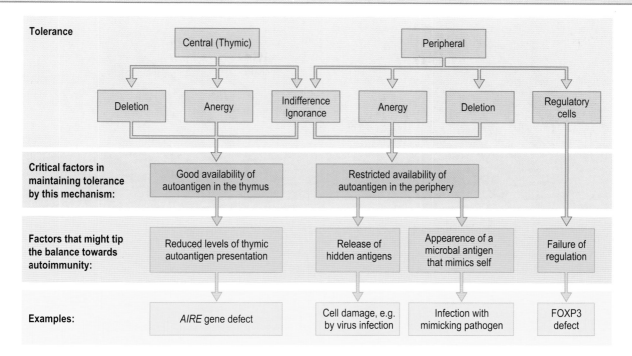

Fig. 9.6 **Mechanisms of making and breaking T cell tolerance.**

Table 9.5 HLA associations with immune-mediated diseases

Disease	HLA allele
Type 1 diabetes	*DQA1*0301/DQB1*0302* (DQ8; susceptibility)
	DQA1*0501/DQB1*0201 (DQ2; susceptibility)
	DQA1*0102/DQB1*0602 (DQ6; protection)
Multiple sclerosis	*DRB1*1501* (DR2; susceptibility)
Rheumatoid arthritis	*DRB1*0404* (susceptibility)
Coeliac disease	*DQA1*0501/DQB1*0201* (DQ2; susceptibility)

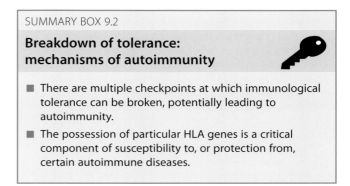

SUMMARY BOX 9.2

Breakdown of tolerance: mechanisms of autoimmunity

■ There are multiple checkpoints at which immunological tolerance can be broken, potentially leading to autoimmunity.

■ The possession of particular HLA genes is a critical component of susceptibility to, or protection from, certain autoimmune diseases.

3. HLA-DQβ57Ala or Ser molecules are poor at presentation of critical islet autoantigen epitopes in the thymus, thus failing to generate regulatory T cell populations that can prevent autoimmunity developing in the periphery. In contrast HLA-DQβ57 Asp molecules are very good at thymic presentation and induction of Tregs.

These possibilities remain to be established from experimental studies. Some clues that options 2 and 3 might be important come from animal studies (see Science Box 9.1).

Autoimmune disease

Mechanisms of immune damage

The scheme shown in Figure 9.8 is an attempt to distil mechanisms of immune damage in autoimmune disease. For the most part these are pathogenic processes, which could apply equally well in physiological immune responses against pathogens.

The central cell in the autoimmune response is likely to be the CD4 T_H cell. This will become activated against an autoantigenic peptide displayed within the binding groove of a class II HLA molecule. Typically, presentation will be by a 'professional' antigen-presenting cell such as a DC, but the target cell itself may express HLA class II molecules and presumably present its own antigens. In autoimmune thyroid disease, for example, this is thought to lead to amplification of the autoimmune response. T_H1 cells secreting IL-2 and IFN-γ are likely to promote cellular immune responses, dom-

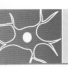
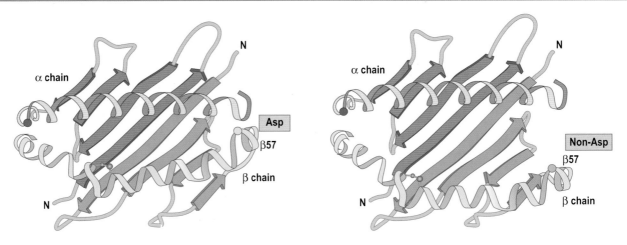

Fig. 9.7 Theoretical shapes of the HLA-DQ molecules associated with type 1 diabetes.
The protective molecule has a more closed groove over peptide pocket 9, since the Asp at position 57 on the β chain is charged and attracted towards the α chain. The susceptibility molecule has no charge at position 57 and is more open over position 9.

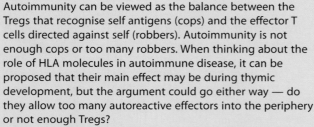

SCIENCE BOX 9.1

Fewer cops, more robbers?

Autoimmunity can be viewed as the balance between the Tregs that recognise self antigens (cops) and the effector T cells directed against self (robbers). Autoimmunity is not enough cops or too many robbers. When thinking about the role of HLA molecules in autoimmune disease, it can be proposed that their main effect may be during thymic development, but the argument could go either way — do they allow too many autoreactive effectors into the periphery or not enough Tregs?

To address this is difficult, but it is made possible by a curious detail in relation to a mouse that spontaneously develops diabetes (the non-obese diabetic, or NOD mouse). The NOD mouse bears many resemblances to human type 1 diabetes; it develops islet destruction through the activation of CD4 and CD8 T cells, as well as B cells, that recognise islet autoantigens such as insulin (see Ch. 13). Intriguingly, it only expresses one MHC class II molecule, called I-Ag7, which has a strong structural similarity with HLA-DQ8; amazingly, there is a non-Asp at position 57 on the β chain of I-Ag7. Researchers were quick to perform transgenic studies on this molecule, and found that mutating the β chain to express Asp at β57 completely prevented diabetes development!

The next set of experiments had even greater complexity and was designed to address the 'cops versus robbers' concept. Using transgenic technology two teams of researchers now made a NOD mouse that over-expressed one type of TCR. The selected TCR came from a CD4 T cell that was known to be able to cause diabetes if injected into the mouse. The NOD-TCR transgenic mice developed diabetes very rapidly. Each team now manipulated the I-A molecule in these mice and looked in the thymus to see whether they could detect effects on thymic selection. Amazingly, one research team, focusing on thymic selection, found that the I-Ag7 molecule is critical for selection of pathogenic cells — without it the number of pathogenic cells allowed into the periphery was vastly reduced and diabetes development was controlled. The other research team, focusing on regulation, found that changing the MHC promoted a population of cells capable of regulating the pathogenic TCR+ cells. So, there is evidence for both sides of the argument.

inated by other CD4 T cells, CD8 T cells and macrophages, while T$_H$2 cells will activate autoantibody production by B lymphocytes. To be damaging, autoantibodies must target surface components and be capable of recruiting effectors such as complement or Fc receptor-bearing killer cells or macrophages. Macrophages and T$_H$1 cells can secrete pro-inflammatory and potentially damaging cytokines, such as IL-1 and TNF-α. If CD8 T cells are to have a role in cellular damage then they must be primed by DCs cross-presenting the same peptide as the target cell presents.

In some autoimmune diseases, neither the CD4 nor CD8 T cell is the prime mediator of damage. In Graves' thyroid disease, for example, hyperthyroidism is mediated by the production of an autoantibody that binds to the receptor for thyrotrophin and provides a stimulatory signal, leading to uncontrolled production and release of thyroid hormones and to thyrotoxicosis. In myasthenia gravis, an autoantibody to the acetylcholine receptor (AChR) acts at the neuromuscular junction to interfere with signal transmission possibly through a complement-mediated mechanism.

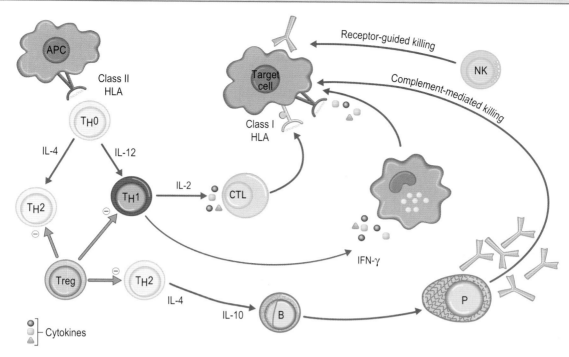

Fig. 9.8 Disease model for development of autoimmune disease.
There is a primary event involving damage to the target cell, fragments of which are presented by professional APCs. This initiates T_H1 and T_H2 cell activation, with recruitment of cytotoxic T cells and B lymphocytes making autoantibodies. Inflammation in the target organ leads to up-regulation of HLA class I molecules, rendering the target cell susceptible to killing by CD8 T cells. Tissue damage can also result from the actions of autoantibodies recruiting complement, or directly by the action of cytokines made by T cells or macrophages.

Defining a disease as autoimmune

There are now over 80 diseases classified as autoimmune, affecting as many as 1 person in every 20 in the UK. Some of the diseases are very clear cut in their autoimmune origin, but others are not. It is useful to have a set of criteria for the diagnosis of a disease as autoimmune, and both major and minor factors can be defined.

Major criteria:

1. Evidence of loss of tolerance: presence of T cell or B cell autoimmunity (e.g. presence of circulating autoantibody).

2. Clinical response to appropriate immune suppression (e.g. anti-B cell therapy for an autoimmune disease mediated by autoantibodies).

3. Passive transfer of the putative immune effector (e.g. autoreactive T cell or autoantibody) causes the disease (hardest criterion to satisfy but most stringent).

Minor criteria:

1. An animal model that resembles the human condition, and in which there is a similar loss of tolerance (see Table 9.6 for examples).

2. Evidence that, in the animal model, passive transfer of the putative immune effectors reproduces the disease in a naïve animal.

3. HLA association.

For examples of how these criteria may be satisfied, see Chapter 13 on endocrine autoimmune diseases.

Therapies

Until recently, the mainstays of treatment for autoimmune disorders have either been replacement therapy for loss of endocrine secretions (insulin, thyroxine), 'blanket' immune suppression using corticosteroids (which appear to have effects on almost every compartment of the immune system, interfering with cell activation and migration) or selectively targeted immune suppression aimed at the T or B cell compartment. These approaches, which are described in more detail in Chapter 22, carry risks: corticosteroids have many side-effects, and, to be effective, immunosuppression is often used at doses that compromise protective immunity while treating autoimmunity. Inevitably there is a weighing of the potential risks and benefits of these therapies: some

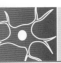
Table 9.6 Animal models of human autoimmune disease

Animal model	Method of induction	Human equivalent
Non-obese diabetic (NOD) mouse	Diabetes arises spontaneously	Type 1 (insulin-dependent) diabetes
Experimental allergic encephalomyelitis (EAE)	Immunisation with myelin basic protein or key peptides	Multiple sclerosis
Adjuvant arthritis	Immunisation with an adjuvant (derived from *Mycobacterium tuberculosis*)	Rheumatoid arthritis
Collagen-induced arthritis	Immunisation with collagen	Rheumatoid arthritis

autoimmune diseases, such as systemic lupus erythematosus, are potentially life threatening, and powerful immune suppression is fully justified. In other situations, the opposite view may be taken: type 1 diabetes and autoimmune hypothyroid disease may be managed with replacement therapy with good life expectancy.

In recent years, the search for more specific immune-based therapies has intensified. The Holy Grail is a therapy in which tolerance to the target organ is restored. There is an expectation that the greater understanding of autoimmunity that has been acquired in recent years will promote this search.

SUMMARY BOX 9.3

Autoimmune disease and therapy

- There are clear criteria for diagnosing a disease as autoimmune.
- Organ or tissue damage in autoimmune disease arises through the effector arms of the immune system.
- Unravelling the complex nature of autoimmunity offers the promise of novel therapies that restore tolerance.

Further reading

Albert LJ, Inman RD 1999 Molecular mimicry and autoimmunity. N Engl J Med 341(27): 2068–2074

Cheng MH, Shum AK, Anderson MS 2007 What's new in the Aire? Trends Immunol 28(7): 321–327

Davidson A, Diamond B 2006 General features of autoimmune diseases. In: Rose NR, Mackay IR (eds) The autoimmune diseases, 4th edn. Elsevier: London

Goodnow CC 2007 Multistep pathogenesis of autoimmune disease. Cell 130(1): 25–35

Kamradt T, Mitchison NA 2001 Tolerance and autoimmunity. N Engl J Med 344(9): 655–664

Moser M 2006 Antigen presentation, dendritic cells and autoimmunity. In: Rose NR, Mackay IR (eds) The autoimmune diseases, 4th edn. Elsevier: London

Walker MR, Nepom GT 2006 Major histocompatibility complex and autoimmunity. In: Rose NR, Mackay IR (eds) The autoimmune diseases, 4th edn. Elsevier: London

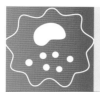

Hypersensitivity reactions and clinical allergy

Hypersensitivity was originally categorised, according to the effector mechanisms thought to be involved, by Gell and Coombs in the 1970s. At that time, several disorders seemed to fit neatly into one or other of the four categories. In the intervening years, the curtain has slowly been drawn back on the complexity of the immune response in many diseases, and few now fit as well into Gell and Coombs' groups as they once did. However, the classification still serves as a useful guide to the mechanisms whereby immunopathology arises and as such it is an appropriate point at which to start the study of clinical immunology.

Hypersensitivity reaction types II, III and IV describe disease mechanisms but do not usefully define a discrete group of disorders. For this reason, although some clinical syndromes involving these reactions will be described, the diseases themselves will be considered in depth in their appropriate chapters. Type I hypersensitivity stands alone in defining a pathogenic mechanism that underlies a group of diseases with a similar demographic, genetic and environmental basis and to which a similar therapeutic strategy is applied. The type I hypersensitivity reaction is central to the group of disorders termed 'allergic' and these will be dealt with in full in this chapter.

For the purpose of host defence, the immune system is charged with damaging and potentially lethal effector cells and molecules. For the most part, these are well controlled. An immune response directed against a pathogen results in clearance of the organism and resolution of any inflammatory process. Under some circumstances, however, the inciting stimulus is a harmless molecule, ignored by the immune systems of the majority but initiating in some people an immune response that leads to tissue damage and even death of the host. These exaggerated, inappropriate reactions come under the umbrella of the term **hypersensitivity reactions**. Understanding the genetic and environmental basis for these diseases is by no means an academic exercise. Allergic disease is common and on the increase. It is estimated that the number of Swedish children with allergic rhinitis, asthma and eczema has doubled in the last 12 years. The economic cost of allergic disease in the USA is estimated at \$12 billion, of which over half goes on treatment.

Type I hypersensitivity: IgE and the mast cell

The interaction of antigen, specific IgE, and the high-affinity receptor for IgE on the mast cell surface results in cell degranulation (Fig. 10.1; see also the electron micrographs of mast cell degranulation, Figs 3.7 & 3.8, p. 34). When this interaction occurs in allergic disease, the antigen is termed an **allergen**. The vasoactive mediators released give rise to vasodilatation and localised oedema. In the skin, where the existence of type I hypersensitivity is usually assessed, this reaction is itchy, has the appearance of a 'wheal' (swelling) and 'flare' (redness) and arises within minutes of the antigen being introduced. The basis for the mast cell reaction and the mediators involved has already been described in Chapter 3 and has been the subject of medical research for many decades (Science Box 10.1). The antigens involved in type I hypersensitivity are usually inert molecules derived from the environment and of no apparent threat to the host organism. The combination of the timing and the innocuous nature of the provoking stimulus in **allergic reactions** has earned this reaction the alternative label of **immediate hypersensitivity**.

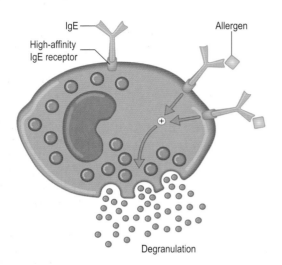

Fig. 10.1 Mast cell degranulation.
The mast cell carries high affinity receptors for the Fc portion of IgE. Allergen specific IgE, occupying these receptors, induces mast cell degranulation immediately allergens are encountered. See also Figures 3.7 and 3.8.

Pathogenesis of allergic disease

There are several components to an allergic response: the allergen, the host's state of reactivity and the genetic and environmental influences on this. In addition, it has become clear in recent years that the manifestations of allergic disease do not equate simply with mast cell degranulation and the immediate hypersensitivity reaction. Allergic disorders are also typified by an aftermath, occurring a few hours after exposure and lasting up to several days. These 'late' immune reactions are the indirect result of mast cell degranulation as well as other mechanisms and have important pathogenic and therapeutic implications.

The allergen

Allergy, derived from the Greek *allos ergos*, meaning altered reactivity, is a term much abused. For our purposes it can be defined as a state of heightened reactivity of the immune system to foreign substances. For the sake of clarity, we will also confine the use of the term 'allergic' to those reactions that are initiated when mast-cell-bound IgE interacts with its target antigen, known as an allergen. The allergic diseases that cause the greatest morbidity and mortality are **asthma**, a chronic lung disease; **allergic rhinitis** (seasonal allergic rhinitis is 'hay fever'); **eczema** and **urticaria** (skin disorders); and **generalised anaphylaxis**.

Passive transfer of allergy to fish: 'Don't do this at home' (you might win a Nobel Prize!)

In one of the classic medical experiments of the last century, the basis for allergic reactions was shown to reside in serum. It is the kind of experiment that would certainly be frowned upon today, but in the early 1920s earned its performers, Carl Prausnitz and Heinz Küstner, the accolade of having an immunological reaction named after them. In the original Prausnitz–Küstner reaction, serum was separated from the blood of Küstner, a professor of obstetrics and gynaecology who was allergic to fish. This was then injected under the skin of the forearm of Prausnitz, a man previously without allergy of any sort. The next day, a fish extract was injected into the same site and for the first time in his life Prausnitz had a positive skin prick test. The factor in serum responsible for this reaction was termed 'reagin'. Finally, in the late 1960s, reagin was identified as a new class of antibody, left undiscovered when IgG, A, M and D were described, because of its very low concentration in normal serum. Two teams identified IgE at almost the same time, one group through studying a patient with high levels caused by allergy, the other following the characterisation of an IgE monoclonal antibody in a patient with a plasma cell tumour (myeloma; see p. 300).

The trend towards self-experimentation in the search for medical advances has lasted into the present century.

In 2005, the Nobel Prize in Medicine was awarded to Barry Marshall and Robin Warren, for their identification of the bacterium *Helicobacter pylori* as the causative agent in gastric and duodenal ulceration. This eventually led to the abandonment of complex surgery for the condition, in favour of the use of antibiotics. Many disbelieved their early assertion that *H. pylori* colonised the stomach and caused inflammation. As a means to convince their peers, Marshall and Warren decided to experiment on themselves. Marshall was endoscoped by Warren to check that his stomach lining was normal and that there was no sign of infection. Marshall then drank a bacterial brew and spent a couple of days feeling fairly unwell with nausea and vomiting. Warren repeated the endoscopy, which showed gastritis and inflammation. As Marshall said subsequently 'After that, people started to pay a bit more attention!'. This is the latest example of a long tradition in self-experimentation for the advancement of medical science, including that of Werner Forssmann, who received the Nobel Prize for Medicine in 1956 after performing a cardiac catheterisation on himself. The work of Marshall and Warren ignited a heated debate about the ethics of such experiments, but one cannot doubt the power of the approach when it works.

Some of the most intense research into the mechanisms of allergic responses has concentrated on the nature of the allergens. Could these molecules have particular features that give them the power to incite these damaging IgE responses? The World Health Organization nomenclature for allergens adopts the first three letters of the name of the genus and the first letter of the species from which the allergen originates, followed by a number according to the order in which the allergen was identified. Some examples are given in Table 10.1.

Several allergens have protease activity, and it is possible that this is an important property for crossing skin or mucosal barriers. Allergens tend to be contained within carrier particles (e.g. pollen grains, house dust mite faecal material) that are small (diameter 2–60 μm) and aerodynamic, which may be important properties in gaining aerial access to nasal and bronchial mucosa. After all, one of the main functions of the mucosa at these sites, particularly in the nose, is to filter inhaled air. Other common features of aeroallergens are that their source may be dominant (e.g. timothy grass pollen is the most prevalent pollen in the air in the UK, and allergy to it is the main cause of hay fever) and that within a pollen the allergen may be a large proportion of the soluble protein.

Table 10.1 Common allergens

Allergen source	WHO nomenclature[1]
Cat (*Felis domesticus*)	Fel d 1
Timothy grass (*Phleum pratense*)	Phl p 1 Phl p 5
Ragweed[2] (*Ambrosia artemisifolia*)	Amb a 1 Amb a 3 Amb a 5
House dust mite (*Dermatophagoides pteronyssinus*)	Der p 1
Latex from the rubber tree (*Hevea brasiliensis*)	Hev b 1
Peanut proteins (*Arachis hypogaea*)	Ara h 1–3

Notes: [1]World Health Organization nomenclature, see http://www.allergen.org/Allergen.aspx; [2]Ragweed is an important allergen in North America.

Inheritance

The tendency to allergic reactions has a strong heritability, and this tendency has been termed **atopy**. Atopy is most easily defined as the presence of a type I hypersensitivity reaction to an allergen, usually demonstrated in the skin prick test (see below); this potentially allergic state need not result in disease. Two, one or no atopic parents pass on the atopic trait to their children with a risk of 75, 50 and 15%, respectively, and between 20 and 30% of the population is atopic.

The nature of what exactly is inherited by atopic individuals and, therefore, what predisposes to allergy is complex (Fig. 10.2). Amongst genes known to be involved are the β chain of the high affinity receptor for IgE (*FcεRI-β*), IL-4 genes, CD14 and HLA-DR alleles. In each case, common polymorphisms predispose to atopy, although the mechanisms are not known with certainty. The presence of T_H2 cells recognising allergens is the pathological hallmark of allergy, and could be promoted by IL-4 gene polymorphisms. Since CD14 constitutes part of the receptor for bacterial cell wall lipopolysaccharide, and infection may have a role in the development of allergy, CD14 polymorphisms affecting sensitivity to pathogens could promote hypersensitivity. Studies on HLA associations with allergy have not been particularly revealing and the most convincing shows that in a North American population IgE and IgG hyperresponsiveness to one of the ragweed antigens is associated with HLA-DR2 in patients with ragweed pollen allergy.

Environment

In monozygotic identical twins (i.e. twins with identical genes) concordance for asthma (i.e. both twins having the

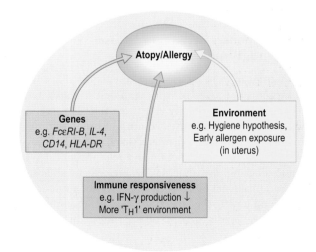

Fig. 10.2 **Multifactorial susceptibility to atopy and allergy.** The manifestation of atopy or clinical allergy in an individual is the end result of numerous different influences. There are genetic components such as linkage to polymorphisms of *FcεRI-B, IL-4, CD14* and *HLA-DR* genes; the nature of host immune responsiveness; and the environment.

disease) is only 20% and environmental factors clearly have a role. The doubling of allergy in Sweden over a 12-year period arose without any fundamental change in the genetic stock of the inhabitants. A graphic illustration of the power of the environment over allergy is provided by the fact that these disorders were much less common in East Germany before reunification with West Germany, but disease rates in children born in the former eastern city of Leipzig are now rising alarmingly.

One possibility is that atopic tendencies arise during fetal or infant life. It has been demonstrated, for example, that high levels of IgE in the cord blood of infants predicts future development of atopy. Moreover, stimulated cord blood T cells from infants who subsequently developed allergic disease produce less IFN-γ than normal; this is one of the cytokines that down-regulate IgE production (see p. 108). Individuals raised at high altitude, where exposure to house dust mite is comparatively low, have a significantly lower incidence of asthma. The peak incidence of allergic rhinitis caused by birch pollen allergy, which is particularly common in Scandinavia, is found amongst children born during the months of birch pollen release (February to April).

The recent increase in asthma incidence in the developed countries has provoked considerable discussion. Some of the favoured explanations are that our use of central heating and double glazing provides the optimal conditions — warmth and humidity — under which the house dust mite (a major allergen in asthma) flourishes. Another favoured explanation is the '**hygiene hypothesis**'. This states that over-zealous attention to cleanliness in developed societies (use of antibiotics, reduced exposure to pathogens which might favour a T_H1-like environment) has resulted in the favouring of a T_H2 response. Some epidemiological studies support this theory. For example, there are considerable differences in the nature of the gut flora between infants in Sweden (high prevalence of allergy) and Estonia (low prevalence).

The late responses in allergic disease: more than IgE and mast cells

In an attempt to examine cells and mediators that result in the symptoms and signs of clinical allergic diseases, models have been developed, mainly in asthma and allergic rhinitis, in which patients are exposed to allergens under controlled conditions. In asthma allergen is inhaled and then measurements are made of lung function and cells are collected from the fluid bathing the mucosa by bronchoalveolar lavage (BAL) and bronchial biopsies taken. Another approach is to perform skin testing (i.e. injection of small amounts of allergen under the epidermis) on allergic individuals and take skin biopsies.

Some important findings, common to these models, have been made since the mid-1980s and reveal clinical allergy to be much more than the sum of allergen, IgE and mast cells. Taking asthma as one of the best studied models, approximately 15 minutes after endobronchial challenge with allergen there is a fall in the 1-second forced expiratory volume (FEV₁) (Fig. 10.3). This 'early' response recovers spontane-

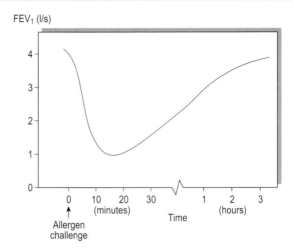

Fig. 10.3 **A patient with allergic asthma is given an endobronchial challenge with allergen and the 1-second forced expiratory volume (FEV$_1$) is measured.**

ously after 1–2 hours and is suppressed by pre-treatment with antihistamines, though not completely because of the numerous other pro-inflammatory mast cell mediators involved. Similarly, in hay fever sufferers, sneezing, increased secretions and nasal congestion occur minutes after nasal challenge with allergen and then subside over the next 2 hours. Again this is sensitive to antihistamines. Further evidence that mast cell products are important in this response comes from the identification of histamine and LTs (leukotrienes B4, C4 and D4, see p. 25) in the nasal secretions. Therefore, it would appear that in immediate hypersensitivity reactions, mast cell activation by allergen-specific IgE is the key pathogenetic event.

However, in most allergic patients challenged with allergen, further symptoms arise some 4–6 hours later, the so-called **late-phase response** (LPR). In the asthmatic model, there is the development of wheezing, **hyperresponsiveness** in the bronchi to challenge with allergen or histamine and reduction in FEV₁. Hyperresponsiveness is one of the key clinical features of allergy, and this constellation of symptoms and signs most closely resembles the clinical picture seen in many asthmatics. In rhinitis there is nasal blockage and in skin allergy there is prolonged oedema, swelling and redness. These features are not responsive to antihistamines but are suppressed by corticosteroids.

For these reasons, the LPR has been studied extensively, since it appears to hold the key to some of the most debilitating aspects of clinical allergy, and several important findings have been made (Fig. 10.4). First, the cells involved have been identified. In studies on skin biopsies after intradermal challenge, neutrophils are prominent in the first 18 hours of the LPR, but numbers have dwindled by 48 hours. Eosinophils are also prominent and may persist for 2–3 days. T lymphocytes, predominantly CD4⁺, accumulate around small blood vessels and persist for 1–2 days. Analysis of BAL fluid in patients with an LPR following endobronchial challenge has revealed similar results. Eosinophils appear in BAL after 6 hours and there is also an expansion of neutrophils and

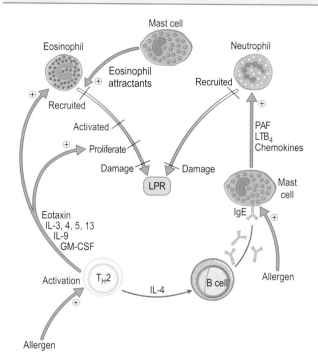

Fig. 10.4 **Advances in understanding the mechanism of the late-phase response (LPR) in type I hypersensitivity.** See text for details.

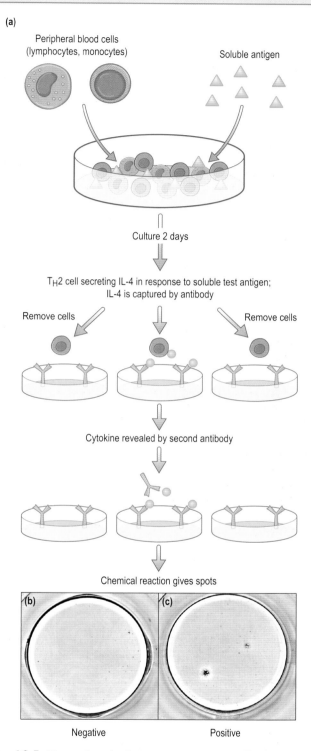

Fig. 10.5 **Measuring the immune response to allergens using the cytokine ELISPOT assay.**
The cytokine ELISPOT is the most sensitive immunological assay currently available, for detection of T cell responses, measuring as few as 1 antigen-specific responder cell amongst 1 million peripheral blood lymphocytes (PBLs). (a) In the figure, PBLs from a patient with diabetes, who has a very rare allergy to injected insulin, have been cultured with insulin. The dark spots seen in panel (c) are a result of the detection of secreted IL-4, indicating a marked T_H2 response to insulin in this patient, and accounting for their allergic disease. Courtesy of Dr Sefina Arif.

CD4 T lymphocytes. Cells are likely to be recruited by release of specific chemotactic factors at the site of allergen-induced inflammation. Platelet activating factor (PAF) and LTs attract and activate eosinophils and neutrophils, respectively. One of the particular features of cellular responses in the LPR in allergy is that, relative to their proportions in the circulation, **eosinophils** are recruited in preference to neutrophils. This has been attributed to the actions of IL-5 and eotaxins, and eosinophil persistence at these sites is thought to be the combined result of the actions of IL-3, IL-4, IL-5, IL-9 and GM-CSF.

Having arrived at the scene of inflammation, what is the contribution of these cells to the pathogenesis of the LPR? The role of neutrophils is not yet clear, though their phagocytic ability and tendency to release proteolytic enzymes on activation could have a role in tissue damage. Because of their selective recruitment, eosinophils have been extensively studied in allergic inflammation, which is often also associated with blood eosinophilia. The magnitude of the eosinophil expansion in BAL fluid correlates well with the degree of bronchial constriction in the asthmatic LPR and several eosinophil granule proteins are damaging to the respiratory epithelium (see p. 31).

Working backwards, it is clear from the list of eosinophil-activating and IgE-promoting cytokines that allergic disease is T_H2 dominated. The regulation of IgE production is under the control of T_H2 cytokines. CD4 T cells from patients with allergic disease are activated when stimulated with appropriate allergens (e.g. Der p 1 in asthmatics with house dust mite allergy; and see Fig. 10.5). During this proliferation,

Table 10.2 Summary of effects of T_H2 cytokines in development of type I hypersensitivity

Cytokine	Allergy-promoting effect		
	IgE production	Mast cell development	Eosinophil development
IL-3		✓	✓
IL-4	✓	✓	
IL-5			✓
IL-9	✓	✓	✓
IL-13	✓		

responding T cells release T_H2 cytokines such as IL-4, IL-5 and IL-13 and, in the presence of B lymphocytes from the same patient, IgE production is stimulated by these T_H2 cells. Recruitment, activation and expansion of eosinophils at sites of allergen exposure is also a result of T_H2 cytokine effects (see above) and both mRNA and protein detection highlights the presence of these in the bronchial mucosa and BAL fluid of asthmatics. These advances in understanding the underlying immunological mechanisms that prevail in type I hypersensitivity, and notably the predominance of T_H2 over T_H1 responses, brings with it the rational design of novel immune-based therapies in allergy (see Table 10.2).

SUMMARY BOX 10.1

Mechanism of hypersensitivity

- Hypersensitivity is the term used to describe exaggerated or inappropriate immune responses that result in tissue damage.
- Hypersensitivity reaction types I–IV is a useful and simple classification.
- Allergy (type I hypersensitivity) results from the activation of mast cells by allergen-specific IgE.
- An allergen is a small protein, which, for reasons unknown, induces a persistent IgE response in some individuals.
- The tendency to allergic reactions (atopy) has both inherited and environmental components.
- T cells, eosinophils and neutrophils are involved in the pathology of clinical allergies such as asthma.

Clinical allergy

Approximately two thirds of atopic individuals, defined by a positive allergen skin test (Fig. 10.6), have clinical allergic disease, which itself has a prevalence of between 15 and 20%;

males and females are equally affected. Allergic reactions range from being a minor irritation to being life threatening. Occasionally they result in death, usually in association with the chronic lung disease asthma and more rarely through wasp and bee stings or allergy to foods. Allergic disease accounts for up to one third of school absences because of chronic illness, and it is estimated that one of the most common forms, asthma, affects 4 million adults and 1 million children in the UK. Asthma as a disease consumes over £800 million of National Health Service resources, £1200 million in lost productivity at work and kills 1000–2000 people in the UK each year, of which 40–45 are children. As many as 5–10% of the population may have an adverse immune response to food and adopt the label of 'food allergic', although this is a difficult clinical area (see Ch. 15).

Diagnosis

The diagnosis of allergic disease is usually made when the history is taken, and at the same time a good guess can be made regarding the nature of the allergens. The timing of the episodes of illness may relate to a seasonal allergy or to exposure to house dust. There is likely to be a family history, and exposure to pets at home or at other people's homes is a frequently recognised trigger.

Skin prick testing against a wide panel of antigens is usually performed and is almost always positive (Fig. 10.6). Skin tests occasionally reveal sensitisation to allergens not recognised by the patient, and this can help in avoidance. The size of the wheal and flare response, relative to the histamine control or other allergens, gives some idea of the importance of each agent. Total IgE levels are raised in the majority of patients. Highly sensitive blood tests for specific IgE against a vast range of potential allergens are now widely available and widely used. In preference, blood tests should be reserved for situations in which the clinical history and skin test results are at variance; when skin testing cannot be performed because of the continuous use of antihistamines, which suppress the reaction, or a co-existing

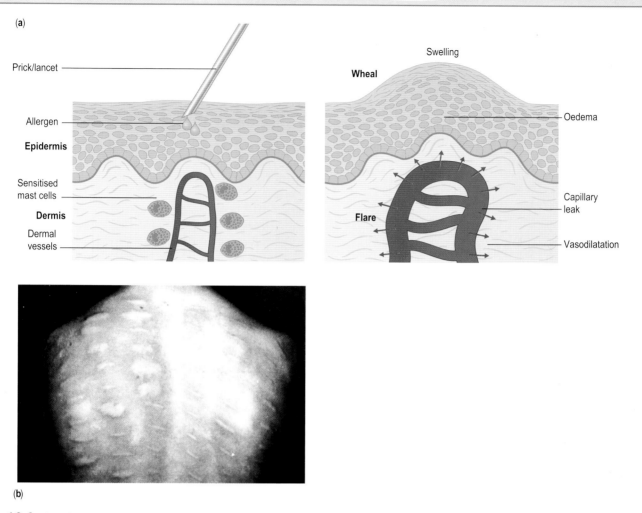

(a)

Prick/lancet

Allergen

Epidermis

Sensitised mast cells

Dermis

Dermal vessels

Swelling

Wheal

Oedema

Flare

Capillary leak

Vasodilatation

(b)

Fig. 10.6 **The allergen skin test (skin prick test).**
(**a**) Method of testing. (**b**) Back of an atopic individual demonstrating wheal and flare responses to skin prick tests administered by subcutaneous scratching with the test allergen. (Please note, this test is typically done on the forearm; it has been performed on this patient's back for illustrative purposes)

severe eczema; and when desensitisation is being considered (see below).

A blood eosinophilia (between 0.4×10^9 and $1.0 \times 10^9/l$) is often observed in allergic disease. Rarely, a provocation test, exposing the patient to the putative allergen, may be required. These are particularly important in the diagnosis of occupational asthma and should be performed under careful supervision.

Treatment: general principles

Although specific therapies tailored to the disease, particularly with regard to asthma, are important, there are some general principles that can be stated. The first line of therapy is allergen avoidance, followed by drugs. In some allergic disease, desensitisation (also termed allergen immunotherapy) is highly effective. Avoidance measures may be as obvious as refraining from cycling through the local park in the hay fever months, or it may be as painful as removing the family pets. Bedding and other furniture is an important

source of house dust mites. Mattresses can be encased in plastic, bedding hot-washed regularly and synthetic rather than natural fibres used where possible. Regular vacuuming and damp-dusting helps maintain areas mite-free, and acaricides (mite-killing compounds) are under development. Drug therapies and the use of desensitisation are discussed below.

Asthma

Asthma is the most common chronic disease of childhood, affecting some 5% of children and 2% of adults. The disorder is generally defined as a clinical syndrome of increased responsiveness of the bronchi to a variety of stimuli, with resultant airway narrowing, which reverses spontaneously or after drug therapy and is associated with cellular inflammation. Most asthma is allergic, although 'intrinsic' non-atopic asthma does occur, particularly in adulthood, and can follow a severe and protracted course.

Pathogenesis

The pathogenesis of asthma undoubtedly combines the mechanisms of type I hypersensitivity and the late-phase response. The commonest allergens involved in the development of asthma are the house dust mites *Dermatophagoides pteronyssinus* and *D. farinae*, and grass pollen. The primary house dust mite allergen appears to be an intestinally derived enzyme with which the mites coat their faecal material. Bronchial hyperresponsiveness results from prolonged damage to, and inflammation of, the respiratory epithelium by mechanisms discussed above. Hyperresponsiveness manifests itself as bronchoconstriction, inflammation and mucus production with airway plugging in response to innocuous triggers that include upper respiratory tract infections, exercise, cold air, smoke and paint fumes.

Clinical and immunological features

The diagnosis of asthma rests upon the taking of a careful history, the principal complaints being cough (often nocturnal in children), wheeze and shortness of breath. Lung function tests (e.g. FEV_1) demonstrate airways obstruction, but these may be normal between attacks. Since bronchial hyperresponsiveness is an important feature, it can be assessed formally, usually as the amount of a stimulus (e.g. histamine or methacholine) to produce a fall (usually of 20%) in a lung function measurement (e.g. the FEV_1). This is termed the PC_{20} (PC, provocative concentration) (Fig. 10.7). Immunological tests (skin prick test, serum IgE levels) are usually performed to aid diagnosis and to add information gained from the history regarding triggers, so that avoidance can be optimised.

Therapy

After allergen avoidance has been optimised, there are several lines of drug therapy. Antihistamines do not have a role in the treatment of asthma. Education is an important component: some of the drugs require inhalation and optimal delivery is an acquired skill. For mild asthma, or the relief of acute shortness of breath or wheeze, an inhaled, short-acting β_2-adrenoceptor agonist (e.g. salbutamol), which relaxes bronchial smooth muscle, is recommended. They are usually inhaled as an aerosol, powder or nebuliser, though they may also be given orally in young children. If asthma is deemed severe, or β_2-agonists are required regularly for symptom relief, then a more regular treatment regimen aimed at prevention is required, usually comprising an inhaled corticosteroid (the inhalation route reduces the dose required, which is important in view of the effects of long-term administration of steroids), to which an inhaled, longer-acting β_2-agonist may be added. Corticosteroids have several well-identified modifying actions in the allergic process: production of prostaglandin and leukotriene mediators is suppressed, inflammatory cell recruitment and migration is inhibited and vasoconstriction leads to reduced cell and fluid leakage from the vasculature. It is known that experimental administration of cysteinyl leukotrienes (cysLTs) to animals and humans can reproduce many of the symptoms of asthma. This has given rise to a relatively new class of 'designer' drug that inhibits cysLT action by blockade of the type 1 receptor (cysLT1; e.g. montelukast). Although there is independent efficacy in asthma, the benefit is variable amongst patients, is less than that offered by steroids and does not appear to be additive with steroids. See Clinical Box 10.1 for other developments.

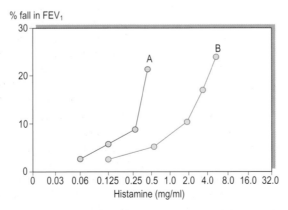

Fig. 10.7 Testing bronchial hyperresponsiveness in asthma.
The percentage fall in FEV_1 in a patient (A) and control (B) after challenge with histamine. The concentration of histamine required to lower the FEV_1 by 20% (PC_{20}) was lower in the patient (0.4 mg/ml) than in the control (4.0 mg/ml) indicating hyperresponsiveness in the patient.

CLINICAL BOX 10.1

Mopping up IgE

Since the degranulation of mast cells following cross-linking of allergen-specific IgE is a major pathological event in allergy, it makes sense to be developing novel strategies to prevent this process. One new idea, already tried in early phase trials in asthma, has been the use of a monoclonal antibody (Mab) directed against IgE. Because of the obvious danger of such a Mab cross-linking IgE on the mast cell surface, and itself causing degranulation, the antibody that has been selected binds to the same part of the Fc region that binds the high affinity IgE receptor (FcεRI). That way, the therapeutic Mab can only interact with soluble IgE, but not IgE that is bound to the mast cell surface. Typically, when administered this achieves a 90–99% reduction in IgE levels in the serum. Several studies have now confirmed that this biologic drug, called omalizumab, has beneficial effects on disease markers in asthma, including reducing the early and late phase responses to inhaled and injected allergen, and down-regulating FcεRI on mast cells and APCs. So far, there have been five therapeutic trials to gauge evidence of clinical benefit, all showing a positive outcome in terms of symptom relief and quality of life measures. Future studies are planned to identify which specific patient groups might get the most benefit — this is especially important, as a course of the drug for one year will cost between £2000 and £10 000 depending on dose, compared with £1000 to £2000 for conventional therapies.

Acute, severe asthmatic attacks are a medical emergency and may require hospitalisation with administration of xanthines (e.g. theophylline) or β₂-adrenoceptor stimulants given intravenously and parenteral corticosteroids.

Allergic rhinitis

Although allergic rhinitis appears a somewhat trivial disorder, it is sufficiently common and disabling to constitute an important cause of morbidity. The annual cost of medical services for allergic rhinitis in the USA is estimated at between $2 and $5 billion. Usually beginning in childhood or teenage years, it affects up to 10% of children and 20% of adolescents, and seasonal allergic rhinitis (hay fever) has a marked effect on school performance and examination achievement in this age group. The main symptoms of rhinitis are nasal congestion, sneezing, often in paroxysms, itching and nasal and post-nasal discharge. Allergic conjunctivitis is a frequent association with itchiness, grittiness and excessive watering of the eyes. As with asthma, the target organ is hyperresponsive, and smoke and paint fumes can trigger symptoms. The rest of the upper airway mucosa may be affected, with itchiness of the palate and pharynx and hearing loss caused by middle ear fluid.

The pathogenesis of allergic rhinitis is similar to that of asthma. Type I hypersensitivity to allergens, particularly grass or other pollens (seasonal), the house dust mite and pet furs (perennial), is the initiating factor, and a late-phase reaction can be demonstrated in many patients on nasal challenge.

The diagnosis of allergic rhinitis or associated disorders is made on the history. Particular attention must be paid to the geographical and temporal relationship of the symptoms. Establishing whether the disorder is seasonal and which season is involved (June–July for grass pollen, July–August for moulds such as *Alternaria*) coupled with skin testing allows the allergens to be identified and hence the diagnosis to be made. Examination, particularly in children, reveals mouth breathing, pale, blue, oedematous nasal turbinates, and frequently a red line across the bridge of the nose caused by the tendency to push the itchy nose upwards. A clear fluid discharge may be visible in the middle ear. Of less value, serum total IgE levels may be raised in 30–40% of children with allergic rhinitis, and a blood eosinophilia may be found. Tests for allergen-specific IgE and skin testing may be useful and are necessary if desensitisation is being considered.

Therapy should include attempts at avoidance of exposure, whilst the main pharmacological therapy centres on the use of antihistamines, which are most effective when given prophylactically, before the pollen season starts. Antihistamines specific for the H₁ histamine receptor have fewer sedative side-effects than previous histamine blockers. Nasally administered sodium cromoglicate (a mast cell stabiliser) and steroids, as well as cysLT1 blockade, form the second-line treatments and when all of these therapies are being used, they constitute the most effective combination. Topical steroids are most effective in treating nasal congestion, a symptom which represents the late-phase reaction. For conjunctivitis, prophylactic oral antihistamines and ocular drops of cromoglicate are the best approach. Desensitisation also has an important place in the management of allergic rhinitis.

Desensitisation

Desensitisation in the context of allergy is also termed **allergen immunotherapy**. It first appeared as a revolutionary treatment for allergy in 1911, but until recently ran a controversial course. The principle, as expounded in the title of the original report, is that allergy can be 'prophylactically inoculated against' in much the same way that measles or mumps can be, by giving the potentially damaging agent (in this case the allergen) in a controlled, safe encounter. Safety emerged as a major issue in the UK in the early 1980s after several deaths following severe generalised reactions to allergen preparations. The Committee on Safety of Medicines issued guidelines in 1986 that restricted the practice to specialist centres with highly trained staff with immediate access to resuscitation equipment. Desensitisation has since emerged from these dark days to represent a major therapeutic track, in particular for patients with seasonal allergic rhinitis.

Desensitisation is currently indicated for disorders in which the hypersensitivity is clearly IgE mediated. Skin tests and allergen-specific IgE detection must be performed to demonstrate this and to confirm that there is IgE production against the allergen preparation to be used in the therapy. Typical indications include life-threatening allergy to insect stings, drug allergy and allergic rhinitis. It comprises an induction course of subcutaneous injections of increasing doses of the allergen extract, given once every 1–2 weeks. Once the maximum dose is achieved (usually after 6–10 weeks), maintenance injections may be required monthly for 2–3 years but may provide benefit for a further number of years. A recent systematic review of 51 published randomised placebo-controlled clinical trials, enrolling a total of nearly 3000 participants, showed a low risk of adverse events with consistent clinical benefit. Indeed, adrenaline (epinephrine) was required in only 19 out of over 14 000 injections and there were no deaths. A variety of immune mechanisms for the beneficial effect has been proposed (Table 10.3). Desensitisation is generally not considered for asthma, and is less effective in those with multiple allergies. A new development has been the concept that the allergen does not need to be injected, but can be absorbed under the tongue. Large-scale clinical trials of sublingual immunotherapy are currently under way, and early results (using GRAZAX® tablets of Phl p 5 from timothy grass) are highly encouraging, with the advantage of the therapy being home-based.

Atopic eczema

The term eczema is derived from Greek and means 'the result of boiling over'. Often used interchangeably with dermatitis,

Table 10.3 Mechanism of action of desensitisation

Mechanism	Explanation
IgG blocking antibodies	During repeated exposure to desensitising allergen, IgG class antibodies develop (especially IgG4); these compete with the pathogenic IgE for allergen binding, and/or prevent IgE-allergen complexes binding to mast cell high affinity IgE receptors
Regulation	Exposure to repeated desensitising allergen induces Treg cells, which recognise allergen but invoke regulatory immune responses, dampening down migration, infiltration and inflammation
Immune deviation	A shift away from T_H2- to T_H1-producing CD4 cells results in the generation of cytokines (e.g. IFN-γ), which are inhibitory to IgE production

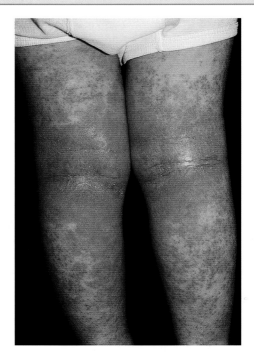

Fig. 10.8 Typical flexor distribution of eczema in childhood.
From White G 2004 Colour Atlas of Dermatology, 3rd edn, Mosby, with permission.

eczema defines an inflammatory skin disorder with many possible causes, the hallmark being a histological process called spongiosis: the accumulation of oedema fluid within and between keratinocytes in the epidermis, giving a 'spongy' appearance. It is common, affecting between 5 and 10% of the population, and 10–20% of children. Some 30% of sufferers go on to develop asthma, and 50% develop allergic rhinitis.

The main symptoms are itching or, in the infant, the appearance of dry, red patches with occasional vesicles overtaken by crusting. In infancy, the cheeks, abdomen and limb surfaces are involved, whilst in older children the classical distribution is on the elbow, knee and wrist flexor surfaces (Fig. 10.8). Prolonged scratching leads to the development of discoloured plaques with a leathery texture (lichenification). In approximately 75% of cases the disorder is self-limiting and clears in the first few years of life.

The diagnosis is made on history, examination and skin testing, with the total serum IgE level also usually raised and IgE directed against airborne and food allergens is a prominent feature.

In contrast with the respiratory allergic disorders, however, the pathogenesis of allergic eczema is less clear. Skin testing evokes a wheal and flare response but not eczematous lesions. After skin prick tests T_H2 cytokines are detectable in the skin, followed some hours later by a mixed pattern that includes T_H2 mediators and IFN-γ. It is possible to replicate eczema-like plaques by patch testing with allergens such as house dust mite extracts in sensitive individuals. (Patch testing, in which the allergen is secured as a disc onto the skin surface of the back for 48 hours, is usually used for the identification

of sensitisers that give rise to contact dermatitis, a type IV hypersensitivity reaction; see below.)

The relationship between diet and eczema is perhaps the most intriguing and controversial aspect of the disease. Well-designed studies in which potential triggers in food (cow's milk, hen's egg protein, peanuts) are avoided appear to bring about an improvement in eczema, but only in children. Skin prick tests against food derivatives are usually unhelpful. More complex and comprehensive avoidance diets run the risk of incomplete nutrition and compliance is a problem. At present, therefore, the best advice to parents of children with eczema appears to be a therapeutic trial of avoidance of the foods listed above, preferably followed by a period of reintroduction, with the diet to be continued if tolerated and of benefit. In addition, topical corticosteroids may be required. New attempts to treat the roots of the disorder have been directed against T cells, including short courses of ciclosporin and topical tacrolimus, both of which act on T cell activation (see p. 315).

Urticaria and angio-oedema

Urticaria (also commonly known as 'hives' or 'nettle rash') is a disorder in which well circumscribed, itchy weals erupt over different areas of the body (Fig. 10.9). It is caused by localised vasodilatation and oedema occurring in the superficial dermis. Angio-oedema is a related disorder in which the oedema forms deeper within the dermis, giving larger areas of swollen tissue. Angio-oedema may also arise as a

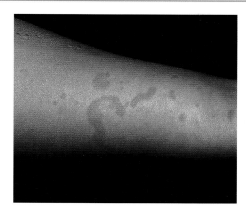

Fig. 10.9 Typical appearance of urticaria.
From White G 2004 Colour Atlas of Dermatology, 3rd edn, Mosby, with permission.

SUMMARY BOX 10.2

Clinical allergy—cont'd

- Eczema results from oedema between and within the keratinocytes of the epidermis (spongiosis). It most commonly presents in children under 5 years of age and may be helped by allergen avoidance.

- Urticaria (itchy wheals) and angio-oedema are both mediated by histamine, are typically acute and may be related to food.

non-allergic disorder as result of failure to inhibit the complement cascade (see p. 279). Both disorders may be caused by an IgE-mediated type I hypersensitivity in which histamine is one of the dominant pathogenic mediators. However, in the majority of cases a cause for the urticaria/angio-oedema is not found. In these the disease may be chronic and idiopathic or secondary to other disease. Rare forms of the disease characterised by IgG autoantibodies against FcεRI-α and against IgE have also been described, and these may respond to plasmapheresis.

Urticaria associated with type I hypersensitivity is typically acute in onset and frequently occurs in children in association with foodstuffs. The first symptoms are tingling and then swelling of the lips and tongue, some of the commoner allergens being seafood, nuts, berries, eggs and chocolate. Insect stings and drug reactions may also produce the migrating wheals of urticaria, as may latex. The diagnosis is frequently made by the patient or on the history, and skin testing may be helpful. Since it is often acute in onset and self-limiting, allergic urticaria is difficult to treat apart from the avoidance of provoking stimuli. Antihistamines are also of benefit in acute urticarial reactions.

SUMMARY BOX 10.2

Clinical allergy

- Diagnosis by skin tests and detection of allergen-specific IgE.

- Treatment starts with avoidance of the allergen, then makes use of drugs and desensitisation.

- Asthma is increased responsiveness of the bronchi to stimuli with resulting airway narrowing. It is treated with β_2-adrenoceptor agonists and corticosteroids are required to control the disease long term.

- Allergic rhinitis affects the upper airways. It can be treated with antihistamines, cromoglicate, corticosteroids and desensitisation.

Anaphylaxis: definition and general considerations

The term anaphylaxis describes 'a serious allergic reaction that is rapid in onset and may cause death'. Classically, it is the clinical manifestation of an acute, generalised IgE-mediated immune reaction involving specific antigen, mast cells and basophils. The reaction requires priming by the allergen, followed by re-exposure. It appears to be a modern phenomenon. For many years an ancient Egyptian hieroglyph was interpreted as showing the Pharoah Menes being killed by a wasp sting in 2600 BC. There is now some doubt as to the original interpretation of the symbols, and a revisionist view is that Menes was in fact a mythical figure killed by hippopotami, and probably not, therefore, as a result of anaphylaxis (see Clinical Box 10.2). To provoke anaphylaxis, the allergen must be systemically absorbed, either after ingestion or parenteral injection and a range of allergens have been identified:

- *foods*: nuts (peanuts, Brazil, cashew), shellfish (shrimp, lobster), dairy products, egg (and more rarely citrus fruits, mango, strawberry, tomato)

- *venoms*: wasps, bees, yellow-jackets, hornets

- *medications*: antisera (tetanus, diphtheria), dextran, latex, some antibiotics.

Anaphylaxis is rare, and the symptom/sign constellation ranges from widespread urticaria to cardiovascular collapse, laryngeal oedema, airway obstruction and respiratory arrest leading to death. A syndrome identical to anaphylaxis may occur in the absence of IgE-mediated responses. In this, the triggering response may occasionally be IgG mediated, as in some drug reactions. The acute formation of large quantities of immune complexes intravascularly, possibly following repeated infusion of blood products, activates complement and gives an anaphylaxis-like state.

Data on the current incidence of anaphylaxis are difficult to acquire, but the following statistics give some flavour of the size of the problem: fatal reactions to penicillin occur once every 7.5 million injections; between 1 in 250 and 1 in 125 individuals have severe reactions to Hymenoptera (bee and wasp) stings, and a death takes place every 6.5 million stings; such stings cause between 60 and 80 deaths per year in America, and 5–10 in the UK. There is controversy as to

The discovery of anaphylactic reactions

There is controversy as to whether the hieroglyphics detailing the death of King Menes of Egypt following an insect sting nearly 4000 years ago are indeed the first report of a fatal anaphylactic reaction. At the turn of the twentieth century, the term anaphylaxis was coined by Portier and Richet. These French biologists, as guests aboard the yacht of the Prince of Monaco cruising in the Mediterranean, became interested in whether it was possible to become protected against the poisonous sting of the Portuguese man-of-war jellyfish. They subsequently investigated whether prior exposure of dogs to sea anemone toxin protected them from the severe reactions associated with the venom when reinjected. On the contrary, the dogs reacted even more severely the second time and died within 30 minutes, hence the term anaphylaxis which derives from the Greek and means 'anti-protection'. It became clear that not only toxic substances produced a severe reaction after reinjection: some of the most important studies on anaphylaxis were performed on individuals given more than one dose of the horse serum antitoxins used to treat tetanus and diphtheria in the 1920s. In the 1960s, it is estimated that between 100 and 500 Americans died of anaphylaxis per year when exposed to a repeated dose of penicillin. Today, penicillin, stings from bees and wasps and, rarely, some food reactions are the most important causes of anaphylaxis; in 2006 a UK West Country woman died of tomato allergy, emphasising the power of the 'anti-protection' reaction.

whether atopy predisposes to anaphylaxis, early studies indicating this to be the case, whereas latterly no association has been found.

Pathogenesis

The molecules that incite anaphylactic responses may be moderately sized proteins (>10 kDa), or they may not be sufficiently large to be antigenic in their own right but behave as haptens (see pp. 297 and 149) — this is often true for drugs. In penicillin allergy, some of the determinants against which IgE responses can be detected by skin testing are common to penicillin derivatives, and the chance of cross-reaction with these is high. Up to 50% cross-reactivity with the cephalosporins has also been described. Animal-derived serum products, such as antilymphocyte globulin and antisera against snake venoms, are potent inducers of anaphylactic responses. The Hymenoptera order of insects contains two families: the Apidae (bees) and the Vespidae (wasps, hornets and the yellow-jackets common in North America). The major sting allergens are the forms of phospholipase A in the venom, although other sting contents may be involved. The IgE responses are not cross-reactive between wasps and bees. As a prelude to **desensitisation** (see Clinical Box 10.3), it is important to establish the nature of the insect from the history if possible, as well as using skin tests and measure-

ment of allergen-specific IgE to identify the allergen to be used in the therapy. Skin testing in these circumstances carries a small risk of anaphylaxis and should be conducted under careful supervision. In some circumstances, carefully monitored challenges with incremental doses of supposed allergens may be required.

At the heart of the pathogenesis of anaphylaxis is the activation of mast cells and basophils, with systemic release of some mediators and generation of others. The initial symptoms may appear innocuous: tingling, warmth and itchiness. The ensuing effects on the vasculature give vasodilatation and oedema. The consequence of these may be no more than a generalised flush, with urticaria and angio-oedema. More serious sequelae are hypotension,

Desensitisation using peptides — a serendipitous finding

As discussed, desensitisation is thought to work, at least in part, by the induction of CD4 Tregs specific for allergen peptides presented by class II HLA molecules. This raises the question as to whether administering the allergen peptides (rather than the whole allergen) would induce Tregs directly and be an effective form of therapy. Indeed, it turns out that this form of 'peptide immunotherapy' shows very encouraging signs in early clinical trials. The story of how the therapy was stumbled upon is an interesting example of serendipity in clinical research. In the early 1990s, an allergy research group in London were trying to induce the late phase response (LPR, which is T cell dependent) in subjects with allergy to the cat fur allergen Fel d 1 by administering short peptides they hoped would correspond to the epitopes recognised by pathogenic, allergen-specific T_H2 cells. The aim of the study was to develop a model of the LPR for use in testing new drugs to prevent it. The study began cautiously with low peptide doses intradermally, and nothing much happened until about 80 micrograms of peptide were given, and a patient developed classic symptoms and signs of the LPR (see p. 136). In effect, the peptide administered into the skin of the arm had diffused into blood and into the lung, where it bound HLA class II-expressing APCs and activated the local T_H2 response. Delighted with the outcome, the group continued the work to extend numbers of subjects and began to prepare their manuscript for publication. At the stage of writing the paper, they uncovered a few additional experiments they would like to perform, and recalled some of the patients from the original study. However, when these subjects were re-challenged with peptide — no LPR! In fact, as subsequent studies showed, the 'treated' patients also had reduced skin prick responses to whole allergen and had generated CD4 T cells capable of regulating T_H2 cells in vitro. In effect, the original dosing with peptide, whilst transiently activating an LPR had also induced Tregs. As a result, peptide immunotherapy is becoming an increasingly active area of clinical research in inflammatory and autoimmune diseases in which a regulated response is a therapeutic goal.

bronchospasm, laryngeal oedema and cardiac arrhythmia or infarction. Death may occur within minutes. Up to 20% of patients treated for the initial episode may have a further serious manifestation of anaphylaxis up to 8 hours later, possibly reflecting the release of mediators from recruited cells, akin to the late-phase response in other allergic conditions.

Clinical features

Early recognition and treatment are essential. Death is quick, and delay increases its likelihood. The main aim is the protection of respiratory and cardiovascular function: 0.5 mg of adrenaline should be given intramuscularly. The effects may be short lived and the therapy may need to be repeated at frequent intervals: as the medical maxim states, the first, second and third lines of treatment of anaphylaxis are adrenaline, adrenaline and adrenaline! Its action is to bronchodilate and vasoconstrict as well as inhibiting mast cell mediator release. Further therapies depend upon the course taken by the patient and the facilities available. Ideally, oxygen should be administered, as well as β-adrenoceptor agonists such as salbutamol or theophylline, followed by histamine H_1-receptor antagonists and corticosteroids once the acute phase is under control. Prolonged hypotension results from vasodilatation and fluid loss into the tissues and should be monitored in a high-dependency unit with the use of plasma expanders and inotropes as required. As an aid to diagnosis if the presentation is unusual, plasma levels of histamine (needs to be done within one hour of onset) or tryptase (from mast cells, see Table 3.4; within 1–6 hours) may be measured.

The best treatment is prevention. Avoidance of triggering foods, particularly nuts and shellfish, may require almost obsessive self-discipline. Patient education is, therefore, important, and many are also instructed in the self-administration of adrenaline (epinephrine) and carry pre-loaded syringes. Desensitisation has a well-established place in the management of this disorder, particularly if exposure is unavoidable or unpredictable, as in insect stings.

SUMMARY BOX 10.3

Generalised anaphylaxis and desensitisation

- Occurs after re-exposure to a systemically absorbed allergen, e.g. food, venom, medication.
- It is caused by activation of mast cells and basophils.
- Symptoms range from urticaria to cardiovascular collapse and respiratory arrest; further episodes can occur up to 8 hours later; death may occur within minutes.
- Treatment involves protecting respiratory and cardiovascular function and administering subcutaneous adrenaline (epinephrine); often repeated at intervals.
- Prevention can involve avoiding the trigger, carrying adrenaline and undergoing desensitisation.

Other types of hypersensitivity

Type II hypersensitivity: antibody targets cell surface antigens

Hypersensitivity reactions types II and III are initiated by the interaction between antibody and antigen but in these cases IgE is not involved. The distinction between the types is based on where the complex of antibody and antigen form: in type II, the target is fixed in the tissues or on the cell surface; in type III the target is soluble and circulating immune complexes are formed.

The consequences of antibody binding to a cell surface antigen are predictable: (1) complement is activated leading to cell lysis, mast cell activation and neutrophil recruitment; (2) the antigen–antibody complex recruits cells directly through Fc interactions (Fig. 10.10). The arrival of cells with cytotoxic capability (neutrophils, eosinophils, monocytes, killer cells) may lead to a mechanism of damage described as antibody-dependent cell-mediated cytotoxicity (ADCC). In addition, there may be other mechanisms through which antibody binding affects function. Antibody binding can lead to modulated expression of cell surface receptors, resulting in reduced ability of the target cell to function normally. This is thought to happen when anti-acetylcholine receptor auto-antibodies bind at the neuromuscular junction and interfere with nerve conduction in myasthenia gravis (see p. 257). Autoantibodies may, on the other hand, stimulate through surface receptors to which they bind, as happens in relation to autoantibodies that bind the thyroid stimulating hormone receptor in Graves' thyroiditis (see p. 197). Other autoanti-

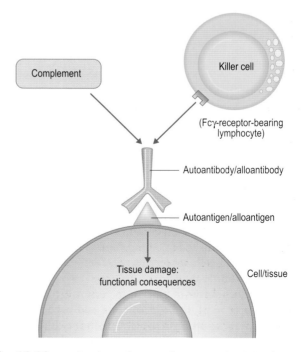

Fig. 10.10 Mechanism of type II hypersensitivity reactions.
See text for details.

bodies may blockade receptors — this is thought to occur in patients with pernicious anaemia who have type I anti-intrinsic factor autoantibodies (p. 212). The diseases that arise as a result of tissue damage in a type II hypersensitivity reaction are varied and the clinical picture depends upon the target tissue and mode of action of the antibody:

- organ-specific autoimmune diseases
  - myasthenia gravis
  - antiglomerular basement membrane glomerulonephritis
  - pemphigus vulgaris and bullous pemphigoid
- autoimmune cytopenias (i.e. blood cell destruction)
  - haemolytic anaemia
  - thrombocytopenia
  - neutropenia
- transfusion reactions
- haemolytic disease of the newborn (rhesus isoimmunisation)
- hyperacute allograft rejection.

The diseases will be described in detail in their respective chapters. In some, the antibodies target self cell surface proteins, resulting in an autoimmune disease. In others, the targets are on exogenous cells, perhaps in an incompatible blood transfusion or organ graft. In some type II hypersensitivity diseases, the pathogenetic mechanisms are known: for example, several forms of haemolytic anaemia follow infectious disease or drug reactions (see p. 294). In these the red blood cell surface antigen may be targeted as a result of cross-reaction with the provoking stimulus. Alternatively, drugs can modify cell surface proteins and render them immunogenic. In haemolytic disease of the newborn (rhesus isoimmunisation; see p. 293), transfusion reactions and hyperacute graft rejection (see p. 155), antibodies against cell surface targets arise during a previous encounter, whether it be a previous pregnancy, in the case of rhesus isoimmunisation, or a previous transfusion or transplant. In other conditions, particularly the organ-specific autoimmune diseases, it remains unknown why the antibodies arise.

Type III hypersensitivity: antigen and antibody interact in the circulation

In type III hypersensitivity, antigen–antibody complexes form. To initiate a type III hypersensitivity reaction, the complexes become deposited in a tissue and there the process of complement and cellular recruitment and activation takes place, with resulting tissue damage.

There are two forms of type III hypersensitivity reaction: complexes may form in the circulation and become deposited in the tissues, or they may actually form within tissues. The latter mechanism is also termed the 'Arthus' reaction, after Maurice Arthus who injected foreign proteins under the skin of animals that he had already immunised with the same protein. The antigen–antibody complexes forming within the tissue incited an erythematous lesion after 3–6 hours.

Immune complex formation in itself is not an exceptional or dangerous occurrence, since immune complexes are carried through the circulation during many diseases ranging from the common cold to cancer. This process is a physiological mechanism for removing antigen. Immune complexes in the circulation recruit complement and are carried to the spleen or liver on complement receptors embedded in the red blood cell membrane (see Ch. 21). Within the tissues, small numbers of complexes being deposited are easily removed. For a type III hypersensitivity reaction to occur, then, something must disturb this homeostatic mechanism. Several factors are known to be capable of predisposing to the excessive and damaging formation of immune complexes, and these relate to the antigen, the host response and the tissue.

Factors influencing immune complex formation and damage

Factors relating to the antigen include **charge** and **persistence**. A charged molecule, such as DNA, is more likely to be attracted to, and become attached to, charged areas within the body, such as the glomerular basement membrane (DNA is an important target antigen of autoantibodies in systemic lupus erythematosus; SLE (see p. 167)). Persistent production of antigen will lead to a continuous supply of complexes, overloading the removal process and amplifying the opportunities for deposition and damage. Examples of antigen persistence include the bacterial proteins continuously cast off the heart valves during infective endocarditis, and similar proteins emanating from infected ventriculo-peritoneal shunts used to relieve high intracranial pressure.

The host response is important in determining the potential pathogenicity of immune complexes. The **isotype** of antibody in a complex influences complement fixation and, thus, its solubility. The integrity of the complement cascade is also an important determinant of whether complexes are solubilised and removed. Function of the classical pathway, which requires C2 and C4, is critical in solubilising antigen–antibody complexes. Genetically determined deficiency of complement component C4 is found in approximately half of patients with SLE, one of the best examples of a disease in which immune complexes contribute to the pathogenesis. C2 deficiency is much rarer, but almost all patients with this defect have an SLE-like syndrome (see p. 279). Patients with SLE also have defective complement receptor expression on their red blood cell surface, further reducing their 'buffering' capacity for immune complexes.

The tissues typically exposed to injury by immune complexes are the renal glomerulus and the joint synovium. These are tissues in which plasma from the blood is ultrafiltrated to form urine and synovial fluid, respectively. The hydrostatic pressure involved in such a process and the filtrative function of the glomerular basement membrane are likely to contribute to the retention and, therefore, the pathogenicity of immune complexes.

Finally, there are the characteristics of the complexes themselves, which determine the extent of tissue damage (Table 10.4). Much of the research in this area has been carried out using animal models, in which a source of foreign antigen is injected as a bolus (see Science Box 10.2).

The variety of factors capable of influencing immune complex deposition is paralleled by the variety of diseases that are known to be immune complex mediated. There are three broad categories of immune complex disease (Table 10.5; Fig. 10.12). In some, the immune complexes formed in the circulation deposit in the tissues, leading directly to nephritis, synovitis or iritis. In a second group, complex deposition is predominantly into the walls of medium or small-sized arterioles, and the vasculitis (see p. 232) that ensues is the cause of organ damage in the kidney, skin or other organs. In others, particularly the type III hypersensitivity lung diseases, antigens and antibody combine within the tissue, resembling an Arthus reaction.

Extrinsic allergic alveolitis

Extrinsic allergic alveolitis (EAA), termed **hypersensitivity pneumonitis**, represents the outcome of an interesting group of occupation and 'pastime-related' diseases. Exposure over many months or years to excessive amounts of inhaled antigen leads to the generation of large concentrations of antibodies within the lung interstitium. At a subsequent exposure, immune complex formation takes place on a massive scale in the alveoli. Typically, patients present 3–6 hours after loading mouldy hay, cleaning the pigeon loft or packing the sugar cane (Table 10.6), with symptoms of fever, chills, malaise and dyspnoea. They may admit to milder episodes leading up to the presenting illness. Symptoms usually remit within 24 hours, but chronic exposure can lead to progressive shortness of breath, with cyanosis, lung

Table 10.4 Factors contributing to immune complex disease

Factors	Mechanisms
Relative proportions of antigen and antibody	Complexes formed in antigen or antibody excess are less likely to deposit
Impaired classical complement pathway function	Classical pathway has key role in solubilising and transporting complexes
Isotype of antibody	Isotype dictates ability to fix complement
Rate of complex formation	If rate of formation exceeds clearance, complex deposition is enhanced

---

SCIENCE BOX 10.2

Serum sickness as a model of immune complex disease

The possibility that antigen–antibody complexes could result in disease was proposed by von Pirquet in 1911. At that time, a common therapy was the injection of hyperimmune antiserum against pathogenic toxins such as those produced by diphtheria and tetanus. These antisera were produced by raising the antibodies in horses, but a high proportion of patients developed reactions after the injections. The reaction typically comprised a transient arthritis, skin rash and fever arising a week after the first injection and then more rapidly after subsequent doses. Von Pirquet showed that the reactions could be induced by normal horse serum not containing the antitoxin, and he proposed that antibodies formed against the foreign proteins in horse serum were responsible for the reaction. Studies some 40 to 50 years later reproduced similar effects after a bolus injection of foreign protein into rabbits (Fig. 10.11). This model is termed **acute** serum sickness and probably represents the processes seen in post-streptococcal nephritis (see p. 225), with antibody levels rising rapidly in response to a large bacterial load. Another model, **chronic** serum sickness, is generated by repeated intermittent injection of foreign antigen and could represent the processes seen in immune complex diseases such as SLE.

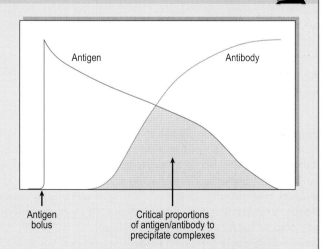

Fig. 10.11 Immune complexes arise in immune complex disease.
See text for details.

Table 10.5 Immune complex mediated disorders

Immune complex deposits	Antigen	Disorder	Pathology
Deposited or formed in tissue	Group A streptococci	Post-streptococcal nephritis	Nephritis
	DNA	Systemic lupus erythematosus (SLE)	Nephritis, serositis
	Bacterial antigens	Subacute bacterial endocarditis (SBE); Shunt nephritis	Nephritis
Vessel deposition	HBsAg	Polyarteritis nodosa	Vasculitis
	DNA	SLE	Vasculitis
	Bacterial antigens	SBE	Vasculitis
Form in tissues	Various microbial and chemical antigens	Extrinsic allergic alveolitis (EAA)	Pneumonitis

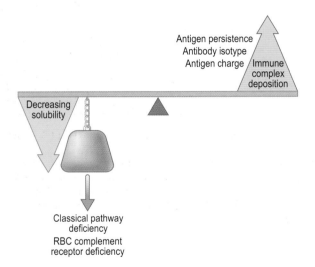

Fig. 10.12 **Factors contributing to immune complex-mediated damage.**

Table 10.6 Antigens involved in extrinsic allergic alveolitis development

Disease	Antigen
Bird fancier's disease	Various avian antigens (pigeons, cockatoos, parakeets, budgerigars)
Farmer's lung	Fungal antigens in mouldy hay
Baggassosis (sugar cane worker's disease)	*Thermoactinomyces sacchari*
Paprika slicer's lung	*Mucor stolonifer*

fibrosis and the development of cor pulmonale. The diagnosis is made on the history and the demonstration of circulating IgG antibodies (called **precipitins**) to the provoking antigen. Farmer's lung has declined in recent years with changes in farming practice, but bird-related pastimes remain popular, hence bird fancier's disease is the commonest form of EAA.

The antigens involved are usually associated with small particles (1 μm) that promote transportation to the alveolar space (contrast with the larger particles seen in bronchial type I hypersensitivity). Although the pathogenesis of the disease is classically a type III hypersensitivity, there is probably a cell-mediated component (see 'type IV hypersensitivity' below), with the documented formation of granulomata. It is not clear why some individuals develop disease whilst others do not, although HLA associations (e.g. with *HLA-DRB1*1305* in pigeon fancier's lung) have been described. Management is predominantly composed of exposure avoidance strategies, as well as oral corticosteroids.

Type IV hypersensitivity: tissue damage by T$_H$1 cells

The description of type IV hypersensitivity is based upon the observation that certain inflammatory conditions associated with tissue damage are characterised by cellular infiltrates, appearing 24 hours after challenge and composed in the main of a combination of lymphocytes and macrophages. If antigen persists, inflammation becomes chronic and the macrophages in the lesion fuse to form giant cells and epithelioid cells.

Some of the best examples of type IV hypersensitivity (also called **delayed type hypersensitivity; DTH**) include reactions to mycobacteria and other similar organisms, which the immune system has difficulty eliminating. Reactions range from the local redness and swelling seen at the site of intradermal tests for tuberculosis immunity (e.g. Heaf test, Mantoux test), in which an extract from the organism is injected, to the caseating necrosis that occasionally results from a host's attempts to deal with *Mycobacterium tuberculosis* infection. Granulomata, which 'wall off' the infective focus, may also arise in response to other infections, such as the parasitic worm infestation of schistosomiasis. Within the granulomata, there is extensive tissue damage, with fibrosis and calcification. This type of reaction can have serious clinical consequences if the site of damage is the lung, liver or bone. In these circumstances, the immune system is caught between the repercussions of not dealing with the infection, and the tissue damage that is caused by activated and differentiated macrophages. Dendritic cells and macrophages are activated by CD4 T_H1 lymphocytes and release powerful hydrolytic enzymes and toxic oxygen metabolites (see Ch. 6). Other factors released within the infiltrate encourage fibrosis and angiogenesis.

Another example of type IV hypersensitivity is that resulting in some individuals from exposure to contact with nickel in jewellery (Fig. 10.13), dichromate in the leather industry or *p*-phenyldiamine in sunscreens and hair dyes. The reaction is confined to the skin and is frequently termed **contact dermatitis**. Typically there is an eczematous reaction with erythema, oedema, vesicles and scaling. Since there are many potential irritants and the lesions usually require 48 hours to appear, the diagnosis of such reactions is often a painstaking piece of detective work. This may be helped by **patch testing** in which potential contact sensitisers are placed in contact with the skin on the back for 48 hours (Fig. 10.14).

Application of sensitising agents to the skin in animal models has allowed some of the pathogenetic aspects of contact dermatitis to be studied. As early as 1942, Landsteiner and Chase demonstrated that cells, but not serum, could transfer contact sensitivity from an affected to an unsensitised animal. Prior to this, Landsteiner had coined the term **hapten** to describe substances incapable, because of their small size, of provoking the formation of antibodies without conjugation to carrier proteins, and this concept is at the heart of the process involved in contact dermatitis. It is believed that the metals or compounds in the sensitising agent become conjugated to tissue proteins.

In vitro, type IV hypersensitivity reactions are recreated in assays in which lymphocytes from a reactive individual are cultured with the provoking agent (mycobacterial extract, schistosomal proteins, nickel). The measurement of T cell proliferation or release of cytokines such as IFN-γ are a useful assessment of the degree of reactivity and of relevance to the pathogenetic processes (Fig. 10.15).

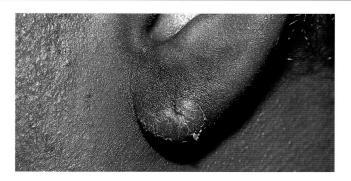

Fig. 10.13 **Example of allergic contact dermatitis to nickel in an earring.**
From White G 2004 Colour Atlas of Dermatology, 3rd edn, Mosby, with permission.

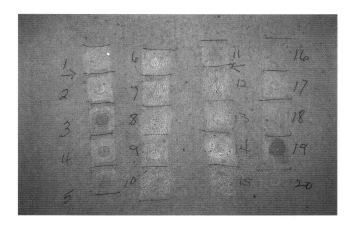

Fig. 10.14 **Patch testing to establish the cause of contact dermatitis.**
Patches containing an array of different potential sensitisers are strapped to the skin on the back of the patient and left for 48 hours. In this case allergens 3 and 19 reacted. From White G 2004 Colour Atlas of Dermatology, 3rd edn, Mosby, with permission.

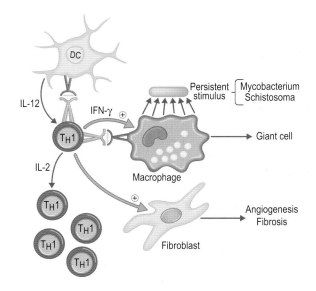

Fig. 10.15 **Diagram illustrating the cellular/molecular basis of a type IV hypersensitivity response.**

SUMMARY BOX 10.4

Other types of hypersensitivity (II–IV)

- Antibody, recruiting complement and cytotoxic cells with Fc receptors can cause tissue damage. This is frequently an autoantibody. The antigenic targets may be tissue fixed (type II) or in the circulation (type III).

- In type II, the target cell surface antigens may be altered self or exogenous cells (e.g. hyperacute graft rejection).

- In type III the immune complex may be deposited in tissues or vessels (SLE) or may form in tissues (farmer's lung).

- Hypersensitivity resulting from T lymphocyte reactions is usually delayed in onset. The central cells in this type IV hypersensitivity are the CD4 T lymphocyte and the macrophage. Granulomata are characteristic and contact dermatitis is a typical clinical example.

Further reading

Ismail T, McSharry C, Boyd G 2006 Extrinsic allergic alveolitis. Respirology 11: 262–268

Deacock SJ 2008 An approach to the patient with urticaria. Clin Exp Immunol 153: 151–161

El-Shanawany T, Williams PE, Jolles S 2008 An approach to the patient with anaphylaxis. Clin Exp Immunol 153: 1–9

Kay AB 2001 Allergy and allergic diseases. First of two parts. N Engl J Med 4; 344: 30–37

Kay AB 2001 Allergy and allergic diseases. Second of two parts. N Engl J Med 11; 344: 109–113

Ogawa Y, Calhoun WJ 2006 The role of leukotrienes in airway inflammation. J Allergy Clin Immunol 118: 789–798

Transplantation

This chapter focuses on the transplantation of organs and tissue from one individual to another. This can be a life-saving procedure, that can at the same time provoke a powerful immune response. The chapter addresses the nature of the immune response to transplants; the impact of this on the recipient; and how modern medical practice tries to get around the problem.

The obvious reason for transplantation is to re-establish a function lost following end-stage disease (or physical loss) of a given organ or tissue. That was not the reason for one of the first grafts on record. To free himself from captivity in Crete, Daedalus aimed to acquire a new function — that of flying — through the xenogeneic transplant of bird feathers. His attempt succeeded and he landed safely in mainland Greece. His son, Icarus, failed in the same attempt. His trans-

plant failed, reportedly from the melting of a thermolabile adhesive — perhaps the first reported case of hyperacute rejection — even though we are now aware of immunological reasons (see Science Box 11.1) for the failure of a **xenograft**, a transplant between members of different species (**xeno = foreign**).

The outcome of an **autograft** is different, as depicted in Byzantine iconography. In one such example, a doubting witness to the Virgin Mary's ascension into heaven finds his arm severed by an impatient Angel. An intervention of the Virgin Mary re-establishes the anatomy and physiology of the severed limb. This successful outcome may not be the result only of the skills of the operator but also of the fact that in this type of intervention, an autograft, a tissue or organ is transplanted within the same individual; in clinical practice the tissue is usually transplanted to a new site. In an autograft, as Hindu physicians knew some 2500 years ago, the graft invariably 'takes'.

During experimental attempts in the early 1950s to transfer kidneys between humans, surgeons were faced with the natural result of an **allograft**, which is a graft between genetically non-identical members of the same species (**allo = different**). The outcome, invariably, was **rejection** of the new organ or tissue. These experimenters noted that rejection can be partly controlled by drastically restraining the immune system with **immunosuppression**. During these initial attempts at kidney transplantation, it was also noted that a **syngraft**, a graft between genetically identical subjects, such as monozygotic twins, would not undergo rejection (**syn = same, identical**).

The study of why genetically different individuals cannot share tissues easily (i.e. we are generally speaking histoincompatible) led to the identification of the proteins encoded by the MHC that are the key to tissue compatibility. As discussed elsewhere (see p. 67, Science Box 5.3), the enormous variability of the MHC molecules within a species must confer some evolutionary advantage. If that species were confronted, say, by a pandemic with a lethal virus, it would be advantageous for some individuals to have a set of MHC molecules — missing in the remaining dying population — that was able to present a peptide of the processed virus to the immune system in such a way that the virus was eliminated and the individuals survived. A downside to this evolutionary advantage is the fact that the tissues of one

Xenogeneic transplantation

The shortage of organs for transplantation has focused research on the possibility of animal donors. A logical source is represented by pigs, since their organs match the human equivalents for size. When transplanted into humans, however, pig organs undergo hyperacute rejection. This is because of the presence of 'natural' anti-pig antibodies in the human circulation, which react with swine endothelial cells lining the blood vessels, activate complement massively and provoke graft destruction within minutes of surgery. Various approaches have been considered to overcome these limitations including neutralisation of the 'natural' antibodies and prevention of complement activation.

In xenogeneic transplants, the endothelial cell damage is ultimately caused by unrestrained complement activation. The activation is unrestrained because pig cell membrane-bound complement inhibitors cannot control activation of human complement. Transgenic pigs, expressing the human complement regulatory protein decay-accelerating factor

(hDAF) have been generated and this has provided some protection against complement mediated hyperacute rejection with pig-to-primate grafts surviving for several days. The antigen recognised by the human anti-swine antibodies has been identified as a single carbohydrate epitope comprising a terminal trisaccharide: galactosyl α-1,3-galactosyl β-1,4-N-acetylglucosaminyl (Gal). By combining organs expressing hDAF with a Gal glycoconjugate — which mops up the xenoantibodies — the survival of pig hearts to baboon has been extended to over 2 months. 'Knock-out' pigs have been subsequently generated in which the gene encoding the enzyme responsible for the production of the damaging epitope, α-1,3-galactosyl transferase, is crippled. In this setting, the pig-to-primate heart graft survives 6 months. These extending survival times, from days to months, are very encouraging — but non-Gal xenoantibodies have also now been detected and the search for ideal xenografting conditions is far from over.

---

individual, which express his or her MHC molecules, are quite different to the tissues of the next individual, and so on. These differences in the tissues are picked up by the immune system and form the basis for the vigorous anti-donor-MHC immune response that can occur when organs are transplanted. The nomenclature used to describe different types of transplant is summarised in the box: 'Nomenclature'.

Nomenclature

- Autograft or autologous transplant: the organ/tissue is transplanted within the same individual. It does not undergo rejection.

- Syngraft or syngeneic transplant: the organ/tissue is transplanted between genetically identical subjects, such as monozygotic twins or inbred laboratory animals. It does not undergo rejection.

- Allograft or allogeneic transplant: the organ/tissue is transplanted between genetically non-identical members of the same species. It is rejected unless immunosuppression is instituted.

- Xenograft or xenogeneic transplant: the organ/tissue is transplanted between members of different species. It is rejected hyperacutely.

On the basis of studies in genetically identical inbred animals some rules of transplantation have been established (Fig. 11.1):

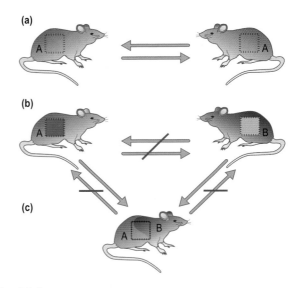

Fig. 11.1 Rules of transplantation.
(**a**) A syngeneic transplantation, within individuals of an inbred strain, always succeeds. (**b**) An allogeneic transplantation, between individuals of different inbred strains, always fails. (**c**) A transplantation from an inbred parent to a hybrid (F1) offspring succeeds, but grafts from the offspring to either parent will fail. Moreover, whilst the immunocompetent cells of AB react with neither of the alloantigens encoded by A or B, the cells of A or B can react against alloantigens present in AB. In the last example, the graft is not rejected itself but provides immunocompetent cells that attack the host, through the recognition of alloantigenic differences, in what is known as graft-versus-host (GVH) reaction. GVH occurs when immunocompetent cells are transferred into an animal that cannot reject them either for genetic reasons, as in the case depicted, or following immunosuppression.

- transplantations within inbred strains will succeed

- transplantation between inbred strains will fail

- transplantations from an inbred parent to a hybrid (F1) offspring will succeed, but grafts from the offspring to either parent will fail.

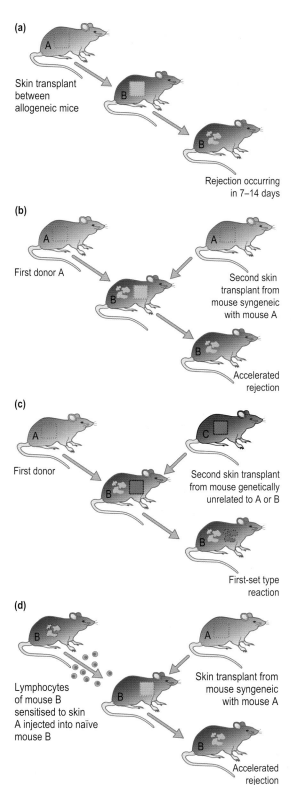

(a)

Skin transplant between allogeneic mice

Rejection occurring in 7–14 days

(b)

First donor A

Second skin transplant from mouse syngeneic with mouse A

Accelerated rejection

(c)

First donor

Second skin transplant from mouse genetically unrelated to A or B

First-set type reaction

(d)

Lymphocytes of mouse B sensitised to skin A injected into naïve mouse B

Skin transplant from mouse syngeneic with mouse A

Accelerated rejection

Using inbred animals it has been possible to define the dynamic process of rejection (Fig. 11.2). Transplanting a segment of skin from mouse A into the genetically unrelated mouse B (allotransplantation), the skin is rejected in 7–14 days (first-set or primary rejection). If mouse B is transplanted again with skin of mouse A, the rejection occurs much more speedily (second-set or secondary rejection). A second-set rejection occurs even if the skin derives not from the very same mouse A but from a mouse of the same inbred strain, a syngeneic mouse. If the transplanted tissue, however, derives from a third-party mouse C, genetically unrelated to both mouse A and B, the skin is eliminated following the pattern of a first-set type of rejection. In common with conventional immune responses, therefore, antigraft immunity has the characteristics of memory and specificity.

SUMMARY BOX 11.2

Introductory points

■ Transplantation is used to replace organs that have undergone an irreversible pathological process, which threatens the patient's life or considerably hampers the quality of life.

■ In humans, the organ usually derives from a genetically unrelated individual (allograft), rarely from a monozygous twin (syngraft); in the future it may derive from a member of a different species (xenograft).

■ An allograft would normally be rejected. This is prevented by immunosuppression. A syngraft is never rejected, while a xenograft is rejected hyperacutely.

Mechanisms of rejection

In an attempt to understand the mechanisms of rejection, tissues of the rejecting organs obtained by biopsy have been analysed. They invariably contain an inflammatory infiltrate predominantly composed of mononuclear white blood cells, i.e. lymphocytes and macrophages. The analysis of such infiltrates with monoclonal antibodies has demonstrated their composition to be heterogeneous, with CD4 cells, CD8 cells, macrophages, B lymphocytes and natural killer cells all being

Fig. 11.2 Types of rejection.
(**a**) Transplantation of a skin graft from mouse A to the genetically unrelated mouse B (allograft) results in rejection of the skin graft. This starts manifesting itself 1 week post-transplant and leads to the elimination of the graft though a process of primary — or first-set — rejection. (**b**) If a mouse B is grafted a second time with skin from mouse A or from a mouse genetically identical to A, the ensuing rejection is accelerated. (**c**) If mouse B is grafted a second time but with skin from a mouse C, unrelated to B or A, the ensuing rejection has the features of a primary rejection. (**d**) The lymphocytes of a mouse that has undergone rejection are able to transfer the memory of sensitisation to a naïve mouse, such that on engraftment of skin a second-set rejection occurs.

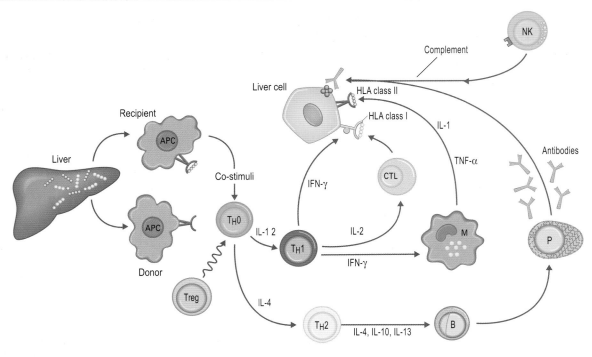

Fig. 11.3 Immune responses to a liver graft.
Intact alloantigens present on donor APCs or allopeptides present in the groove of the recipient's HLA molecules are presented to an uncommitted T helper (T_H0) lymphocyte. T_H0 cells become activated and, according to the nature of the alloantigen and the presence in the microenvironment of IL-12 or IL-4, differentiate into T_H1 or T_H2 cells to initiate a series of immune reactions. These are determined by the cytokines produced: T_H2 cells secrete mainly IL-4 and IL-10 and direct alloantibody production by B lymphocytes; T_H1 cells secrete IL-2 and IFN-γ, which stimulate cytotoxic T lymphocytes (CTL), enhance expression of class I and induce expression of class II HLA molecules on hepatocytes and activate macrophages. Activated macrophages release IL-1 and TNF-α. If T regulatory (Treg) lymphocytes do not oppose, a variety of effector mechanisms are triggered: liver cell destruction could derive from the action of CTL; cytokines released by T_H1 cells and recruited macrophages; complement activation; and/or engagement of FcR-bearing natural killer (NK) cells by the alloantibody bound to the hepatocyte surface.

represented. Therefore, the analysis of the infiltrate characterising cellular rejection (see below) that occurs 7–14 days post-operatively does not suggest the involvement of a single type of immunocompetent cell, or indeed a single mechanism, in the development of rejection.

There is evidence to suggest that the mechanisms prevailing during physiological immune responses also apply to graft rejection (Fig. 11.3). As in classical immune responses, it is the balance between the different components of the immune system that decrees the magnitude and manifestations of the rejection process. Once a virgin (or naïve) helper CD4 cell designated T_H0 has recognised an alloantigen, presented by a professional antigen-presenting cell such as a dendritic cell, which is singularly competent in providing the co-stimulation signals needed to arouse virgin cells, it can become either a T_H1 or a T_H2 cell according to the microenvironment it encounters and the nature of the alloantigenic stimulus. If the surrounding medium is rich in IL-12, a macrophage-derived cytokine, the virgin T_H0 CD4 cell will commit itself to the T_H1 phenotype and function and orchestrate the activation of CD8 cytotoxic T cells and of macrophages through the release of IL-2 and IFN-γ. If, however, the prevailing cytokine is IL-4, the virgin cell will differentiate into the T_H2 phenotype, and through the secretion of IL-4

and IL-10 will direct the activation of B lymphocytes and antibody production. The study of proteins and RNA transcripts within the graft during cellular rejection has consistently shown the presence of IL-2 and IFN-γ and of granzyme B, a specific marker of cytotoxic T cells, but not of IL-4, suggesting the execution of a T_H1-directed programme during rejection episodes. IFN-γ would recruit and activate macrophages and enhance MHC expression on the graft, making it particularly susceptible to the cytotoxic action of CD8 cells; IL-2 would, in turn, favour the activation of cytotoxic T cells. There is some evidence indicating the involvement of cells of the T_H2 phenotype in the induction of graft tolerance.

Alloantigen recognition

So, what is it about an allograft that induces such a potent immune response? The antigens recognised during rejection are referred to as **alloantigens** and, as mentioned earlier, the key alloantigens are those encoded by the MHC. In humans these are known as HLA molecules. The physiological function of such molecules is to present peptide antigen to a complementary T cell receptor. The key question arises as to how MHC-derived alloantigens are recognised. Two possibilities exist (Fig. 11.4). First, the recipient's immune system could recognise an intact MHC molecule (**direct allorecognition**). Second, a peptide (allopeptide) derived from the foreign MHC molecule could be presented within the groove of the recipient's own MHC molecule (**indirect allorecognition**). It has been established that cells capable of recognising intact donor-MHC molecules outnumber those recognising processed allopeptides by 1000–10 000.

Classification of rejection reactions

In clinical practice, the vast majority of transplanted organs are allogeneic and, in spite of immunosuppression therapy, tend to undergo episodes of rejection of different severity. Rejection can be classified according to the timescale of its appearance and to the immune mechanisms involved (Table 11.1).

Hyperacute rejection

Hyperacute rejection is mediated by preformed antibodies in the recipient that are directed against antigens of the donor organ; it occurs within minutes to a few hours after implantation, depending on the concentration and type of the 'anti-donor' antibody present in the recipient. Transplants across the ABO blood group barrier provide examples of hyperacute rejection, which can be particularly dramatic

Table 11.1 Classification of rejection

Type	Time after transplantation	Probable mechanism
Hyperacute	Minutes	Preformed antibodies
Accelerated acute	1–5 days	T lymphocytes
Acute	From 2nd week	T lymphocytes
Chronic	Months to years	Antibodies, complement, adhesion molecules

when an organ from a group A or B donor is transplanted into an O recipient, whose circulation contains anti-A and anti-B antibodies (isohaemagglutinins). Remember that ABO blood group antigens are abundantly expressed on endothelial cells. Hyperacute rejection can also be mediated by antibodies directed against donor HLA class I molecules, the origin of which can be traced to previous leukocyte-containing blood transfusions, previous transplants or pregnancies. The recipient's preformed antibodies bind to the endothelium in vessels and activate complement and the clotting cascade, leading to the formation of thrombi and necrosis of the implanted organ. In addition to antibodies and complement, a heavy polymorphonuclear leukocyte infiltration characterises hyperacute rejection.

The approach to managing hyperacute rejection is preventative — there is the need to identify whether preformed antibodies against donor antigens are present in the recipient (see section below on presensitisation) and thus avoid transplanting in this context. A further approach is to exploit a phenomenon known as **accommodation**. This has been described after the transplantation of an ABO-incompatible organ, when temporary depletion of the natural antibodies (immediately before the transplant and subsequently for a period of several days) may result in long-term graft survival, despite the return of the antibodies in the presence of their specific target antigens.

Acute rejection

Acute rejection is mediated by T lymphocytes and becomes apparent some 7 days post-operatively. The recipient's T cells recognise alloantigens mainly through the mechanism of direct allorecognition (see above). Lymphocyte- and monocyte-rich cell infiltrations characterise this type of reaction. An accelerated form of acute rejection that occurs within 1–5 days post-transplant is probably mediated by T lymphocytes that have been previously sensitised to alloantigens (e.g. through transfusions, pregnancies).

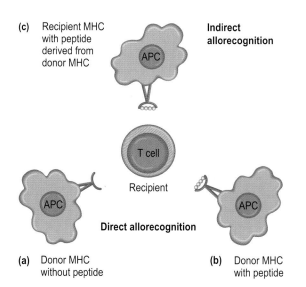

(c) Recipient MHC with peptide derived from donor MHC

Indirect allorecognition

APC

T cell

Recipient

APC

APC

Direct allorecognition

(a) Donor MHC without peptide

(b) Donor MHC with peptide

Fig. 11.4 **Types of allorecognition.**
The recipient's T cells have the potential of recognising HLA molecules as they are (**a**) or loaded with 'carry-over' peptides (**b**), the latter generated through the processing of antigens that occurred in the donor until the day of donation. The carry-over peptide magnifies the range of alloantigens to be recognised by the recipient's immune system. (a) and (b) depict the two forms of direct allorecognition. (**c**) An alloantigen, typically an HLA molecule, can be taken up and processed by the recipient's APC and then its peptides be presented to autologous T cells. This exemplifies indirect allorecognition.

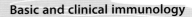

The therapeutic approach to acute rejection is immune suppression, which is discussed below.

Chronic rejection

Chronic rejection appears months or years after successful transplantation. It is the major cause of long-term graft loss, but its pathophysiology is poorly understood. It is thought that an early damage to the vascular endothelium, whether or not immune in nature, is a predisposing factor to this late complication. The endothelium may be further damaged by antibodies to alloantigens, deposition of immune complexes, activation of complement, exposure of collagen and activation of the clotting cascade. This would favour endothelial cell proliferation and narrowing of the vascular lumen. Cell infiltration is not a major feature of chronic rejection, although macrophages are deemed to play an important role through cytokine release (IL-1, IL-6, TNF-α). Adhesion molecules are up-regulated on endothelial cells.

No tests can predict the development of the chronic rejection and no drugs can control or reverse it.

Graft-versus-host reactions

A singular immunological condition arises when grafts containing immunocompetent cells are engrafted into immunologically incompetent recipients. Immunocompetent cells from the graft recognise alloantigens of the recipient and the recipient develops a disorder known as the graft-versus-host (GVH) reaction. This reaction is common after transplantation of bone marrow, even when the matching between donor and recipient has been stringent. When GVH becomes symptomatic the term graft-versus-host disease (GVHD) is more appropriate. GVHD has been described not only following bone marrow transplantation but also, occasionally, after liver transplantation and even after blood transfusions. GVHD can be divided into two distinct entities: acute disease, occurring in the first 1 or 2 months after transplantation, and chronic disease, developing at least 2 or 3 months after transplantation. In humans, GVHD typically affects the skin, liver, intestinal tract and immune system and appears within days or weeks after bone marrow transplantation. In mild GVH reactions, patients manifest erythema of the palms, soles and ears. Hepatic signs of mild reactions are limited to asymptomatic hyperbilirubinaemia, and gastrointestinal involvement is indicated by mild diarrhoea. In the case of severe GVHD, the skin lesions can include a necrolytic disorder, characterised by blister formation and desquamation. Severe liver abnormalities include jaundice, elevation of alkaline phosphatase, which denotes cholestasis, and of transaminases, a sign of liver cell damage. Severe gastrointestinal GVHD includes abdominal pain and diarrhoea, with life-threatening electrolyte abnormalities. These manifestations are the result of injury to the epithelial cells of the target organs. Mild GVH may resolve spontaneously or with mild immunosuppressive treatments. Severe GVH is usually unresponsive to treatments and has a fatal outcome. The chronic form of the disease shares certain clinical characteristics with systemic sclerosis (see p. 186).

The most effective prophylaxis of acute GVHD is a combination of methotrexate and ciclosporin. Treatment of established acute GVHD is with methylprednisolone, ciclosporin/tacrolimus, at times associated with T cell depletion with the anti-CD52 monoclonal antibody Campath-1.

The problem of donor organs

Current transplantation medicine is highly advanced, with most organ grafts providing excellent function and either saving lives or significantly reducing morbidity. Organs have been traditionally provided by the cadaveric donor, usually following a road traffic accident. Despite brain death the donor can be maintained on life support systems for hours/days whilst the ethical and practical issues of donation are addressed (e.g. HLA matching, see below). However, the organ supply through this route does not match demand. Additional options have therefore been introduced in recent years. One option in some centres is the non-beating heart donor; here, a sudden death is followed by immediate (20–30 minutes) removal of organs. There has also been an increase in living related donors — siblings, parents, and even spouses.

Tissue typing

Matching for molecules of the HLA system is the ideal criterion for selection of donors for allografts. How well this aim is achieved is in some ways dictated by the demand, the organ for grafting and the type of donor. Transplantation of kidneys, the most commonly performed type of graft, provides a good example of 'ideal' practice. Kidneys are reasonably robust — therefore up to 48 hours of cold ischaemia (i.e. the period in which the explanted organ is preserved in the cold) can elapse between explant and reimplantation of kidneys without major prejudice to their viability or function. With cadaveric donation, therefore, there is sufficient time for HLA typing and matching. HLA types are routinely determined for HLA-A, HLA-B and HLA-DR, using rapid DNA-based techniques (see p. 59). Thus it is possible to type a donor, find the best country-wide match using national databases, and transport the kidney. Potential kidney recipients are usually on life-preserving haemodialysis and can therefore wait for a good organ match. The benefit of HLA matching has been clearly demonstrated in large series of kidney transplants. Although it is also apparent in heart transplants that HLA matching is beneficial, it is generally precluded by time constraints (a period of 4 hours of cold ischaemia is the longest considered safe in heart transplantation) and the urgent clinical need — better to graft the heart and use stronger anti-rejection drugs than wait for matching.

Therefore, a full work-up is logistically feasible for the transplantation of kidneys but not yet for heart and other organs. In the context of renal transplantation, the clinical benefits of matching have been demonstrated unambiguously in a large prospective study based on cadaveric donors. The 1-year graft survival was 88% for HLA-matched kidneys and 79% for mismatched kidneys. This advantage was heightened beyond the first year after transplantation (Fig. 11.5). Increasing degrees of HLA-A, HLA-B and HLA-DR antigen matching improves graft survival in a gradual fashion (Fig. 11.6).

The analysis of some 8000 patients who underwent cardiac transplantation also demonstrates an impressive correlation between matching for HLA-A, HLA-B and HLA-DR and graft survival.

For living related donation of kidneys, good HLA matching will be an ideal but not an absolute requirement. In this context, some compensation is achieved by the excellent graft function obtained when using a healthy donor and very short ischaemia time (because donor and recipient are in the same hospital).

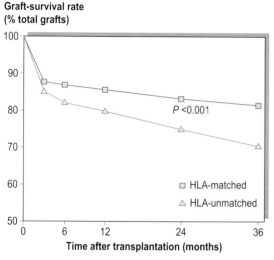

Fig. 11.5 **Tissue typing and graft survival.**
Effect of matching for HLA-A, HLA-B and HLA-DR on graft survival. Graft-survival rates in HLA-matched compared with those in HLA-unmatched cadaveric renal transplants (modified from Takemoto 1992 New England Journal of Medicine, 327: 834–839).

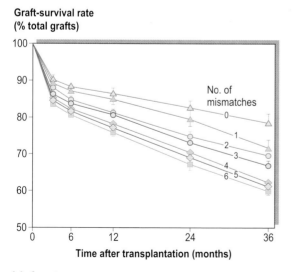

Fig. 11.6 **Influence of the number of matches on graft-survival rates in cadaveric renal transplants.**
The survival rate falls with the number of mismatches of HLA-A, HLA-B and HLA-DR antigens (modified from Terasaki 1991 Clinical transplants. Los Angeles CA, UCLA Tissue Typing Laboratory, pp. 409–430).

Presensitisation

The presence of antibodies that react with antigens of the graft may have disastrous results. Hyperacute reactions, which are mediated by complement-fixing antibodies, are virtually irreversible. The existence of presensitisation is tested for by incubating the serum of the recipient and the lymphocytes of the donor. Binding of antibodies in the recipient serum is analysed using flow cytometry (see p. 89). Presensitisation is considered an absolute contraindication in renal transplantation, where a positive cross-match is usually predictive of hyperacute rejection. If the clinical need dictates, removal of preformed antibodies can be achieved by plasma exchange, immune suppression or removal of B lymphocytes using anti-CD20 monoclonal antibody (see p. 308). Currently, presensitisation is not routinely evaluated in cardiac and liver transplantation.

SUMMARY BOX 11.3

Mechanisms of rejection

- There are different types of rejection. Hyperacute rejection results from preformed antibodies to HLA class I antigens or antigens of the ABO blood group. Acute and accelerated acute rejections are caused by cellular allorecognition of the graft. The mechanisms of chronic rejection are unknown.

- The transfer of immunocompetent allogeneic cells into an immune depressed individual leads to these rejecting the recipient (graft-versus-host reaction; GVH). This is known as graft-versus-host disease (GVHD) when accompanied by clinical manifestations.

- Good HLA matching prolongs graft survival. Pre-operative matching is routinely done for renal transplants, but not for liver, heart and lung transplants because of the short periods for which the latter organs maintain their function when explanted. This limitation will soon be remedied by use of rapid molecular HLA typing techniques.

- Presensitisation, i.e. the presence of preformed antibodies to HLA class I or ABO antigens in the recipient's blood, is tested for in renal but not other types of transplantation. This policy is currently under review.

Immunosuppressive therapy

Drugs

The action of the immunosuppressive drugs discussed here is not specifically 'anti-rejection'. These drugs are widely used in a range of conditions in which a 'dampening down' of the immune system is required. However, several of them, most notably ciclosporin A, have transformed clinical transplantation and for this reason it is appropriate that the pharmacological approach to controlling rejection be discussed here (Table 11.2). In Chapter 22, these drugs and their modes of action are discussed in greater detail.

Azathioprine

The antimetabolite azathioprine acts as a purine antagonist and functions as an effective antiproliferative agent. It was for two decades the keystone to immunosuppressive therapy in humans.

Corticosteroids

Corticosteroids have multiple effects on the immune system, including a decrease in the numbers of circulating B lymphocytes and inhibition of monocyte trafficking, T cell proliferation and cytokine gene expression (i.e. transcription of IL-1, IL-2, IL-6, INF-γ and TNF-α). Side-effects of these drugs on skin, bones and other tissues continue to present problems in clinical transplantation. Glucocorticoids are important adjuncts to immunosuppressive therapy in transplantation. **Prednisone** is given immediately before or at the time of transplantation, and its dosage is gradually reduced. **Methylprednisolone** is administered immediately upon diagnosis of beginning rejection and continued once daily for 3 days. Although azathioprine and prednisone can be used successfully to control graft rejection, both of these agents act non-specifically on the immune system.

Table 11.2 Mechanisms of action of immunosuppressive drugs

Agent	Mode of action
Azathioprine	Inhibits purine synthesis
Corticosteroids	Block cytokine gene expression
Ciclosporin A; tacrolimus	Block Ca^{2+}-dependent T cell activation pathway
Sirolimus	Blocks IL-2 triggered proliferation and CD28/CTLA-4 mediated co-stimulatory signals

Ciclosporin A

Ciclosporin A, the first calcineurin inhibitor to be used in clinical practice, is a small fungal cyclic peptide that has had a major impact on clinical transplantation since the early 1980s, significantly increasing graft-survival rates and reducing the incidence of severe GVHD following bone marrow transplantation. The major effects of ciclosporin A on T cells is through the inhibition of IL-2 secretion. Another possible mode of action of ciclosporin A is the stimulation of production of cell growth-inhibitory cytokines, such as TGF-β. Because TGF-β inhibits both T cell proliferation and the generation of cytotoxic lymphocytes, a heightened production of TGF-β may contribute to the immunosuppressive activity of ciclosporin A. A common, dose-dependent and partially reversible side-effect of ciclosporin A is nephrotoxicity.

Tacrolimus

Tacrolimus is a macrolide antibiotic isolated from a Japanese soil fungus, *Streptomyces tsukubaensis*, with similar immunosuppressive effects, mechanisms and renal side-effects to those of ciclosporin. Due to their similar mechanism of action ciclosporin and tacrolimus are collectively referred to as calcineurin inhibitors (see p. 315).

Sirolimus

Sirolimus, previously known as rapamycin, is a macrocyclic lactone that inhibits biochemical pathways that are required for cell progression through the late G1 phase or entry into the S phase of the cell cycle and is therefore labelled as antiproliferative. As a major side-effect, sirolimus causes hypertriglyceridaemia.

Antibodies

Antibodies can be used to target specific immune cells thought to be involved in rejection. The function of the targeted cells is abolished or lessened either through antibody-directed cell lysis or modulation of surface molecules. Polyclonal and monoclonal antibodies can be made that react with cell surface molecules expressed by all lymphocytes, by T cells but not B cells, by some T cells, for example CD4 or CD8 subsets, or by activated but not resting T cells, for example those expressing IL-2 receptor (CD25).

Monoclonal antibodies have the advantage of monospecificity and can be purified to homogeneity. Not all monoclonal antibodies specific for the same molecule may have the same effects in vivo since (1) they may react with different epitopes and deliver a different signal to the cell, and (2) antibodies with specificity for an identical epitope, but with different Fc regions, may have different properties.

Polyclonal antilymphocyte and antithymocyte globulin

Since the early 1980s, antilymphocyte globulin (ALG) and antithymocyte globulin (ATG) have been used by many transplant centres for the treatment of rejection episodes. These polyclonal antisera are composed of multiple antibodies specific for a variety of lymphocyte cell surface molecules. Both ALG and ATG are prepared by injecting lymphocytes or thymocytes into horses, rabbits or goats to produce anti-lymphocyte serum, from which the globulin fraction is then separated. The thymus is greatly enriched in T cells. One problem is variation between different preparations of anti-sera. The main adverse effect is fever, which results from the release of pyrogens owing to the rapid breakdown of lymphoid cells.

Monoclonal anti-CD3

The mouse monoclonal antibody OKT3, which recognises the human CD3 molecule, has been used to treat recipients of allografts in clinical transplantation. Intravenous administration of OKT3 clears T cells from the circulation very efficiently, presumably by opsonisation. An increase in the number of circulating lymphocytes that are unreactive with OKT3 but are reactive with antibodies directed at other T cell markers is also observed, suggesting that one mode of action of OKT3 is modulation of the CD3 molecule from the surface of T cells. The major disadvantages of anti-CD3 monoclonal antibody treatment are its side-effects and the development of anti-mouse Ig antibodies in approximately 75% of patients. As a result, OKT3 therapy can only effectively be used to treat a rejection episode after transplantation.

Monoclonal anti-CD4 and anti-CD8

Monoclonal antibodies specific for the two major subsets of T cells are also available. The immunosuppressive properties of monoclonal antibodies specific for the human CD4 molecule, OKT4, have been tested in a primate model; however, the results obtained were not very encouraging. Nonetheless, clinical trials of anti-CD4 monoclonal antibody therapy are currently in progress.

Monoclonal antibodies specific for activation antigens

When T cells respond to antigen and become activated, they express the IL-2 receptor. Targeting this receptor may allow more selective immunosuppressive therapy. This antibody is used in islet transplantation (see p. 163).

Side-effects of antibody therapy

Significant untoward events are associated with clinical use of OKT3 and antilymphocyte ALG/ATG. Soon after administration, some patients experience a syndrome of fever and myalgia that is believed to be caused by systemic release of cytokines. The second major adverse event is development of lymphomas. These account for about 65% of all tumours that develop in transplantation recipients, and they occur in 1–2% of all recipients of transplanted organs. Like other immunosuppressive drugs, immunosuppressive antibodies also increase the risk of infectious complications in recipients.

Immunosuppressive regimens

Typical immunosuppressive regimens involve the use of multiple immunosuppressive drugs acting at different levels of T cell activation. A standard regimen includes tacrolimus and corticosteroids.

Antilymphocyte antibodies are used in some centres before transplantation to prevent the activation of anti-graft immune responses or during episodes of rejection. The treatment is effective but is accompanied by an increased incidence of lymphoproliferative disorders and possibly of infections. The administration of the murine anti-CD3 antibody OKT3 is associated with an early cytokine-mediated set of manifestations that include fever, chills and, in some cases, hypotension, pulmonary oedema, encephalopathy and nephropathy; these together constitute a capillary leak syndrome.

Furthermore, because of its murine nature, OKT3 is the target of the recipient anti-murine Ig immune response that can reduce the antibody efficacy during the first cycle of treatment and prevent its use in future episodes of rejection. Attempts are being made to 'humanise' murine monoclonal antibodies, such that the murine antigen-recognising elements of the immunoglobulin are inserted onto a human immunoglobulin background.

Common complications of allotransplantation

As a consequence of the vigorous immunosuppression required to avoid allograft rejection, a number of complications, including infections and malignancies, commonly arise after transplantation. Bacterial, fungal or viral infections are frequent and may be life threatening early after surgery. After the first post-operative month, those opportunistic infections that typically emerge when the cellular immune system is impaired start appearing. Agents frequently responsible include cytomegalovirus (see below), herpes viruses, fungal organisms (*Aspergillus* and *Nocardia* spp., cryptococcal infection), mycobacteria and parasites (*Pneumocystis*, *Toxoplasma* spp.).

Cytomegalovirus infection

This is the most frequent and pathologically important post-transplant infection. Cytomegalovirus (CMV) belongs to the β herpes virus group, has a worldwide distribution and its spread normally requires repeated or prolonged intimate exposure. Transfusions containing viable leukocytes also transmit CMV. CMV infection probably lasts for life and usually remains latent. In patients with impaired T cell immunity (e.g. the recipients of organ transplants), CMV frequently reactivates. Primary CMV infections also occur in recipients of organ transplants and derive from the graft itself. Reactivation of latent virus or, occasionally, reinfection with a new strain accounts for the infection in CMV-seropositive transplant recipients.

Chronic antigen stimulation provided by the allograft in association with immunosuppression appears to be an ideal setting for CMV activation and CMV-induced disease. In renal, cardiac, lung, liver and bone marrow transplant recipients, CMV is responsible for several manifestations including fever, leukopenia, hepatitis, pneumonitis, oesophagitis, gastritis and colitis, typically starting 1 month after surgery. CMV retinitis can appear later. The transplanted organ is peculiarly susceptible to CMV, with hepatitis arising after liver transplantation and CMV pneumonitis after lung transplantation. A number of measures are implemented to reduce the impact of CMV infection in transplantation, including using blood and organs from seronegative donors for seronegative recipients and matching of organ or bone marrow transplants by CMV serology.

Ganciclovir, a guanosine derivative, is used in the treatment of CMV infection, since it is a selective inhibitor of CMV DNA polymerase.

Malignancies

With the improved survival of patients receiving an allograft, an increase in the incidence of malignancies has also been observed. The use of multiple immunosuppressive drugs has been implicated as a strong contributing factor for this increased susceptibility to malignancy. The most common cancers seen after organ transplantation are lymphoma, skin cancer and Kaposi's sarcoma. The increased incidence of malignancy is a major factor in the increased morbidity and late failure rates in transplant recipients. That immunosuppression has a key role in predisposing to malignant tumours is demonstrated by the relatively common occurrence of malignancies such as Kaposi's sarcoma and lymphomas in patients with AIDS. Immunosuppressive therapy is likely to favour growth of neoplastic cells by reducing mechanisms of immune surveillance. The overall incidence of skin cancer in kidney transplant patients is about 100 times higher than in control populations, with cutaneous carcinomas accounting for about 50% of cancers and the incidence increasing with time after renal transplantation.

The development of **lymphoproliferative diseases** is also dependent on immunosuppression, induced by drugs such as ciclosporin, tacrolimus and OKT3. In the setting of allotransplantation, these disorders are particularly aggressive, with a high incidence of central nervous system and extranodal involvement; they are mainly classified as B cell-derived, large-cell non-Hodgkin's lymphomas and can be polyclonal or monoclonal. Their outcome is poor, unless immunosuppressive therapy can be stopped. The origin of these lymphoproliferative diseases has been ascribed to the effect of the oncogenic Epstein–Barr virus over B cells constantly stimulated by the allograft. Immunosuppression would play a catalysing role.

Clinical transplantation

Kidney transplantation

The indications for kidney transplantation include end-stage renal disease caused by type 1 diabetes mellitus, chronic glomerulonephritis, polycystic kidney disease, nephrosclerosis, systemic lupus erythematosus, interstitial nephritis, IgA nephropathy and Alport's syndrome. The use of ciclosporin has improved cadaveric graft-survival rates to over 80% at 1 year and to 70% at 5 years. Graft loss from rejection is much slower after the first year. Donors can be cadavers or volunteer blood-related living donors: in Europe up to 85% of kidneys come from cadavers.

Preservation for at least 48 hours is achieved by flushing the kidney with appropriate solutions and by storage in ice. The surgical procedure differs according to the age of the recipient. In adults, the renal graft is placed extraperitoneally in the iliac fossa; in small children, it is placed retroperitoneally.

HLA matching is routinely practised for selection of donors for renal allografts, and potential recipients are normally screened for preformed antibodies to HLA class I antigens. The histological appearance of acute renal rejection, typically occurring 7–14 days post-transplant, is shown in Figures 11.7 and 11.8.

The failure of transplanted kidneys after several years of adequate function is attributed to 'chronic rejection'. This is characterised by the development of nephrosclerosis, with proliferation of the vascular intima of renal vessels, and intimal fibrosis, resulting in decrease in the lumen of the vessels (Fig. 11.9). Current modes of treatment have little effect on the progression of chronic rejection, which remains the most common cause of failure of long-term allografts.

Amongst other complications, dyslipidaemia is frequently observed, with cardiovascular disease being the most common cause of long-term mortality in these patients. The

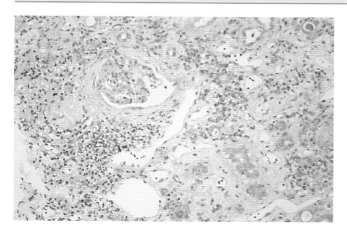

Fig. 11.7 **Mononuclear cells, including lymphocytes, macrophages and plasma cells, infiltrate the renal interstitium and tubular epithelial cells (lymphocytic tubulitis) in acute cellular rejection.**
(Courtesy of Dr P. J. O'Donnell.)

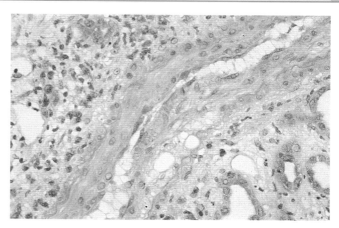

Fig. 11.9 **A medium calibre artery shows considerable luminal narrowing due to intimal fibrosis, mucoid change and smooth muscle proliferation in chronic renal rejection.**
(Courtesy of Dr P. J. O'Donnell.)

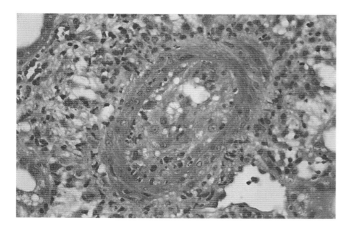

Fig. 11.8 **A small artery shows oedema and mononuclear cell infiltration of the intima with disruption of the endothelial lining in acute vascular rejection of the kidney.**
(Courtesy of Dr P. J. O'Donnell.)

original disease recurs in 10 to 20% of grafts, recurrent glomerulonephritis in the transplanted kidney being common. The nephritides that recur most commonly are membranous glomerulonephritis, mesangiocapillary glomerulonephritis and IgA nephropathy.

Liver transplantation

The indication for liver transplantation is irreversible liver disease. The aetiology of this can differ in children and adults. Indications common to both age groups include end-stage cirrhosis and fulminant liver failure of whatever origin. Biliary atresia, inherited or genetic metabolic disorders associated with liver failure are characteristic of childhood, while chronic hepatitis C, alcoholic cirrhosis and primary biliary cirrhosis are typical of adults. Following the introduction of calcineurin inhibitors, 1-year survival rates approach 85% while the 5-year survival rates are approximately 75%. Donors are selected on the basis of negativity for bacterial or fungal infections and exclusion of hepatitis B and C viruses and human immunodeficiency virus (HIV). Compatibility for ABO blood groups is assessed even though ABO-incompatible donors are used in emergencies. Tissue typing for HLA matching is not routinely performed, and presensitisation is not an exclusion criterion in liver transplantation (see Clinical Box 11.1). There are studies to demonstrate, however, that histocompatibility testing and assessment of presensitisation would also improve the outcome in liver transplantation.

Liver preservation can last up to 24 hours with the use of graft preservers such as 'University of Wisconsin solution', which is rich in lactobionate and raffinose.

Acute rejection of the transplanted liver occurs in the majority of patients, beginning 1 to 2 weeks after surgery and is accompanied by increases in serum bilirubin and aminotransferase levels. These elevations, however, lack specificity. Liver biopsy is often performed to establish the correct diagnosis. The histological appearance shows mononuclear cell portal infiltration, bile duct injury and endothelial inflammation ('endothelialitis') (Figs 11.10 & 11.11).

Chronic rejection is characterised by progressive cholestasis, focal parenchymal necrosis, mononuclear infiltration, vascular lesions and fibrosis (Fig. 11.12).

Recurrence of the initial condition is almost invariable for hepatitis B and C. Diseases with a putatative immune pathogenesis, such as primary biliary cirrhosis, sclerosing cholangitis and autoimmune hepatitis, have also been reported to recur occasionally.

Pancreas transplantation

Pancreas transplantation has not yet become a standard mode of treatment. It is a life-enhancing not a life-saving procedure, as the transplantation of other organs is. The

News in liver transplantation

A number of new approaches are currently being implemented in liver transplantation.

'Split' livers. This refers to the use of one liver for two recipients. This procedure helps in tackling organ shortage and in shortening the time on the waiting list. The operation is technically demanding and requires the simultaneous work of two transplant teams.

Auxiliary orthotopic transplantation. This refers to the transplantation of a segment of donor liver in a recipient who has undergone hemi-hepatectomy to make room for the graft. Orthotopic means that the graft is placed in its correct anatomical location. This procedure is used to offset enzymatic liver defects that are not accompanied by structural hepatic damage (e.g. Crigler–Najjar syndrome, propionic acidaemia, urea cycle defects) but are responsible for lethal systemic effects. In this setting, if the donor's liver fails, the recipient's own organ can function as a backup until a new liver is found. Auxiliary transplantation is also used as a temporary measure in fulminant liver failure, where the recipient's liver has the potential of regeneration and full functional recovery. This avoids life-long immunosuppression.

Living related donors. The donor of the liver segment is typically a first-degree living relative. The operation can be carefully planned and it is usually performed when the recipient is still in relatively good condition. When the organ donation comes from a blood relative — and not from a spouse — rejection is less frequent and less severe. This procedure avoids damage to the liver resulting from preservation but does present some risks for the donor.

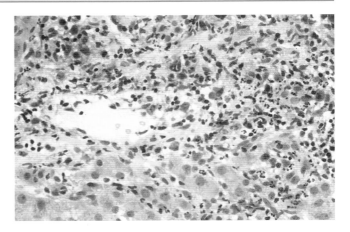

Fig. 11.11 Magnified view of endothelitis affecting a portal vein radicle.
(Courtesy of Professor B. Portmann.)

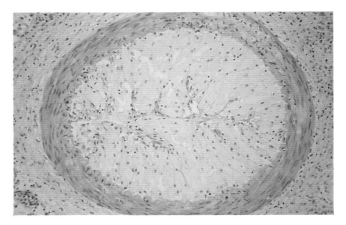

Fig. 11.12 Arterial damage typical of chronic liver rejection.
The arteriole is occluded by 'foamy' cells, inflammatory cells and fibrin. (Courtesy of Professor B. Portmann.)

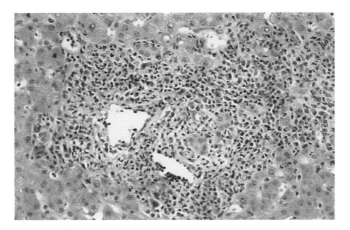

Fig. 11.10 Mononuclear cells including lymphocytes, lymphoblasts and macrophages infiltrate a portal tract during acute liver rejection.
Lymphocytes damage the endothelial lining of portal vein radicles. Bile duct epithelial cells are swollen and damaged. (Courtesy of Professor B. Portmann.)

main indication is insulin-dependent diabetes, where the graft would improve not only the metabolic imbalance but also help in preventing late diabetic complications. It has been typically performed in nephropathic diabetic patients in association with a kidney allograft, the logic being that the immunosuppression is being given anyway, so why not add in another, much needed organ replacement. Transplantation of the pancreas as a whole or as a segment has proved highly successful in curing diabetes, and reduces the progression of diabetic complications.

The transplantation of isolated islets of Langerhans has been repeatedly attempted with relatively unrewarding results until a decade ago. But in recent years, scientists at the University of Alberta in Edmonton, Canada, have devised a new procedure called the Edmonton Protocol to treat patients with type 1 diabetes. Islets are isolated by ductal perfusion with cold, purified collagenase and transplanted immediately into the recipient's liver. Immunosuppression consists of a glucocorticoid-free regimen comprising sirolimus, tacrolimus and the anti-CD25 monoclonal antibody known as Daclizumab. One year after transplantation 84% of patients remain insulin free and after three years, 89% of patients are still producing insulin.

Heart transplantation

The indication for heart transplantation is a cardiac disease unresponsive to conventional medical or surgical treatment and likely to cause the patient's death within 6–12 months. Cardiomyopathy and congenital uncorrectable defects are the main indications in children, while coronary heart disease and dilated cardiomyopathy are the main indications in adults. Since the introduction of calcineurin inhibitors, 1-year survival approaches 90%, while 5-year survival exceeds 70%. The cardiac transplant recipient can achieve approximately 70% of the maximal cardiac output.

Tissue typing for HLA matching is not routinely performed because of time constraints. Criteria for optimising heart transplantation focus on organ size, ABO matching and avoidance of transferring organs from a CMV-positive donor to a CMV-negative recipient. Assessment of pre-sensitisation is not routinely performed, though studies have demonstrated that patients with preformed antibodies directed at one or more of the HLA antigens have a poorer overall rate of graft survival than non-sensitised recipients.

Histology plays a key role in the diagnosis of acute rejection and repeated endomyocardial biopsies are normally performed for monitoring ongoing rejection. The prolongation of isovolumic relaxation time, measured by echocardiography, is also compatible with rejection. Biopsies, taken every 1 to 2 weeks early after transplantation, and with gradually widening intervals thereafter, demonstrate changes

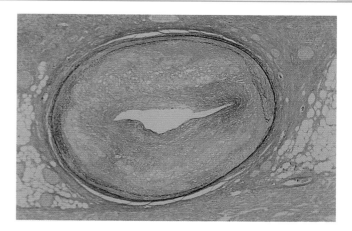

Fig. 11.14 The principal manifestation of chronic rejection in heart transplantation is coronary graft vascular occlusive disease.
This is characterised by intimal thickening, which tends to be more diffuse and concentric than conventional atherosclerosis. The thickening seen here is concentric and muscular elastic in nature. (Courtesy of Dr N. Cary.)

suggestive of rejection (Fig. 11.13). An accelerated coronary vascular disease appears later and is referred to as chronic rejection, even though the involvement of the immune system in its causation still remains to be demonstrated. This diffuse vascular process affects both distal and proximal coronary vessels so that conventional modes of intervention such as angioplasty or coronary artery bypass grafting are ineffective (Fig. 11.14).

Lung transplantation

End-stage pulmonary disease represents the indication for lung transplantation. The most common diagnoses that have required lung allograft include chronic obstructive pulmonary disease, emphysema caused by α_1-antitrypsin deficiency, idiopathic pulmonary fibrosis, cystic fibrosis and primary pulmonary hypertension. Lung transplantation improves lung function in patients with restrictive or obstructive disease and alleviates pulmonary hypertension in patients with pulmonary vascular disease.

ABO group compatibility and lung size are the only factors that are routinely matched between the donor and recipient.

A majority of recipients have early episodes of acute rejection that are characterised by non-specific manifestations, including cough, dyspnoea, fever, radiographic infiltrates and worsening of pulmonary function and oxygenation. A quarter of patients develop chronic rejection, characterised by airflow limitation and histologically by obliterative bronchiolitis and vascular sclerosis (Fig. 11.15). The lung as an allograft is especially susceptible to infections.

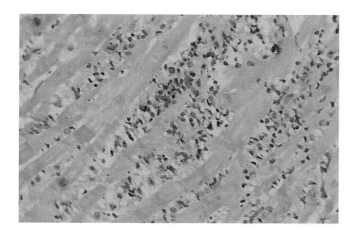

Fig. 11.13 Focus of acute cellular rejection in a heart-transplant recipient.
A mononuclear cell infiltrate composed of lymphocytes and macrophages characterises an episode of acute cellular rejection. (High magnification — courtesy of Dr N. Cary.)

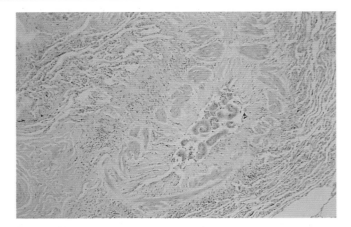

Fig. 11.15 The principal manifestation of chronic rejection following lung transplantation is the development of obliterative bronchiolitis.
This is characterised by occlusion of bronchioles by fibrous connective tissue. In its developing phases this may show inflammatory infiltration. In this case there is subtotal obliteration of the bronchiolar lumen due to a thick layer of pale-staining submucosal fibrosis, seen here between the partially detached bronchiolar epithelium (artefact) and the darker-staining smooth muscle bundles. (Courtesy of Dr N. Cary.)

Haematopoietic stem cell transplantation (HSCT)

Cytokine-mobilised peripheral blood stem cells have largely replaced bone marrow as the source of cells in autologous transplantation because of more rapid neutrophil and platelet recovery and faster immune reconstitution. Allogeneic peripheral blood stem cells similarly lead to faster hematologic recovery: however, their effects on GVHD, relapse, survival, and immune reconstitution are less certain. Peripheral blood stem cells transplantation (PBSCT) and bone marrow transplantation involve the transfer of pluripotent haematopoietic stem cells capable of regenerating all cellular elements of the blood and immune system. It has become the conventional form of treatment for congenital immunodeficiency diseases, selected malignancies and aplastic anaemia for patients who have an HLA-identical sibling or an identical twin. For patients who lack an HLA-matched sibling, a closely HLA-matched unrelated individual or an imperfectly HLA-matched relative may act as donors.

The reason why HLA matching needs to be especially stringent in HSCT is because the recipient is either immunodeficient or needs to be 'conditioned', i.e. undergo profound chemoradiotherapy to eliminate residual disease and create space for the new marrow. This results in ablation of the recipient's immune system. The immunoincompetent recipient is, therefore, at high risk of developing life-threatening GVHD.

Donor selection is done in sequential steps starting from the search for the best match, namely a genotypically identi-cal sibling. Information regarding genotypic identity for HLA class I and II determinants can be readily obtained within families by determining the HLA class I and class II antigens of the four parental haplotypes and analysing their segregation in the family. If genotypically identical siblings are unavailable, the second best choice is to obtain bone marrow from HLA-haploidentical relatives. Parents and off-spring are always HLA haploidentical. The degree of disparity between HLA-haploidentical donor–recipient pairs depends on the similarity of the non-shared haplotypes. The risk of GVHD increases progressively with the number of HLA disparities in the recipient compared with the donor. Bone marrow can be obtained from unrelated donors, if neither genotypically identical siblings nor haploidentical relatives are available. In this case, the donors are HLA phenotypically identical unrelated volunteers. Serologic typing alone does not ensure that the individuals share the same HLA genes. DNA-based techniques now permit molecular typing and a high degree of matching. Patients who are truly highly matched appear to have better outcomes. Worldwide, approximately 30–40 000 HSCTs are performed yearly, with an annual increase of 10–20% each year. More than 20 000 people have now survived 5 years or longer after HSCT.

The indications for bone marrow transplant are numerous and are increasing. Allogeneic bone marrow transplantation has been successful in treating children with a range of congenital immunodeficiency disorders (see Ch. 19). In **aplastic anaemia**, marrow transplantation is the preferred method of treatment if an HLA-identical sibling is available, and in this setting 85% long-term survival is achieved. In children with homozygous **beta-thalassaemia**, allogeneic bone marrow transplantation has led to disease-free 1-year survival of 75%. Non-transplanted patients undergo iron overload and usually die in their twenties.

In **haematological malignancies**, long-term survival and cure rates of up to 70% have been reported. In **acute lymphoblastic leukaemia**, bone marrow transplantation is indicated in those 50% of children who are not cured by a primary chemotherapy regimen. Interestingly, patients with leukaemia treated with bone marrow transplantation experience the beneficial graft-versus-leukaemia (GVL) effect (see Clinical Box 11.2) that occurs in association with GVHD.

In **chronic myelogenous leukaemia** (CML), allogeneic transplantation with marrow from an HLA-matched sibling donor is the treatment of choice for patients who are in the stable phase. If the patient with CML has no HLA-identical family donor, transplantation should be undertaken only when the clinical condition deteriorates, in order to justify a riskier procedure. Long-term disease-free survival has been achieved in patients with both **Hodgkin's disease** and **non-Hodgkin's lymphoma**. In both conditions, the results are better when the treatment is performed soon after a relapse, at a time when the disease is minimal. Under these circumstances, a disease-free survival of up to 70% can be achieved. A lower mortality rate is associated with the use of an autologous graft, and this is the preferred mode of treatment in most centres. Though autologous HSCT does not cure **multiple myeloma**, event-free survival rates and overall survival

Graft-versus-leukaemia

Patients with leukaemia treated with bone marrow transplant are said to have a lower rate of leukaemic relapses if their transplant is accompanied by GVHD. Those patients who receive bone marrow depleted of T lymphocytes — and do not experience GVHD — appear to suffer from an increased rate of relapses. The beneficial anti-tumour effect associated with GVHD is known as the graft-versus-leukaemia effect (GVL). The mechanisms at the basis of GVL are unknown.

rates are prolonged approximately 1 year compared with survival rates achieved by chemotherapy. Bone marrow transplantation is being tested in non-haematological malignancies, where extremely aggressive, bone marrow impairing chemotherapeutic regimens may be desired to treat the original malignancy. Anecdotal successes have been reported in neuroblastoma, breast cancer, testicular tumours and gynaecological cancers.

Before HSC are infused, the recipient must undergo chemotherapy and/or radiotherapy — **conditioning** — to suppress the immune system, to create space in the bone marrow and to eliminate malignant cells in cases where malignancy was the reason for the transplantation. The major complications of marrow transplantation are graft rejection, **GVHD**, opportunistic infection and recurrence of malignancy. In the setting of recipients receiving marrow from an HLA-identical sibling, this complication is fortunately rare. Predisposing factors include previous blood transfusions and insufficiently aggressive conditioning regimens. A complication peculiar to bone marrow transplantation is **veno-occlusive** disease of the liver, which consists of three main symptoms: jaundice, tender hepatomegaly and ascites. It is present in up to 50% of the patients. Progressive liver failure can develop and a fatal outcome is not unusual.

Clinical transplantation

- Graft-versus-host disease is typically seen in bone marrow transplantation, where the grafted tissue comprises immunocompetent allogeneic cells. GVHD can be observed in other settings when the organ transplanted contains a sufficient number of immunocompetent cells.

- Indications for clinical transplantation expand steadily. This expansion is challenged by organ shortage.

- Organ shortage is currently tackled by effective use of available resources (e.g. organ-sharing programmes, use of split livers, donations from relatives). 'Humanised' xenogeneic grafts should soon alleviate this problem.

Transplantation: an outlook

Organ transplantation faces a number of problems, ranging from organisational to philosophical. Organs are in short supply, and graft failure of non-paired organs is synonymous with death if a new organ is not found promptly. The rate of malignancies is increased by the aggressive immunosuppressive regimens needed for long-term graft survival. The concept of heart-beating cadaveric donors sounds like an oxymoron and poses ethical problems. Only grafts from living donors are culturally acceptable in some societies. Moreover, several cases are known to have occurred in which poverty and not a close family link was the reason to part with one kidney. Can any of these issues be addressed in the near future?

The organ shortage will soon be tackled by the use of organs obtained from genetically 'humanised' animal donors. Additionally, the manufacture of artificial devices to pump blood around the body or to control sugar levels may provide an answer to shortage of hearts and pancreata. The possibility of more specific modes of treatment to silence allorecognition is being vigorously explored, although current evidence suggests that effective immune intervention needs to be tailored to an individual patient, raising economical question marks over the large-scale feasibility of such an approach. The prospect of subduing universal mediators of inflammatory damage, such as complement and cytokines, with specific antagonists appears to be more promising in the short term. Ethical issues will remain. The question asked will probably be: 'Do we have the right to use animals as a source of spare parts for our own survival?'.

An alternative approach to address the shortage of organs and tissues is the pluripotent stem cell approach. Stem cells have the potential for differentiation into any type of functional tissue that might be required — heart muscle, liver cell, insulin-producing cell. This might, in the future, allow for a limitless supply. There is at least one important caveat — namely that unless the issue of tissue compatibility can be addressed, stem cell-derived transplants will face the same problems of rejection as any other donor organ does currently. One approach to this, that is possible but highly challenging, is to derive autologous stem cells, so that the resulting graft tissue becomes an autograft — the ultimate in designer medicine.

Further reading

Lechler RI, Sykes M, Thomson AW, Turka LA 2005 Organ transplantation – how much of the promise has been realized? Nat Med 11: 605–613

Gokmen MR, Lombardi G, Lechler R 2008 The importance of the indirect pathway of allorecognition in clinical transplantation. Curr Opin Immunol 20: 568–574

Rheumatic diseases

This chapter describes a number of diseases with a proved or supposed immune pathogenesis; they are variably referred to as **rheumatic**, **connective tissue** or **collagen diseases**. Rheumatic denotes the migratory nature of the pain (ρέω, reads reo, Greek for flowing), whilst the terms 'connective tissue' and 'collagen' indicate the components typically affected. In these disorders, collagen may have dual relevance: as a target for autoimmune reactions and as a component of connective tissue produced in excess. Clinical manifestations centre around the joints and muscles, but other systems are involved to differing degrees in the different conditions. In systemic lupus erythematosus, for example, systemic manifestations frequently predominate over those localised to the joints, whereas a disease such as ankylosing spondylitis is mainly focused on a particular region, in this case the sacroilium.

Systemic lupus erythematosus

Systemic lupus erythematosus (SLE, also often shortened to **lupus**) is a multisystem disease that follows a fluctuating course, with exacerbations and spontaneous remissions. It is identified by its clinical features and by a variety of circulating autoantibodies. In particular, autoantibodies directed against components of the cell nucleus play a pivotal diagnostic — and pathogenic — role. SLE affects 40 in 100 000 North European or American Caucasians. The incidence appears to be higher in Afro-Caribbean populations and higher still in Orientals. Nine of ten SLE patients are women, 80% of them being of childbearing age. Possession of certain HLA class II alleles — *DRB1*0301 (DR3)* in Caucasians, *DRB1*1501 (DR2)* in Orientals — confers susceptibility to the disease. The role of genes in the causation of the disease is indicated by the higher concordance for SLE in monozygotic when compared with dizygotic twins.

Pathology

Renal failure is a major cause of morbidity and mortality in SLE, and its pathogenesis is discussed in full in Chapter 16. A renal biopsy is taken when the information it can provide is useful for treatment. The localisation and type of immune complex, as well as the activity and chronicity of the histological lesions are all important for grading lupus nephritis, guiding treatment and assessing prognosis. Detection of immune complexes, also called immune deposits, is carried out on frozen tissue sections using a direct immunofluorescence technique. In between one half and all cases of active SLE, such immune deposits can also be seen at the dermoepidermal junction in the skin.

Pathogenesis

Akin to other autoimmune diseases, the pathogenic scenario for SLE sees environmental factors interacting with susceptibility genes to produce an overactive, autoaggressive immune response: the main effectors of tissue damage are autoantibodies and immune complexes. To examine the genetic link first; HLA class II gene products have been implicated in predisposition to SLE, presumably acting at the level of T helper lymphocyte recognition of a 'lupus peptide', but the relative risks associated with possession of *DRB1*0301* and *DRB1*1501* are small. More relevant, at least in Caucasians, is possession of the HLA class III allele *C4AQ0*. This is a silent allele encoding for the production of quantity 0 (Q0) of the A isotype of the C4 molecule, which belongs to the classical pathway of the complement system (see p. 15). This allele is part of an extended lupus-predisposing HLA haplotype *B*0801 DRB1*0301 DQB1*0201 C4AQ0* (*B8 DR3 DQ2 C4AQ0*). Normal levels of functioning C4 are essential in maintaining immune complexes in solution and in preventing their tissue deposition. It is not surprising, then, that possession of a C4A non-coding gene predisposes to an immune complex disease such as SLE. Intriguingly, well-defined clinical manifestations in lupus such as dermatitis, or possession of autoantibodies such as anticardiolipin antibody, also tend to be associated with HLA alleles, but these are different alleles from those actually predisposing to SLE, arguing in favour of heterogeneity of the disease. There is a strong association between the rare disorder of complement C1q deficiency and SLE. Certain polymorphisms of genes encoding Fc receptors, especially FcγIIA and FcγIIIA, predispose to lupus, possibly coding for receptors inefficient at the removal of immune complexes. Amongst the predisposing factors, femaleness undoubtedly plays a major role (see Science Box 12.1).

No definite environmental factors have been identified, with the exception of drugs known to provoke SLE (see below) and ultraviolet light, especially UV-B radiations. Three quarters of lupus patients are photosensitive. A role for a virus, frequently suggested but never actually demonstrated, as the cause of this autoantibody-dominated disease has received some support by the finding that the lupus-specific anti-Sm (Smith protein) autoantibody (see Table 12.2) reacts with the p24 gag protein of retroviruses and that anti-Ro, (Ro, Robert) another autoantibody typical of SLE, also recognises a nucleocapsid protein on vesicular stomatitis virus (see Science Box 12.2).

With these strong similarities between viruses and the targets of autoantibodies found in SLE, a process involving molecular mimicry between organisms and self (see p. 123) is one of the most frequent explanations for how the disease may arise. Autoantibodies found in SLE are produced by B lymphocytes that have undergone gene rearrangements and somatic mutations typical of an antigen-driven response. A generalised B lymphocyte dysregulation appears also to be

---

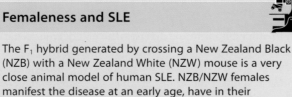

SCIENCE BOX 12.1

Femaleness and SLE

The F₁ hybrid generated by crossing a New Zealand Black (NZB) with a New Zealand White (NZW) mouse is a very close animal model of human SLE. NZB/NZW females manifest the disease at an early age, have in their circulation antinuclear and anti-dsDNA antibodies (autoantibodies typical of SLE) and develop a lethal immune complex-mediated nephritis. Artificial control of sex hormones — by drug treatment or by castration — has a profound effect on the expression of the disease. Male hormones tend to suppress the disease, improve survival and decrease the severity of nephritis when they are administered to females. In contrast, female hormones accelerate the course of the disease.

SCIENCE BOX 12.2

A man and his dog

In the debate over the contribution of environmental factors to the aetiology of SLE it is worth noting that dogs owned by lupus patients have significantly higher levels of anti-dsDNA autoantibodies (the diagnostic test in SLE) compared with 'control' dogs. The sharing of this serological lupus hallmark has led to the suggestion that a common environmental factor, possibly a transmissible agent, is involved in causing SLE in the two species. The debate has expanded as to the origin, human or canine, of this potential transmissible agent, and it has been concluded, with some reason, that a canine source was more likely in view of the higher chance of dogs biting and licking their owners than the reverse.

---

involved, leading to vast amounts of autoantibodies being produced. These autoantibodies damage cells and tissues, either through direct binding to cell-surface membranes or by forming immune complexes that become deposited.

The damaging role of antiplatelet autoantibodies in the thrombocytopenia seen in SLE patients is well established, while antineuronal autoantibodies have been implicated in neurological manifestations of lupus and antilymphocyte antibodies in lymphopenia. Circulating anticardiolipin autoantibodies are additional pathogenic agents; they react with phospholipid moieties (one of the main ones being cardiolipin) and are involved in causing both arterial and venous thrombosis and in spontaneous abortion (see Clinical Box 12.1). Immune complexes of autoantibody and autoantigen lodge in highly vascularised tissues such as the renal glomerulus. Pathogenicity of these complexes increases with increasing ability of the antibody to fix complement: complex size, charge and clearance (dependent on functional C4 and complement receptors) are all of importance in influencing deposition in the tissues. As we have seen, C4 concentration is often reduced. CR-1 (complement receptor 1) numbers are reduced on the erythrocyte surface of lupus patients: this defect, usually acquired but occasionally inherited in SLE, prevents delivery of the full immune complex load to the mononuclear phagocyte system within the liver and spleen. The cationic nature of DNA in immune complexes in lupus facilitates binding to capillary walls within the glomerulus (see Ch. 16).

Clinical features

SLE is a multisystem disease and can affect virtually all organs and systems (Fig.12.1): whilst some manifestations are common, others are rare. Therefore, joints, skin and blood are affected in 80–100% of patients, kidneys, CNS and cardiopulmonary system in over 50%; while thrombosis, a typical lupus manifestation associated with possession of the anticardiolipin antibody, is present in 10% of patients. The

Antiphospholipid antibody syndrome

This syndrome, characterised by both venous and arterial thromboses, was described by G. R. V. Hughes in 1983 in a patient with SLE. It is now clear that it can occur in isolation as the primary antiphospholipid antibody syndrome. Venous thrombosis can manifest itself as deep-vein thrombosis and thrombosis of retinal, renal or hepatic veins (Budd–Chiari syndrome). Arterial thrombosis can induce limb ischaemia, strokes, amaurosis and myocardial infarction, and Addison's disease through adrenal thrombosis. Heart-valve disease is present in a quarter of patients and women have a much increased risk of spontaneous abortion. Thrombocytopenia is common (platelets have surface phospholipids). The serum of these patients contains antiphospholipid autoantibodies, deemed responsible for the clinical manifestations of the syndrome. The mechanisms through which these antibodies provoke damage, however, have not been clarified, even though reactivity to cell membranes — platelets, endothelial cells — and clotting factors has been documented.

severity of clinical manifestations is variable and exacerbations typically alternate with periods of relative quiescence. Systemic manifestations, including fatigue, malaise, fever, anorexia, nausea and weight loss, are present in the great majority of patients.

The diagnosis of SLE is made using the criteria set by the American Rheumatism Association (Table 12.1).

Musculoskeletal features

Arthralgias and arthritis, frequently migratory in nature, affect virtually all patients, with the degree of pain being disproportionate to the physical signs of synovitis. Joints in the hands (proximal interphalangeal and metacarpophalangeal) are affected, while the spine is spared. Erosions are rare.

Cutaneous features

A malar (butterfly) erythema over cheeks and bridge of the nose is typical but only occurs in one third of the patients (Fig. 12.2). More frequent is a maculopapular rash in sun-exposed areas (neck, extensor surfaces of arms and legs) that accompanies disease flare-ups. Alopecia, usually patchy but extensive at times, is also frequently seen. A characteristic

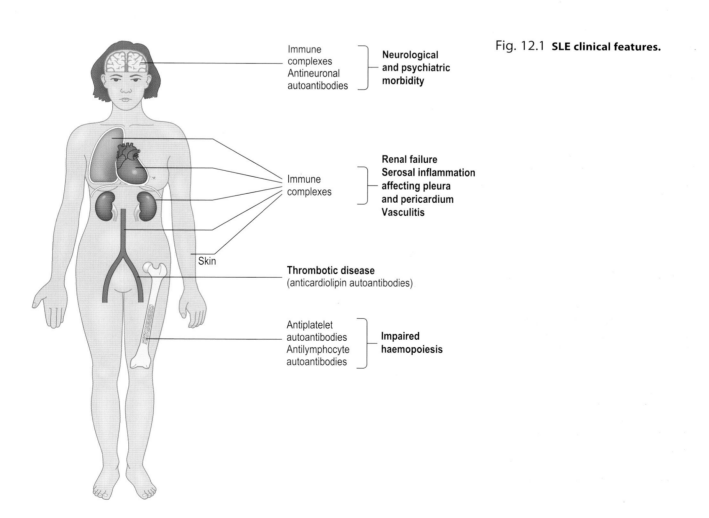

Fig. 12.1 **SLE clinical features.**

Table 12.1 Diagnosis of SLE using the criteria set by the American Rheumatism Association[a]

	Criteria	Description
1.	Malar rash	Fixed erythema, flat or raised over the malar eminences
2.	Discoid rash	Erythematous raised patches with adherent keratotic scaling and follicular plugging; atrophic scarring may occur
3.	Photosensitivity	
4.	Oral ulcers	Includes oral and naso-pharyngeal, observed by physician
5.	Arthritis	Non-erosive arthritis involving two or more peripheral joints, characterised by tenderness, swelling or effusion
6.	Serositis	Pleuritis or pericarditis documented by rub or ECG, or evidence of pericardial effusion
7.	Renal disorder	Proteinuria greater than 0.5 g in 24 hours, or 3+, or cellular casts
8.	Neurological disorders	Seizures without other cause or psychosis without other cause
9.	Haematological disorders	Haemolytic anaemia or leukopenia (less than $4 \times 10^9/l$) or lymphopenia (less than $1.5 \times 10^9/l$) or thrombocytopenia (less than $100 \times 10^9/l$) in the absence of offending drugs
10.	Immunological disorders	Anti-dsDNA or anti-Sm antibodies or false positive serology for syphilis for at least 6 months
11.	Antinuclear antibodies	An abnormal titre of antinuclear antibodies (ANAs) by immunofluorescence or an equivalent assay at any point in time in the absence of drugs known to induce ANAs

[a]If four of these criteria are present at any time during the course of disease, a diagnosis of systemic lupus erythematosus can be made with 97% specificity and 97% sensitivity.

photosensitive, erythematous, papulosquamous rash, which becomes hypopigmented and leaves no scars, defines sub-acute cutaneous lupus (SCLE). Patients with this condition tend to have arthritis and fatigue but rarely renal or CNS involvement. Some such patients are negative for antinuclear antibody, while all tend to have anti-Ro (SS-A) antibody.

Renal features

Most patients have immunoglobulin deposits present in their glomeruli, and a clinically relevant glomerulonephritis is present in some 50% of patients, ranging from a mild focal proliferative disease to aggressive diffuse proliferative disease requiring vigorous treatment with corticosteroids and cytotoxic drugs. Urinalysis shows haematuria, proteinuria and renal casts. Of importance in monitoring renal disease are persistently abnormal urinalysis, elevated serum levels of

antibodies to double-stranded (ds) DNA and low levels of complement factors, especially C4, all of which presage development of nephritis.

Neurological features

Any area of the central nervous system can be affected in SLE, with manifestations ranging from psychosis, through seizures to organic brain syndromes. A mild cognitive dysfunction is frequent, as are depression and anxiety. Micro-focal scarring located in the subcortical white matter is associated with the presence of lupus neuropathy. These lesions are normally undetectable, or give non-specific alterations, even under magnetic resonance imaging. Some 50% of patients with neurological involvement have antineuronal autoantibodies in their serum and cerebrospinal fluid, but the pathogenicity of these is as yet unproved.

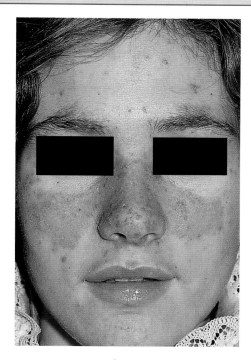

Fig. 12.2 Butterfly rash.
A malar erythema over cheeks and bridge of the nose is typical of SLE (from Forbes & Jackson 2003 Color and Atlas Text of Clinical Medicine, 3rd edn, Mosby, with permission).

Cardiopulmonary features

Pericarditis is the most frequent cardiac manifestation of lupus. At times it is the presenting manifestation and is typically mild but can occasionally result in tamponade. Valvular abnormalities can be identified by ultrasound in a quarter of patients, probably representing the echocardiographic counterpart of the ovoid vegetations found at post-mortem examination of lupus patients, known as Libman–Sacks verrucous endocarditis. Antiphospholipid antibodies are associated with this condition. Pleural effusion is also a common finding. A corticosteroid-responsive lupus pneumonitis, characterised by fleeting infiltrates, interstitial pneumonitis and pulmonary hypertension, can occasionally occur in SLE.

Vascular features

These complications tend to be thrombotic in nature, affecting vessels of any size and are usually associated with antiphospholipid antibodies. Retinal vasculitis is a serious **ocular** manifestation, requiring aggressive immunosuppression. Up to 10% of lupus patients develop **Sjögren's syndrome** (see p. 185).

General laboratory findings

The most frequent laboratory alteration that is identified is normochromic normocytic anaemia of chronic disorders.

Table 12.2 Antinuclear antibodies in connective tissue diseases

Pattern	Antigen	Disease association
Homogeneous	DNA–histone complex	SLE; other rheumatic diseases
	Histones	Drug-induced SLE
Speckled	Sm (Smith) protein complexed to six small nuclear RNAs (U1 to U6)	SLE
	RNP (ribonucleoprotein) complexed to U1 RNA	Mixed connective tissue disease; SLE; Sjögren's syndrome
	Ro (Robert) (SS-A) protein complexed to RNAs Y1 to Y5	Sjögren's syndrome; SLE
	La (Lane) (SS-B) phosphoprotein complexed to RNA polymerase III transcripts	Sjögren's syndrome; SLE
	Jo-1, histidyl transfer RNA synthetase	Polymyositis; dermatomyositis
	Scl-70, DNA topoisomerase 1	Systemic sclerosis
	Centromere; proteins in kinetochore	CREST syndrome
Peripheral (membranous-rim-like)	Double-stranded DNA(?)	SLE
	Nuclear envelope proteins	
	Lamins A and C	SLE; systemic sclerosis
Nucleolar	RNA polymerase; PM-Scl; periribosomal particle	Systemic sclerosis
Crithidia luciliae kinetoplast	Double-stranded DNA	SLE

SCIENCE BOX 12.3

Immunofluorescence

The detection of antinuclear antibodies (ANAs) and their pattern definition is classically done by immunofluorescence. This technique permits the detection of antigens in tissues or on cell surfaces using antibodies specifically directed to these antigens. Alternatively, when a preparation is known to contain a given antigen, immunofluorescence can be used to identify its complementary antibody. To ascertain whether a lupus patient is 'ANA positive', serum is applied to nuclei-containing tissues, typically of rodent origin, or to a smear of a cell line culture characterised by large nuclei. The use of this latter substrate enables a good definition of the ANA pattern. If the patient is ANA positive, the autoantibody will bind to the nuclei. To reveal this binding, a second antibody is added. The second reagent has been raised in an animal against human immunoglobulin and is tagged with a fluorescent label. This second antibody will bind and ANA will then be seen by placing the preparation under a fluorescence microscope. This technique is known as **indirect immunofluorescence** (**I-IFL**; Fig. 12.3), since the autoantibody is revealed through a two-step procedure. Indirect immunofluorescence is the standard technique for the detection of a wide variety of autoantibodies.

In a patient with lupus nephritis, a kidney biopsy is frequently obtained for diagnostic reasons. The glomeruli of such bioptic renal material contain antigen–antibody complexes. By applying a fluorescent antibody directed against human immunoglobulin — similar to that used in the second step of ANA detection — to a frozen section of the kidney biopsy, it is possible to reveal glomerular immune complex. This one-step technique is known as **direct immunofluorescence** (**D-IFL**; Fig. 12.4).

Central to immunofluorescence are fluorochromes and the fluorescence microscope. Fluorochromes are substances emitting light of characteristic colour — green for fluorescein,

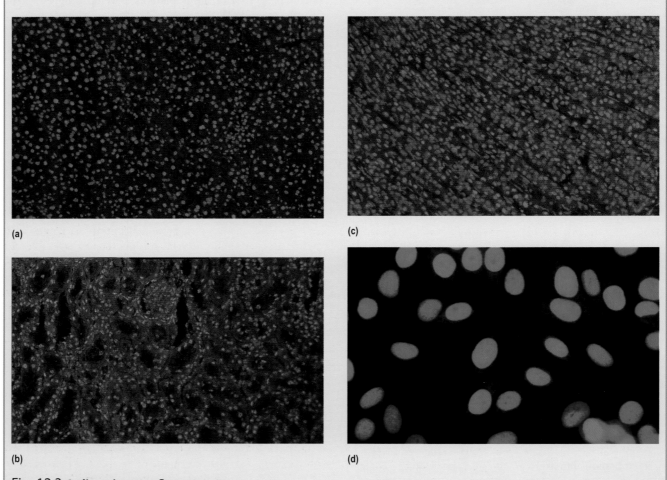

(a)

(b)

(c)

(d)

Fig. 12.3 Indirect immunofluorescence.
The patient's serum is applied to a frozen tissue section containing the relevant antigen. The method is described in the immunofluorescence box. The appearance of antinuclear antibody on rat liver (**a**), kidney (**b**), stomach (**c**) and HEp-2 cells (**d**) is shown.

(*continued*)

Immunofluorescence—cont'd

red for rhodamine and phycoerythrin — at a wavelength lower than that used to excite them. They are used to label antibodies. The fluorescence microscope provides the light source to excite the fluorochromes and the optical devices to visualise the fluorescent image.

Immunofluorescence is also commonly used to identify cell types within a suspension using an antibody directed to a surface structure unique to that cell type (e.g. CD3 for total T lymphocytes, CD4 for helper T lymphocytes, CD8 for cytotoxic T lymphocytes). Fluorescence microscopy has largely been replaced by cytofluorimetry (see p. 89) for cell counting and analysis.

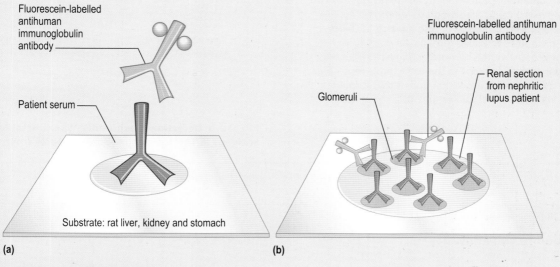

Fig. 12.4 **Direct immunofluorescence.**
A fluorescein-labelled antihuman immunoglobulin antiserum is applied to a frozen section of a kidney biopsy obtained from a lupus patient suffering from glomerulonephritis (see Figs 16.9 and 16.10).

Occasionally a Coombs-positive haemolytic anaemia is observed. Leukopenia (probably autoantibody mediated), especially lymphopenia, and thrombocytopenia are frequent. Urinalysis can show haematuria, proteinuria and renal casts in the presence of glomerulonephritis. The erythrocyte sedimentation rate is typically elevated, while C-reactive protein (CRP) tends to be normal. This last finding is intriguing, since CRP is usually elevated in inflammatory states.

Immunological laboratory findings

The sero-immunological hallmark of SLE is **antinuclear antibody** (ANA) (see Table 12.2). In the absence of ANA, the diagnosis of SLE is put into question, even though some 5% of patients may have an ANA-negative serology. It is safe to consider that, over time, all patients with SLE will have ANA in their serum. ANA is currently detected using the technique of indirect immunofluorescence (see Science Box 12.3), where diluted patient's serum is applied to a tissue — or cell preparation — in which nuclei are prominent. Frozen tissue, especially liver, of rodent origin and cell lines of human origin, such as the HEp2 cell line derived from a laryngeal tumour, are used as substrate to detect ANA. Four ANA patterns (see Table 12.2) can be readily recognised in immunofluorescence: homogeneous, speckled, peripheral and nucleolar, the presence of the first three, alone or in association, being most relevant to the diagnosis of SLE. The homogeneous pattern is caused by an antibody directed against the DNA-related proteins called histones; the **speckled** pattern corresponds to a variety of antibodies directed against other antigens in the nucleus. These have become known collectively as the **extractable nuclear antigens** (ENA) and are normally detected by immunodiffusion (see Science Box 12.4) or ELISA techniques. Anti-ENA antibodies are frequently named after the patient whose serum was used to identify them. Therefore, there is anti-Sm (Smith), found almost exclusively in SLE, and anti-RNP (ribonucleoprotein), more typically associated with mixed connective tissue disease (see below) than with SLE. Other antinuclear antibodies seen in SLE are anti-Ro (Robert) also called SS-A (for Sjögren's syndrome antigen A) and anti-La (Lane) or SS-B (Sjögren's syndrome antigen B). Other anti-ENA autoantibodies are anti-Jo-1, anti-Scl-70 and anticentromere, which are associated mainly with polymyositis, systemic sclerosis and CREST syndrome, respectively (see below). The **peripheral** pattern of ANA staining is traditionally said to correspond to anti-dsDNA, but this is controversial. Antibodies to proteins of the nuclear envelope, such as

Detection of antibodies to extractable nuclear antigens (ENAs)

Although the use of ELISAs has become widespread, in many laboratories ENAs are still detected using a technique developed some four decades ago. This is immunodiffusion in agarose gels. A gel is poured and wells cut into it as shown in Figure 12.5. The central well is filled with the extract containing the antigens, in this case a nuclear preparation. Test serum is placed in an outer well, adjacent to a serum known to contain the autoantibody of interest (in this case antibodies to the ENA called Sjögren's syndrome A; SSA). When the antigen and serum diffuse towards each other, antigen–antibody complexes form at the point of equivalence between the two, appearing as a white line. Certainty that the white line in the test sample represents anti-SSA comes from the fact that it joins that formed by the anti-SSA in the known serum sample (the so-called line of identity).

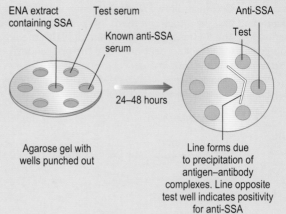

Fig. 12.5 Detection of antibodies to extractable nuclear antigens (ENAs) by immunodiffusion in agarose gels.

There before you know it

Taking advantage of the US Department of Defense Serum Repository, which contains some 30 million specimens from 5 million US Armed Forces personnel, Melissa Arbuckle and collaborators were able to investigate the autoimmune serology in 130 lupus patients before they developed clinically overt disease. At least one SLE antibody preceded the diagnosis in 88% of patients at a mean of 3.3 years before diagnosis, with ANA appearing first, followed by anti-Ro/anti-La, antiphospholipid, anti-dsDNA and, lastly, by anti-Sm and anti-RNP. The highly diagnostic anti-dsDNA was detectable at a mean of 2.2 years before the diagnosis, but ANA could be detected even 10 years before clinical symptoms. The editorial note accompanying this article in the *New England Journal of Medicine* raised two questions: 'Could this observation provide a clue to pathogenesis?' and 'Do the results of this study help the clinician determine whether a disease associated with ANA is present or likely to develop?'. The answer given to the first question is that we now have a better idea of the sequence in SLE autoantibody production, even though the pathogenetic events — environmental factors acting on a genetically predisposed background — most likely occur before the earliest detection of autoantibodies. As far as helping the clinician the answer was also diversified. The knowledge of the sequential autoantibody formation may help the clinician in reaching an earlier diagnosis, but if, on the other hand, it leads to earlier and not selective testing of patients, it may increase the number of worried ANA-positive individuals who are anticipating SLE that never develops.

lamins, are also responsible for the peripheral pattern. The **nucleolar** pattern is rare in SLE, being more associated with systemic sclerosis.

In summary, ANA is a very sensitive test for SLE, being present in virtually all patients and frequently at high titres; its disease specificity is relatively low since it is frequently found in other rheumatic diseases, as well as in autoimmune liver disease, during viral infections and, occasionally, at low titres, in normal subjects, especially when the very sensitive HEp2 cells are used as detection substrate (see Science Box 12.5). It has a tendency to increase in prevalence with age in healthy adults. Transfer of autoantibodies from the mother to a fetus can occur (see Clinical Box 12.2).

While the disease specificity of ANA is low, that of anti-dsDNA autoantibodies is high. The DNA used in the assay must be double stranded: autoantibodies to single-stranded (ss) DNA exist in many diseases and are specific for none. The prevalence (70%) of anti-dsDNA autoantibodies is much higher in SLE, giving a higher diagnostic sensitivity than the similarly disease-specific anti-Sm autoantibodies (30%). Anti-dsDNA autoantibodies are usually detected by very analytically sensitive techniques, such as radioimmunoassay (RIA) or enzyme-linked immunosorbent assay (ELISA). They can also be detected by immunofluorescence staining of an organelle called a kinetoplast in the flagellate *Crithidia luciliae*, which contains dsDNA. Within SLE, dsDNA anti-

CLINICAL BOX 12.2

Neonatal SLE

This rare condition can affect babies born to women suffering from SLE. It is characterised by a cutaneous rash appearing shortly after birth, especially if there is exposure to UV light in the nursery. Another typical manifestation is congenital heart block, which can be fatal. The disease disappears within 6 months after birth, with the disappearance of maternal immunoglobulin from the newborn's circulation. Placental transfer of anti-Ro, one of the numerous autoantibodies characteristic of SLE, is pathogenic in this condition. Intriguingly, however, anti-Ro antibodies do not appear to cause cardiac dysfunction in adults.

Drug-induced lupus

A variety of drugs including procainamide, hydralazine, quinidine, minocycline, chlorpromazine, isoniazid, practolol, methyldopa and several others can cause manifestations closely mimicking SLE. ANA appears in over half of patients treated with procainamide and in a quarter of patients taking hydralazine within months of commencement of treatment. Some 10–20% of ANA-positive individuals go on to experience systemic complaints and joint pain. The ANA is directed against histones; anti-dsDNA is usually absent and complement levels are normal. Other lupus manifestations may occur, even though renal and neurological manifestations are rare. Cessation of treatment is generally followed by abatement of symptoms; on occasional instances, corticosteroids may be temporarily required. ANA may remain present for years.

Treatment

Treatment is dictated by the type of manifestation. Non-steroidal anti-inflammatory drugs and aspirin should be used for arthritis, myalgias and mild serositis. Anti-malarial drugs, such as hydrochloroquine, can be effective in cutaneous manifestations, with frequent checks for retinal toxicity. Corticosteroids alone or in association with cytotoxic drugs, such as cyclophosphamide and azathioprine/mycophenolate mofetil, are used in case of severe, life-threatening manifestations. The addition of cytotoxic drugs is considered useful in controlling the rate of flare-ups and in decreasing the dose of steroids. Since SLE is characterised by an abundance of autoantibodies, produced by lymphocytes of the B cell lineage, the chimeric monoclonal antibody Rituximab, which depletes B cells by targeting the pan-B-cell surface marker CD20, has been experimentally used with promising results. Controlled trials are needed to validate its efficacy.

bodies tend to associate with the presence of glomerulonephritis. Their levels are used by some clinicians to monitor disease activity.

The range of autoantibodies seen in SLE is outlined in Table 12.3.

Immune complexes (IC) are frequently present in the circulation, but no single test is available to measure their levels satisfactorily. Different tests measure immune complexes through their different properties: such as their ability to fix complement, to bind Fc receptors, or according to their molecular weight. Tissue immune complexes, readily visualised by electron microscopy and by their characteristic granular pattern by light microscopy along the glomerular basement membrane, are presently of more value in diagnosis and management. **Antiphospholipid antibodies** are present in a minority of lupus patients (10–15%), but their presence is associated with defined clinical manifestations (see above). Anticardiolipin antibodies, detected in an ELISA, and lupus anticoagulant, identified by its ability to prolong the partial thromboplastin time, belong to the antiphospholipid antibody family and are both responsible for thrombosis. Antiphospholipid antibodies account for the false positive VDRL results (Venereal Disease Research Laboratory; a test for syphilis) observed at times in lupus patients. Assessment of the **complement** profile is of importance in management. Serial determinations of CH_{50}, a functional assay measuring complement haemolytic activity, and of the individual factors C3 (common pathway) and C4 (classical pathway), inform on how much immune complexes are consuming complement (for complement assays see p. 271). However, since complete or partial congenital deficiency of certain complement components, especially C4 and C2, is associated with SLE, a low or very low CH_{50} in a patient with mild SLE may reflect congenital deficiency rather than active disease. A test of elevated sensitivity and specificity for SLE has recently been proposed consisting of the ratio between the erythrocyte bound C4d, an activation fragment of C4, typically increased in SLE and the erythrocyte complement receptor 1, typically decreased. The EC4d/CR1 ratio is reported to have a sensitivity of 81% and a specificity of 91% for SLE.

SUMMARY BOX 12.1

Systemic lupus erythematosus

- Antinuclear antibodies of homogeneous and/or speckled pattern are present in virtually all patients. These antibodies have high sensitivity but low specificity, being found almost invariably in SLE but also in several other connective tissue and autoimmune diseases.

- Anti-dsDNA and anti-Sm antibodies are specific for SLE but are not universally present, occurring in 70% and 30% of the patients, respectively.

- SLE is associated with the HLA-*DRB1*0301* (DR3) (Caucasians) and *DRB1*1501* (DR2) (Orientals) alleles within class II, and with the *C4AQ0* silent allele within class III HLA genes.

- Immunoglobulin, complement and dsDNA (immune complexes) gathered in a granular fashion are present in the glomerular basement membrane of patients with lupus nephritis.

(continued)

Table 12.3 Autoantibody spectrum in SLE

Autoantibody	Prevalence (%)	Comments
Antinuclear (pattern: homogeneous, speckled or membranous)	95	The absence of this antibody questions the diagnosis of SLE
Anti-dsDNA	70	High specificity for SLE; high titres associated with low complement levels and glomerulonephritis
Anti-Sm	30	High specificity for SLE
Anti-RNP	30	More common in the so-called mixed connective tissue disease
Anti-SS-A(Ro)	20	More common in Sjögren's syndrome; associated with neonatal lupus
Anti-SS-B(La)	10	More common in Sjögren's syndrome; frequently associated with SS-A/Ro
Antiphospholipid	30	Anticardiolipin is the best defined amongst the antibodies of this group; responsible for thrombosis, recurrent abortions and for the antiphospholipid syndrome
Antierythrocyte	50	Directed to red cell-surface antigens; occasionally results in haemolytic anaemia
Antilymphocyte	50	Responsible for lymphocytopenia; up to 90% react also with neuronal cells
Antiplatelet	>10	Responsible for thrombocytopenia
Antineural cells	50	Possibly responsible for CNS manifestations
Rheumatoid factor	25	

SUMMARY BOX 12.1

Systemic lupus erythematosus—cont'd

- Immune complexes can derive from the circulation or originate from a 'planted' antigen (e.g. dsDNA).
- Active disease is characterised by decreased complement levels, especially those of C4, and by increased levels of anti-dsDNA.
- Antiphospholipid antibodies are associated with thromboembolic episodes and recurrent abortions.
- Autoantibodies against lymphocyte, platelet, erythrocyte and neuronal cells may be directly involved in cell injury.

Rheumatoid arthritis

Rheumatoid arthritis (RA) is a multisystem chronic inflammatory disease, principally affecting peripheral joints in a symmetric fashion and commonly leading to cartilage destruction, bone erosions and joint deformities. Its course is variable; extra-articular manifestations, such as vasculitis and subcutaneous nodules, are present in 20–25% of the patients. Women are affected more than men, with a female : male ratio of 3 : 1; the disease onset reaches its apex between 35 and 50 years. RA has a worldwide distribution, with a prevalence of approximately 1%.

Pathology

Hyperplasia and hypertrophy of the synovial lining are, with microvascular injury, early findings in the course of the disease. With time, the oedematous synovial tissue protrudes into the synovial cavity in what is known as pannus. A mononuclear infiltrate surrounds vessels and consists of T lymphocytes, macrophages and B lymphocytes. All these cells reveal their active involvement in the chronic inflammatory process through the expression of activation and commitment markers. Amongst T lymphocytes, CD4 cells vastly outnumber CD8 cells; with cells expressing the uncommon γδ T cell receptor forming a discrete component of the infiltrate. In contrast to the synovial membrane infiltrate, the inflammatory cells present in the exudate contained in the articular cavity are mainly polymorphonuclear leukocytes. The **rheumatoid nodule**, an extra-articular manifestation of RA (see below and Figs 12.6 & 12.7), contains a centre of fibrinoid necrosis, probably a remnant of focal vasculitis, surrounded by palisading macrophages and an outer zone of granulation tissue.

Pathogenesis

There is a clear genetic component to the pathogenesis of RA, as indicated by its familial clustering and by the higher concordance for the disease in monozygotic than in dizygotic twins. This genetic susceptibility is in part conferred by HLA class II alleles *DRB1*04 (DR4)* and *DRB1*01 (DR1)*. In a pathogenic scenario (see p. 131), these class II molecules would present an arthritogenic (i.e. arthritis-inducing) peptide autoantigen to CD4 T cells, which are particularly well represented and in a state of activation within the rheumatoid synovium. These helper T cells would in turn activate CD8 cytotoxic T cells, macrophages and B lymphocytes. Macrophage activation is indicated by elevated levels of monocyte-derived cytokines, such as TNF-α and IL-1, within the synovium, synovial fluid and circulation (see Science Box 12.6).

Intrasynovial B lymphocytes produce **rheumatoid factors**. These are autoantibodies directed against the Fc portion of IgG. These autoantibodies can belong to any of the three main Ig classes, G, A or M, but the 'classical' rheumatoid factor is a pentameric IgM. Rheumatoid factors react against

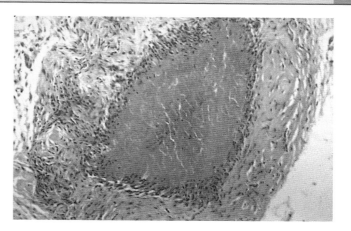

Fig. 12.6 Rheumatoid nodule.
A centre of fibrinoid necrosis is surrounded by palisading macrophages and an outer zone of granulation tissue.

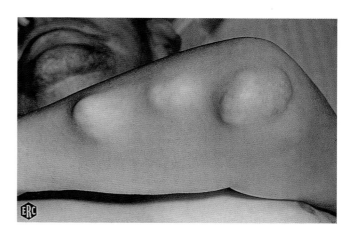

Fig. 12.7 Rheumatoid nodule.
On the extensor surfaces is a typical extra-articular manifestation of RA (courtesy of Dr J. Goodwill).

IgG molecules that are abnormal in their carbohydrate moieties, a feature that probably renders them immunogenic. The resulting immune complex is likely to participate in the perpetuation of inflammatory processes (see Science Box 12.7). As a consequence, the level of complement is reduced through activation and consumption within the inflamed

---

SCIENCE BOX 12.6

Evidence for the involvement of IL-1 and TNF-α as mediators of joint tissue damage in rheumatoid arthritis

1. High levels of these cytokines, or their mRNA, are present in the rheumatoid synovium at sites of active tissue destruction.

2. Synovial fluids containing these cytokines are injurious to normal cartilage in vitro.

3. This damage can be prevented by specific cytokine inhibitors or antagonists.

4. Recombinant IL-1 and TNF-α produce damage to normal cartilage in vitro and in vivo.

5. Progression of tissue damage in patients with RA is in part prevented by treatment with inhibitors of TNF-α and IL-1.

joint. The anaphylotoxins C5a and C3a are released in abundance, inducing the release of histamine and attracting polymorphonuclear leukocytes towards the articular cavity. Here, polymorphs engulf immune complexes, release lysosomal enzymes, produce reactive oxygen species and, in concert with locally generated leukotrienes and prostaglandins, participate in the destructive inflammatory process of the joint.

Attempts at identifying environmental factors provoking RA have met with limited success. Mycoplasma, rubella virus, cytomegalovirus and herpes virus have been incriminated in turn as aetiological agents. More recently, parvovirus B19 has been added to the list of possible offenders, because of the anecdotal appearance of RA following infection with this organism in a few patients. Epstein–Barr virus (EBV) has long been associated with RA: renewed interest has been generated by the observation that the EBV glycoprotein gp110 shares five amino acid residues (QKRAA) with the HLA class II susceptibility gene products. The *E. coli* dnaJ protein, a bacterial heat-shock protein, also contains the QKRAA sequence and suggested a link between gut bacteria and chronic arthritis. In both cases a mechanism of molecular mimicry has been invoked, but how this would operate in the development of RA remains to be established.

In addition to IgG and heat-shock protein (see Science Box 12.8) as autoantigens, collagen type II could also be important: autoantibodies to this connective tissue protein are present in elevated titres in the serum of patients with RA.

Clinical features

The onset of this chronic polyarthritis is normally insidious with a symmetrical involvement of several joints, typically of the hands, wrists, knees and feet, though inflammation can affect any articulation involving two joint surfaces. The proximal interphalangeal and metacarpophalangeal joints (Fig. 12.8) are the most frequently affected. Pain is a major complaint and is aggravated by movement. On examination, swelling and warmth — both resulting from synovial inflammation — are evident. Morning stiffness lasting for longer than 1 hour is characteristic of RA. To minimise pain, patients tend to maximise the joint space by keeping the joints in flexion. With time, characteristic deformities develop, such as the swan-neck deformity (hyperextension of the proximal interphalangeal joints with compensatory flexion of the distal interphalangeal joints (Fig. 12.9) and the boutonnière deformity (flexion of the proximal interphalangeal joints and extension of the distal interphalangeal joints. The extent of cartilage loss and bone erosion is well documented by radiography (Fig. 12.10).

Extra-articular manifestations are associated with elevated levels of rheumatoid factor; rheumatoid nodules, usually asymptomatic, develop as tissue swellings in one third of the patients, usually on extensor surfaces and typically on the forearm (see Fig. 12.7). Other sites for nodules include the pleura, sclera and myocardium. **Rheumatoid vasculitis** can affect almost every organ and in its most severe form produces polyneuropathy. Cutaneous vasculitis

---

SCIENCE BOX 12.7

Does rheumatoid factor cause arthritis?

This question recurs frequently and remains usually unanswered. Some forgotten experiments conducted several decades ago have the answer to this question. At a rheumatological meeting held in the late 1950s, it was reported that the 'transfusion of high-titre rheumatoid factor plasma into normal recipients was carried out. No symptoms appeared in the recipients. Simultaneous injection of high-titre rheumatoid plasma and living rheumatoid peripheral leukocytes did not change the recipient response pattern . . .'

The authors concluded — with some reason — that under their experimental conditions, the rheumatoid factor was devoid of intrinsic pathogenicity. Two additional points are of note. First, that the 'volunteer' population included carcinoma patients, laboratory workers and prison inmates. Second, that amongst the mainly technical and congratulatory debate following this presentation a discordant voice questioned who should be used as volunteers and whether this type of experiment is ever justified in human beings.

SCIENCE BOX 12.8

Mycobacterium tuberculosis and rheumatoid arthritis

M. tuberculosis has been the focus of recent interest in RA for a number of reasons. First, large sequences are shared in common between mycobacterial and human heat-shock proteins; second, mycobacterial heat-shock proteins are important in the induction of so-called 'adjuvant arthritis', an animal model of RA; third, the inflamed synovium is infiltrated by a relative abundance of γδ T cells. It appears that T cells bearing this less common form of the TCR have a

great cytotoxic potential and also frequently react with heat-shock proteins. Since heat-shock proteins are expressed on stressed cells, it is possible that after an initial encounter with *M. tuberculosis* γδ T cells specific for its heat-shock proteins may expand and cross-react with stressed, endogenous cells expressing heat-shock proteins. How this inflammatory process becomes focused onto the synovium remains to be established.

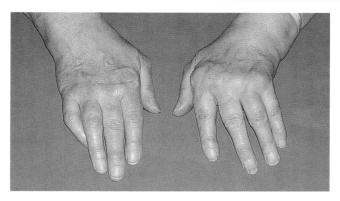

Fig. 12.8 Symmetrical involvement of joints in RA.
Advanced symmetrical involvement of joints of the hands (proximal interphalangeal and metacarpophalangeal joints) is typical of rheumatoid arthritis. Note the ulnar deviation (from Forbes & Jackson 2003 Color and Atlas Text of Clinical Medicine, 3rd edn, Mosby, with permission).

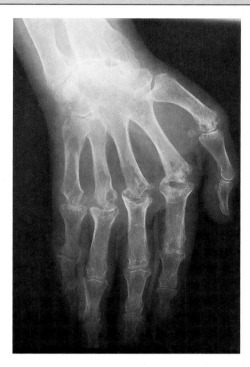

Fig. 12.10 Radiogram of the hand of a patient with advanced RA.
Cartilage loss and bone erosion are clearly documented (from McRae & Kinninmonth 1997 Orthopaedics and Trauma — An Illustrated Colour Text, Churchill Livingstone, with permission).

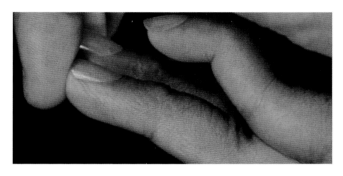

Fig. 12.9 Swan-neck deformity.
Hyperextension of the proximal interphalangeal joints with compensatory flexion of the distal interphalangeal joints (from Forbes & Jackson 2003 Color and Atlas Text of Clinical Medicine, 3rd edn, Mosby, with permission).

manifests itself with small brown lesions in the nail bed; ischaemic lesions leading to ulceration can also develop, especially on the legs. Pulmonary manifestations are more frequent in males and include pleuritis and pulmonary fibrosis. Pericarditis can occur and, like pleuritis, tends to be asymptomatic in life and a very common finding at autopsy. The presence in RA of splenomegaly, neutropenia and, at times, anaemia and thrombocytopenia define **Felty's syndrome**. This syndrome tends to affect patients with high titres of rheumatoid factor and other manifestations of extra-articular disease. Sjögren's syndrome (see p. 185) is present in 30% of the patients.

The guidelines used for classification of RA are given in Table 12.4.

Laboratory findings

Normochromic, normocytic anaemia is common. Both erythrocyte sedimentation rate and C reactive protein are elevated, reliably reflecting the severity of disease; for this reason they are commonly used to monitor disease progres-sion. The rheumatoid factor (RF) measured routinely belongs to the IgM class and because of its pentameric structure is easily revealed in agglutination assays (see Science Box 12.9).

IgM rheumatoid factor is present in three quarters of patients with RA (termed 'seropositive'). Virtually all patients seronegative by the conventional agglutination assays actually have monomeric rheumatoid factors of the IgG, IgA or IgM class. High titres of classical rheumatoid factor are particularly associated with extra-articular manifestations, and high titres at the onset of the disease tend to presage a poor prognosis. In recent years it has been shown that autoantibodies directed to the unusual amino acid citrulline, a post-translationally modified arginine residue, are specifically present in the sera of RA patients. A major target of these antibodies is the citrullinated form of filaggrin, a keratin-related protein. The antibodies against citrullinated peptides are collectively referred to as anti-CCP (cyclic citrullinated peptides): they are present in the majority of patients with RA, they can predict RA in pre-symptomatic patients and can also predict radiographic joint damage in known rheumatic patients. Antinuclear antibodies, usually at low titres, are frequently found in RA. Circulating levels of complement components (C3, C4) tend to be paradoxically elevated because of their behaviour as acute-phase reactants. Within affected joints, complement is always reduced, reflecting the local activation of the complement system induced by immune complexes.

Table 12.4 Guidelines for classification of RA[a]

Criteria	Description
1. Morning stiffness	Stiffness in and around the joints lasting 1 hour before maximal improvement
2. Arthritis of three or more joint areas	At least three joint areas, observed by a physician, simultaneously have soft tissue swelling or joint effusions, not just bony overgrowth; the 14 possible joint areas involved are right or left proximal interphalangeal, metacarpophalangeal, wrist, elbow, knee, ankle and metatarsophalangeal joints
3. Arthritis of hand joints	Arthritis of wrist, metacarpophalangeal joint or proximal interphalangeal joint
4. Symmetric arthritis	Simultaneous involvement of the same joint areas on both sides of the body
5. Rheumatoid nodules	Subcutaneous nodules over bony prominences, extensor surfaces or juxta-articular regions, observed by a physician
6. Serum rheumatoid	Demonstration of abnormal amounts of serum rheumatoid factor by any method for which the result has been positive in less than 5% of normal control subjects
7. Radiographic changes	Typical changes of RA on posteroanterior hand and wrist radiographs, which must include erosions or unequivocal bony decalcification localised in or most marked adjacent to the involved joints

[a]Four of seven criteria are required to classify a patient as having rheumatoid arthritis.

SCIENCE BOX 12.9

Agglutination

The detection of rheumatoid factor is conventionally carried out using an agglutination test. A range of inert particles including blood cells, latex or gelatin can be coated with antigen, which in the case of rheumatoid factor is IgG. Agglutination is a sensitive, semi-quantitative technique in which the reaction between antibody and antigen can be titrated to a visible end-point. The ability of pentameric IgM antibodies to agglutinate is some three orders of magnitude higher than that of IgG antibodies. Agglutination 'suffers' from the prozone phenomenon, in which very high titres of antibody can produce false-negative results: hence the need for the antibody under investigation to be tested at different dilutions. Antigenic determinants recognised by the rheumatoid factor are exposed on the particles and the addition of rheumatoid factor to the carriers results in agglutination (see Figs 12.11–12.13).

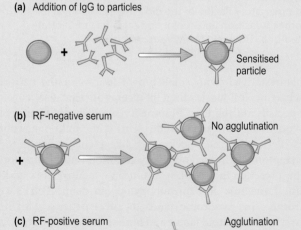

(a) Addition of IgG to particles

Sensitised particle

(b) RF-negative serum

No agglutination

(c) RF-positive serum

Agglutination

Fig. 12.11 **Basics of testing for rheumatoid factor.**
(**a**) IgG is adsorbed onto inert particles, such as latex or red blood cells. The addition of a negative-control serum results in no agglutination (**b**) while the addition of a rheumatoid factor-positive serum results in agglutination (**c**).

Agglutination—cont'd

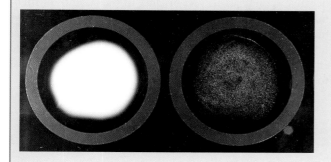

Fig. 12.12 **Detection of rheumatoid factor (RF) using sensitised latex beads.**
Left: RF-negative serum. Right: RF-positive serum.

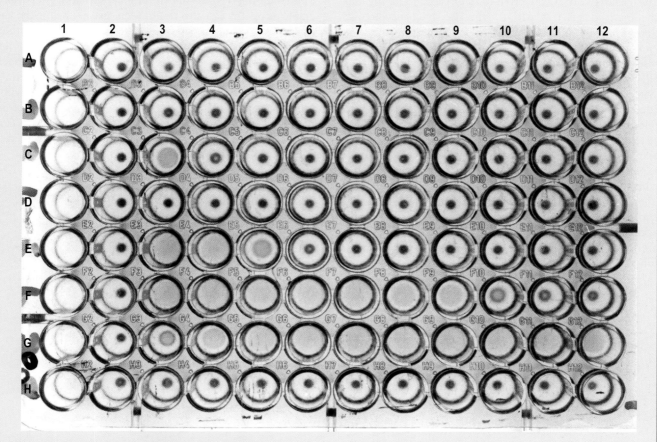

Fig. 12.13 **Titration of rheumatoid factor (RF) in a 96-well titration plate.**
Lane 1, diluent; lane 2, unsensitised gelatin particles; lanes 3–12, particles sensitised (i.e. coated) with IgG. The addition of sera in all the wells of lane 2 gives no agglutination and this negative reaction is seen as a tight button at the bottom of the wells. Wells in lane 3 receive patient sera diluted 1:20. The sera are then double-diluted so that in lane 12 all the sera are diluted 10 240-fold. Rows A, B, D and H contain negative sera. Rows C, E, F and G contain RF-positive sera with titres of 1:20 (C), 1:40 (E), 1:1280 (F), 1:10 240 (G). In well G3 and to a lesser extent G4, it is possible to see a prozone phenomenon. This describes a suboptimal agglutination due to excess of antibody. To ascertain whether a given value is due to a low amount of antibody or to an excess of it, the serum must be tested at different dilutions against a fixed amount of antigen, in this case a fixed amount of antigen-coated particles. The prozone phenomenon can be seen in other immune reactions such as precipitation reactions.

Treatment

This is mainly empirical and follows a gradual approach. A first line of medication is represented by non-steroidal anti-inflammatory drugs (NSAIDs), which tend to control symptoms by blocking cyclooxygenase-2 (Cox-2) and the production of prostaglandins, prostacyclins and thromboxanes. Gastrointestinal intolerance is a frequent side-effect of NSAIDs and cardiovascular complications of Cox-2 inhibitors. To a second line of medications belong drugs thought to modify the disease course. They include agents such as anti-malarials, methotrexate, D-penicillamine and gold salts, with little anti-inflammatory activity but with the ability to ameliorate the course of the disease in a majority of patients. This group of drugs is referred to as disease modifying anti-rheumatic drugs (DMARDs). The use of corticosteroids, though symptomatically effective, is generally avoided, in view of the fact that they do not alter the course of the disease but are associated with important long-term side-effects (although a recent study, yet to be confirmed by others, suggests that early introduction of steroids does alter the course of RA). Cytotoxic drugs — azathioprine and cyclophosphamide — are also usually avoided in view of their potential side-effects, apart from in patients with severe extra-articular manifestations. Currently moving from the experimental phase to the clinic are biological DMARDs comprising monoclonal antibodies and cytokine antagonists. There are three products against TNF-α, one against IL-1 and one against the B cell marker CD20. These biological agents are usually very effective; possible side-effects of the anti-cytokine products are lymphoma and reactivation of tuberculosis (see Ch. 22).

Seronegative spondylarthritides

This group of disorders is collectively referred to as the seronegative spondylarthritides because of the absence of rheumatoid factor. They also share other features such as the involvement of sacroiliac and peripheral joints; the association with the HLA class I antigen B27; and the tendency to enthesitis (enthesis being the site of attachment of tendons to bone).

Ankylosing spondylitis

This condition typically affects the axial skeleton, but peripheral arthropathy can also occur. Men, usually below the age of 40, develop the disease three times more frequently than women (Fig. 12.14). Approximately 90% of the patients are HLA-*B*27* positive, while the prevalence of this antigen in the general population is 7%. Of all the adult HLA-*B*27*-positive individuals, 1–2% have ankylosing spondylitis (AS). AS shows familial aggregation; the concordance in monozygotic twins is approximately 60%, indicating that both genetic and environmental factors must be involved.

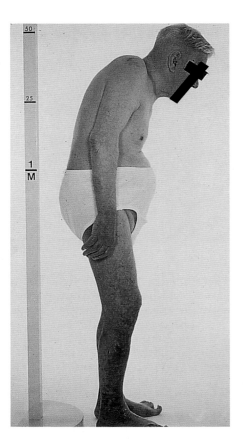

Fig. 12.14 Patient suffering from advanced ankylosing spondylitis.
(From Forbes & Jackson 2003 Color and Atlas Text of Clinical Medicine, 3rd edn, Mosby, with permission.)

SUMMARY BOX 12.2

Rheumatoid arthritis

■ RA is characteristically associated with the HLA-*DRB1*04 (DR4) and DRB1*01 (DR1)* alleles.

■ Pentameric IgM rheumatoid factor is the serological hallmark of RA.

■ Rheumatoid factor levels are particularly elevated in the presence of extra-articular manifestations such as vasculitis.

■ Mononuclear cells, especially CD4 T lymphocytes, predominate in the synovial infiltrate, while polymorphonuclear leukocytes are the dominant cells in the synovial fluid.

■ Levels of complement factors (e.g. C3, C4) are low intra-articularly, reflecting complement consumption, and are high in the bloodstream, indicating an acute-phase reaction.

■ Disease activity is monitored by the measure of erythrocyte sedimentation rate or C-reactive protein.

Pathology

The lesion of sacroiliitis — first manifestation of the disease — is characterised by subchondral granulation tissue containing a mainly mononuclear cell inflammatory infiltrate. Inflammatory granulation is present also in the spine at the junction of the annulus fibrosus with the vertebral bone. Outer fibres are replaced by bone; these bony excrescences (syndesmophytes) ultimately join vertebral bodies, resulting in the radiological picture of the 'bamboo spine' (Fig. 12.15). In the peripheral joints the inflammation is similar to that of rheumatoid arthritis but less vigorous. Non-specific inflammatory changes are seen in the iris of those 20% of patients that suffer from uveitis.

Pathogenesis

It is believed that a form of molecular mimicry triggers the onset of AS (see Science Box 12.10).

Clinical features

The onset of AS tends to be insidious with a dull lumbar pain; this persists over 3 months and is accompanied by morning stiffness, relieved by exercise. Arthritis of the peripheral joints is seen in one third of the patients. Amongst extra-articular manifestations, iritis is the most troublesome: it tends to be unilateral and accompanied by photophobia and pain. Inflammation of the colon and ileum is frequent but usually asymptomatic. The course of the disease is very vari-

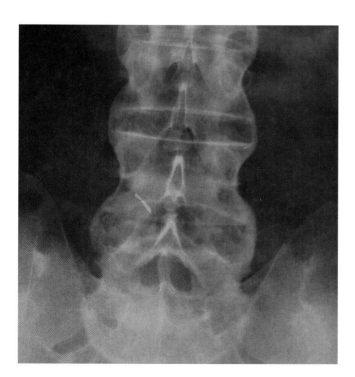

Fig. 12.15 Spine radiogram showing the 'bamboo spine' typically seen in ankylosing spondylitis.

SCIENCE BOX 12.10

The arthritogenic peptide model of ankylosing spondylitis

HLA-B*27 is an HLA class I molecule and as such binds antigenic peptides and presents them to CD8 cytotoxic T cells (CTL). An 'arthritogenic peptide' model sees AS as being the result of a CTL-mediated response to a peptide only found in joint tissues and presented by HLA-B*27 molecules. The theory suggests that under normal conditions the concentration of the self peptide is too low to trigger T cell recognition. Infection with microorganisms containing sequences shared by the arthritogenic peptide would activate T cells and lead them to recognise the arthritogenic peptide even at its normally low concentration (another example of molecular mimicry operating in autoimmune disease).

---

able, the onset in adolescence being associated with poorer prognosis.

Laboratory findings

Patients with AS tend to have elevated levels of IgA and, when the disease is active, elevated erythrocyte sedimentation rates and levels of C-reactive protein. Rheumatoid factor and antinuclear antibody are consistently negative. The clinical need to assess the HLA-B*27 status of a patient with symptoms and signs of AS is controversial. This HLA molecule is present in some 90% of Caucasoid patients and in a lesser proportion of patients of a different ethnic origin. Presence of B27 is neither pathognomonic of the disease nor necessary for making the diagnosis. In patients who have not yet developed clear radiological changes, however, it may be of diagnostic help.

Other seronegative arthritides

A large proportion of these conditions comprises reactive arthritides, the prototype of which is the **Reiter's syndrome**. The diagnostic triad of urethritis, conjunctivitis and arthritis defines this syndrome, even though the diagnosis can be made when just two of these are present, or when balanitis and buccal ulcerations are additional manifestations. The term 'reactive' in the description implies that they follow an infection, frequently unnoticed by the patient and also distant in time and space from the 'reactive' joints. Venereal and enteric infections are typically involved, with microorganisms such as *Chlamydia trachomatis* being the paradigm of venereal infection while a variety of *Shigella*, *Salmonella*, *Yersinia* and *Campylobacter* spp. may be responsible for the enteric infections. HLA-B*27 is present in up to 85% of patients with reactive arthritis; the male/female ratio is 1:1 in post-enteric infection cases, while venereally acquired

Basic and clinical immunology

reactive arthritis is thought to be mainly a male disease, even though the disease in women can be under diagnosed as a result of clinically unapparent urethritis and cervicitis.

Pathology and pathogenesis

The synovial histology is that of inflammatory arthritis with a mononuclear cell infiltrate where T lymphocytes and monocytes predominate. Enthesitis is common, as is the microscopic inflammatory involvement of colon and ileum. Almost all the elements to draw a pathogenic scenario are available. There are well-defined environmental factors: the microorganisms (which, interestingly, are mainly intracellular parasites) responsible for the initial infection. There is a well-defined genetic factor: the HLA-B*27 molecule. As for AS, the assumption must be that cells harbouring the infectious agent process and present it as small peptides in the B27 peptide-binding groove as the target of harmful CD8 cytotoxic T lymphocytes. The unanswered question is why the immune reaction should just be confined to the joints, and only some of them at that, in view of the fact that HLA class I molecules are present on virtually all nucleated cells. Intriguingly, though, there is now evidence to show that antigens from *Chlamydia*, *Yersinia* and *Salmonella* spp. can actually be found in the joints in reactive arthritis, possibly accounting for the localisation of the injurious immune response. Moreover, there is the pivotal observation that synovial T lymphocytes can proliferate in response to antigens of the triggering microorganism. A critique to the above pathogenic scenario has been that not all the patients have HLA-B*27; however, a number of HLA-B*27-negative patients are HLA-B*07 positive, and these two HLA molecules have much of their amino acid sequences in common. Lastly, the importance of the HLA-B*27 gene in the causation of these arthritides and AS is emphasised by a B27-transgenic rat model (see Science Box 12.11). This animal develops inflammatory disease of the axial joints, gut and male genital tract. Any triggering microorganism remains to be defined.

Clinical features

The manifestations can vary from a transient monoarthritis to an asymmetrical additive polyarthritis with prominent constitutional symptoms like fever, malaise, fatigue and weight loss. An infection preceding the onset of arthritis can be found by taking a careful history in the majority of patients, but not in a considerable minority, even though a history of a new sexual partner is at times elicited. Dactylitis, also referred to as 'sausage digit' is typical of reactive arthritis and is caused by diffuse swelling. Urogenital ulcers can occur any time during the course of the disease and ocular manifestations can range from conjunctivitis to the much more severe anterior uveitis. The laboratory findings are few: elevated erythrocyte sedimentation rate during acute phases of the disease, mild anaemia, the presence of HLA-B*27 in 80% of patients and, in some, increased levels of antibodies

against the triggering infectious agent. The infection has usually subsided by the time arthritis appears. The treatment is based on non-steroidal anti-inflammatory drugs, occasionally on the local use of corticosteroids for tendinitis and enthesitis. In the case of uveitis, treatment involves vigorous systemic use of corticosteroids.

SUMMARY BOX 12.3

Ankylosing spondylitis and other seronegative arthritides

- AS is characteristically associated with HLA-B*27, being present in ~90% of patients.
- Elevated IgA levels are common; antinuclear antibodies and rheumatoid factor are usually absent.
- Reactive arthritis is also characteristically associated with HLA-B*27 (~80% of patients).
- An enteric or venereal infection precedes joint manifestations.
- Increased levels of antibodies against the triggering infectious agent are often found.

Sjögren's syndrome

Sjögren's syndrome (SS) is a chronic inflammatory condition affecting lacrimal and salivary glands, leading to dry eyes and mouth (also referred to as keratoconjunctivitis sicca and xerostomia). There are two forms: primary, when the disease

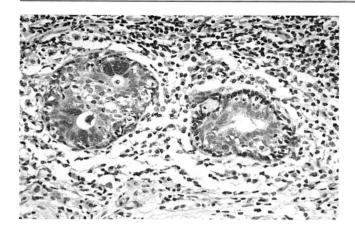

Fig. 12.16 **Sjögren's syndrome.**
The histology of the parotid gland reveals a dense
mononuclear cell infiltrate (courtesy of Dr J. Salisbury).

occurs alone, and secondary, when it is associated with rheumatoid arthritis, SLE and, less frequently, with systemic sclerosis. SS affects middle-aged women (nine females for one male) and has a strong association with the HLA-*B*8-DRB1*03 (B8 DR3)* haplotype. The histology of lacrimal and salivary glands reveals a mononuclear cell infiltrate (Fig. 12.16), mainly composed of T and B lymphocytes, with a predominance of CD4 T lymphocytes, all expressing markers of activation. Hypergammaglobulinaemia is frequent and usually polyclonal. Rheumatoid factors of the pentameric IgM type are present in 90% of the patients while anti-cyclic citrullinated peptides antibodies are rare. Antinuclear antibodies of the speckled and homogeneous type are found in two thirds of patients. More specific to SS are autoantibodies to the extractable nuclear antigens, anti-SS-A (anti-Ro; see above) and anti-SS-B (anti-La), which are present in at least half of the SS patients, in a small proportion of lupus patients (frequently with symptoms of SS) and in virtually no other condition. The production of SS-associated autoantibodies is controlled from genes within the HLA region, especially by the heterodimer HLA-*DQA1*0501/DQB1*0201*. Possession of specific amino acid sequences in the second hypervariable region of the HLA-DQα and HLA-DQβ chain gene products promotes both SS-A and SS-B autoantibody production. The molecular targets of these autoantibodies have also been identified. SS-A recognises polypeptides complexed with Y1–Y5 RNAs. SS-B is a phosphorylated protein complexed with small RNA polymerase transcripts. The pathogenesis of SS is open to conjecture. Whether activation of B lymphocytes, as suggested by the production of a variety of autoantibodies and the presence of hypergammaglobulinaemia, is a key defect is not established. However, in favour of this view is the tendency for the disease to culminate in monoclonal gammopathy, and the fact that patients with SS have a 40-fold increase in the incidence of lymphoma. However, CD4 T cells predominate in the inflammatory infiltrate, and culture of these from SS patients has led to the isolation of an A-type retrovirus (see

Science Box 12.12), indicating the possibility that infection of regulatory T cells could be an important disease trigger.

The **clinical features** of SS include dry eyes with a gritty feeling under the eyelids, symptomatically treated with artificial tears. A reduction in tear flow is documented through the Schirmer's test, while the detection of punctate corneal ulcerations by slit lamp examination after Bengal staining is highly diagnostic. Dry mouth, accompanied by a high incidence of caries, requires fastidious oral hygiene; dysphagia for dry food is the result of involvement of glands of the gastrointestinal tract; dryness of the vagina is accompanied by dyspareunia. Extraglandular manifestations include fatigue, low-grade fever, arthralgias and myalgias. The erythrocyte sedimentation rate is frequently elevated, and mild anaemia can be observed.

Systemic sclerosis

Systemic sclerosis (scleroderma) is a chronic, disabling condition of unknown aetiology, characterised by fibrosis of the skin, blood vessels and internal organs, including lung, heart, gastrointestinal tract and kidney. It is subdivided into: (1) a more severe diffuse cutaneous form that rapidly involves the skin extensively and the internal organs; and (2) a limited cutaneous form, in which the skin thickening is limited to the distal extremities and face. This form can be part of the so-called **CREST syndrome**, the acronym standing for calcinosis, Raynaud's phenomenon, oesophageal involvement, sclerodactyly and telangiectasia. Systemic sclerosis can also affect the visceral organs alone, sparing the skin (systemic sclerosis without scleroderma). Females are affected three times more frequently than males, with a peak incidence in the third to fifth decade. Occurrence of multiple familial cases and a loose association with the HLA antigens have been described.

Pathology

Bundles of collagen bind the skin to the underlying tissue. In early lesions of systemic sclerosis, a mononuclear cell infiltrate consisting of T cells, monocytes, plasma cells and mast cells is seen. The epidermis is thin. In the oesophagus, a thin mucosa, frequently ulcerated, covers abundant collagen deposition in the lamina propria, submucosa and serosa. Similar changes can be seen in other gastrointestinal tract segments, with accompanying mononuclear cell infiltrate. In the lung, a thickening of the alveolar membrane characterises alveolar fibrosis. The alterations of the synovial membrane are similar to those of other inflammatory arthritides, with oedema and an infiltrate of mononuclear cells. Interstitial fibrosis is seen in muscles and myocardium, the fibrosis at times involving the conduction system resulting in conduction defects. The lesions of primary biliary cirrhosis can be noted in the liver, when systemic sclerosis is associated with this liver disease. IgM, complement and fibrinogen can be detected by immunofluorescence in affected renal vessels. These vessels show thickening of the intima of interlobular arteries and fibrinoid necrosis of the intima and media of afferent arterioles.

Pathogenesis

The pathogenic process can be divided into two phases. The first phase, characterised by endothelial injury, is followed by a second phase where fibrosis predominates.

In the early phase, it is thought that activated cytotoxic T/NK cells release granzyme B that damages endothelial cells; endothelial cells are also targeted by antibodies that mediate damage by antibody-dependent cellular cytotoxicity (see p. 113). TNF-α derived from activated macrophages can also induce endothelial damage. The binding of the von Willebrand factor released by damaged endothelium leads to activation of platelets, with the consequent release of platelet-derived growth factor (PDGF; a factor mitogenic for fibroblasts) and TGF-β, which stimulates collagen production by fibroblasts. Both these 'fibrogenic' cytokines are also secreted by activated macrophages and fibroblasts, while activated T lymphocytes produce TGF-β. The state of activa-

tion of T cells is demonstrated by elevated circulating levels of soluble IL-2 receptor and IL-2. Lymphocytes from patients proliferate in the presence of laminin and type IV collagen, components of the endothelial cell membrane. Fibroblasts in the skin lesions express elevated levels of messenger RNA for collagen I and III; when fibroblasts are isolated from affected skin, they continue to produce an abundance of collagen.

Clinical features

Raynaud's phenomenon is usually the first manifestation of systemic sclerosis, frequently preceding other symptoms by months or years. It is typically triggered by cold and reveals itself as pallor and/or cyanosis of the fingers followed by rubor (redness) on rewarming. This phenomenon is present in virtually all patients with systemic sclerosis and may remain a solitary manifestation. The initial skin lesions are characterised by oedema, either localised to the hands or diffuse in character, followed by an indurative phase when the skin becomes firm and bound to the subcutaneous tissue. This can limit extension of digits, leading to flexion contractures. The involvement of the face results in effacing of wrinkles and microstomia, which can interfere with eating (Fig. 12.17). The skin tends to lose hair and become dry and coarse. In a third stage, the skin undergoes softening. Arthritic symptoms, at times resembling those of RA, and an inflammatory myopathy are frequent manifestations affecting the musculoskeletal apparatus. Pulmonary fibrosis is frequent, but it is also frequently asymptomatic. Pulmonary hypertension develops in 10% of patients. Pleuritis, pericarditis and cardiac fibrosis are frequent post-mortem findings.

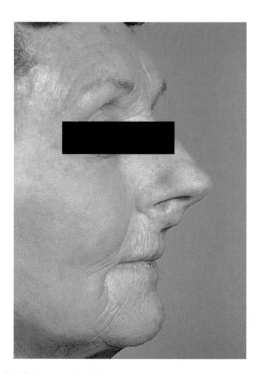

Fig. 12.17 Systemic sclerosis.
Typical facies with tight skin, partial effacing of wrinkles and microstomia (courtesy of Dr J. Goodwill).

Renal involvement is somewhat unusual but can be fatal. SS can be superimposed onto systemic sclerosis.

Laboratory findings

Laboratory tests reveal elevated erythrocyte sedimentation, anaemia and hypergammaglobulinaemia. Low titres of rheumatoid factor are present in a quarter of the patients and antinuclear antibodies are usually present. A speckled pattern is frequently seen, the target antigen being the nuclear enzyme DNA topoisomerase 1 (also known as Scl-70). Antitopoisomerase 1 autoantibodies are present in 20–40% of the patients and tend to be more frequent in the diffuse cutaneous form of the disease and with pulmonary interstitial fibrosis. In contrast, anticentromere autoantibodies are associated with the localised form of the disease or with the CREST syndrome, being rare in the diffuse form. Antinucleolar autoantibodies are considered to be specific for systemic sclerosis, above all when they are an isolated finding. Their targets comprise RNA polymerase I, II and III, and an antigen referred to as PM-Scl. Antibodies to PM-Scl give a homogeneous nucleolar pattern and are associated with polymyositis and renal involvement.

Treatment

The treatment of systemic sclerosis is symptomatic. Raynaud's phenomenon is treated by keeping warm and controlling stress. The renal hypertensive crises are successfully treated with drugs blocking the renin–angiotensin system (captopril, enalapril). Oesophageal and intestinal hypomotility can be improved with metoclopramide.

SUMMARY BOX 12.5

Systemic sclerosis

- Associated with speckled antinuclear antibody.
- Antitopoisomerase 1 autoantibody, also called anti-Scl-70, is present in 20% of patients and tends to be associated with pulmonary interstitial fibrosis.
- Antinucleolar antibodies are present in 30% of patients and are specific for systemic sclerosis.
- Anticentromere antibody is associated with the CREST syndrome.
- A serine protease, TNF and antiendothelial cell antibodies are all involved in damaging endothelial cells.
- The fibrogenic cytokines PDGF and TGF-β promote collagen deposition.

Polymyositis and dermatomyositis

The inflammatory processes involving the skeletal muscle are classified into three main groups: polymyositis (PM), dermatomyositis (DM) and inclusion body myositis (IBM). DM is associated to malignancies.

Pathology

The histological examination of a skeletal muscle biopsy, required for diagnosis in a majority of patients, shows an inflammatory infiltrate, consisting of lymphocytes, macrophages, plasma cells and occasional eosinophils and neutrophils, associated with local or diffuse degeneration of muscle fibres. The inflammatory infiltrate can also be observed around vessels, while signs of muscle fibre degeneration tend to co-exist with signs of regeneration. In IBM, vacuolated fibres with β-amiloid deposits are noted.

Pathogenesis

In 75% of patients with PM and IBM there is an association with the class II HLA alleles *DRB1*0301* and *DQB1*0201*, while in juvenile DM there is an increase in *DQB1*0501*; electron microscopic examination has repeatedly suggested the presence of viral particles within muscle fibres, though no virus has ever been isolated. A polymyositis-like condition can be induced in animals by Coxsackie virus, and a mild form of myopathy can accompany human infections with Coxsackie and influenza viruses. The strongest evidence that a virus is linked to PM and IBM is provided by the observation that some individuals infected with HIV develop PM or IBM. A similar disorder has also been noted in primates infected with the simian immunodeficiency virus.

In PM and IBM the damage is thought to be CD8 T cell mediated. This is suggested by the fact that CD8 cells prevail in the inflammatory infiltrate and that muscle fibres aberrantly express MHC class I molecules, normally absent from the sarcolemma of normal muscle fibres. A possible damaging role for humoral immunity is suggested in DM by the finding of IgG, IgM and the membrane attack complex of the complement system (C5b-9) in vessels of the skin and muscle.

Clinical features

Primary idiopathic polymyositis affects twice as many women as men, usually has an insidious onset and is characterised by weakness in proximal limb muscles (PM and DM), manifesting itself as difficulty in climbing or descending stairs, rising from a chair or from the squatting position, or combing hair. The distal muscles are affected in IBM with impairment of fine-motor movements, such as buttoning a shirt, knitting or writing. The additional cutaneous lesions of primary idiopathic dermatomyositis may precede or follow muscular symptomatology, and typically include a lilac (heliotrope) rash either limited to eyelids and knuckles or occasionally extending to large areas of the body. Malignancies associated to DM are those of the lung, ovary, breast, stomach and myeloproliferative disorders. The paediatric forms are associated with vasculitis of skin, muscles and gastrointestinal tract, while those associated with connective tissue disorders are most frequently linked to SLE, RA and mixed connective tissue disease (see below). The diagnosis is supported by increased levels of the muscle enzymes creatine kinase and transaminases and by typical electromyographical and histological changes.

Laboratory findings

In addition to the characteristic enzymatic profile, erythrocyte sedimentation rate is normally increased, rheumatoid factor is found in half and antinuclear antibody in up to three-quarters of the patients, frequently showing a speckled pattern. An antigenic target for this antibody has been identified as histidyl-transfer RNA synthetase or Jo-1, which is typically found in polymyositis when there is an interstitial pulmonary involvement. Other antinuclear autoantibodies are seen when polymyositis is associated with other connective tissue diseases. The treatment is based on the vigorous use of corticosteroids, at least in the severe cases, with decreasing levels of creatine kinase reflecting the effectiveness of the treatment. Cytotoxic drugs (azathioprine, methotrexate and cyclophosphamide) are used to spare corticosteroids and/or supplement their action. Intravenous immunoglobulin has also been used with anecdotal reports of success.

SCIENCE BOX 12.13

Connective tissue diseases and HIV

In trying to understand the pathogeneses of 'immune-mediated' diseases such as the rheumatic disorders, it is useful to observe their course during infection with HIV, when the CD4 lymphocytes — key regulatory cells in immune homeostasis — are gradually being removed (see Ch. 20). Patients with RA who acquire HIV infection suffer from a much milder form of the disease, strengthening the notion that CD4 lymphocytes play a key role in the pathogenesis of RA. Patients with reactive arthritis such as Reiter's syndrome, however, who contract HIV infection see the course of their disease worsen significantly. Why the depletion of CD4 T cells should exacerbate the course of reactive arthritis is far from clear. What this does tell us is that the pathogenesis of these two types of arthritis is likely to be different.

---

and impaired diffusing capacity of the lung are those of systemic sclerosis, as indeed is the renal involvement. Constitutional symptoms such as fever and lymphadenopathy and an association with Sjögren's syndrome have been occasionally reported.

The usefulness of observing the course of 'immune-mediated' diseases during HIV infection is discussed in Science Box 12.13.

SUMMARY BOX 12.6

Polymyositis and dermatomyositis

- Lymphocytes, macrophages and plasma cells infiltrate degenerating muscle fibres.
- Class II HLA alleles *DRB1*03* (DR3) and *DRB3*01* (DR52) are frequently present.
- Antinuclear autoantibody, often speckled, is present in three-quarters of the patients; rheumatoid factor in half.
- An antigenic target for the antinuclear autoantibody is tRNA synthetase, also called Jo-1.
- Anti-Jo-1 is typically found in patients with polymyositis who also have interstitial pulmonary involvement.

SUMMARY BOX 12.7

Mixed connective tissue disease

- Antinuclear antibody with a speckled pattern is typically found in this condition.
- This antinuclear antibody is directed against ribonucleoprotein (anti-RNP).

Mixed connective tissue disease

Mixed connective tissue disease (MCTD) is described as an 'overlap' syndrome, which borrows elements from several other connective tissue diseases. Elevated titres of a speckled pattern antinuclear antibody directed against ribonucleoprotein (anti-RNP) is the distinguishing feature that makes MCTD a separate diagnostic and pathological entity. The majority of the patients are female and typically experience the Raynaud's phenomenon. The cutaneous manifestations can be those of lupus, or those of dermatomyositis (typically the heliotrope rash). The arthritis tends to be non-deforming, even though it may acquire the features of RA. The skeletal muscle involvement is that of polymyositis, with mononuclear cell inflammatory infiltrate and increase in the circulating levels of creatine kinase. The oesophageal dysmotility

---

Further reading

Rahman A, Isenberg DA 2008 Systemic lupus erythematosus. N Engl J Med 358: 929–939

Crow MK 2008 Collaboration, genetic associations, and lupus erythematosus. N Engl J Med 358: 956–961

Levine JS, Branch DW, Rauch J 2002 The antiphospholipid syndrome. N Engl J Med 346: 752–763

Firestein GS 2003 Evolving concepts of rheumatoid arthritis. Nature 423: 356–361

McInnes IB, Schett G 2007 Cytokines in the pathogenesis of rheumatoid arthritis. Nature Reviews 7: 429–442

Hansen A, Lipsky PE, Dorner T 2005 Immunopathogenesis of primary Sjogren's syndrome: implications for disease management and therapy. Curr Opin Rheumat 17: 558–565

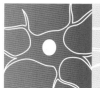

Endocrine autoimmune disease

This chapter highlights the consequences of a malfunction in the immune system that leads to the generation of an autoimmune attack on the hormone-producing endocrine organs. The general principles underlying the development of autoreactive T and B cells were discussed in Chapter 9. Here we will examine specific genetic and environmental constellations that give rise to autoimmune endocrine disease. In some disorders the resultant loss of hormone secretion can have immediate life-threatening consequences; in others, increased hormone production can lead to disease; in most, the disorders lead to chronic morbidity and reduced mortality.

The autoimmune response that targets an endocrine organ is similar to that giving rise to diseases in the gastro-intestinal tract such as pernicious anaemia and autoimmune hepatitis (see Ch. 16). Collectively these are termed the **organ-specific autoimmune diseases**, setting them apart from the **non-organ-specific disorders** that affect multiple tissues and sites (see Ch. 12). Tissue damage is almost always target cell-specific and the resulting organ failure or dysfunction gives rise to a clinical syndrome that reflects the specific hormone deficiency. For example, the target of the auto-immune attack in type 1 diabetes is the β cell, which makes insulin. Once most β cells have been destroyed, insulin is deficient and high blood sugar (diabetes) ensues.

In recent years there have been considerable advances in our understanding of the underlying mechanisms of autoimmune disease at the genetic, environmental and immunological levels; this has given rise to some exciting options for immune-based therapies to cure or prevent these disorders.

The diseases to be discussed are those most commonly encountered in clinical practice (type 1 diabetes, thyroiditis) as well as rarer diseases with severe consequences affecting the adrenal and reproductive glands, and a very rare auto-immune syndrome affecting multiple organs. The sections will focus on immunological features of the disease that may be of clinical use, the underlying disease mechanisms, and possible therapeutic avenues, building on the basic principles and disease models in Chapter 9.

Several of the endocrine autoimmune disorders share common features. Some are more common in women, strongly implying a hormonal influence on their development. The disorders frequently 'run' in families but there is usually not a simple pattern of heritability. Rather, the diseases are polygenic. A common genetic thread is the involvement of HLA genes. The major clue that a disease is autoimmune is usually given by the existence of circulating serum autoantibodies and these provide powerful diagnostic and predictive tools.

Type 1 diabetes

Diabetes is a state of high blood sugar (hyperglycaemia) that can have many underlying causes. The autoimmune form of the disease, Type 1 diabetes represents 10–15% of all diabetes. In this case, the hyperglycaemia results from insufficient insulin secretion by β cells in the islets of Langerhans of the pancreas. After diagnosis, patients require multiple insulin injections daily to sustain life. The diagnosis is usually a clinical one, with a typical patient having pro-dromal symptoms of weight loss, thirst, excessive drinking and urination over several weeks or months. A random blood test reveals a high level of glucose (>7 mmol/l on 2 occasions), which is diagnostic. A fasting blood glucose above 11.1 mmol/l is also diagnostic. If the diagnosis is in doubt, a further test involves giving an oral glucose challenge (75 g) and diabetes is diagnosed if the 2-hour glucose level is above 11.1 mmol/l. A sustained high blood glucose level promotes severe metabolic disturbances that can lead to coma and death, but improvements in clinical care and a

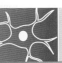

greater awareness of the disease have made this a very rare outcome.

Although it is true to say that the advent of injected insulin earlier in the twentieth century restored health in what had always been an acutely fatal disease, this treatment does not hold all the answers. Insulin-treated type 1 diabetes is still associated with excessive morbidity and mortality rates. These result from a series of conditions termed 'diabetic complications', which include cardiovascular disease, renal failure and severe sight impairment and are the indirect result of chronic impairment of blood glucose control. In economic terms, diabetes as a whole consumes approximately 8–10% of the acute services budget in developed countries, through its contribution to the burden of arterial disease, blindness and renal failure.

Type 1 diabetes affects all age groups. It has a peak onset around puberty and the incidence within Europe ranges from 5 to 50 cases per 100 000 of the population per year, along an approximate north–south gradient from Finland to Greece. In the UK and USA, the incidence is approximately 20 cases per 100 000 per year and the prevalence 1/250. Worryingly, type 1 diabetes is on the increase in all age groups, but especially in the very young. Unlike some other autoimmune diseases, type 1 diabetes affects the sexes equally.

Type 1 diabetes arises on a very distinctive genetic background. Some 90% of cases are sporadic, whilst the remainder occur within families that already have a diabetic member. There are at least 18 genetic loci known to contribute to the disease, called *IDD1–18* and for some of these, the actual genes involved have been identified (Table 13.1). It is estimated that 50% of the genetic susceptibility maps to *IDD1*, which is the HLA class II region on chromosome 6. Some of the HLA-DQ molecules encoded confer susceptibility, whilst others confer protection. The other main gene loci identified so far are *IDD2* (the insulin gene, *INS*) and *IDD12*, the gene encoding CTLA-4 (see p. 111). Together, these genes give major clues as to the likely sequence of events leading to diabetes, and have allowed a very clear pathogenetic model of the disease to be built up, as well as contributing to the potential use of genetic screening for at-risk individuals (see below).

Pathology of the islet in type 1 diabetes

Healthy human islets of Langerhans are composed of a core of some 80% β cells (making the glucose-regulating hormone insulin), with a mantle of other endocrine cell types, producing glucagon (α cells), somatostatin (δ cells) and pancreatic polypeptide (PP cells) making up the remainder. Histologically, the islets of Langerhans at diagnosis of type 1 diabetes have a mixture of appearances: (i) a proportion are small, have lost all β cells and have no inflammatory cells; (ii) others have numerous intact β cells that are surrounded by infiltrating activated T (CD4 and CD8) and B lymphocytes and APCs (an appearance termed **insulitis**); and (iii) some islets appear normal with no or few infiltrating cells. These appearances probably reflect three stages of a sequential process during which the immune cells travel between islets in a 'seek, destroy, move on' operation. Throughout the pancreas β cells have disappeared whilst α, δ and PP cells remain untouched. Overall, these characteristics suggest a slowly evolving disease, in which inflammatory cells flit from islet to islet, with the single mission of targeted β cell destruction (Fig. 13.1).

Clinical and immunological features

Type 1 diabetes is a diagnosis made on clinical grounds, based on the history and biochemical tests. Immunological tests, in the form of autoantibody detection, are used only in specific circumstances (see Clinical Boxes 13.1 and 13.2).

Table 13.1 Major genes involved in type 1 diabetes susceptibility

	Genetic locus	Phenotype	Speculated disease mechanism	Relative risk* conferred by allele
IDD1	HLA class II region	Expression of HLA molecules (DR4, DR3, DQ8, DQ2)	These HLA molecules promote selected presentation of autoantigens	Varies according to allele, but in the range 1–10
IDD2	Insulin gene	Reduced expression of proinsulin in thymus	Allows thymic escape of autoreactive T cells	2–3
IDD12	CTLA-4 gene	Increased expression of soluble forms of CTLA-4	Results in poor regulation of T cell activation	1.2

*Relative risk (RR) of carrying gene A for the disease = [patients with A × controls lacking A] ÷ [patients without A = controls with A].

Normal islet

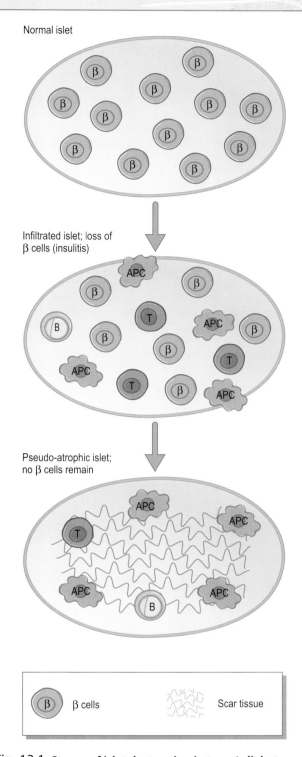

Infiltrated islet; loss of β cells (insulitis)

Pseudo-atrophic islet; no β cells remain

β cells

Scar tissue

Fig. 13.1 Stages of islet destruction in type 1 diabetes.
The normal islet has a full complement of β and other endocrine cells, and no infiltrating immune cells. Insulitis is present at the early stage of the disease — there is loss of some β cells and islet infiltration by T cells, B cells and APCs. The final stage for the islet is that β cells have been replaced by scar tissue, and there are few if any immune cells left. The non β cells remain.

CLINICAL BOX 13.1

Clinical uses of islet cell autoantibodies

So, under what circumstances are islet cell autoantibodies such as IAA, GADA and IA-2A useful in a clinical setting? The first use is for diagnosis, the second for prediction (see Clinical Box 13.2). Although in most cases type 1 diabetes is diagnosed clinically because of the symptoms, occasionally the disease evolves slowly. This is especially true in adults, who, because of their age, are assumed to have type 2 diabetes (the form associated with obesity and insulin resistance, and typically seen in the over 35 years age group). However, in some of these adults, there is a gradual requirement for insulin injections and, more importantly, GAD65 autoantibodies (GADA) are detected in the serum. This condition is therefore termed **Latent Autoimmune Diabetes in Adults** (LADA, also called type 1½ diabetes by some!), and GADA is therefore a useful diagnostic tool in patients presenting at this age. A further point of note is that LADA may be the underlying form of diabetes in as many as 10–20% of all adults presenting with apparent type 2 disease. This is an active research area, but to date it appears that in most immunopathogenic respects, LADA is similar to type 1 diabetes.

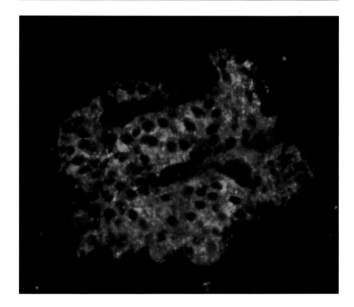

Fig. 13.2 Indirect immunofluorescence study of a section of healthy human pancreas stained with serum from a patient with type 1 diabetes mellitus.
The autoantibodies present in the patient's serum have stained the islet cells with a distinctive pattern, called islet cell autoantibody (ICA; see Indirect immunofluorescence technique described on p. 173).

The islet cell autoantibodies are the defining immunological feature of type 1 diabetes (Fig. 13.2). There are four proteins that constitute the major target autoantigens for these autoantibodies; insulin, glutamic acid decarboxylase-65 (GAD65), a tyrosine phosphatase called IA-2 and the zinc transporter molecule ZnT8. Insulin and ZnT8 are specific for the β cells.

CLINICAL BOX 13.2

The era of screening and intervention trials in type 1 diabetes

Advances in the use of genes and autoantibodies to predict diabetes makes it feasible to consider interfering in the disease process. The roadmap to diabetes development in Figure 13.3 shows how this might work. First, the assumption is made that the healthy individual starts life with 100% β cell mass. At this stage the disease risk can be estimated from a family history of diabetes, or from genes (e.g. HLA). These are common genes and their predictive power is low. Therefore, any disease intervention at this stage (**primary prevention**) would have to be very safe, since it would be applied to many who would not get the disease. Examples could include dietary modulation or vaccination against candidate viruses.

When the disease trigger is applied, the progressive loss of β cells commences. At this stage, there is silent autoreactivity manifested by islet cell autoantibodies. These can be combined with genes to predict future diabetes. At this stage **secondary prevention** (secondary because the disease process has already commenced) could be contemplated. However, not all of those with autoantibodies progress to

diabetes (see Fig. 13.4), so therapies attempted under these circumstances should have a good safety profile. Examples of agents that have been tried at this stage in large multi-centre studies are nicotinamide (protects β cells from chemical damage) and injected and oral insulin (designed to 'rest' β cells and/or induce tolerance; see Ch. 9). Nicotinamide and injected insulin both failed, but oral insulin appeared to enhance survival in a subgroup of patients, so this trial is being repeated.

Finally, clinical disease develops when approximately 10–20% of β cells remain. If these remaining cells could be salvaged, diabetes is more easily controllable, and the risk of serious diabetic complications lessened. Since the disease has now been diagnosed, there is no risk of treating individuals without diabetes, and therefore therapies with higher toxicities could be contemplated at this stage (**tertiary prevention**). Several agents have shown promise recently, including a monoclonal antibody against CD3 on T cells, and a peptide designed to induce islet-specific tolerance (see Ch. 22).

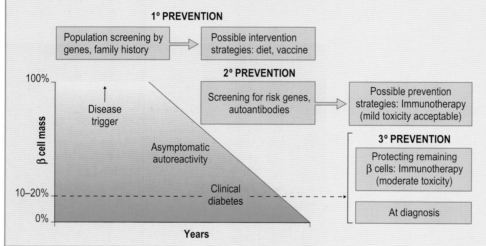

Fig. 13.3 **Roadmap to diabetes development, showing options for prediction and therapy at different stages of disease and pre-disease.**

GAD65 and IA-2 may also be found in other islet cell types and in the nervous system (Table 13.2). Although the individual autoantibodies may only be present in a half to two thirds of patients, typically 90% of patients will have at least one of these autoantibodies at diagnosis. Interestingly, these autoantigens may be present in the thymus during T cell development.

Islet cell autoantibodies are emerging as being especially important in disease **prediction**. From studies on individuals at risk of developing type 1 diabetes (e.g. first-degree relatives of patients) it has become clear that apparently healthy people can have islet cell autoantibodies — up to 10% of relatives are positive for IAA, GADA or IA-2A when tested. Does this mean they will develop diabetes in the future? By making the studies prospective and following

antibody-positive individuals for 5–10 years, a very clear pattern of disease risk has emerged (see Fig. 13.4). Some of these relatives do indeed progress to diabetes, the risk escalating with the number of autoantibodies present. Thus it would appear that the breadth and intensity of the auto-immune response determines whether anti-islet immunity develops into clinical disease. These pioneering studies have now been translated into the general population (this is important for screening purposes, as 90% of new diabetic patients do not have relatives with the disease). Although far fewer of the general public are autoantibody-positive, those that are have a disease risk determined by the number of autoantibodies present. The era of accurate diabetes prediction has made it feasible to design intervention trials, aimed at modifying the autoimmune response in such a

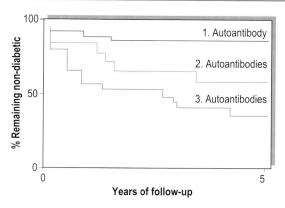

Fig. 13.4 Using islet cell autoantibodies to predict future type 1 diabetes.
A cohort of healthy first-degree relatives of patients with type 1 diabetes are screened for autoantibodies (IAA, GADA, IA-2A) and then classified according to the number of different antibodies they possess. During follow-up to see whether they develop diabetes it becomes clear that the risk goes up with the number of autoantibodies present.

way as to prevent diabetes development in at-risk subjects (Science Box 13.1).

How does the β cell die?

Although islet autoantibodies are highly predictive of diabetes, it is now thought extremely unlikely that they actually cause the disease; for example, it is possible to have the autoantibodies without disease, and pregnant mothers with circulating IgG islet autoantibodies that cross the placenta into the foetal circulation do not give birth to diabetic babies. On the basis of the features of the insulitis, most scientists in this field believe that autoreactive CD4 and CD8 T cells are directly responsible for β cell death. Although it is clearly unethical to adoptively transfer T cells from a diabetic patient to a healthy individual in order to prove this, occasionally such 'experiments' are carried out inadvertently (see Science Box 13.2).

The predominance of CD8 T lymphocytes in the insulitis supports the proposal that β cells are probably damaged in a cell-mediated cytotoxic reaction. However, it is clear from animal models of type 1 diabetes that both CD4 and CD8 T cells are required for disease. It thus seems likely that CD4 T lymphocytes recognising islet autoantigens such as insulin,

Table 13.2 Features of islet autoantigens in type 1 diabetes

Antigen/ Autoantibody	Islet specific?	Present in thymus during T cell ontogeny?	Function	Proportion of patients positive at diagnosis	Other features
Insulin autoantibodies/ IAA	Yes, and β cell specific	Yes	Regulates glucose	50–60% overall, but higher in children	
Glutamic acid decarboxylase autoantibodies/ GADA	No, present in other islet cells and CNS	Yes	Catalyses synthesis of GABA[1], a negative neurotransmitter; probably regulates insulin release	65–75% overall, higher in adults	Also a target autoantigen in stiff man syndrome (SMS)
Islet tyrosine phosphatase autoantibodies/ IA-2A	No, present in other islet cells and CNS	Yes	Unknown	50–60% overall but higher in children	
Zinc transporter 8/ZnT8	Yes, and β cell specific	Not yet known	Zinc transport	50–60%	

[1]GABA; γ-amino butyric acid.

Identification of glutamic acid decarboxylase as an autoantigen: serendipity in medical research

Throughout the 1980s, it was known that sera from up to 80% of diabetic patients could react against an autoantigen present in the islets of Langerhans. The only thing known with certainty about the protein was its molecular weight: 64 kilodaltons. Since islets are tiny structures, hidden inside the pancreas, identifying the protein was a difficult challenge. The search became known as the '64K question', and was nearly 10 years old, when a stroke of luck led to the answer. A patient at the San Raffaele Hospital, Milan, was diagnosed as having a rare neurological condition, known as stiff man syndrome (SMS). This disease is all in the name: patients are characteristically rigid in the back and limbs. This particular patient also had type 1 diabetes and ICA. A worldwide search across four continents revealed 33 patients with SMS, six of whom had type 1 diabetes and 18 of whom had ICA. Since the patients had a neurological condition, scientists checked whether there were any autoantibodies reacting against brain tissue. Lo and behold, in 22 patients, antibodies were

detected reacting with GABA-secreting neurons in the cerebellum and, of these patients, 30% had type 1 diabetes and 95% had ICA. Since brain tissue was easily accessible for study, it was not long before the antigen was identified as GAD, the enzyme responsible for catalysing the conversion of glutamate to GABA. It soon became clear that it was the same antigen being detected in the islet and that anti-64K antibodies were in fact anti-GAD antibodies. Not all aspects of the story have become clear, however. For example, in both type 1 diabetes and SMS there are antibodies to GAD. Yet, whilst diabetes is common in SMS patients, SMS is exceptionally rare in diabetics. Moreover, the anti-GAD antibodies in SMS may actually be pathogenic, since plasmapheresis is an effective therapy. How is it that diabetics with anti-GAD do not become stiff? It appears that a subtle difference in the GAD-binding site in SMS and diabetic sera may account for the difference.

Proof that T cells cause type 1 diabetes?

As discussed in the text here and in Chapter 9, the 'gold-standard' for proving that a particular immune cell or antibody is responsible for an autoimmune disease is to transfer it from a diseased subject to a healthy one. Clearly, scientists would have difficulties getting the ethical committee to approve such a study! However, there are occasions when transfer of immune cells is carried out, and the experiment is performed inadvertently. The best example is bone marrow transplantation (BMT). There are now several cases in the medical literature that read roughly as follows. A young girl develops leukaemia and, although for several years the disease is held in remission by conventional chemotherapy, she eventually relapses and the only prospect of cure is BMT, preferably from a closely related sibling. The girl is lucky — she has a brother with a perfect HLA match. The only problem is that he has had type 1 diabetes for the last 5 years. The doctors test his blood, and find no evidence of islet autoantibodies. They reason that whatever process caused his diabetes has 'burned out' and, since his sister is at

death's door, they go ahead with the BMT. Before this, they take several steps to ensure that the girl's leukaemic cells are completely eradicated — in effect, they wipe out her whole immune system (a process termed conditioning). The BMT is a success. In the ensuing weeks and months, the new bone marrow cells are engrafted, and she is cured of her leukaemia. Until . . . 2 years later, she develops . . . type 1 diabetes! Whatever immune cell caused her diabetes, it cannot have been her own, since they had all been removed during the conditioning. The only conclusion is that during her BMT, some T cells were transferred from her brother and these turned out to be islet destructive. The adoptive transfer experiment was done, albeit unintentionally.

The reporting of several of these cases has led to steps to reduce the risks of transferring potentially damaging T cells during BMT. Nowadays, when such BMTs are performed, the marrow is depleted of mature T cells using monoclonal antibodies.

GAD65, IA-2 and ZnT8 become activated in the local lymph nodes, activate cytotoxic CD8 T cells recognising related targets on β cells, which travel to the islets and initiate the destructive process. Autoreactive CD4 T cells make the same journey, and in conjunction with local APCs and B cells, the autoimmune response is established in the tissues and proceeds from islet to islet until the β cell is eradicated. Since the whole process requires presentation of autoantigens by class II HLA molecules, this model is in keeping with the strong association between type 1 diabetes and class II HLA genes. As yet, however, it is not clear how class II HLA molecules influence disease. As discussed in Chapter 9, they could favour presentation of epitopes that are critical to disease development; these could be from autoantigens or from mimicking viruses (Table 13.3). Alternatively, certain class II HLA molecules could be poor at presentation of peptides that are important for generating T cells that regulate the immune system and prevent autoimmunity.

Table 13.3 Homology between GAD65 and the PEVKEK enterovirus sequence

Protein	Amino acid sequence
P2-C non-structural protein of the enterovirus coxsackie B4	35-KIL**PEVKEK**HEFLN-48
Glutamic acid decarboxylase-65	257-KMF**PEVKEK**GMAAL-270

Why does the β cell die?

Armed with fairly good evidence that the β cell is destroyed by T cells, the question arises as to why? Why does the immune system turn its array of cytotoxic cells and molecules on the innocent β cell? Various disease models can be proposed, and have to take into account the genetic influences discussed earlier. In addition, it is known that the environment has a role to play in diabetes development. Evidence for this comes from several sources, one of the most powerful being a large number of studies of monozygotic (identical) twins. In a disease in which both nature (i.e. genes) and nurture (i.e. environment) have a contribution, the twins can indicate the relative influence of each. If a disease is genetically determined, then identical twin pairs should be 100% concordant (i.e. both twins in the pair have the disease). In type 1 diabetes, the concordance rate is about 35%, indicating the strong influence of non-genetic (i.e. environmental) factors.

Numerous environmental influences have been proposed, but top of the list are viruses. In light of these findings, at least two of the autoimmunity models described in Chapter 9 could be at play in the development of type 1 diabetes. These are molecular mimicry and bystander activation, as illustrated in Figure 13.5. Bystander activation may be sufficient to generate T cells that recognise β cell antigens. Molecular mimicry could assist this, if antiviral T cells cross-react with β cell antigens.

The pathogenic scenario painted in Figure 13.5 is very attractive. But it begs the question, 'Why does this only seem to happen to people with a particular genetic background of HLA, INS and CTLA-4 genes?'. The argument must be that in some way the genes make this pathogenic scenario more likely to happen. There are several examples of ways in which this could happen:

- Thymic deletion of T cells capable of recognising β cells may be incomplete. This could result from the effects of HLA genes in the thymus or the *INS* gene (see Table 13.1).

- Peripheral regulation of T cells capable of recognising β cells may be suboptimal. This could result from the effects of the *CTLA-4* gene (see Table 13.1).

- Peripheral activation of T cells capable of recognising β cells has a lower threshold. This could result if the HLA genes associated with diabetes enhance autoantigen presentation.

SUMMARY BOX 13.1

Type 1 diabetes mellitus

- Type 1 diabetes is a common and debilitating autoimmune disease, characterised by β cell destruction, anti-islet cell autoantibodies and a major role for T cells in tissue damage.

- The autoantibodies are highly predictive of disease and make future prevention of diabetes a real possibility.

- Although parts of the jigsaw puzzle are known, the exact cause of the disease is open to speculation.

- The strongest speculation suggests that a virus initiates β cell damage and that the genes that confer susceptibility to diabetes allow this to escalate into an autoimmune attack.

Autoimmune thyroid disease

Autoimmune disease affecting the thyroid gland is common, affecting approximately 1–2% of the UK population, with a similar incidence in the USA. Two pieces of evidence put the frequency of subclinical disease at around 15%: thyroid autoantibodies are frequently detected in healthy individuals, particularly women, and a lymphocytic thyroid infiltrate has been noted in analysis of post-mortem specimens from individuals who died without any known evidence of thyroid disease. Some estimates suggest that 1–2% of adolescents, 3–4% of the middle-aged population and more than 20% of the elderly have autoimmune thyroid disease.

Autoimmune thyroid disease is broadly classified into two categories on the basis of the effect on gland function: autoimmune **hypo**thyroidism includes **Hashimoto's thyroiditis** and **primary (atrophic) hypothyroidism**; **hyper**thyroidism is seen in **Graves' disease**. All three disorders share some common features. The diseases are all more common in women by 4–6 times, run in families and tend to be influenced by HLA genes, though this is weak in comparison to type 1 diabetes (relative risk for a single allele is usually around 2–4). There are also environmental factors influencing the development of autoimmune thyroid disease. One of the best known is the dietary intake of iodine: the higher this is in a population, the more frequent is autoimmune thyroid disease. Other predisposing factors are stress and smoking.

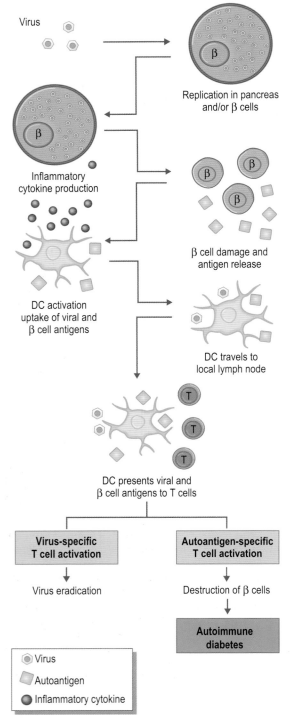

Fig. 13.5 Disease model for the development of type 1 diabetes.

A virus infection in the pancreas has two effects: (i) cells are damaged, releasing β cell antigens, and (ii) local dendritic cells are activated by the damaged cells and by virus RNA/DNA. The dendritic cells take samples from the inflamed tissue to the local lymph node. There, they process and present antigens that will include viral and β cell proteins. T cells are activated to eradicate the virus. Inadvertently, T cells are activated against β cells and the slow process of β cell damage starts. The virus is eradicated, and all evidence of the initiating virus is long gone by the time the patient presents with clinical diabetes.

From an immunological viewpoint, thyroid autoimmunity represents several landmarks. It was the first condition in which autoantibodies were defined (anti-thyroglobulin antibodies in 1956), and hence in some ways the 'first' autoimmune disease. It is the commonest group of autoimmune diseases and, if type 1 diabetes is the prototype of an autoimmune disease caused by T cells, then Graves' is the equivalent caused by autoantibodies.

Hashimoto's thyroiditis

Hashimoto's thyroiditis (increasingly the term **autoimmune thyroiditis** is being used) is a chronic disease typically characterised by enlargement (goitre) and dense lymphocytic infiltration of the thyroid gland. It is four times more common in women and has an incidence of approximately 0.5% in the general population; the incidence peaks in middle age. Patients usually complain of goitre as the main symptom, with an enlarged, firm, sometimes nodular thyroid gland on examination. At presentation, patients may still be euthyroid, but with time the pathological processes result in loss of thyroid tissue and hypothyroidism. Symptoms and signs of hypothyroidism may be seen at the first consultation (fatigue, cold intolerance, dryness of skin, anorexia, weight gain, menstrual disturbance, huskiness of voice, mental slowing, abnormal reflexes). Much less commonly, a period of temporary thyrotoxicosis lasting weeks or months is encountered. The diagnosis of Hashimoto's disease is made mainly on the history and examination, and serum thyroid autoantibodies (see later) may also be of use.

There is a weak HLA association with Hashimoto's thyroiditis but it is not consistent in different racial groupings.

Pathology

Histologically, there is evidence of loss of colloid in the thyroid follicles, occasionally some fibrosis and a lymphocytic infiltrate including numerous plasma cells. At its most florid, the infiltrate is organised, with the formation of lymphoid follicles and germinal centres. Within the infiltrating cells, some 20% may be macrophages, 30% B lymphocytes or plasma cells and the remainder T lymphocytes in the ratio CD4 : CD8 of up to 4 : 1.

Pathogenesis and immunological features

As in type 1 diabetes, autoimmune thyroid disease is characterised by the presence of autoantibodies. There are two main autoantibodies found in Hashimoto's thyroiditis, which are common to all types of autoimmune thyroid disease (Table 13.4). Antibodies to **thyroid peroxidase (TPO)**, the enzyme involved in iodination of thyroglobulin, are found at high titre (i.e. autoantibody activity remains after dilution of serum in excess of several thousand times) in the circulation. TPO has been identified on the apical border of the thyrocyte as it abuts the thyroid follicular space full of colloid, and it appears that circulating antibodies can gain access to and

Table 13.4 Characteristics of thyroid autoantibodies

Autoantibody	Method of detection	Percentage positive			Other features
		General population	Hashimoto's thyroiditis and primary hypothyroidism	Graves' disease	
Antithyroglobulin (TG)	Particle agglutination, ELISA[a]	3%	40–70%	20–40%	
Anti-thyroid peroxidase (TPO)	Particle agglutination, ELISA[a]	10–15	80–95	50–80	
Anti-TSH receptor (stimulating TRAb)	Sensitive radioimmunoassay detects the antibody, but a bioassay is needed to show the stimulatory effects (some TRAbs do not stimulate)	1–2	6–60	70–100	Mimics TSH; causes thyrotoxicosis; autoantibodies (stimulate) crosses placenta and causes disease in newborn ('neonatal thyrotoxicosis')

ELISA: enzyme-linked immunosorbent assay.

SCIENCE BOX 13.3

Spectacular success of a humanised mouse in uncovering the pathogenesis of Hashimoto's thyroiditis

As stated in the text, until recently it was not clear which part of the immune system actually caused the cell damage that led to hypothyroidism in Hashimoto's thyroiditis, although many scientists and clinicians in the field thought that it must be a result of the action of TPO autoantibodies.

To test the hypothesis that T cells alone are capable of causing the disease, a group of UK researchers engineered a mouse so that the only T cell receptor it was capable of expressing came from a human T cell that recognised a peptide of TPO and had originally been isolated from a diseased human thyroid gland. The human T cell receptor turned up on both CD4 and CD8 mouse T cells and, amazingly, the mouse spontaneously developed infiltration

of the thyroid gland, with hypothyroidism and weight gain, just as seen in human disease. These effects did not require the presence of B cells, indicating that the T cell alone is capable of causing this disease.

One highly intriguing aspect of the work is that the TPO epitope recognised by the T cell clone is cryptic. In other words, although some antigen presenting cells (APCs) will not present this peptide from whole TPO, others can, including the thyrocyte itself. The scientists involved in the work speculated that the 'cryptic' epitope might not be very efficiently generated by APCs in the thymus, leading to incomplete deletion of autoreactive T cells, which are then easily activated in the periphery.

bind their target here. Such antibodies could therefore kill thyroid cells directly and also interfere with the catalytic function of thyroid peroxidase, contributing to the generation of hypothyroidism. Antibodies to **thyroglobulin (Tg)** were the first autoantibodies ever described in a human autoimmune disease, in 1956. Anti-Tg antibodies are considered unlikely to have a pathogenic role in Hashimoto's thyroiditis. Both antithyroglobulin and anti-thyroid peroxidase antibodies are usually detected by particle agglutination (see p. 180) using gelatin coated with purified thyroglobulin, or by enzyme-linked immunosorbent assay (ELISA).

For many years, TPO autoantibodies were considered to have a major and important role in thyroid gland damage. Recently, however, a new piece of research has strongly indicated that autoreactive T cells, recognising TPO, are actually responsible for cytotoxic reactions (see Science Box 13.2). The other cell involved in the thyroid autoimmune response and worthy of mention is the thyrocyte itself. Under inflammatory conditions it expresses HLA molecules, adhesion molecules and CD40, equipping it to play a potentially important role in disease (see Science Box 13.3 and Fig. 13.6).

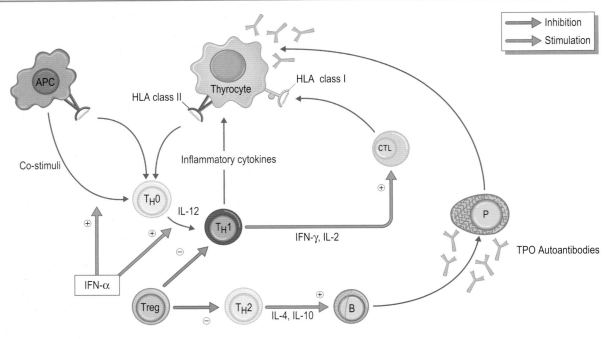

Fig. 13.6 Disease model for development of thyroiditis.
Presentation of autoantigens by professional APCs initiates the process, which has both T$_H$1 and T$_H$2 elements. Once the process is established, the thyrocyte itself up-regulates immune molecules such as HLA class II and becomes capable of perpetuating the inflammation, presenting self thyroid autoantigens to infiltrating T cells. Thyrocyte damage is probably a result of the combined effects of CD4 and CD8 T cells and autoantibodies. The autoimmune process may be accelerated by external agents such as IFN-α. Treg cells may be defective since the disease is linked to polymorphisms of the *CTLA-4* gene, a negative regulator of T cells.

Treatment of hypothyroidism is with thyroxine replacement therapy.

Graves' disease

Graves' disease is characterised clinically by hyperthyroidism and goitre. Patients typically present with the symptoms or signs of hyperthyroidism (palpitations, tachycardia, arrhythmias, heat intolerance, increased appetite with weight loss, diarrhoea, weakness and proximal myopathy, nervousness and tremor). One characteristic feature of Graves' disease is worthy of note: eye disease characterised by protrusion of the eyeball and lid retraction resulting from tissue inflammation in the retro-orbital space. Laboratory findings are of elevated thyroid hormones — thyroxine (T4) and triiodothyronine (T3) — with suppressed levels of thyroid-stimulating hormone (TSH). Whilst untreated Graves' disease is life threatening, current pharmacological and surgical approaches have rendered the disease eminently treatable. The main drugs used (carbimazole and propylthiouracil) are designed to inhibit synthesis of the thyroid hormones.

Graves' disease has a peak incidence in the third and fourth decades and is found in approximately 0.1–0.5% of the general population. Predispositions to Graves' disease include living in an area of high iodine intake, female sex (female : male ratio 7 : 1) and possession of HLA-DR3, which confers a relative risk of approximately 4. Concordance for the disease in monozygotic twins is approximately 50%. Stress has frequently been invoked as a precipitating factor in Graves' disease, and indeed it is curious that in the early 1990s both the US President (George Bush Snr) and his wife should have been diagnosed as having Graves' disease within months of each other and within months of his inauguration as President. More intriguing still is the powerful effect of two immune therapies on induction of Graves' disease: both interferon-α therapy and use of the powerful T cell depleting drug Campath-1H provoke Graves' thyroiditis (see below).

Pathology

The predominant features are of increased size and vascularity, with hyperplasia and hypertrophy of the endocrine tissue. In contrast with Hashimoto's thyroiditis, the lymphocytic infiltration is less florid, formation of lymphoid follicles is less common and destruction of normal thyroid gland is not seen.

Pathogenesis and immunological features

The key feature distinguishing Graves' disease is the presence of autoantibodies that stimulate glandular function, resulting in hyperthyroidism (see Table 13.4). The history of the dis-the antibody competed with TSH for binding to the TSH receptor, identifying the mechanism by which this autoantibody, now termed the **TSH receptor autoantibody** (**TRAb**), is pathogenic in Graves' disease. The autoantibody may be detected by one of two techniques: a radioligand assay in which it competes with radiolabelled TSH for receptor binding or in a bioassay assessing stimulatory effects of the antibody on cultured thyroid cells.

What, then, could account for the development of these pathogenic autoantibodies in Graves' disease? (Fig. 13.8). Several theories exist, but none has yet been proven unequivocally. Like type 1 diabetes, Graves' disease and autoimmune hypothyroidism are also associated with polymorphisms in the *CTLA-4* gene. It seems probable, therefore, that Graves' disease has a similar underlying basis, with the tendency to generate anti-thyroid T cell autoimmunity being promoted by particular HLA-DR and HLA-DQ molecules, and facilitated by poor regulatory function in the periphery. These suggestions get strong support from the effects of IFN-α and Campath-1H in precipitating Graves' disease. IFN-α, given as an antiviral agent (e.g. to patients who fail to clear hepatitis C virus) would have powerful effects on bystander activation as it mimics the effect of activated DCs. Campath-1H, a monoclonal antibody targeted at a T cell determinant, was given as an experimental drug to patients with the autoimmune disease multiple sclerosis. Approximately one third developed Graves' disease. The best explanation for this effect is that Campath-1H had an unexpectedly powerful effect in depleting regulatory T cells, allowing autoreactivity to take hold.

Clinical features

The diagnosis of Graves' disease is made mainly on clinical grounds, with the support of an isotope scan showing diffuse uptake. The hyperthyroidism is usually controlled pharmacologically, and response to therapy is associated with a decline in TSH receptor autoantibodies. The agents used, carbimazole and propylthiouracil, inhibit the synthesis of thyroid hormones, but their use also appears to decrease the rate of relapse, implying that they have a direct and beneficial effect on the autoimmune process. In studies in which TSH receptor autoantibodies have been measured, persistence or reappearance during treatment frequently heralds relapse. Surgery or thyroid ablation using radioiodine may then be required.

Graves' disease is frequently (approximately 8%) complicated by a thyroid eye disease, an ophthalmopathy that occurs only rarely in association with Hashimoto's thyroiditis. Patients may complain of protuberance of the eyes, discomfort, pain, double vision and even visual loss. Magnetic resonance imaging shows enlargement of the extra-ocular muscles and increase in the volume of intra-orbital fat. There is lymphocytic infiltration of the periorbital tissue and it is thought that pre-adipocytes in this location express the TSH receptor and become targeted by the same immune process as the thyroid gland.

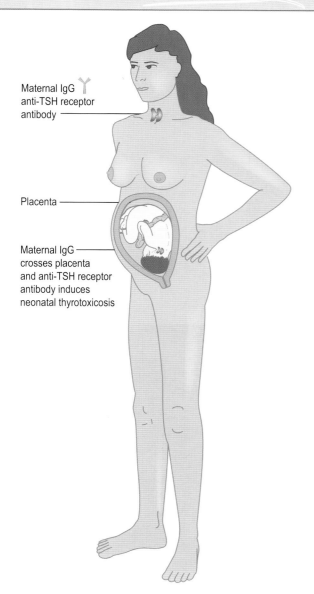

Maternal IgG anti-TSH receptor antibody

Placenta

Maternal IgG crosses placenta and anti-TSH receptor antibody induces neonatal thyrotoxicosis

Fig. 13.7 An experiment of nature.
TSH receptor autoantibody produced in the mother is of the IgG class and passively crosses the placenta, giving rise to thyrotoxicosis in the newborn.

covery of these autoantibodies began in the 1950s with the identification of a serum factor distinct from TSH that promoted synthesis and release of thyroid hormones. This 'long-acting thyroid stimulator' was found initially in roughly three quarters of the patients studied, but refinement of its detection showed it to be present in almost all patients. In the 1960s, this thyroid stimulator was identified as an immunoglobulin, and evidence that it belonged to the IgG class derived from an experiment of nature: babies born to mothers with high circulating levels of the antibody exhibited transient hyperthyroidism as a result of transfer across the placenta (Fig. 13.7). In the 1970s came the demonstration that

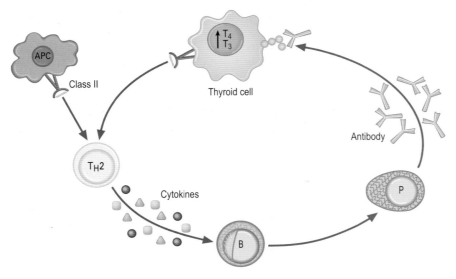

Fig. 13.8 The mechanism of thyroid dysfunction in Graves' disease.
A T$_H$2 response is initiated and induces production of a stimulatory autoantibody against the TSH receptor.

Fig. 13.9 Anti-adrenal cortex antibodies.
The antibodies are identified by indirect immunofluorescence on a section of human adrenal gland, using serum from a patient with idiopathic Addison's disease. (Original magnification ×40; courtesy of Dr Ted Davies, King's College Hospital, London.)

Addison's disease

Failure of the adrenal cortex (termed Addison's disease) was once attributable almost entirely to tuberculosis. With the decline of this disease, a form of Addison's disease has emerged that has no known aetiology, except for an association with autoimmunity. Although rare (a prevalence of 40–50 cases per million) autoimmune Addison's disease is of great clinical importance since it is lethal if undiagnosed. In 40% of patients it is part of a polyglandular autoimmune syndrome in which several such disorders occur together in the same individual (see below). The disease is slightly more common in women (male : female ratio 1 : 2) and is associated with HLA-DR3 and HLA-DR4 heterozygosity in a similar way to type 1 diabetes: HLA-DR3 and HLA-DR4 alone carry a relative risk of around 5, but when together this increases to 25.

Pathology

Lymphocytic infiltration may be seen if analysis is performed early, otherwise there is notable scarring and atrophy of the adrenal cortex.

Pathogenesis and immunological features

Autoantibodies to adrenal cortical cells (Fig. 13.9) are seen in most patients at diagnosis. They are rare in the general population, but if detected are highly predictive of the onset of Addison's disease: 45% of such asymptomatic individuals have overt disease in 30 months. The major target of these autoantibodies is 21α-hydroxylase, an enzyme found in the

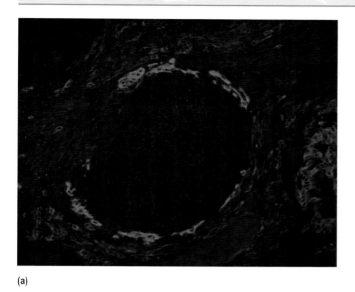

(a)

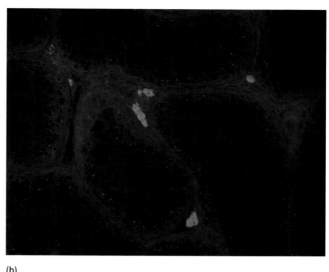

(b)

Fig. 13.10 **Steroid cell autoantibodies (SCA).**
These are identified by indirect immunofluorescence: (**a**) on a section of human ovary using serum from a patient with premature ovarian failure, the cells stained are the theca cells of the Graafian follicle; and (**b**) on a section of human testis showing staining of the Leydig cell cytoplasm. (Original magnification ×40; courtesy of Dr Ted Davies, King's College Hospital, London.)

zona glomerulosa and responsible for side chain cleavage in the production of steroid enzymes.

Clinical features

Patients may present in Addisonian crisis with hypotension, salt and water loss, hyperkalaemia, hypercalcaemia and hypoglycaemia. Prodromal symptoms are lassitude, dizziness and increased pigmentation. Long-term management involves replacement with glucocorticoids and mineralocorticoids.

Autoimmune gonadal failure

Premature ovarian failure (POF) has many causes but the identification of autoantibodies in some women with the condition indicates that at least some of the disease burden is autoimmune. Like Addison's disease, POF may also occur in the context of a polyglandular disease. In men, but much more rarely, there may be an autoimmune reaction directed against the Leydig cells in the testis that results in testicular failure.

Pathology

Analysis of the ovaries in POF has demonstrated lymphocytic infiltration in some cases and merely fibrosis in others. Little is known about the immunopathology of testicular failure.

Pathogenesis and immunological features

Both premature ovarian failure, occurring sporadically or as part of a polyglandular syndrome, and testicular failure may be characterised by autoantibodies to cell components in the target organ, often referred to as steroid cell antibodies (SCA) (Fig. 13.10). The targets of SCA are enzymes involved in the synthesis of steroid sex hormones (e.g. P450 side chain cleavage enzyme). When present at high titre in an asymptomatic patient, these autoantibodies are associated with a high risk of premature ovarian failure.

Autoimmune polyendocrine syndromes (APS)

One of the themes of this chapter has been the genetic and familial nature of some of the autoimmune disorders affecting endocrine organs. A different type of disease clustering is sometimes seen in which an individual develops numerous autoimmune diseases and has numerous autoantibodies. These clusters have become better characterised in recent years, and at least 3 polyendocrine autoimmune disorders have now been defined (Table 13.5). Early on in the study of these disease clusters, there was a prediction that perhaps a single gene might predispose to autoimmunity — this has indeed been borne out, with some very enlightening discoveries that are highly compatible with the disease model elaborated in Chapter 9.

APS type 1 is associated with a defect in the autoimmune regulator (*AIRE*) gene. The function of the *AIRE* gene product, and how it may give rise to autoimmunity, has been discussed in Chapters 7 and 9. Likewise, the important role of the gene product of *Foxp3* in the function of $CD4^+CD25^+$ Tregs makes the development of an autoimmune syndrome in patients with defective Foxp3 an understandable outcome (p. 112).

Table 13.5 Features of autoimmune polyendocrine diseases

Feature	APS type I	APS type II	IPEX
Prevalence	Rare	Common	Very rare
Age of diagnosis	Infancy	Infancy to adulthood	Neonatal period
Major gene defect	Autosomal recessive inheritance of defect in *AIRE** gene	Polygenic	X-linked inheritance of defect in *Foxp3* gene
Immunodeficiency	Susceptibility to candida	None	Severe autoimmunity due to loss of Tregs
Commonest disease manifestations	Candidiasis, Addison's disease	Addison's disease, type 1 diabetes, autoimmune thyroiditis	Neonatal diabetes

APS = Autoimmune polyendocrine syndrome; IPEX = Immune dysregulation, enteropathy, polyendocrinopathy, X-linked syndrome.
AIRE = Autoimmune regulator gene.

SUMMARY BOX 13.3

Autoimmune disease of the endocrine system

- Autoimmune diseases of endocrine organs such as the adrenal gland and ovary are rare.
- Autoimmune diseases of the endocrine organs may occur in clusters, giving rise to autoimmune polyendocrine syndromes (APS).
- Studying APS has been highly instructive regarding the immune pathways that lead to autoimmunity and autoimmune disease.

Further reading

Cheng MH, Shum AK, Anderson MS 2007 What's new in the Aire? Trends Immunol 28: 321–327

Di Lorenzo TP, Peakman M, Roep BO 2007 Systematic analysis of T cell epitopes in autoimmune diabetes. Clin Exp Immunol 148: 1–16

McLachlan SM, Rapoport B 2004 Autoimmune hypothyroidism: T cells caught in the act. Nat Med 10: 895–896

Peakman M, Roep BO 2006 Secondary measures of immunologic efficacy in clinical trials. Current Opinion in Endocrinology & Diabetes 13: 325–331

Staeva-Vieira T, Peakman M, von Herrath M 2007 Translational mini-review series on type 1 diabetes: immune-based therapeutic approaches for type 1 diabetes. Clin Exp Immunol 148: 17–31

Tree TI, Peakman M 2004 Autoreactive T cells in human type 1 diabetes. Endocrinol Metab Clin North Am 33: 113–133, ix–x

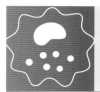

Liver diseases

14

The liver is the target organ of several immune-mediated disorders. These illustrate a variety of tissue-damaging mechanisms. Autoimmune hepatitis and the autoimmune form of sclerosing cholangitis provide examples of organ-specific autoimmune disease; primary biliary cirrhosis is so strongly associated with the presence of autoantibodies to mitochondria that the diagnosis of the disease is questioned in the absence of the autoantibody (Table 14.1). Several viruses home to the liver. Some produce liver damage through their cytopathic properties (e.g. hepatitis A virus) while others (e.g. hepatitis B virus) are not directly cytopathic but render liver cells targets to the immune system, which eliminates virus-infected cells. The hepatitis C virus is currently the focus of lively debate since it has been suggested as the aetiological agent of some forms of autoimmune hepatitis, in addition to being the causal agent of a viral hepatitis.

Autoimmune hepatitis

Autoimmune hepatitis (AIH) is a rare condition characterised by active inflammation, liver cell necrosis and fibrosis, which may lead to hepatic failure, cirrhosis and ultimately death. It is currently diagnosed on the basis of a histological picture of interface hepatitis (Fig. 14.1) and elevated levels of serum immunoglobulins and of non-organ-specific and liver-specific autoantibodies.

Autoimmune hepatitis has been divided into two main subgroups according to the type of autoantibody detected. Type I is associated with smooth muscle antibody (SMA) and/or antinuclear antibody (ANA) and type II with anti-liver/kidney microsomal (LKM) antibody. Type II patients often have IgA deficiency and usually a more severe course of the disease with rapid progression to cirrhosis despite immunosuppressive treatment. The LKM antibody (LKM-1) found in type II AIH is directed against cytochrome P4502D6, a drug metabolising enzyme with genetic polymorphism. Although these autoantibodies are non-organ-specific and may be found in other diseases, when present at high titre they are important diagnostic markers of AIH.

There is a strong genetic influence upon the development of AIH. Patients are usually female and frequently possess the haplotype HLA *A1-B8-MICA*008-TNFA*2-DRB3*0101-DRB1*0301-DQB1*0201* and null (i.e. non-productive) C4 complement genes. It has been shown that susceptibility to type I AIH is conferred by the possession of either *DRB1*0301* or *DRB1*0401* genes, while predisposition to type II AIH is imparted by *DRB1*0701*.

Pathology

A liver biopsy is required to establish the diagnosis. The typical histological picture is that of interface hepatitis (Fig. 14.1), which is characterised by a portal mononuclear cell infiltrate that erodes the triad limiting plate and spills over into the parenchyma (periportal hepatitis or piecemeal necrosis) where inflammatory cells surround dying hepatocytes. Plasma cells are abundant. Histological signs of cirrhosis can be found in up to 50% of the diagnostic biopsies.

Pathogenesis

T-regulatory function
Using various in vitro assays, impaired non-antigen-specific T cell suppressor function has been demonstrated in patients with AIH and in their first-degree relatives: this defect segregates with the possession of the HLA haplotype B8/DR3. In addition, it has been shown that patients with AIH have a specific defect in a subpopulation of suppressor T cells controlling the immune response to liver-specific membrane antigens.

Table 14.1 Characteristics of immune-mediated liver diseases

	Autoimmune hepatitis		Primary biliary cirrhosis
	Type I	**Type II**	
Age/sex	Juvenile: F >> M Mature: F = M	Juvenile F >> M Mature F = M	Middle age (F : M, 9 : 1)
Diagnostic antibodies	ANA, SMA	LKM-1	AMA
HLA association	Juvenile: *DRB1*0301* Mature: *DRB1*0301* and *DRB1*0401*	*DRB1*0701*	*DRB1*0801*
Target antigens of pathogenic immune responses	ASGPR[1], LSP[2]	ASGPR, LSP, CYP2D6[3]	PDH[4]

[1]Asialoglycoprotein receptor.
[2]Liver-specific lipoprotein.
[3]Cytochrome P4502D6.
[4]Pyruvate dehydrogenase.

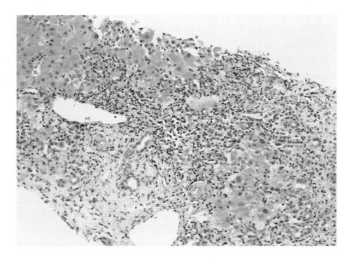

Fig. 14.1 Histological picture of interface hepatitis.
This is typically found in autoimmune hepatitis. The main features are a dense mononuclear cell infiltrate in the portal tract that erodes the triad's limiting plate, invading the parenchyma (interface hepatitis). Courtesy of Dr Alberto Quaglia.

Autoantibodies against liver-specific membrane antigens

Patients with AIH have high serum antibody concentrations to a macromolecular complex called liver-specific lipoprotein (LSP); the titre closely correlates with the extent of histological liver damage. Within anti-LSP reactivity, there are antibodies directed against a single antigen, the human asialoglycoprotein receptor (ASGPR), titres of which also correlate with disease activity. ASGPR is a well characterised

SCIENCE BOX 14.1

T cell cloning

Cloning, i.e. the generation of millions of daughter cells from a single progenitor, has been successfully achieved in AIH by exploiting the ability of activated T lymphocytes expressing the IL-2 receptor to proliferate in the presence of IL-2.

Liver-specific CD4 T cell clones, obtained both from the peripheral blood and the liver biopsies of patients with AIH have been shown to direct autologous B lymphocytes to produce liver-membrane-specific autoantibodies and antibodies to the ASGPR. It is likely that these autoantibodies target the liver cell membrane and recruit mediators of damage.

plasma membrane protein exclusively found on hepatocytes and a likely target of immune attack (see Science Box 14.1). The question as to whether these autoantibodies exert a pathogenic role is, at least in part, answered by the finding that hepatocytes isolated from diagnostic liver biopsies of patients with AIH are coated in vivo with antibodies (Fig. 14.2).

Mechanism of liver damage

Liver damage in AIH is likely to be orchestrated by CD4 T lymphocytes recognising a self antigenic peptide, possibly derived from ASGPR (Fig. 14.3). The model proposed in Figure 14.3 is supported by a number of observations:

- hepatocytes from patients with active AIH express class II HLA antigens (Fig. 14.4), not normally expressed on liver cells and can, therefore, present autoantigenic peptides
- CD4⁺ and activated lymphocytes are present in areas of piecemeal necrosis
- liver-specific autoantibodies are present in the circulation of these patients in high titres and coat their liver cells, which then become susceptible to damage by killer lymphocytes
- T regulatory cell number and function are impaired.

Clinical features

The onset of disease tends to be insidious in most cases, although the presentation may be that of an acute, even fulminant, hepatitis particularly in young patients. The course is variable, but the disease is usually controlled by a lifelong treatment with immunosuppressive drugs. Alterations of liver function tests do not necessarily reflect the extent of the histological lesion. An increase of aspartate aminotransferase (AST) is common, as is an elevation of globulins and in particular of IgG with values frequently exceeding 20 g/l (normal upper limit 15 g/l). Diagnostic autoantibodies (ANA, SMA, LKM-1) are present at titres of ≥1/40 in adults and ≥1/20 in children (Fig. 14.5). The condition is treated with a combination of corticosteroids and azathioprine, the dosages of which are guided by the levels of AST.

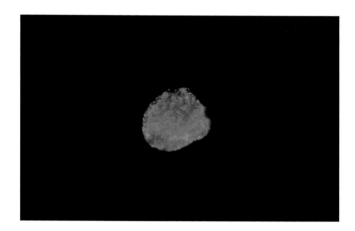

Fig. 14.2 Direct immunofluorescence of a hepatocyte isolated from a patient with AIH.
A fluorescent antihuman IgG was applied to a monodispersed suspension of liver cells. The picture shows the hepatocyte coated by antibodies.

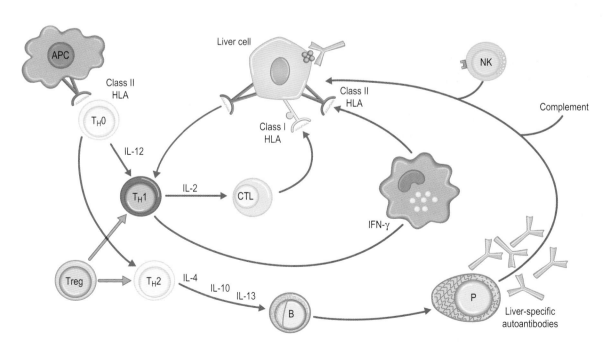

Fig. 14.3 Model of immune attack on the liver cell in autoimmune hepatitis. Liver pathogenic scenario.
A peptide from a normal component of the liver cell — possibly the ASGPR — is presented to a T helper 0 (T$_H$0) lymphocyte either directly or by an APC within the groove of class II HLA molecules. Impaired regulatory T cells permit T$_H$2 lymphocytes to direct autoantibody production by B lymphocytes with engagement of Fc-receptor expressing natural killer (NK) cells.

Autoimmune hepatitis—cont'd

■ Autoimmune hepatitis is characterised by the histological picture of interface hepatitis.

■ Hepatocytes are coated with IgG in vivo probably produced under the direction of autoantigen-specific CD4 T lymphocytes.

Autoimmune sclerosing cholangitis

Autoimmune sclerosing cholangitis is a rare disorder of unknown aetiology, characterised by chronic inflammation and fibrosis leading to narrowing and dilatation of the intrahepatic or extrahepatic bile ducts, or both. The condition is associated in the majority of cases with chronic inflammatory bowel disease, particularly ulcerative colitis.

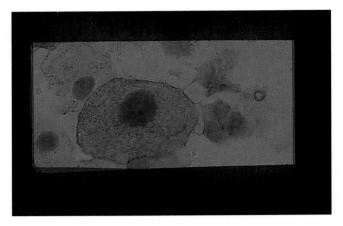

Fig. 14.4 Direct immunoperoxidase staining of a hepatocyte isolated from a patient with AIH with anti-HLA class II antibody.
The positive peripheral staining indicates that HLA class II molecules — absent from the hepatocytes of healthy individuals — are present on the membrane of the cells of this patient enabling them to present autoantigens to the immune system.

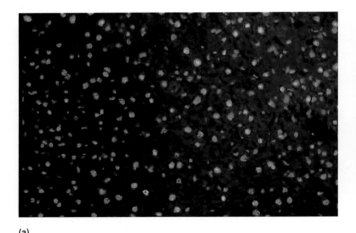

(a)

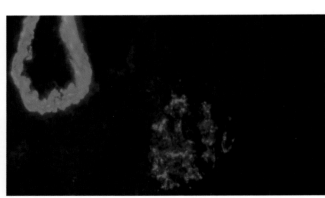

(b)

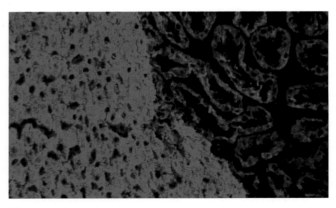

(c)

Fig. 14.5 Indirect immunofluorescence pattern of ANA, SMA and LKM-1 autoantibodies.
This is of diagnostic value in AIH. (**a**) ANA stains the nuclei of hepatocytes homogeneously. (**b**) SMA stains the smooth muscle structures contained in the wall of a renal artery. Frequently the glomeruli are also stained by SMA. (**c**) LKM-1 reacts with renal tubules, mainly proximal, and the cytoplasm of hepatocytes. (Substrate: rat liver and kidney, original magnification ×40.)

Patients may present with clinical, biochemical, immunological and histological features indistinguishable from those of type I autoimmune hepatitis, though they have more frequently an atypical peri-nuclear anti-neutrophil cytoplasmic antibody. This pANCA is atypical in that its target antigen appears to be nuclear and not cytoplasmic. The correct diagnosis can be made only by demonstrating the characteristic bile duct abnormalities by specialised imaging such as endoscopic retrograde cholangio-pancreatography (ERCP; Fig. 14.6) or magnetic resonance cholangiography.

SUMMARY BOX 14.2

Autoimmune sclerosing cholangitis

- Rare disorder characterised by chronic inflammation and fibrosis.
- Often associated with chronic inflammatory bowel disease.
- Indistinguishable from type I autoimmune hepatitis unless specialised imaging such as endoscopic retrograde cholangiopancreatography or magnetic resonance cholangiography is performed.

Primary biliary cirrhosis

Primary biliary cirrhosis (PBC) is a chronic liver disease of unknown aetiology characterised by slowly progressive intrahepatic cholestasis caused by an inflammatory destruction of small intrahepatic bile ducts. It is 10 times more common in women than in men and is most common in women over the age of 50. The clinical course of PBC is variable, ranging from a few years, in rapidly progressive cases, to a normal life-expectancy in a proportion of asymptomatic cases. It has long been recognised that the disease is characterised by the presence of high-titre antimitochondrial antibodies (AMA) in over 90% of the patients (Fig. 14.7) and elevated serum IgM (Table 14.1). The predisposing role of the HLA system to the disease has not been fully clarified, although a weak but significant association with HLA-*DRB1*08* has been reported.

Pathology

The histological picture is characterised by lymphocyte infiltration and destruction of small and medium size bile ducts, ductular proliferation, periductular granulomas, fibrosis and ultimately cirrhosis. The histological alterations are frequently patchy and for this reason the result of a liver biopsy is considered consistent with, rather than diagnostic of, PBC.

Pathogenesis

Several types of antimitochondrial autoantibodies (AMA) have been described in PBC including M2, M4, M8 and M9. The AMA which serves as the diagnostic marker for PBC is the subtype anti-M2. The molecular targets of AMA-M2 have been characterised (see Science Box 14.2) and their use for classification and staging of PBC is in progress. AMA are strong disease predictors since their accidental detection is virtually always followed by the development of the disease. This, however, may take up to 20 years to manifest itself.

The few available immunohistochemical studies agree that in PBC T lymphocytes in the portal lymphoid infiltrates greatly outnumber other lymphoid cells, and these T cells exhibit markers of activation. CD4 helper T cells predominate overall but are localised mainly in the portal infiltrates, whereas those T cells that surround and/or invade the walls

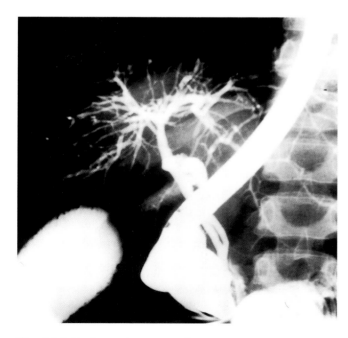

Fig. 14.6 Endoscopic retrograde cholangiopancreatographic picture showing the bile duct alterations (narrowing, strictures and dilatations) of sclerosing cholangitis.

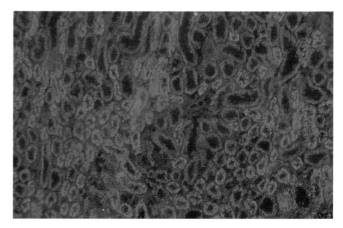

Fig. 14.7 Indirect immunofluorescence pattern of AMA. Note the stronger staining of the distal tubules (smaller than the proximal), which are particularly rich in mitochondria. (Substrate: rat kidney.)

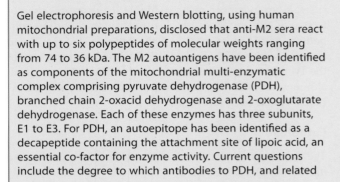

SCIENCE BOX 14.2

Mitochondrial autoantigens

Gel electrophoresis and Western blotting, using human mitochondrial preparations, disclosed that anti-M2 sera react with up to six polypeptides of molecular weights ranging from 74 to 36 kDa. The M2 autoantigens have been identified as components of the mitochondrial multi-enzymatic complex comprising pyruvate dehydrogenase (PDH), branched chain 2-oxacid dehydrogenase and 2-oxoglutarate dehydrogenase. Each of these enzymes has three subunits, E1 to E3. For PDH, an autoepitope has been identified as a decapeptide containing the attachment site of lipoic acid, an essential co-factor for enzyme activity. Current questions include the degree to which antibodies to PDH, and related enzymes, account for the mitochondrial reactivity defined by immunofluorescence and the cell-surface expression of M2 autoantigens. The reasons for the localisation of the lesions of PBC to intrahepatic biliary ductules is unclear since mitochondrial autoantigens are not tissue specific. Based on available evidence the following suggestions have been proposed to explain hepatobiliary localisation of the injury: (1) there are allelic forms of PDH specific to the hepatobiliary cells; (2) bile favours penetrance of immune effector agents such as antibodies or T cells; and (3) the biliary tract is colonised by a microorganism displaying epitopes, cross-reactive with human pyrunate dehydrogenase enzymes.

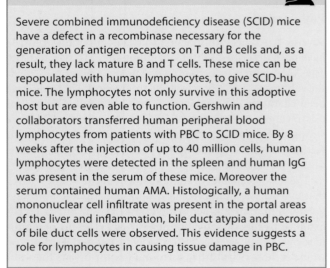

SCIENCE BOX 14.3

Man or mouse?

Severe combined immunodeficiency disease (SCID) mice have a defect in a recombinase necessary for the generation of antigen receptors on T and B cells and, as a result, they lack mature B and T cells. These mice can be repopulated with human lymphocytes, to give SCID-hu mice. The lymphocytes not only survive in this adoptive host but are even able to function. Gershwin and collaborators transferred human peripheral blood lymphocytes from patients with PBC to SCID mice. By 8 weeks after the injection of up to 40 million cells, human lymphocytes were detected in the spleen and human IgG was present in the serum of these mice. Moreover the serum contained human AMA. Histologically, a human mononuclear cell infiltrate was present in the portal areas of the liver and inflammation, bile duct atypia and necrosis of bile duct cells were observed. This evidence suggests a role for lymphocytes in causing tissue damage in PBC.

Clinical features

PBC is often asymptomatic, the earliest symptom usually being pruritus and fatigue. Jaundice, darkening of the skin in exposed areas and manifestations resulting from impaired bile excretion follow. The latter range from steatorrhoea to impaired absorption of lipid-soluble vitamins, leading to osteomalacia (from vitamin D malabsorption), bruising (vitamin K) and occasionally night blindness (vitamin A). Whilst the physical examination can be rather unremarkable, laboratory investigations tend to be informative. Alkaline phosphatase is elevated early in the course of the disease, and AMA at a titre >1:40 is present in over 90% of patients.

Serum bilirubin rises over time, an increase in AST levels is frequently seen but it is never dramatic, hyperlipidaemia is common.

Treatment

No treatment is able to alter the natural history of the disease. Ursodeoxycholic acid has been reported to ameliorate inflammation and fibrosis. The symptomatic treatment is directed at alleviating pruritus, steatorrhoea and at replacing fat-soluble vitamins. End-stage disease is treated with liver transplantation.

of bile ducts, which are likely to be the actual effectors, are of the cytotoxic (CD8+) phenotype. Immunohistochemistry has also been applied to the identification of HLA-encoded molecules on hepatocytes and bile duct cells, since this may give clues to the pathogenesis. Bile duct epithelium normally expresses HLA class I molecules; in PBC, HLA class II molecules also become expressed on biliary epithelial cells, presumably under the influence of cytokines, including INF-γ. Bile duct damage may derive from different effector mechanisms. Given that HLA class I molecules are constitutively expressed on biliary epithelial cells and that CD8 T cells are identifiable histochemically at sites of damage, a cytotoxic T cell response to a mitochondrial peptide, associated with a class I HLA molecule on the biliary epithelial surface, is one possibility. An alternative (or co-existing) process would be an induction of CD4 helper T lymphocytes, with release by activated cells of cytokines with tissue-damaging potential (see Science Box 14.3).

SUMMARY BOX 14.3

Primary biliary cirrhosis

- Antimitochondrial antibody is present in over 90% of patients.
- A multi-enzymatic complex comprising pyruvate dehydrogenase, branched chain 2-oxacid dehydrogenase and 2-oxoglutarate dehydrogenase contains the target antigens of antimitochondrial (M2) antibody.
- Serum IgM is typically elevated.
- Bile ducts are infiltrated by lymphocytes and destroyed.

Viral hepatitis

This section will deal with the immunological aspects of viral hepatitis; the virological and clinical features are comprehensively discussed in other texts. The list of hepatitis viruses grows steadily and currently extends from A to G. We will concentrate on those types of viral hepatitis in which the immune system is thought to contribute to the liver damage or to exercise control over the virus.

Hepatitis A

The liver damage in acute hepatitis A has long been thought to derive from a direct cytopathic effect of the virus. However, it is now believed that a T cell-mediated immune attack on virus-infected cells plays a major additional pathogenic role, similar to that in hepatitis B. Infection with hepatitis A virus (HAV), however, does not become chronic, suggesting that the interaction between virus and host is different from that observed in HBV infection, and that the immune system is generally very efficient at controlling HAV.

Hepatitis B

The liver damage caused by the hepatitis B virus (HBV; Fig. 14.8) varies greatly in severity: it can be mild and transient, severe and prolonged, or fulminant. The mechanisms responsible for determining the course and outcome of hepatitis B are not known. However, many investigations have suggested that HBV is not directly cytopathic, but that liver damage derives from the host immune response to the virus-infected hepatocytes. A normal immune response would lead to self-limiting acute hepatitis, an impaired immune response to chronic hepatitis, and a hyperactive response to fulminant hepatic failure. During viral infections, T lymphocytes recognise viral antigens on the surface of the infected cell in association with HLA molecules. Following infection of the liver cell, viral peptides can bind to HLA class I molecules, which carry the viral antigens to the cell surface where the complex becomes a target for CD8 cytotoxic T lymphocytes.

It is not clear why certain patients progress to chronic infection while others clear HBV after acute infection (see Science Box 14.4), though a combination of host, infective agent and environmental factors certainly combine to determine the outcome of the infection. In chronic hepatitis B, defective viral particles are produced in great numbers, and there are data to indicate that spontaneous mutations in the genome are associated with the development of particularly aggressive forms of chronic hepatitis or fulminant hepatic failure. Control of the virus is mainly associated with T_H1 immune responses, while T_H2 responses are more frequent in viral persistence.

Hepatocellular carcinoma, the most frequent primary malignant tumour of the liver, is associated with HBV infec-

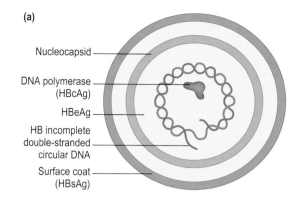

(a)

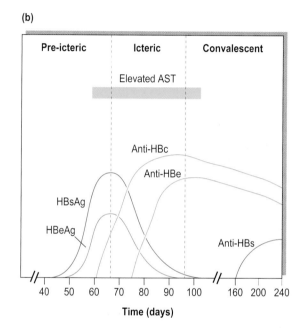

(b)

Fig. 14.8 Hepatitis B virus infection.
(**a**) The constituents of the hepatitis B virion. This DNA virus is composed of a surface coat and of a core. Other key components are DNA and DNA polymerase. (**b**) The dynamics of HBV serological markers during acute hepatitis. Serum hepatitis B surface antigen (HBsAg) and hepatitis e antigen (HBeAg) precede jaundice and aspartate aminotransferase (AST) increase. Antibodies against core (anti-HBc) are the first to appear, belonging to the IgM class first and then the IgG. Anti-HBe appears later followed by production of anti-HBs. This last is deemed to be protective and is a marker of acquired immune status.

tion. There is an effective vaccination against HBV that has been shown to prevent all the pathologies related to the virus, including hepatocellular carcinoma.

Hepatitis C

Like hepatitis B, hepatitis caused by the C virus (HCV) can be acute and self-limiting or, more frequently, progress to chronic liver damage. The mechanisms leading to hepatocyte injury remain to be elucidated. Like HBV, HCV is not directly cytopathic and the liver damage results from the immune

SCIENCE BOX 14.4

Control of HBV in acute hepatitis

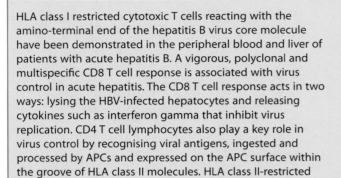

HLA class I restricted cytotoxic T cells reacting with the amino-terminal end of the hepatitis B virus core molecule have been demonstrated in the peripheral blood and liver of patients with acute hepatitis B. A vigorous, polyclonal and multispecific CD8 T cell response is associated with virus control in acute hepatitis. The CD8 T cell response acts in two ways: lysing the HBV-infected hepatocytes and releasing cytokines such as interferon gamma that inhibit virus replication. CD4 T cell lymphocytes also play a key role in virus control by recognising viral antigens, ingested and processed by APCs and expressed on the APC surface within the groove of HLA class II molecules. HLA class II-restricted

CD4 T cell lymphocytes recognising an immunodominant 20 amino acid sequence located within the amino-terminal part of the core molecule have been identified in the peripheral blood of patients with self-limiting acute hepatitis B. Moreover, CD4 T lymphocytes, obtained from liver biopsies and cloned in vitro, are capable of providing help to B cells for anti-HBc production. It is conceivable that the vigorous virus-specific CD4 and CD8 cell responses act in concert in the control of HBV during acute hepatitis B. Virus-specific T cells persist for long periods after clinical recovery, indicating that the virus persists at low levels. Viral control, and not viral elimination, defines clinical and serological recovery.

elimination of virus-infected cells. There is great interest in findings suggesting a connection between HCV and autoimmune hepatitis. LKM-1 — the diagnostic marker of AIH type II — has been found in the serum of several patients chronically infected with HCV; this has led to the proposal that the virus is the trigger of 'autoimmune hepatitis'. The additional finding that HCV and the target of LKM-1 (the cytochrome P4502D6) share sequences in common, appeared to sanction a link between virus and autoimmune disease, the autoimmune response being triggered through molecular mimicry. The enthusiasm generated by the above observations was tempered by the finding that no sign of infection with HCV is present in patients suffering from the classical AIH type II. It appears that a proportion of patients with HCV infection develop LKM-1; but LKM-1 is present, without signs of HCV infection, in most patients with type II AIH.

Further reading

Vergani D, Mieli-Vergani G 2007 Autoimmune hepatitis. In: Textbook of hepatology: from basic science to clinical practice. 3rd Edn ed. UK: Blackwell Publishing; 1089–1101

Krawitt EL 2006 Autoimmune hepatitis. N Engl J Med 354: 54–66

Vergani D, Mieli-Vergani G 2006 Primary sclerosing cholangitis. In: Rose NR, Mackay IR, eds. The autoimmune diseases. 4th edn Amsterdam: Elsevier; 767–777

Kaplan MM, Gershwin ME 2005 Primary biliary cirrhosis. N Engl J Med 353: 1261–1273

Viral hepatitis: http://www.cdc.gov/ncidod/diseases/hepatitis/index.htm

SUMMARY BOX 14.4

Viral hepatitis

- Liver damage may result from host immune responses to virus-infected hepatocytes.
- Defective interfering particles (HBV) or frequent mutation (HCV) may allow persistence of infection and lead to chronic hepatitis.
- HAV infection is controlled by the immune system and does not become chronic.
- HCV may trigger autoimmune reactions.

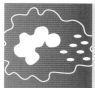

Gastrointestinal diseases

The gut presents a peculiar challenge to immunity — close proximity to billions of microorganisms. This chapter starts by discussing the specialised immune system that the gut operates in order to cope with this daily confrontation. The following sections detail what happens when this malfunctions, giving rise to a range of autoimmune and inflammatory diseases.

The mucosal immune system of the gastrointestinal tract

There are two major factors at play when considering the lymphoid system of the gastrointestinal tract as distinctive. The first is functional, the second anatomical. Antigens ingested orally tend to elicit qualitatively different immune responses to antigens arriving by other routes. Most strikingly, mucosal tissues are associated with high levels of production of IgA, the major externally secreted immunoglobulin. There is also a tendency for antigens administered orally to induce tolerance rather than active immune responses. This may be an important protective mechanism: many foreign animal and vegetable proteins will be encountered in the gut, along with antigens deriving from colonising bacteria, and it would be dangerous to the host to mount massive immune responses to these. The distinctive anatomy of the lymphoid system of the gastrointestinal tract is revealed by histological analysis, which shows lymphocytes scattered in the lamina propria, in the epithelial layer of the luminal surface, in

Peyer's patches (pp. 6–7), and in mesenteric lymph nodes (Fig. 15.1).

Peyer's patches are collections of lymphoid tissue organised into follicles similar to those found in other lymphoid sites but lacking a capsule or afferent lymphatics. They are separated from the intestinal lumen by a layer of epithelial cells amongst which are notable the microfold (M) cells. These cells bind invasive pathogens, particulate antigens and sample the intraluminal milieu. Peyer's patches contain large germinal centres, with aggregates of IgA^+ B lymphocytes separated by the T cell areas. The lamina propria contains mainly CD4 T lymphocytes, but also many B cells and plasma cells and some CD8 cells. Intraepithelial T cells are usually $CD8^+$ and some bear the unconventional $\gamma\delta$ TCR (p. 52). The diversity of TCR chain usage in the intraepithelial T cells appears less than in other sites, and it has been speculated that the gut could be a site of extra-thymic T cell maturation.

Autoimmune atrophic gastritis — Pernicious anaemia

Clinical and immunological features

Pernicious anaemia (PA) is a megaloblastic anaemia caused by a deficiency of vitamin B_{12} resulting from malabsorption. Impaired absorption is the result of defective intrinsic factor (IF) secretion. This is due to atrophy of the gastric mucosa caused by autoimmune reactions to gastric parietal cells and their products. Were B_{12} absorption to cease abruptly, 3–6 years would be required for a normal individual to become deficient.

Pernicious anaemia is the most common form of vitamin B_{12} deficiency in temperate climates; it affects both sexes equally, is more common in individuals of northern European descent and is rare under the age of 30, the average presenting age being 60 years.

It shows family clustering and is frequently associated with other organ-specific autoimmune diseases, such as Graves' disease, myxoedema, Addison's disease (idiopathic adrenocortical insufficiency), vitiligo and hypoparathyroidism. Pernicious anaemia is also frequently present in patients

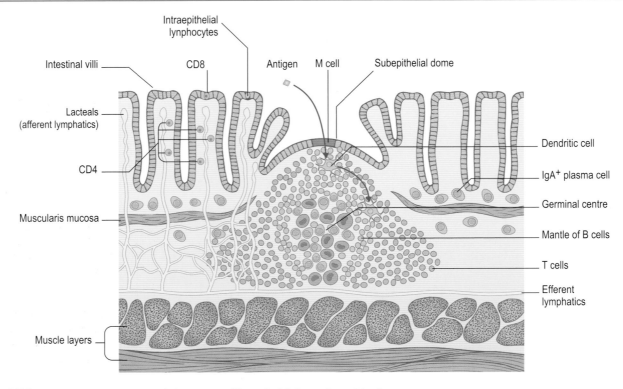

Fig. 15.1 Anatomical structure of the mucosal lymphoid tissue found in the gut.
Note the presence of intraepithelial T and B lymphocytes abutting the mucosal surface, the high density of plasma cells, particularly IgA$^+$ ones, the open, unencapsulated architecture of the Peyer's patch lymphoid follicle, and the rich draining lymphatics. Antigen enters through the M cell, is processed by APC and presented to T cells within the Peyer's patch. Antigen-specific effector CD4 cells and CD8 cells migrate into lamina propria and epithelium.

with common variable immunodeficiency. A genetic predisposition, indicated by familial occurrence of the disease, is not accounted for by HLA genes, since the reported associations are weak and inconstant.

The most characteristic abnormality in PA is gastric atrophy affecting the acid- and pepsin-secreting portion of the stomach. Chronic atrophic gastritis can be classified into two types according to whether or not the lesion affects the gastric antrum. Autoimmune gastritis involves the fundus and body of the stomach and spares the antrum and is associated with PA. Non-autoimmune gastritis involves the antrum as well as the fundus and body, and is usually associated with *Helicobacter pylori* infection.

Pathogenesis

Virtually all patients have gastric parietal cell antibody detected by indirect immunofluorescence. This antibody stains in the cytoplasm of gastric parietal cells (Fig. 15.2) targeting antigens in the secretory canaliculi, which are the intracellular channels carrying hydrochloric acid into the gastric lumen (Fig. 15.3) and its major target is the α subunit of the gastric proton pump (H$^+$, K$^+$, ATPase), an enzyme composed of two transmembrane components, the α and β subunits.

In addition, there are at least two types of antibody against intrinsic factor: **blocking** and **binding** antibodies (Fig. 15.4); the blocking type reacts with the combining site for vitamin

B$_{12}$ on IF and is found in most patients (over 70%), while the binding antibody reacts with other epitopes on IF (whether this is free or complexed to vitamin B$_{12}$) and is present in some 60% of patients. Both inhibit absorption of vitamin B$_{12}$ and are more frequently found in gastric juices than in serum. In animal models of autoimmune gastritis, the disease is transferred with the transferral of proton pump specific CD4 cells, but not CD8 or autoantibodies. The nature and specificity of T cell responses in humans remain to be clarified.

Clinical features and laboratory findings

The main symptoms of pernicious anaemia are those of severe anaemia. The patient is pale and slightly jaundiced, reflecting an increase in indirect bilirubin resulting from ineffective erythropoiesis.

The laboratory findings show macrocytosis (mean corpuscular volume, MCV, greater than 100 fl), and a low reticulocyte count. In the blood film, haemoglobinised macro-ovalocytes are seen, and the neutrophils are typically over segmented: finding six nuclear lobes is highly suggestive of megaloblastic anaemia. Measurement of vitamin B$_{12}$ will demonstrate a deficiency and a Schilling test will pinpoint the diagnosis. This test consists of two parts. In the first part, the patient is given radioactive vitamin B$_{12}$ orally and the absorption measured as radioactivity present in the urine of the next 24 hours. This part of the test is abnormal in perni-

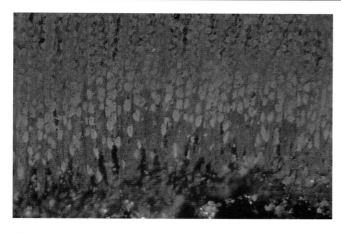

Fig. 15.2 Indirect immunofluorescence pattern of antigastric parietal cell antibody.
The staining in parietal cells is intracytoplasmic. This reflects the intracellular distribution of canaliculi containing the gastric proton pump. (Rat stomach, original magnification ×40.)

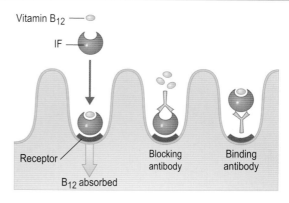

Fig. 15.4 Absorption of vitamin B_{12}.
Vitamin B_{12} binds to intrinsic factor (IF) and is absorbed after binding to a receptor in the ileal mucosa. Anti-IF **blocking** antibody prevents vitamin B_{12} from binding to IF, whilst the **binding** type prevents vitamin B_{12}–IF complex from binding to its receptor. Both prevent vitamin B_{12} absorption.

cious anaemia where absorption is impaired. The test returns to normal in the second part when radiolabelled B_{12} is given with intrinsic factor, a manoeuvre that overcomes defective absorption. Vitamin B_{12} replacement therapy is used to correct the anaemia.

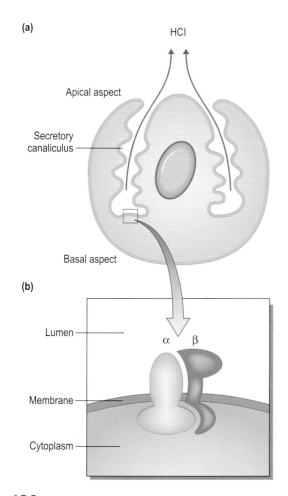

Fig. 15.3 Gastric parietal cells.
(**a**) Stimulated gastric parietal cell displaying the secretory canaliculus. (**b**) Within this structure resides the gastric proton pump whose α and β subunits contain the targets of antigastric parietal cell antibody.

SUMMARY BOX 15.1

Pernicious anaemia

- Pernicious anaemia is a megaloblastic anaemia caused by vitamin B_{12} malabsorption.
- Antigastric parietal cell antibodies are present in virtually all the patients and target the gastric proton pump.
- Blocking and binding antibodies to intrinsic factor prevent absorption of vitamin B_{12}. They are of diagnostic importance in pernicious anaemia but are not found in all patients.

Coeliac disease

Coeliac disease is a disorder of the small intestine characterised by malabsorption, villous atrophy (Fig. 15.5) and intolerance to gluten, a protein found in wheat, barley and oats. It is also called **gluten-induced enteropathy** since the disease improves when treated with a gluten-free diet but relapses if gluten is reintroduced. It is either limited to the intestine or associated with a vesicular skin disease known as **dermatitis herpetiformis** (see p. 245).

The incidence of coeliac disease in siblings is many times higher than in the general population: 3–20% of first-degree relatives are affected by the condition. This strong genetic predisposition is in part accounted for by the association of the disorder with the haplotype HLA-*B*8*, HLA-*DRB1*03* (DR3) or HLA-*DRB1*07* (DR7), and by the even closer association with the HLADQ2 allele (HLA-*DQA1*0501*, *DQB1*0201* (see Science Box 15.1).

The fact that 70% — and not 100% — of monozygotic twins are concordant for coeliac disease implies that non-genetic (environmental) factors are involved in the pathogenesis of the disease.

Pathology

Jejunal biopsy specimens (Fig. 15.5b) show the classical lesion characterised by blunting and flattening of the mucosal surface, with villi either absent or broad and short. The crypts are elongated, a sign of a marked increase in epithelial cell turnover, and the lamina propria is infiltrated by a variety of mononuclear cells including plasma cells, CD4 T lymphocytes, macrophages, mast cells and basophils. IgA plasma cells are increased in number and predominate, but there is also a disproportionate increase in IgG plasma cells. The surface epithelium is altered, with sparse brush border, cuboidal rather than columnar cells and an increase in intraepithelial T lymphocytes, especially CD8 T lympho-

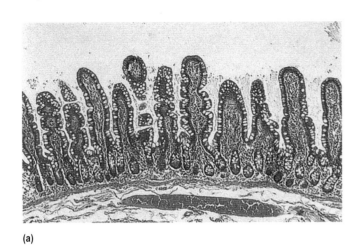

(a)

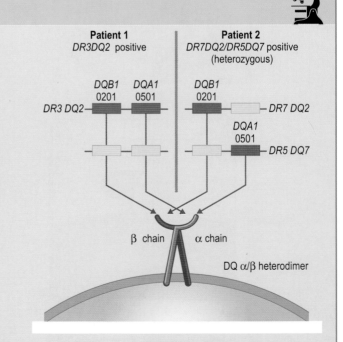

(b)

Fig. 15.5 Coeliac disease.

(a) Histology of normal jejunal mucosa. (b) Atrophic jejunal mucosa in coeliac disease: note the virtual absence of villi, elongated crypts and mononuclear cell infiltrate. LP; Lamina propria (from Young et al 2006 Wheater's Functional Histology, 5th edn, Churchill Livingstone, with permission).

SCIENCE BOX 15.1

HLA-DQα/β heterodimer

The strongest predisposition to coeliac disease is conferred by possession of the haplotype HLA-*DR3DQ2* (*DQA1*0501, DQB1*0201*). Patients with the disease who are negative for this are frequently heterozygous HLA-*DR7DQ2/DR5DQ7* (*DQA1*0501, DQB1*0301*). Therefore, as shown in Figure 15.6, the same *DQA1* and *DQB1* genes can be present in individuals with coeliac disease who have different HLA haplotypes. If the patient is *DR3DQ2* positive, *DQA1* and *DQB1* are in the *cis* position while they are *in trans* if the patient is *DR5DQ7/DR7DQ2* heterozygous. Therefore, most patients may express the same HLA-DQα/β heterodimer, *cis*-encoded in *DR3DQ2*-positive individuals and *trans*-encoded in *DR5DQ7/DR7DQ2* heterozygotes (*trans*-complementation). Binding of gliadin peptides to this heterodimer may be crucial to the pathogenesis of coeliac disease. (The use of the old HLA notations in this box reflects their preferential use by workers in the field of coeliac disease.)

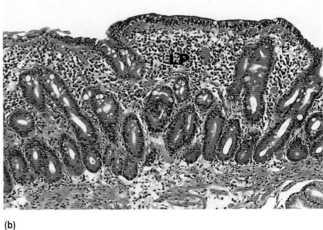

Fig. 15.6 Expression of the DQα/β heterodimer.

The DQ α/β heterodimer can be encoded by the haplotype *DR3DQ2* or by the heterozygous *DR7DQ2/DR5DQ7* status.

cytes. The histological lesions, including the infiltrate, regress with a gluten-free diet.

Pathogenesis

The **immunological** theory rests on the fact that the ingestion of gliadins in susceptible individuals leads to a CD4 infiltration in the lamina propria, an increase in intraepithelial CD8 T lymphocytes and evidence in the mucosa and serum of gliadin-specific reactivity. These patients have antigliadin antibodies in their serum, mostly belonging to the IgA class. Antiendomysium antibody, which also belongs to the IgA class, has been shown to be of diagnostic importance. The target antigen of antiendomysium is tissue transglutaminase (tTG), an enzyme expressed on the subepithelial layer of the intestinal epithelium: antibodies to tTG of the IgA class are the hallmark of the disease. They are readily detectable by ELISA, as opposed to antiendomysium, which are detectable by immunofluorescence. In IgA-deficient coeliac patients, the diagnostic antibody is anti-tTG of the IgG class.

A pathogenic scenario has recently been delineated (Fig. 15.7). Proteins found in wheat, barley and rye such as gliadins, hordeins and secalins contain a 33-amino-acid (33-mer) peptide that, against expectations, survives the action of low pH and digestive enzymes, reaching the small intestine intact. The 33-mer contains repeat epitopes recognised by CD4 T cells, especially after undergoing deamination by tissue transglutaminase. These deaminated epitopes fit perfectly well in those HLA class II molecules that characterise coeliac disease. The presentation of these deaminated epitopes to CD4 T cells is probably the starting point of coeliac disease and the trigger to its relapses. Importantly, the 33-mer peptide can also be generated by in vitro microbial digestion, offering a possible tool for devising tolerance-restoring interventions. Also, the 33-mer peptide, resistant to enzymatic attack in humans, can be digested by microbes, raising the possibility of alternatives to gluten-free diets (i.e. diets that contain the pre-digested peptide). Knowledge of the 33-mer sequence may also enable the production of genetically modified foods containing a non-immunogenic form of the peptide.

Clinical features

Most patients with coeliac disease present with the typical picture of a malabsorption syndrome characterised by failure to thrive when gluten is introduced in the diet, weight loss, abdominal distension and bloating, diarrhoea, steatorrhoea and abnormal tests of absorption function. Patients can present, however, with isolated abnormalities: iron-deficiency anaemia or a metabolic bone disease can be the initial features in the absence of overt diarrhoea and steatorrhoea.

In the absence of a specific diagnostic test, the diagnosis rests on:

- evidence of malabsorption
- typical histological picture of the jejunal mucosa with blunting and flattening of the villi
- Clinical and histological improvement on a gluten-free diet.

In ambiguous cases, the patient may be challenged with oral administration of gluten. The diagnosis is settled if this manoeuvre promptly results in diarrhoea and steatorrhoea.

Management and prognosis

Treatment with a gluten-free diet is effective in about 80% of patients, but this may take up to 24 months to work. Although normal health and life expectancy is usually restored by a gluten-free diet, it is of note that coeliac disease is associated with an increased incidence of intestinal carcinoma and lymphoma.

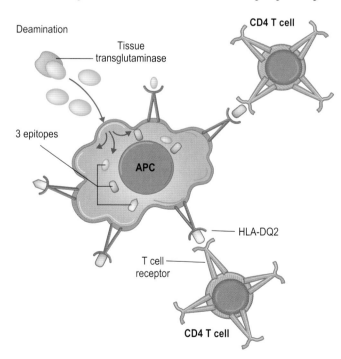

Fig. 15.7 **33-mer.**
A 33-amino-acid (33-mer) peptide contained in gliadin reaches the small intestine intact. Here it undergoes deamidation by tissue transglutaminase. Antigen-presenting cells take up the deamidated peptide that is processed into three epitopes. These are expressed within HLA-DQ2 molecule and are recognised by CD4 T cells. Upon antigen recognition, CD4+ T cells become activated and release cytokines that amplify the immune response, which finally results in villous atrophy.

SUMMARY BOX 15.2

Coeliac disease

- Coeliac disease is a disorder of the small intestine with malabsorption and intolerance to gluten.
- High serum levels of anti-tissue transglutaminase, antigliadin and antiendomysium antibodies, all belonging to the IgA class, are present.
- Mononuclear cell infiltrate is seen in the lamina propria.
- The heterodimer HLA-DQB1*0201/DQA1*0501 is present in the vast majority of patients.
- Association is also seen with dermatitis herpetiformis.

Inflammatory bowel disease

Inflammatory bowel disease (IBD) may be divided into two major groups:

- ulcerative colitis
- Crohn's disease.

Ulcerative colitis is confined to the colon and affects the mucosal layer only, whilst Crohn's disease may affect any part of the gastrointestinal tract, classically the ileocaecal region, with a transmural inflammation. Clinically these disorders are characterised by recurrent inflammation of intestinal segments with diverse clinical manifestations, often resulting in a chronic, unpredictable course.

Both conditions affect the sexes similarly but are more common in whites than blacks and more frequently seen in Ashkenazi Jews. In most populations, there is no clear association with the genes of the HLA region. Both appear to be more common in industrialised nations, to be steadily rising in their incidence, especially Crohn's disease, and to share a peak occurrence between 15 and 35 years of age. Family clustering and higher concordance in monozygotic than in dizygotic twins suggest genetic components for both disorders. The genetic component is stronger in Crohn's disease where twin concordance is 50% while in ulcerative colitis is 10%. Through microsatellite marker investigations a mutation in the *NOD2* (nucleotide-binding oligomerisation domain 2) gene on chromosome 16 has been identified as a predisposing factor in Crohn's disease. Individuals who are homozygous for the mutation have a relative risk of developing Crohn's of 38.0, but even they do not necessarily develop the disease indicating that predisposition to Crohn's disease, and to IBD in general, is due to several genes, a view corroborated in animal models.

The role for a specific infective agent has not been established, although the atypical mycobacterium *Mycobacterium paratuberculosis* has been incriminated in Crohn's disease. In genetically engineered animal models of IBD, the disease becomes apparent only upon colonisation with the bacterial microflora. Animals reared in germ-free environments either do not develop the disease or develop it in a milder form. The disease improves with the administration of antibiotics.

Pathology

The inflammatory reaction of ulcerative colitis involves principally the colonic mucosa leading to the macroscopic appearance of an ulcerated, hyperaemic, usually haemorrhagic colon. The surface mucosa is destroyed and the submucosa is heavily infiltrated with polymorphonuclear neutrophils. Small crypt abscesses are characteristic, though not specific.

The earliest pathological manifestations of Crohn's disease — a hyperaemic ileum with swollen and reddened mesentery and mesenteric lymph nodes — are not unique to Crohn's disease. In contrast to ulcerative colitis, the mucosa can have a normal appearance or, in more advanced cases, assume a cobblestone pattern. Ulcerations penetrate the submucosa and muscularis, resulting in fissures and fistulae.

The inflammatory process is continuous in ulcerative colitis but is frequently discontinuous in Crohn's disease, with skip areas interrupting the affected segments. Granulomas are not found in ulcerative colitis but are present in Crohn's disease, albeit in only 50–60% of the cases.

Pathogenesis

The current view on pathogenesis is that an exaggerated response to commensal microflora causes IBD, with a T_H1 profile in Crohn's disease and a T_H2 profile in ulcerative colitis. In Crohn's disease, there is an overproduction of IL-12 by macrophages and of IFN-γ by T lymphocytes. Crucial to the argument that IL-12 is involved in the development of the disease is the fact that patients treated with antibody specific for the p40 chain of IL-12 (IL-12p40) experience a prompt and marked improvement of the inflammatory process. The evidence that ulcerative colitis is a T_H2-mediated disease is less strong, though there is an increase of the T_H2 cytokine IL-5. Favouring a T_H2 pattern is the fact that ulcerative colitis is associated with the production of various autoantibodies, such as perinuclear anti-neutrophil cytoplasmic antibody (pANCA; see p. 233) and anti-tropomyosin. However, IL-4, the definitive T_H2 cytokine, is not increased. Evidence is accumulating that a defect in regulatory cells, such as $CD4^+CD25^+$, plays a permissive role in both types of inflammatory bowel disease.

Clinical features

In ulcerative colitis, bloody diarrhoea and abdominal pain with fever and weight loss in the more severe cases are the main symptoms. The laboratory findings are mostly non-specific, reflecting blood loss and inflammation, and include anaemia, leukocytosis, elevated sedimentation rate and C-reactive protein levels. Seventy percent of patients with ulcerative colitis, but not with Crohn's disease, have been reported to have in their sera an anti-neutrophil cytoplasmic antibody (ANCA) that gives a characteristic perinuclear staining (pANCA; see p. 233). This autoantibody differs from that found in Wegener's granulomatosis (see p. 232) and can also be seen in primary sclerosing cholangitis, a hepatobiliary disease with a probable immune pathogenesis and frequently associated with ulcerative colitis.

In Crohn's disease the major clinical manifestations include fever, abdominal pain, diarrhoea (often without blood) and fatigability. Typical laboratory findings include anaemia (chronic disease, iron deficiency, vitamin B_{12} deficiency, folate deficiency), leukocytosis, thrombocytosis, elevation of the sedimentation rate, hypoalbuminaemia and electrolyte imbalance in the presence of severe diarrhoea. The measurement of C-reactive protein appears to be of use in monitoring the progress of the disease.

Diagnosis

In both inflammatory bowel diseases, the key diagnostic procedures are radiologic, endoscopic and histologic.

Management and prognosis

The bowel inflammation is controlled with sulfasalazine or the newer 5-amino-salicylic acid (5-ASA) compounds, antibacterial drugs for complications of Crohn's disease and IBD, adrenocortical steroids, and the immunosuppressive compounds 6-mercaptopurine (6MP), azathioprine and ciclosporin. Tumour necrosis factor (TNF) alpha blocking drugs are able to provide an alternative treatment for patients who do not respond to corticosteroid or immunosuppressive drug treatment (see Ch. 22).

SUMMARY BOX 15.3

Inflammatory bowel disease

- Mucosal inflammation of the colon occurs in ulcerative colitis and transmural inflammation of the intestinal wall in Crohn's disease.
- Levels of C-reactive protein reflect disease activity.
- Monocyte/macrophage-produced IL-1 and IL-6 may be important in the pathogenesis of both conditions.
- Anti-neutrophil cytoplasmic antibody (perinuclear pattern) is found in 70% of patients with ulcerative colitis.

Allergic food reactions

The topic of allergic food reactions is undoubtedly one of the most confused of clinical immunology. The term 'allergic' is frequently used inappropriately to describe all conditions where reproducible reactions are triggered by food ingestion, disappear on an elimination diet and recur on a blind challenge. 'Food intolerance' is the appropriate term to define the entirety of these conditions.

Pathogenesis

Allergic food reactions should be confined to those cases where an immune mechanism can be demonstrated. Most instances of food intolerance are not explained by a clear immunological mechanism, being caused by toxic (spices, sulphites) and pharmacological (caffeine, sodium nitrite) stimuli or by enzymatic deficiencies (lactose deficiency in some cases of milk intolerance). In these non-immune food reactions, however, many of the manifestations may be accounted for by activation of the alternative complement pathway. It is postulated that this pathway is triggered by non-immune stimuli such as food contaminants, leading to formation of anaphylotoxins such as C5a.

Clinical features

Suspected food allergy is extraordinarily common in early childhood, with at least one fourth of all parents reporting one or more adverse food reactions. True food allergy can, however, be confirmed in 5% to 10% of these children with a peak prevalence at 1 year of age. Importantly, most food allergy is lost over time.

In the first year of life, food intolerance is relatively common, with cow's milk being the most frequent initiating stimulus. It appears as gastrointestinal symptoms and possibly wheezing. In adults the foods most frequently involved in intolerance are milk, eggs, fish, nuts, wheat and chocolate. These food reactions frequently have an allergic pathogenesis. Symptoms include urticaria, angio-oedema, asthma, anaphylaxis and, less frequently, nausea and vomiting. Such manifestations, but even more those comprising the oral allergy syndrome — swelling of the lips within minutes of food ingestion and tingling in the mouth and throat — closely correlate with the presence of specific IgE and implicate a type I hypersensitivity as the mechanism responsible for the clinical manifestations. Young patients with true IgE-mediated food allergies have a very high chance of developing additional food allergies as well as inhalant allergies.

Diagnosis

Involvement of type I hypersensitivity can be documented by the detection of specific IgE using the RAST or, less expensively, with a skin prick test (see p. 139). The prick test, unfortunately, is only as good as the test antigen it uses. Therefore, while antigenic preparations from eggs, milk or shellfish may provoke a positive skin reaction in sensitised individuals, highly purified preparations from apple rarely do, even if a hypersensitive subject gives strikingly positive reactions when challenged with cruder preparations from apple juice or apple peel. The main diagnostic procedure in food intolerance is an elimination diet from which suspect foods are gradually removed until symptoms disappear. A positive diagnosis is made when symptoms reappear upon reintroducing a specific food. This challenge should be done in a double-blind manner using placebo controls. The challenge should be avoided, however, if the food is suspected to have caused systemic anaphylaxis in the past. The management of food intolerance consists of avoidance of the offending food.

SUMMARY BOX 15.4

Allergic food reactions

- Food intolerance occurs where reproducible symptoms are triggered by food ingestion.
- There are some IgE-mediated food reactions appropriately termed food allergies.
- Some cases of non-immune food intolerance may be caused by activation of the complement alternative pathway.
- Elimination of the offending food 'cures' both allergic and non-allergic food reactions.

Further reading

Green PH, Cellier C 2007 Celiac disease. N Engl J Med 357: 1731–1743

Bouma G, Strober W 2003 The immunological and genetic basis of inflammatory bowel disease. Nat Rev Immunol 3: 521–533

Strober W 2006 Immunology. Unraveling gut inflammation. Science 313: 1052–1054

Xavier RJ, Podolsky DK 2007 Unravelling the pathogenesis of inflammatory bowel disease. Nature 448: 427–434

Bischoff S, Crowe SE 2005 Gastrointestinal food allergy: new insights into pathophysiology and clinical perspectives. Gastroenterology 128: 1089–1113

Immune-mediated nephritis and vasculitis

glomerulonephritis (GN), which accounts for approximately one third of patients with terminal renal failure, of which there are an estimated 4000 new cases per year in the UK in the 4–70 year age group. This chapter focuses on the role of the immune system in kidney damage and highlights the major diseases and mechanisms that are involved.

There are several key elements in understanding immune pathology in the kidney, including a grasp of the anatomy and histology, a three-dimensional mind's-eye view of the glomerulus and Bowman's capsule (Fig. 16.1) and an idea of the structure and function of the **glomerular basement membrane** (GBM), which lies between the endothelial and epithelial cells. The GBM, which is composed of 3 layers, can be damaged by components of the immune system, and this is an important pathological process in several of the diseases to be discussed. The mesangium is the group of support cells and structures at the core of the glomerulus. **Mesangial cells** are derived from the blood vessel walls and are smooth-muscle like. They can also participate in immune responses by secretion of cytokines. Monocytic cells may also be present in the mesangium, and both these and mesangial cells can have a role in phagocytosis, antigen presentation and cytokine secretion within the glomerulus. Finally, perhaps the most daunting task in understanding renal disease is coming to grips with the terminology. The histopathological and clinical descriptions may give little clue as to the pathogenesis of a renal lesion, or to the underlying disease, and the same description may apply to more than one disorder.

Physiological and clinical considerations

The kidney has several physiological functions, but the role of the specialised structure termed the glomerulus is filtration: the formation of urine with regulation of the internal balance of water, plasma proteins, salts and pH. Several disorders result in damage to this filtration unit, and many of these involve the immune system in the damaging process. These disorders are under the umbrella diagnosis of

Clinical terms in nephritis

Patients with renal impairment present to their doctor with a variety of symptoms and signs, depending on the degree of renal damage and the rapidity of onset and progression. Symptoms include blood in the urine, oedema, oliguria or anuria, and, rarely, loin pain. Clinical examination may reveal hypertension, particularly if glomerular damage has led to chronic renal failure. Urine analysis is performed for evidence of protein loss, red and white blood cells and urinary casts. Casts are made from a conglomeration of cells and Tamm–Horsfall protein, a viscous product of the distal

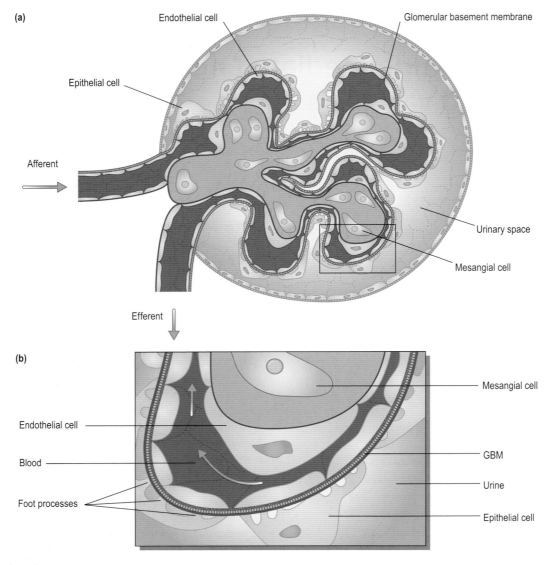

(a) Endothelial cell Glomerular basement membrane
Epithelial cell
Afferent
Urinary space
Mesangial cell
Efferent

(b) Mesangial cell
Endothelial cell
Blood
GBM
Urine
Foot processes
Epithelial cell

Fig. 16.1 The glomerulus.
(**a**) Structure of a normal glomerulus. (**b**) Enlargement showing the capillary loop; note the appearance of three distinct layers within the glomerular basement membrane.

tubule. Red cell casts indicate glomerular bleeding, white cell casts glomerular or tubular inflammation.

The magnitude, and to some extent the selectivity, of protein loss reflects the extent of damage to the filtration system. The greater the damage, the more protein is lost and the higher the molecular weight of the proteins in the urine. The broad clinical division of renal disease is into **nephritic** (typically 1–2 g protein lost per 24 hours) and **nephrotic** (>3.5 g/24 hours) syndromes. The onset of the syndrome may be **acute** or **chronic**, or in some cases **rapidly progressive**.

Histopathological terms in nephritis

Glomerulonephritis denotes evidence of pathological glomerular inflammation. This is frequently shortened to GN and often is blended with a clinical term defining the chronicity of the disorder (acute, chronic or rapidly progressive). Additional terms indicate the histopathological appearance of GN (e.g. cell proliferation, changes to the GBM), which is obtained from examination of renal biopsies examined at the light and electron microscopic levels. Under light microscopy, there may be evidence of proliferation of cells, frequently within the mesangium or the epithelial cells lining Bowman's capsule (termed **proliferative** GN). Fibrin deposition is often a feature. The formation of a crescent of proliferating epithelial cells within the urinary space gives rise to the term **crescentic** GN, which indicates severe renal damage and is frequently associated with a rapidly progressive clinical course. Thickening of the GBM caused by subepithelial 'spikes' may be seen by light microscopy and indicates an inflammatory process with immune complexes present and is described as a **membranous nephropathy**. Other terms

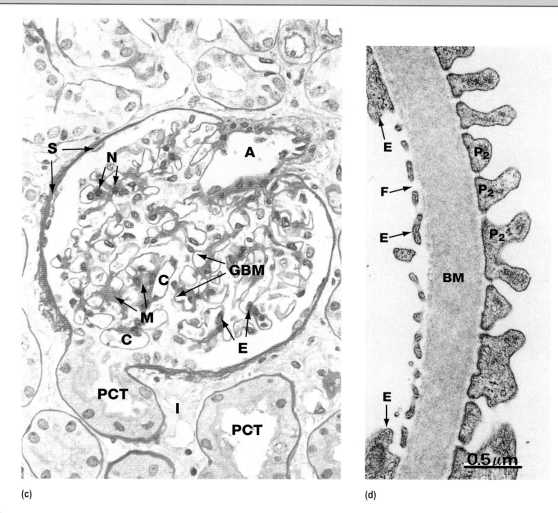

(c)

(d)

Fig. 16.1 The glomerulus—cont'd.
(**c**) Normal glomerulus showing afferent and efferent arterioles at the hilum and the origins of the proximal tubules (from Young et al 2006 Wheater's Functional Histology, 5th edn, Churchill Livingstone, with permission). Note the architecture of the mesangium and the glomerular basement membrane (PAS stain 370×). (**d**) Electron micrograph of normal glomerular basement membrane. Note the epithelial foot processes, electron-dense material in the membrane and thin endothelial cells of the glomerular blood vessels (from Young et al. 2006, with permission). Note: S, squamous cell; A, arteriole; N, mesangial cell nucleus; C, glomerular capillary; GBM, glomerular basement membrane; M, mesangium; E, endothelial cell; PCT, proximal convoluted tubule; I, interstitium; F, fenestrations; BM, basement membrane; P_2, podocyte secondary foot processes.

are often used to describe the distribution of the lesions within the glomerulus or kidney: focal, affecting only certain glomeruli; diffuse, affecting the majority; and segmental, affecting only certain mesangial lobules within a glomerulus. Sclerosis (scarring) may be a histological feature of some forms of GN.

Electron microscopy is used to identify large, electron-dense deposits within the GBM, representing complexes of antigen and antibody. Deposits may be subendothelial, intra-membranous or subepithelial and may also be found in the mesangium.

Mechanisms of immune-mediated renal damage

There are two major mechanisms of renal damage in which the immune system has a prime role, both of which

are discussed in Chapter 10. In a process analogous to a type II hypersensitivity reaction, autoantibodies directed against normal constituents of the GBM bind their target, recruit damaging effector molecules (complement) and cells (phagocytes) and the result is damage to the glomerulus and glomerular filtration. In a variant of this process, antigens may become 'planted' on the GBM and behave as integral components, with the antibodies directed against these self or exogenous targets causing glomerular damage. One mechanism of planting antigens relates to charge: the GBM is anionic and has an affinity for cationic molecules.

The second mechanism of glomerular damage is a type III hypersensitivity **immune complex** disease, with complexes of antigen and antibody forming, or being carried, in the circulation and deposited in the GBM. Once deposited, complexes can recruit complement, with the formation of membrane attack complexes and chemotactic factors.

Immune complex glomerular damage is, therefore, a combination of complement and cell-mediated attack, with the major cell types involved being the polymorphonuclear and mononuclear phagocytes.

Immune complexes that are particularly prone to cause renal damage are those formed by **cryoglobulins**. These are immunoglobulins with a tendency to precipitate at low temperatures (i.e. below 37°C). Cryoglobulins are generated secondary to neoplasms of the lymphoid system or during periods of prolonged immune stimulation (e.g. chronic infection or inflammatory conditions such as the connective tissue diseases).

In addition to the hypersensitivity-type reactions, renal damage may arise as a result of a more widespread process of inflammation of blood vessels, termed **vasculitis**, which is a multisystem disease involving several organs. Different sized vessels are affected in the different vasculitic disorders; not all have renal involvement. However, renal damage is prominent and life threatening in medium-sized vessel disease (e.g. **polyarteritis nodosa**) and small vessel disease (e.g. **Wegener's granulomatosis, microscopic polyarteritis**), and for this reason both will be discussed in detail below.

Immunological diagnosis of renal disease

Direct immunofluorescence studies of a renal biopsy in a patient with suspected immune-mediated renal damage is an important diagnostic test. Staining for deposition of IgG, IgA and IgM, as well as C3, is usually performed. So-called 'linear' staining usually indicates binding of antibody to antigens present along the length of the GBM, whilst 'granular' staining is associated with the presence of immune complexes. In renal diseases in which antibodies are generated against normal constituents of the GBM or other relevant targets, these can be detected in serum by sensitive tests such as enzyme-linked immunosorbent assays (ELISA) or radioimmunoassays (RIA). Although immune complexes have an important role in the pathogenesis of some forms of GN, the measurement of circulating immune complex levels is of little value: small amounts of complexes may cause clinically important GN, whilst high concentrations of complexes may be innocuous. Complement is consumed during the inflammatory process, and measurement of C3 and C4 is an important part of disease monitoring.

In renal damage secondary to a systemic illness, other diagnostic tests are important. For cryoglobulins to be detected reliably, blood samples must be taken, transported and the serum separated at 37°C. Autoantibody tests for systemic lupus erythematosus or other connective tissue disorders may also be indicated in renal disease of unknown aetiology, and, if a vasculitis is suspected, detection of autoantibodies to cytoplasmic constituents of neutrophils (antineutrophil cytoplasmic antibodies, ANCA) by indirect immunofluorescence, ELISA or RIA is required.

SUMMARY BOX 16.1

Nephritis and immune response

- Immune-mediated damage to glomerular structures is a common cause of glomerulonephritis, and hence renal failure.
- Pathological damage to the glomerulus is defined histologically; the terms used are not disease or mechanism specific.
- The major pathogenic processes in immune-mediated glomerulonephritis include the effects of immune complexes of antigen, antibody and complement, and the results of blood vessel inflammation, termed vasculitis.
- Immunological diagnoses rest upon analysis of renal biopsies by direct immunofluorescence, and detection of circulating autoantibodies.

Antibody-mediated nephritis: fixed glomerular antigens

Antiglomerular basement membrane disease

Anti-GBM disease is a syndrome of rapidly progressive severe GN with cell proliferation and the formation of crescents (Figs 16.2 & 16.3), in association with antibody to the GBM demonstrated by direct immunofluorescence (Fig. 16.2). That it is caused by antibody to the GBM was demonstrated in 1967, when antibody eluted from diseased kidneys and injected into primates was shown to cause nephritis.

The disease is rare, being responsible for only 3–5% of cases of GN, and it is most common in males of the 20–40 year age group, although there is a further incidence peak in women over 50 years of age. Approximately 80% of patients carry either the *HLA-DRB1*1501* or *HLA-DRB1*04* genes compared with 20–30% in the general population (see Science Box 16.1).

In 50% of cases, anti-GBM disease is associated with haemoptysis resulting from pulmonary haemorrhage and this is known as **Goodpasture's syndrome** after the author of the first case description in 1919. It seems probable that antibody binding to autoantigens within the lung requires a precipitating event that enhances accessibility to the alveolar basement membrane. Frequently, therefore, Goodpasture's syndrome is preceded by an infection of the respiratory tract that could cause antigen exposure, and the syndrome is also more frequent in cigarette smokers, presumably through a similar mechanism.

Pathology

The pathological changes are initially focal and segmental but typically become diffuse throughout the kidney and each

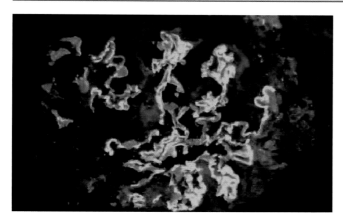

Fig. 16.2 Anti-GBM disease.
Immunofluorescence examination of renal biopsy using fluorescein conjugated antiserum to human IgG raised in rabbits. The 'crushed ribbon' pattern of linear fluorescence along the glomerular basement membrane is typical of anti-GBM disease (from Underwood 2004 General and Systemic Pathology, 4th edn, Churchill Livingstone, with permission).

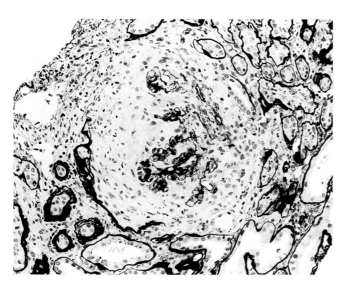

Fig. 16.3 Anti-GBM nephritis, showing collapsed glomerular tuft and a large cellular crescent.
(PASM ×220.) (Courtesy of Dr F. Dische and M. Norman.)

SCIENCE BOX 16.1

Restricted epitopes on the GBM antigen

Anti-GBM disease is associated with possession of the HLA gene *DRB1*1502*, which has a distinctive amino acid sequence around position 71, on one of the α-helices overhanging the antigen-binding groove. This strongly suggests that an autoantigenic peptide critical in the development of anti-GBM disease binds avidly to this region in the antigen-binding groove. Interestingly, the epitope targeted by anti-GBM antibodies is also highly restricted: a single monoclonal anti-GBM antibody can block anti-GBM binding by patient's serum. This region on α3(IV)NC1 has been termed the 'Goodpasture epitope'. It is formed of nine amino acids that are discontinuous, yet combine in 3-dimensions to form an epitope for high affinity IgG autoantibodies that are pathogenic in this disease (Fig. 16.4). Further studies will be required to establish whether there are indeed T cell epitopes in this region, and how they interact with HLA-DRB1*1502 molecules.

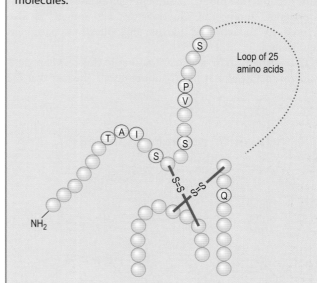

Fig. 16.4 The 'Goodpasture epitope'.
This is the region of the α3(IV)NC1 molecule in the GBM that autoantibodies bind to in patients with anti-GBM disease. It is a classic example of a discontinuous epitope — the key amino acids (marked in pink) that interact with the antibody are not adjacent to each other, but are separated by other residues, and even a whole loop of the protein. For a key to amino acids see Appendix 4.

glomerulus. There is proliferation of cells, particularly of the epithelium, with influx of inflammatory cells, and a typical lesion is the crescent at one pole of the glomerulus (Fig. 16.3). Therefore, this is a **diffuse, proliferative GN with crescents**. Electron microscopy shows discontinuities in the GBM, but electron-dense deposits are rarely seen. Direct immunofluorescence is characteristic (see below).

Pathogenesis and immunological features

The direct immunofluorescence examination of a renal biopsy demonstrates linear deposition of IgG (and occasion-ally IgA and IgM) and C3 along the GBM, with the appearance of a crushed ribbon (Fig. 16.2). ELISA and RIA are able to demonstrate anti-GBM antibodies in the circulation of over 90% of patients and the levels of these are useful for monitoring therapy. These antibodies therefore represent important markers for diagnosis and management.

The fact that autoantibodies to the GBM are pathogenic in anti-GBM disease is strongly supported by the reproduction of the disease in animal transfer studies; the recurrence of anti-GBM disease in transplanted kidneys if circulating antibody remains; and the almost 100% relationship between anti-GBM antibody in the circulation and the disease.

The autoantigen associated with anti-GBM disease and targeted by the pathogenic autoantibodies is the non-collagenous (NC1) globular domain of the carboxy-terminal of the α3 chain of type IV collagen (α3(IV)NC1). This rather ponderous description is given more substance when the constituents of the GBM are viewed (Fig. 16.5). Within the network of type IV collagen fibres, the non-collagenous globular domains of each fibril associate with each other. In fact, >99% of patients develop antibodies against a single epitope from this region. The so-called 'Goodpasture epitope' is made up of nine discontinuous amino acids (see Science Box 16.1).

The α3 chain of collagen has a restricted distribution, but other fluorescence staining may be seen within the kidney around the tubular basement membrane in up to 70% of patients. Rarely, the 'Goodpasture autoantigen' is also targeted in the choroid plexus and intestinal basement membrane.

The mechanism by which antibodies to the GBM are generated in this disease is poorly understood. The fact that the antibody response is IgG and that there is an association with possession of *HLA-DRB1*1501* implies T cell-directed autoimmunity. There is a cellular infiltrate in anti-GBM disease, but T lymphocytes (mainly CD4+) and macrophages are usually scanty. Studies on peripheral blood have shown T_H1 cells that react with α3(IV)NC1. Difficulty in witnessing the disease in evolution hampers studies of the pathogenesis. Anecdotal reports suggest that anti-GBM disease follows upper respiratory tract infection, but whether this induces disease (e.g. by exposing 'hidden' epitopes of α3(IV)NC1 to which there is poor tolerance), or exacerbates pre-existing subclinical disease is unclear. Additional insight into how loss of tolerance to collagen as an autoantigen leads to renal disease is discussed in Clinical Box 16.1.

Clinical features

Rapidly progressive GN is the most common presentation, with the lung haemorrhage occasionally of life-threatening proportions. The disease usually presents with severe renal impairment, and many patients progress to require dialysis and, subsequently, transplantation. Since the continued presence of circulating anti-GBM antibody threatens recurrence in the donor kidney, treatment is aimed at trying to preserve as much renal function as possible but also at eradicating the autoantibody. With prednisolone, cyclophosphamide and plasma exchange, antibody usually becomes undetectable in the circulation after 2 months. If the patient has become anuric, dialysis may be continued long term in the absence of immune suppression (unless there is pulmonary haemorrhage) until anti-GBM antibody disappears of its own accord. Around 80% of patients survive the acute presentation, fol-

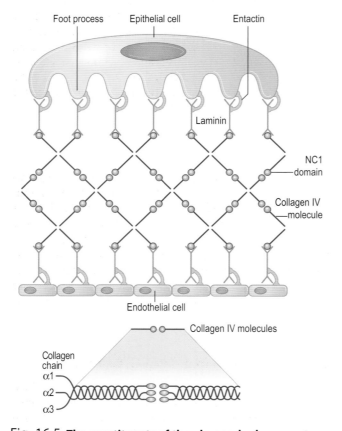

Fig. 16.5 The constituents of the glomerular basement membrane. See text for details.

CLINICAL BOX 16.1

Failed thymic deletion and autoimmunity

A form of hereditary nephritis, called Alport's syndrome, has revealed an interesting twist in the tale of anti-GBM disease. Alport's syndrome is characterised by progressive renal impairment and nerve deafness, affecting males predominantly. Electron microscopy reveals an abnormal glomerulus, with a thin, or thick, lamellated GBM. Type IV collagen, the main constituent of the GBM, has five chains normally, α1–5(IV), and genetic analysis shows that patients with Alport's syndrome have a structural abnormality in the α5(IV) chain gene. In some patients, it has been necessary to restore renal function with a kidney graft. Although this procedure is often successful, it is occasionally thwarted by the development of a form of anti-GBM nephritis affecting the new kidney, with the α5(IV) chain as the target. It is assumed that thymic or peripheral T and B cell tolerance to α5(IV) autoantigens is not generated in these patients, in whom this collagen chain is either abnormal or absent. The α5(IV) chain in the normal GBM of the donor kidney is viewed as 'foreign', therefore, and becomes the target of an autoimmune attack.

lowing which the prognosis can be good. Renal grafting, if required, is usually successful providing anti-GBM antibody has disappeared, which is the case in most patients 1 year after presentation.

It has become increasingly clear that about 30% of patients with anti-GBM disease also have anti-neutrophil cytoplasmic antibodies (typically directed against myeloperoxidase, see below), and therefore these autoantibodies should be measured routinely. Such patients tend to be in the older age group and have additional systemic manifestations of vasculitis (see below).

Other autoantibodies to fixed renal antigens

Several autoantigen–autoantibody reactions involving structures other than the 'Goodpasture antigen' have been described, and although the number of patients affected is much smaller, it indicates the existence of other primary autoimmune renal diseases. **Antitubular basement membrane** antibodies, which give a linear immunofluorescence staining pattern of the tubular basement membrane akin to that of anti-GBM antibodies, are associated with a rare, primary form of **tubulointerstitial nephritis**. There is an interstitial lymphocyte and macrophage infiltrate, with sparing of the glomeruli. Patients present with acute or chronic renal impairment, and the disease typically resolves with a course of corticosteroids.

SUMMARY BOX 16.2

Antibody-mediated nephritis

- The development of autoantibodies to antigens in the glomerular basement membrane results in the organ-specific autoimmune disease anti-GBM nephritis, which has devastating consequences for renal function.
- The immunological hallmarks of anti-GBM nephritis are the linear deposition of IgG on the GBM, seen by direct immunofluorescence, the presence of circulating anti-GBM autoantibodies and the HLA-DRB1*1501 HLA type.

Glomerulonephritis associated with immune complexes

In addition to the damaging effects of antibody binding directly to the GBM, glomerular inflammation can also arise when immune complexes, composed of antibody and antigen, are deposited within this region. Several glomerular diseases have been shown to have characteristic **granular immune deposits** visible using direct immunofluorescence and electron microscopy of renal biopsies. The initial assumption was made that such complexes were forming in the circulation or other tissues and then being deposited in the kidney,

resulting in immunological 'holes' in the glomerulus. Subsequent studies made 'holes' in these hypotheses, and it is now clear that in some circumstances the antigens alone become 'planted' within the GBM, following which the antibodies may bind. For example, components of bacteria that are implicated in post-infective glomerulonephritis have been shown to be capable of direct binding to the GBM, where they may be targeted by antibacterial antibodies. Similarly, autoantigens that are important in SLE may embed preferentially in the GBM (e.g. DNA and histones, both of which have cationic charge) where autoantibodies may bind and lead to local damage.

The tendency at present, therefore, is to have a broad classification of 'GN associated with immune complexes present in the glomerulus', without stating categorically how or where the immune complexes arise. In some diseases, there is good evidence that immune complexes are deposited. In others, the antigens are probably 'planted', while in another group it seems probable that the antigens are fixed in the tissues and that the granular appearance may relate to the discontinuous localisation of the targets. An algorithm for guiding diagnosis of immune complex and antibody-mediated GN is shown in Figure 16.6.

Post-streptococcal glomerulonephritis

Glomerulonephritis arising in association with certain organisms and infectious episodes has been recognised for many years. The best known is post-streptococcal glomerulonephritis; this usually follows infection of the throat or skin and most frequently affects children of school age. Haematuria, oliguria and proteinuria arise 14–21 days after the infection. The most frequent organism responsible is the Group A, type 12, β-haemolytic streptococcus.

Pathology

The typical histological appearance of post-infective glomerulonephritis is one of increased cellularity in the mesangium and capillary loops and polymorphonuclear cells in the capillary lumen (Fig. 16.7a). The distribution of lesions is typically diffuse throughout the kidney and the glomeruli, giving the term **diffuse proliferative GN**. Occasionally crescents form. Direct immunofluorescence studies demonstrate granular deposits (Fig. 16.7b) containing IgG and C3, and electron microscopy shows these to be subepithelial in location (Fig. 16.7c).

Pathogenesis and immunological features

For many years, certain features of this syndrome provided strong circumstantial evidence of a circulating immune complex-mediated disease. In particular, the timing of renal disease after the infection was very similar to that of 'serum sickness' arising after a bolus injection of a foreign protein

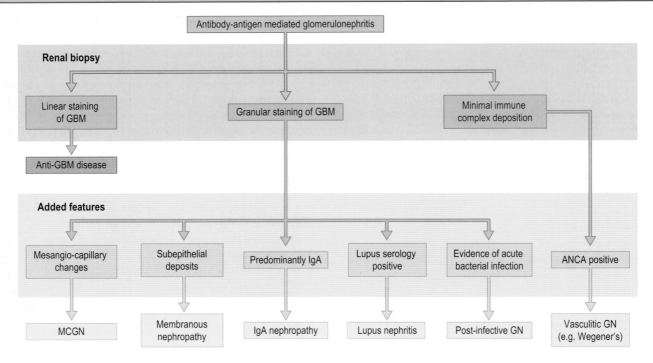

Fig. 16.6 Algorithm for diagnosing glomerulonephritis caused by antibodies or immune complexes, using renal biopsy and additional tests.

(see p. 147). This would be consistent with the generation of large amounts of bacterial antigens followed by the production of specific antibodies, with deposition of immune complexes once the critical ratio of antigen : antibody was reached. Circulating complement components (e.g. C3) are low, implying activation and consumption.

More recently, however, this view has been questioned. As stated above, haematuria may occur before antibody production, implying that bacterial antigens target and damage the kidney. If such antigens are planted in the glomeruli, antibody-mediated damage may follow once antibacterial titres rise. A further suggestion has been that M proteins in streptococci can mimic glomerular autoantigens, and that this is actually an example of molecular mimicry (see p. 126). Support for this proposal comes from the fact that monoclonal antibodies raised against streptococcal antigens have been shown to bind glomerular components, and vice versa.

Clinical features

The diagnosis of post-streptococcal GN is usually a clinical one, reinforced by evidence of a streptococcal focus and a raised titre of antistreptolysin antibodies (ASO titre). Complement levels are reduced in the acute phase. The overall prognosis is good, with children faring better than adults. Most patients recover renal function after the initial illness, and relapse is rare. However, although children have a better rate of recovery, some 30% of patients overall have a slowly progressive loss of renal function over 10 or more years, and

this disease is an important cause of chronic renal failure presenting in adulthood.

Treatment of the acute disease involves antibacterial agents to clear residual infection and dialysis if required.

Membranous glomerulonephritis

Membranous GN represents 25% of causes of nephrotic syndrome (and is the commonest cause in adults) and 10% of all renal disease. It develops secondarily as a result of a wide variety of underlying conditions or treatments, or primarily in so-called idiopathic disease:

- infection: malaria, hepatitis B and C infection
- neoplasia: carcinoma, lymphoproliferative diseases
- drugs/toxins: penicillamine, gold
- connective tissue disease: systemic lupus erythematosus.

The descriptive term 'membranous' comes from the histopathological, immunofluorescence and electron microscopic features of the disease. These demonstrate little inflammatory change but marked abnormalities in the GBM (see below).

Pathology

There is a diffuse thickening of the GBM seen on light microscopy (Fig. 16.8), and special stains reveal that this

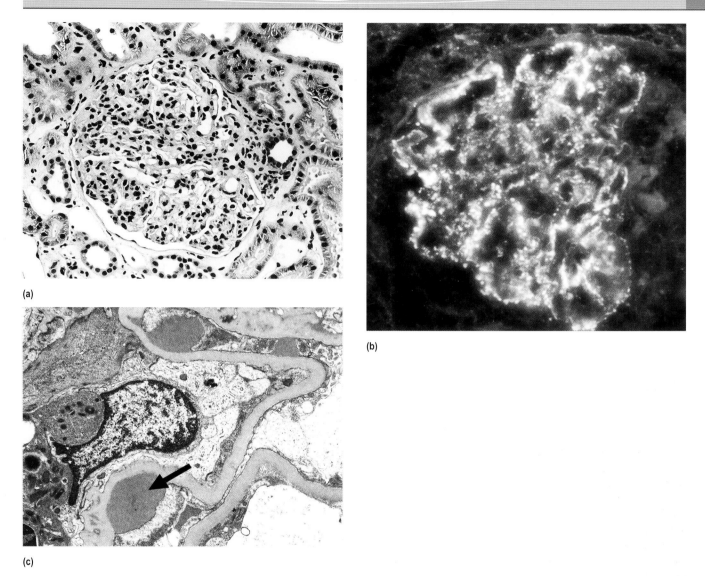

(a)

(b)

(c)

Fig. 16.7 Post-streptococcal proliferative glomerulonephritis.
(**a**) Light microscopy showing an enlarged, intensely hypercellular glomerular tuft, containing neutrophils (H&E ×300). (**b**) Direct immunofluorescence examination of a renal biopsy, showing granular deposits of IgG along the GBM. (**c**) Electron micrograph of a subepithelial deposit (arrow). (Courtesy of Dr F. Dische and M. Norman.)

is due to 'spikes', giving a comb-like appearance to the GBM. Direct immunofluorescence demonstrates granular deposits of IgG, C3 and occasionally IgA and IgM. Electron microscopy shows that the immune deposits are subepithelial deposits (i.e. between the epithelial cell and GBM).

Pathogenesis and immunological features

The pathological appearances of membranous GN strongly suggest the presence of immune complexes giving rise to renal damage. The important question arises as to whether the antigen–antibody complexes involved are deposited direct from the circulation, or whether the antigenic components are 'planted' or fixed and become sitting targets for

antibodies. This factor may well vary according to the underlying disease process.

Behind this theory, of a GN mediated by antibody to an antigen fixed in the glomerulus, is an animal model of membranous GN, first described in 1951. **Heymann's nephritis** (induced by immunisation with kidney extract) has many similar features to membranous GN: it is non-inflammatory, gives rise to the nephrotic syndrome and is characterised pathologically by immune deposits localised to the epithelial side of the GBM. The ability to induce the disease in rats is MHC dependent (an interesting fact, since there is some evidence that membranous glomerulopathy in humans is associated with HLA-DR3 alleles) and disease can be transferred passively using serum from affected animals. Depletion of complement, but not neutrophils, reduces renal damage.

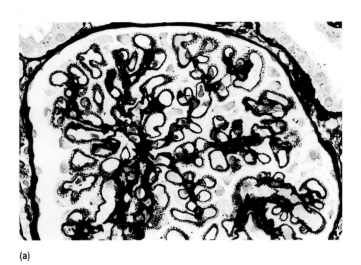

(a)

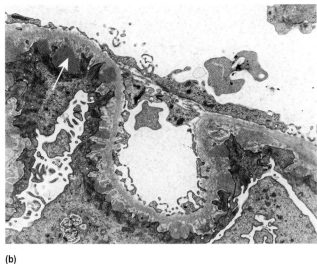

(b)

Fig. 16.8 **Membranous glomerulonephritis.**
(**a**) Glomerular basement membrane thickening showing subepithelial spikes (PASM ×590). (**b**) Electron micrograph of subepithelial deposits and spikes (arrowed). (Courtesy of Dr F. Dische and M. Norman.)

Clinical features

Membranous GN presents as persistent proteinuria or nephrotic syndrome. The majority of cases are idiopathic, and although some 25% of patients may remit, one third of patients progress to end-stage renal failure in 10 years. Corticosteroids have been used extensively in this disease, but its tendency to remit spontaneously has meant that the success of the steroid-based approach is still not completely clear. The cytotoxic agents cyclophosphamide and chlorambucil have been frequently used in the past, and more recently success has been reported with ciclosporin and mycophenolate mofetil.

Minimal change glomerulonephritis

Minimal change glomerulonephritis takes its name from the fact that there are few evident structural or pathological changes in renal biopsies in this group of patients. Despite this, the disease has a sufficient number of telling features to suggest that it has an immune pathogenesis. In addition, it is common: minimal change GN is responsible for 75% of childhood presentations of nephrotic syndrome, and for 30% amongst adults.

Pathology

There are no abnormalities on conventional histological or immunofluorescence analysis. The characteristic change on electron microscopy is the loss of clear definition of the epithelial foot processes, which may appear fused (a lesion termed effacement).

Pathogenesis and immunological features

The cause and disease process are not known, but several features indicate an immune component. First, its onset may be associated with an immune event (e.g. an infection, allergic reaction or routine immunisation). Other diseases occasionally associated with minimal change GN are neoplastic disorders, most notably Hodgkin's disease. Intriguingly, successful chemotherapeutic or radiotherapeutic treatment for the Hodgkin's disease clears the renal lesion, suggesting that a soluble factor produced as a consequence of the neoplasm has a pathogenetic role. Indeed, this, and the responsiveness to steroids (see below), are major pieces of evidence that have led to a prevailing hypothesis that a secreted immune cell product (i.e. cytokine), as yet unknown, causes the ultrastructural changes in the glomerulus.

Clinical features

Minimal change GN usually presents as nephrotic syndrome. If the disease is secondary to a systemic illness, then it usually resolves with treatment of the primary disease but may also relapse accordingly. Overall, the prognosis of the renal lesion is excellent. Most patients with idiopathic disease respond dramatically to a course of corticosteroids, though a proportion, particularly those with relapsing nephrotic syndrome, may require more potent immunosuppressives, such as the cytotoxic agent cyclophosphamide.

Mesangiocapillary glomerulonephritis

Frequently shortened to MCGN, this syndrome also goes under the description **membranoproliferative GN**. It is typical of childhood and probably represents around 10% of renal disease. The distinctive features of MCGN are its histopathology (increased cellularity) and the location of the immune complexes in the subendothelial space. Type I MCGN is four times more common than type II. The identification of IgG and C3 within the glomerulus suggests involvement of immune complexes in the disease, but the underlying processes are unknown. Most cases are idiopathic, but MCGN can arise secondary to SLE, chronic infection (bacterial endocarditis, shunt nephritis, leprosy) and neoplasia.

Pathology

The typical light microscopic appearance in type I MCGN is of mesangial proliferation with capillary thickening. Electron microscopy shows evidence of mesangial and subendothelial immune complexes, showing as granular IgG (80%) and C3 (all cases) deposits on direct immunofluorescence. In type II MCGN, mesangial proliferation is less marked, and the deposits typically appear 'dense' on electron micrographs, trail ribbon-like along the GBM, are intramembranous (i.e. within the GBM) and are composed of IgG (less than half the cases) and C3 (all cases). The descriptive terms used in this syndrome, therefore, refer to the mesangial proliferation and the tendency of the complexes to be most closely associated with the capillary endothelium.

Pathogenesis and immunological features

Type I MCGN has all of the hallmarks of an immune complex disease, but the underlying pathological process remains undefined, as it does for type II. There is an intriguing association between type II MCGN and a disorder called partial lipodystrophy (a condition characterised by loss of subcutaneous fat). In addition, 60% of patients with type II MCGN (and 10% of patients with type I) have a circulating IgG autoantibody directed against the alternative complement pathway C3 convertase, C3bBb. This autoantibody, termed **C3 nephritic factor** (C3Nef), stabilises C3bBb by inhibiting its breakdown by factors H and I and in so doing facilitates exhaustive complement activation. The disease is typically **hypocomplementaemic**, with low C3 levels that tend to be prolonged, in contrast with the short-lived reduction seen in post-streptococcal GN. The role of C3Nef in the pathogenesis of MCGN is unclear. Hypocomplementaemia could contribute to immune-complex deposition, but C3Nef may also occur in the absence of nephritis, and at present the autoantibody does not appear to have a pathogenetic role. Passive transfer studies are difficult to conduct in a manner that conclusively proves the role of C3Nef, since other as yet unidentified serum factors that could have a role in causing MCGN will be transferred with the antibody.

The nature of the deposits in MCGN is not known, but the possibility that they derive in part from circulating factors (e.g. antibody, antigen) comes from the fact that

recurrence of MCGN-type lesions in transplanted kidneys is common (90% of patients with type II and 30% of those with type I).

Clinical features

The disease affects adolescents and young adults and typically presents as nephritis or nephrotic syndrome. One third of cases remit spontaneously; a further third develop end-stage renal failure and a third follow a relapsing remitting course. Whilst any underlying contributory disease should be treated, therapy of MCGN itself remains largely unrewarding, and corticosteroids do not appear to be of benefit.

Glomerulonephritis associated with IgA deposits

This form of GN goes under several other terms, including **IgA nephropathy** and **Berger's disease**. It is probably the most common cause of GN in the Western world (25–30% of all causes; affects 1–2 adults per 10 000 per year). IgA nephropathy is typically not severe, but its frequency means that it contributes 20% of the cases of end-stage renal failure. Males in adolescence or early adulthood are most frequently affected. IgA nephropathy is characterised by mesangial deposition of IgA (Fig. 16.9), in association with C3 and evidence of alternative complement pathway activation. IgA nephropathy may occur as a primary disease, or secondary to a number of infective, inflammatory and neoplastic diseases, including HIV, coeliac disease and lung cancer. There

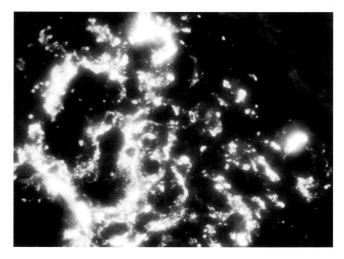

Fig. 16.9 **IgA nephropathy.**
Direct immunofluorescence examination of a renal biopsy from a patient with IgA nephropathy, using fluorescein-conjugated antiserum raised in rabbits against human IgA and demonstrating mesangial deposits of IgA (×640). (Courtesy of Dr F. Dische and M. Norman.)

is an increasing recognition of a genetic component to the disease, including polymorphisms in genes associated with renal and immune function (e.g. angiotensinogen, IL-1, IL-6 genes).

Pathology

Changes in the kidney are focal or diffuse, with proliferation of cells in the mesangium. Occasionally there are crescents. The hallmark of the lesions is the deposition of IgA, usually with IgG and C3 and typically in the mesangium.

Pathogenesis and immunological features

In association with the renal IgA deposits, IgA concentration in the circulation is increased in up to 50% of patients, with IgA-containing complexes in an equivalent proportion. Considerable interest has focused on the antigenic content of the complexes and, particularly, the possibility that these are components of gut pathogens or dietary proteins, given the mucosal origin and function of IgA. It has also been proposed that the deposited IgA molecules are themselves defective in their degree of glycosylation, perhaps leading to increased tissue deposition.

External targets have also been suggested as being the main components of the IgA complexes deposited in the mesangium, the list of offenders including hepatitis B surface antigen, cytomegalovirus proteins and common bacteria. Reports regarding such antigens would fit with the typical history, where IgA nephropathy follows an episode of upper respiratory tract infection, but are controversial and the studies difficult to reproduce.

Whilst the molecular mechanisms of the disease remain enigmatic, there is strong evidence from transplantation studies that the aetiology of IgA nephropathy relates to circulating antibody, with or without complexed antigen. First, IgA deposits reappear in 50% of transplanted kidneys, although the lesions are usually benign. Second, when kidneys that contain IgA deposits have been unwittingly transplanted into patients with other causes of renal failure, the kidney clears! Therefore, there is strong evidence that something in the milieu of the patient with IgA nephropathy favours the formation of the mesangial deposits characteristic of the disease.

HLA studies have revealed no consistent, marked associations with class I or class II alleles.

Clinical features

Patients usually present with haematuria, frequently macroscopic and recurrent, and this is sometimes accompanied by proteinuria. Renal failure may develop slowly in a small proportion (10–20%) over 10–20 years. In therapeutic terms, it appears that neither cure nor prevention are yet possible in IgA nephropathy. Since many of the cases pursue a benign course, treatment protocols are dependent upon the severity of the GN. Corticosteroids may be of some benefit, but this remains controversial, as does the question of whether tonsillectomy can be of benefit.

Glomerulonephritis in SLE

SLE is a multisystem inflammatory disease of connective tissue, characterised by autoantibody reactions to a range of tissue components (see Ch. 12). Glomerulonephritis represents a common and life-threatening complication of the disease. Some 50–60% of patients have proteinuria; 90% have abnormalities on conventional histological analysis of renal biopsies; and almost 100% have abnormalities by electron microscopy and immunofluorescence. It appears that most of the different histological patterns of GN we have discussed may be seen in SLE (Table 16.1), and that the pattern can be different even in sequential biopsies from the same patient. Equally, the clinical presentation is varied with hypertension, proteinuria, haematuria, nephrotic syndrome or end-stage renal failure.

Pathology

In general terms, deposition of IgG, IgM and IgA, along with C3, C4 and C1q and the membrane attack complex, is seen in the subendothelial part of the GBM and in the mesangium. The typical granular appearance on immunofluorescence is shown in Figure 16.10. The variable pattern of abnormalities seen in SLE has invoked the use of a classification system, which is a useful index of the degree of damage (Table 16.2).

Pathogenesis and immunological features

Elution of immune deposits from diseased kidneys shows that a proportion of the complexes are made of DNA–anti-DNA, but these form a minority. The titres of anti-nuclear and anti-DNA antibodies, levels of circulating immune complexes and the degree of complement activation show only rough correlations with the degree of nephritis, arguing against them being the single pathogenic mechanism. In addition, there is evidence that nephritis typical of SLE can

Table 16.1 Renal immunofluorescence patterns seen in glomerulonephritis associated with SLE

Pathology	Direct immunofluorescence
Little or no change by light microscopy	GBM and mesangial deposits of IgG, IgA, IgM and C3
Focal or diffuse proliferative GN	GBM and mesangial deposits of IgG, IgA, IgM and C3
Membranous GN	GBM and mesangial deposits of IgG, IgA, IgM and C3
Tubulointerstitial nephritis	IgG, IgA, IgM and C3 deposits in tubular basement membrane

Table 16.2 Standardised (2004) criteria for pathological glomerular changes in SLE (lupus nephritis)

Class	Name	Renal pathology
I	Minimal mesangial nephritis	Normal light microscopy. Mesangial deposits visible by immunofluorescence only
II	Mesangioproliferative lupus nephritis	Mesangial proliferation visible by light microscopy
III	Focal lupus nephritis	Glomerulonephritis with lesions in <50% of glomeruli
IV	Diffuse lupus nephritis	Glomerulonephritis with lesions in >50% of glomeruli
V	Membranous lupus nephropathy	May occur in conjunction with class III or IV lesions
VI	Advanced sclerosing lupus nephritis	Most glomeruli (>90%) are sclerosed and 'end-stage'

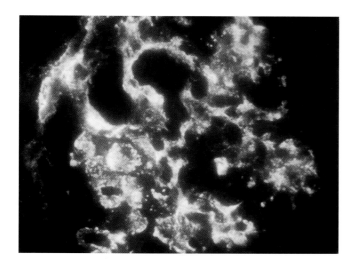

Fig. 16.10 Systemic lupus erythematosus.
Direct immunofluorescence examination of a renal biopsy from a patient with SLE using fluorescein-conjugated antiserum raised in rabbits against human complement component C1q. The staining pattern is granular along the GBM and within the mesangium. (Courtesy of Dr F. Dische and M. Norman.)

present years before these serological abnormalities that are typical of the disease are detectable. However, complement levels and erythrocyte complement receptors (CR-1) are reduced, contributing to potential immune complex disease. In terms of genetic influences on lupus nephritis, the strongest and most consistent association is with polymorphisms in Fc receptors, supporting the view that impaired clearance of immune complex is a major factor in the renal complications. There is some evidence of cross-reactivity between anti-dsDNA antibodies and GBM components, and also the possibility that additional GBM autoantigens, such as actinin and laminin, are targeted by autoantibodies. The severity of infiltration of the kidney by T cells correlates well with renal

function, though it is not yet clear how T cells contribute to renal damage.

An attractive theory at present is that autoantigens are 'planted' in the glomeruli and that the critical damaging antigen–antibody interactions take place there. DNA-associated proteins such as histones are an example of cationic molecules that bind to the GBM, and to its collagen V components in particular.

Clinical features

Mild forms of GN associated with SLE are usually managed with corticosteroids, while more severe disease requires the addition of azathioprine or cyclophosphamide. Surprisingly, the long-term survival of renal function appears to be associated with the degree of interstitial scarring, rather than with the severity of glomerular damage. Of the newer agents, mycophenolate mofetil is an increasingly used alternative to cyclophosphamide.

SUMMARY BOX 16.3

Glomerulonephritis associated with immune complexes

- Inflammation of the glomerulus may arise after deposition of immune complexes on or in the GBM, or after in situ formation of immune complexes involving fixed antigens.

- The renal damage is associated with recruitment of complement and inflammatory cells into the glomerulus.

- There are a variety of pathological processes that can result in this form of GN, involving bacterial antigens, autoantigens, possibly tumour antigens and also unidentified antigens. Different antigen–antibody complexes have distinct characteristics in terms of where they are deposited in the GBM and mesangium.

Renal disease associated with vasculitis

Systemic vasculitis is a manifestation of several disorders and involves a necrotising (i.e. necrosis-inducing) inflammatory process taking place within blood-vessel walls. This leads to organ damage through loss of the blood supply. Any organ may be affected, and the distribution of the disease may be influenced by the size of the vessels involved. The best working classification of vasculitic disorders is that based on the size of the vessels affected. The kidney is typically damaged when small (e.g. **Wegener's granulomatosis** and **microscopic polyarteritis**) or medium-sized (e.g. **polyarteritis nodosa**) vessels are targeted in the vasculitis. Vasculitis is also a manifestation of **cryoglobulinaemia**.

Wegener's granulomatosis

This is an inflammation of the lining of the blood vessels (systemic vasculitis) associated with granulomatous lesions in the upper and lower respiratory tract usually preceding the onset of GN. The characteristics of the renal lesion are that it is typically acute in onset and crescentic. The syndrome was first described by Friedrich Wegener in 1936, but entering into the definition in the last 20 years has been the presence in the serum of an autoantibody directed against components in the cytoplasm of neutrophils. Two major forms of **anti-neutrophil cytoplasmic antibody** (ANCA) exist, and the one that clearly binds diffusely throughout the cytoplasm (cytoplasmic or **cANCA**; Fig. 16.11) is present in almost 100% of patients with Wegener's granulomatosis (i.e. disease sensitivity 100%). It is rarely found in association with other diseases and has a specificity for Wegener's granulomatosis of approximately 90%. This makes it one of the most clinically useful of the antibody tests performed in modern clinical immunology laboratories. As discussed, it may be found in patients with anti-GBM disease. Vasculitis due to cANCA is, however, rare with estimates of prevalence of around 1 in 40 000 of the population.

Pathology

Typically, there is a focal, proliferative GN, often associated with necrosis and crescent formation (Fig. 16.12). There are few or no deposits and few or no infiltrating cells; the EM appearance is of a damaged and disrupted GBM. Wegener's may manifest elsewhere, such as in the respiratory tract,

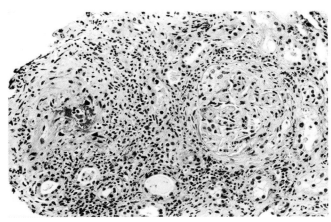

(a)

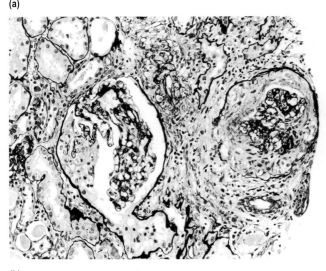

(b)

Fig. 16.12 Wegener's granulomatosis.
(**a**) Renal lesions in Wegener's granulomatosis, demonstrating intense cellular infiltration and glomerular cellularity.
(**b**) Crescent formation. (Courtesy of Dr F. Dische and M. Norman.)

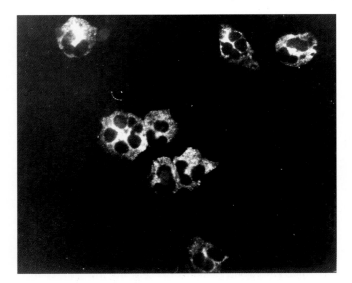

Fig. 16.11 cANCA in Wegener's granulomatosis.
Indirect immunofluorescence examination of normal neutrophils, incubated with serum from a patient with Wegener's granulomatosis and then with fluorescein-conjugated antiserum raised in rabbits against human IgG. The cytoplasmic staining pattern is caused by the presence of anti-neutrophil cytoplasmic antibody (cANCA).

where granuloma formation is associated with zones of necrosis, infiltration by lymphocytes and macrophages, and multinucleate giant cells.

Pathogenesis and immunological features

cANCA is usually identified by indirect immunofluorescence on normal, alcohol-fixed neutrophils (Fig. 16.11) and also by ELISA. The molecular target of the autoantibody has been identified as **proteinase 3** (PR3), an antimicrobial agent of 29 kDa found in the primary granules of neutrophils. There has been much debate about the role of the antibodies in the disease process (see Science Box 16.2).

Clinical features

Males are more commonly affected, and it is a disease of the late middle aged and elderly. In the past, granulomatous lesions in the respiratory tract, presenting as epistaxis or haemoptysis, might have gone undiagnosed for some time in the absence of renal disease. However, cANCA measurement is now widely available. It is a feature of Wegener's granulomatosis that the first manifestations of the disease, or a relapse, are frequently preceded by an infection, and some two thirds of patients are chronic nasal carriers of *Staphylococcus aureus*.

Aggressive use of corticosteroids with cyclophosphamide has led to a considerable improvement in the outcome of a disease associated with an 80% 1-year mortality rate in early series in the 1950s. Nowadays, 80% achieve remission, although some 40% follow a relapsing-remitting course. The level of cANCA appears to be a useful guide to the management of the disease, with rising titres closely correlated with relapse.

Microscopic polyarteritis

This condition is a small-vessel vasculitis, and the histological appearance of the vessels affected is the same as that seen in Wegener's granulomatosis. Microscopic polyarteritis is associated with the presence of ANCA, but of a different type to that seen in Wegener's granulomatosis.

Pathology

Focal necrotising GN is seen, with crescent formation. Necrotising vasculitis is seen systemically in microscopic polyarteritis. Granulomata are not seen. Vessel lesions may be associated with immune deposits containing IgG and C3, but occasionally the evidence for immunological involvement in the vasculitis is lacking, with few or no immune deposits, and this may be described as 'pauci-immune'.

Pathogenesis and immunological features

The distinctive immunological feature of microscopic polyarteritis is a form of ANCA, present in some 60% of patients. This gives a different pattern to the cANCA associated with Wegener's granulomatosis, since the staining is concentrated around the nucleus, so-called perinuclear or pANCA. In fact the main pANCA target autoantigen, myeloperoxidase (MPO), is cytoplasmic and its perinuclear localisation in the immunofluorescence test used is an artefact of the alcohol fixation.

Clinical features

Response to treatment involving immunosuppression with corticosteroids and cyclophosphamide is very dramatic in these disorders.

SCIENCE BOX 16.2

The role of cANCA in necrotising vasculitis

There is now good evidence that the ANCA autoantibodies in patients with vasculitis are pathogenic, i.e. they alone can cause disease. Perhaps the best evidence comes from two case reports. In one, a neonate developed pulmonary haemorrhage and nephritis following transplacental transfer of maternal MPO-ANCA. In the other, a boy with X-linked agammaglobulinaemia who regularly received immunoglobulin-replacement therapy developed uveitis and vasculitic lesions in the retina, associated with cANCA in the serum. Given the unlikelihood of a patient with this form of immunodeficiency being able to generate any antibody-mediated immune response, the batch of immunoglobulin that he had most recently received was also checked for cANCA — and was positive. These reports indicate the potential power of ANCA alone in causing vasculitis. The other apparent co-factor in Wegener's granulomatosis, infection, would certainly have been an ever-present complication of this boy's immunodeficiency. So, the

questions that remain to be answered regarding ANCA and vasculitis are: what induces ANCA production; how is ANCA causing vasculitic lesions; and what is the basis of the association between diseases such as Wegener's granulomatosis and infection? The second and third of these questions are perhaps the only ones to yield to a working hypothesis. In this, it is suggested that ANCA is indeed a key component in the development of vasculitis. The proposal is that there are at least two pathogenetic requirements to initiate vasculitic lesions: the presence of ANCA and an infection (Fig. 16.13). The release of endogenous mediators such as IL-8/CXCL8 from endothelial cells in response to local bacterial infection has an activating effect on neutrophils, which leads to a small degree of granule release, exposing contents such as PR3 transiently on the neutrophil surface. ANCAs bind to their antigens exposed on the neutrophil surface leading to more robust activation and granule release. Normally, the neutrophil would have completed the

(continued)

SCIENCE BOX 16.2

The role of cANCA in necrotising vasculitis—cont'd

process of transendothelial migration before any granule release — but here in the presence of ANCA it is happening on the endothelial cell surface, leading to necrotising damage to endothelia on vessel walls, and hence vasculitis. There are then at least two ways in which tissue damage may become extended: (1) neutrophil granule proteins (PR3, MPO) will be released into the circulation and may bind

endothelium through charge interactions, leading to further proteolytic damage as well as immune complex formation in situ; and (2) the granule proteins may also be carried as immune complexes with ANCA. The final and difficult question is how ANCAs arise, and, as yet, there is no clear answer.

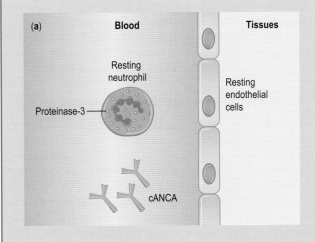

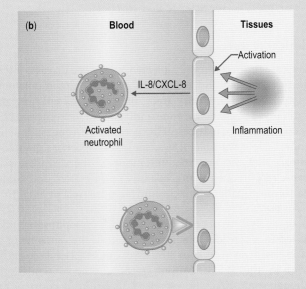

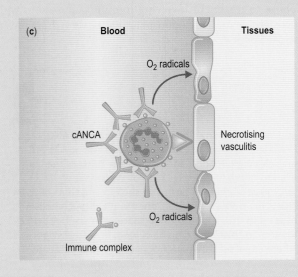

Fig. 16.13 **Schematic representation of a possible pathogenic scenario for the role of ANCA in vasculitis.**
(a) The normal situation. **(b)** Neutrophils activated by an inflammatory focus in the tissues up-regulate adhesion molecules from intracellular granules and are transiently adherent to the vessel wall. Also exposed by this degranulation are other contents, such as proteinase 3 (PR3; the target of cANCA) not normally expressed on the surface of resting cells. **(c)** In the presence of cANCA, there is major release of toxic neutrophil granule contents prematurely onto the vessel wall, causing endothelial cell damage. In addition, adherent neutrophils expressing surface PR3 become further activated by autoantibody binding, releasing toxic oxygen metabolites and causing vessel damage. Immune complexes composed of cANCA and PR3 may establish secondary inflammatory foci at a distance from this site by an immune complex-mediated mechanism.

Table 16.3 Summary of the characteristics of the nephritic disorders

Disorder	Glomerular pathology	Direct immunofluorescence	GBM deposits seen by EM	Immunopathology	Other features
Antibody mediated					
Anti-GBM nephritis	Diffuse proliferative ± crescents	Linear IgG, C3 along GBM	None	Circulating antibody to NC1 domain of α3 chain of type IV collagen	Association with *HLA-DRB1*1502* and haemoptysis (Goodpasture's syndrome)
Associated with immune complexes					
Post-streptococcal GN	Diffuse proliferative ± crescents	Granular IgG, C3 along GBM	Subepithelial	? Circulating immune complexes, 'planted' bacterial antigens, or cross-reactive antibacterial antibodies	
Membranous GN	Thickened GBM	Granular IgG, C3 along GBM	Subepithelial	? Circulating autoantibodies to fixed renal antigen or 'planted' antigen	Association with HLA-DR3
Minimal change GN	Minimal (foot process effacement)	Negative	Negative	? Soluble 'immunological factor' causes damages	
Mesangiocapillary GN (I and II)	Mesangial proliferation and capillary thickening	Granular C3 and IgG along GBM	Subendothelial (type I) and intramembranous (type II)	? Immune complex mediated	Type II associated with partial lipodystrophy and C3Nef

(continued)

Table 16.3 Summary of the characteristics of the nephritic disorders—cont'd

Disorder	Glomerular pathology	Direct immunofluorescence	GBM deposits seen by EM	Immunopathology	Other features
Associated with immune complexes—cont'd					
IgA nephropathy	Mesangial	IgA, C3 proliferation	Negative	? Immune complexes or antibodies to 'planted' antigens	
SLE nephritis	Variable	Granular IgG, IgM, C3, C4 along GBM	Subendothelial and/or subepithelial	? Immune complexes deposited or autoantibodies to 'planted' autoantigens	
Associated with vasculitis					
Wegener's granulomatosis	Focal proliferative GN with crescents	Negative	Negative	Immune damage to vessel walls ± immune complex involvement	cANCA
Microscopic polyarteritis	Focal necrotising GN with crescents	Negative	Negative	? Immune damage to vessel walls ± immune complex involvement	pANCA; idiopathic rapidly progressive GN is similar but restricted to kidney
Cryoglobulinaemia	Similar to mesangiocapillary GN	IgG, IgM, C3 along capillary wall	Subendothelial	Immune complexes deposited	

Glomerulonephritis associated with cryoglobulinaemia

Cryoglobulins are immunoglobulins that form precipitates at low temperatures. Precipitates can thus form at temperatures below the core of 37°C as the circulation enters a peripheral region such as the limbs. The condition of cryoglobulinaemia may be primary, or it may be secondary to disorders including lymphoproliferative disease, the connective tissue diseases and chronic viral infection (especially with hepatitis C virus). Perhaps the most important practical consideration is that cryoglobulins can precipitate at room temperature. When this happens in a blood sample, the precipitate will be removed with the cells and clot on centrifugation. Therefore, under normal blood-taking conditions, cryoglobulins will not be detectable in a serum sample: blood must be collected at 37°C and maintained at this temperature until serum has been separated.

Cryoglobulins are classified according to their properties. Type I are monoclonal, type II mixed mono- and polyclonal and type III polyclonal. The pathogenic cryoglobulins are usually those with polyclonal/mixed origin, with some rheumatoid factor activity (i.e. immunoglobulins form complexes by binding to other immunoglobulins).

Pathology

The most typical pathological lesion is that of mesangiocapillary GN. Immunofluorescence shows granular staining of cryoglobulin and complement along the capillary wall, and deposits seen on electron micrographs are typically subendothelial.

Pathogenesis and immunological features

The reason for the generation of immunglobulins with the property of precipitating at low temperature is not known. The association with chronic infection suggests that chronic antigen stimulation may be one factor in exposing such responses. Once present, cryoglobulins have the capacity to precipitate in the cold extremities, lodging in vessel walls and activating complement, with resulting recruitment of neutrophils and vessel damage. Systemically, levels of classical pathway complement components are low.

Clinical features

The clinical features are dependent upon the underlying cause. Treatment is usually directed against the primary disease, but if the effects of the cryoglobulins need to be controlled, plasmapheresis and cytotoxic chemotherapy may be required. The renal lesions do not tend to be rapidly progressive in most cases, and this systemic therapy may be sufficient to maintain renal function.

The major immunological features of immune-mediated renal disease are distilled in Table 16.3.

SUMMARY BOX 16.4

Renal vasculitis

- The kidney is particularly sensitive to inflammatory processes involving damage to blood vessels.
- In some cases of vasculitis associated with renal damage, the mechanisms are well defined (e.g. cryoglobulinaemia, Wegener's granulomatosis). In the diagnosis of both of these conditions, the immunology laboratory is prominent. Measurement of ANCA is important.

Further reading

Berger SP, Daha MR 2007 Complement in glomerular injury. Semin Immunopathol 29: 375–384

Falk RJ, Jennette JC, Nachman PH 2004 Primary glomerular disease. In: Brenner & Rector's The kidney, 7th edn. Saunders: London

Lionaki S, Jennette JC, Falk RJ 2007 Anti-neutrophil cytoplasmic (ANCA) and anti-glomerular basement membrane (GBM) autoantibodies in necrotizing and crescentic glomerulonephritis. Semin Immunopathol 29: 459–474

Pressler BM, Falk RJ, Preston GA 2006 Kidney disease: Goodpasture's, lupus nephritis, ANCA-associated glomerulonephritis. In: Rose NR, Mackay IR (eds) The autoimmune diseases, 2nd edn. Elsevier: London

Immune-mediated skin disease

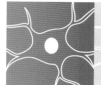

The skin is an important homeostatic organ, regulating amongst other things body temperature and salt and water content. In immunological terms, it forms a major, innate, physical barrier to infection. In recent years it has become clear that the skin also has a specialised contingent of immune cells. The Langerhans cell plays an important role in immune surveillance within the skin. The mast cell is also a resident here and has important immunological functions and involvement in allergy (see Ch. 10). There are also skin-specific homing receptors (cutaneous lymphocyte antigen; CLA) to allow infiltration by lymphocytes, and it is now clear that keratinocytes, the major cellular component of skin, are capable of important immunological functions such as cytokine and chemokine secretion. In this chapter the role of these cells and molecules in maintaining normal immune function is discussed, along with several diseases in which they are dysregulated and involved in damaging inflammatory and autoimmune responses.

Normal and diseased skin

Immunobiology of the skin

To understand the role of the skin and its immune system in disease, it is necessary to revise the histology and physiology of the organ, with particular attention to the site and function of the immune cells. By convention, skin has three layers, the epidermis, dermis and fat (Fig. 17.1). The epidermis is a stratified layer of squamous epithelial cells, the predominant member being the keratinocyte. These cells arise from the basal layer of the epidermis, which abuts onto the basal lamina, or basement membrane zone (BMZ). The keratinocyte migrates upwards from the basal layer, gradually acquiring increasing amounts of the fibrous protein keratin and gradually becoming more flattened in shape. At the surface, keratinocytes have become a dead envelope of keratin, the so-called 'horny layer' (stratum corneum), with important barrier functions. At intervals throughout the epidermis, occasional Langerhans cells may be seen. The BMZ is composed predominantly of laminin, fibronectin and collagen type IV and divides the epidermis from the dermis. Within the dermis lie the blood and lymphatic vessels, as well as the skin adnexal structures (sweat and sebaceous glands, hair follicles).

Immune cells are found predominantly in the dermis, particularly around the post-capillary vessels in what has been termed the **dermal perivascular unit** (Fig. 17.1). Here, in close proximity to the endothelium lie mast cells, macrophages, T cells and dendritic cells, some of which are similar to Langerhans cells. At this site, immune cells are perfectly poised to respond to signals arising from epidermal injury or infection, and to regulate post-capillary endothelial adhesion molecules. Some 10^9–10^{10} T lymphocytes are found in the skin of an adult, and 90% of these are in the dermal perivascular units.

Examination of the epidermis in inflammatory skin conditions has shown that the **keratinocyte** expresses class II MHC molecules and ICAM-1 under stress. The keratinocyte is also capable of phagocytosis, since this is the process involved in the acquisition of melanin pigment from melanocytes. Following stimulation of healthy skin keratinocytes in vitro, several cytokines may be produced: IL-1, IL-6, IL-8, IFN-α and IFN-β, TNF-α and colony-stimulating factors for myeloid cells (G-CSF, GM-CSF). It is, therefore, possible to envisage roles for keratinocytes in attracting and anchoring immune cells (IL-8, CSFs, ICAM-1, as well as chemokines such as CCL-27, RANTES and MCP-1 that attract lymphocytes, neutrophils, eosinophils and dendritic cells); cell activation (IL-1, IL-8, TNF-α); in exerting cytotoxicity against

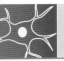

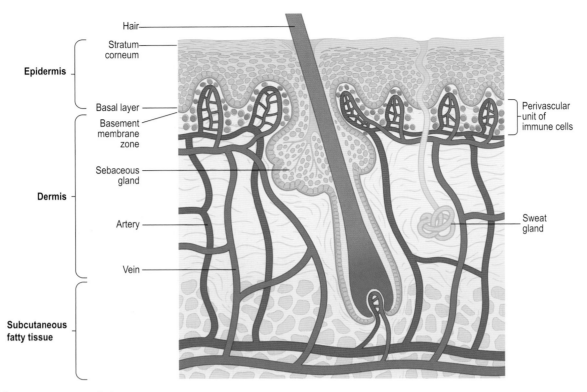

Fig. 17.1 The structure of skin.

microbial organisms (IFN-α/β, TNF-α); and even in antigen processing and presentation (class II MHC molecules).

Langerhans cells are bone-marrow derived and have a dendritic morphology (i.e. have many processes to provide an extensive area of contact). Like DCs these cells express class II MHC molecules constitutively. Also like DCs, once they have become activated and trapped relevant antigens, they undergo rapid migration to the local lymph node to process and present peptide antigens to T lymphocytes.

T lymphocytes in the skin bear the αβ or γδ TCRs in roughly the same proportions as in blood. The CD4 : CD8 ratio within the skin approximates one, with most CD4 T lymphocytes bearing the CD45R0 (memory) phenotype. Skin T cells also predominantly (90%) express CLA, a marker found on <5% of T cells at other sites.

Cell adhesion in the skin

Adhesion between cells and between cells and the extracellular matrix is critical to the maintenance of an intact skin barrier. This barrier is frequently broken in immune-mediated skin disease and, therefore, of great relevance to immunological skin disease. Recent advances in skin biology have identified the multiple, complex mechanisms and structures used to maintain skin integrity.

The major adhesion organelles between keratinocytes in skin are termed **desmosomes**. Desmosomes are structures that anchor keratin filaments within keratinocytes to the plasma membrane, and also project outside the cell to adhere to each other on adjacent cells (Fig. 17.2). The desmosomes

are comprised of glycoprotein molecules, some of which belong to the **cadherin** family of cell–cell adhesion structures and include desmoglein and desmocollin (often termed **desmosomal cadherins**). Cadherins are calcium-dependent transmembrane cell-adhesion molecules that operate in a process termed 'homophilic adhesion' (i.e. one cadherin on a cell binds to the same molecule on another cell).

In addition, there are structures that are responsible for adherence of basal layer keratinocytes to the BMZ and thence to the dermis. This is known as the **adhesion complex**. It includes a structure termed the **hemidesmosome**. Hemidesmosomes are present just beneath the plasmamembrane of the basal layer keratinocytes and serve to anchor these cells, and hence the epidermis, to the lamina densa of the BMZ. The lamina densa is further anchored into the dermis through **type VII collagen**.

Terminology in skin disease

The classics scholar *cum* physician is ideally placed to become a dermatologist. The descriptive terms used to define skin lesions and the diseases associated with them are best addressed ahead of the immunology (Table 17.1).

Skin diseases and immunology: general considerations

Skin diseases in which there is an immune component to the pathogenesis fall into several categories. There are the allergic

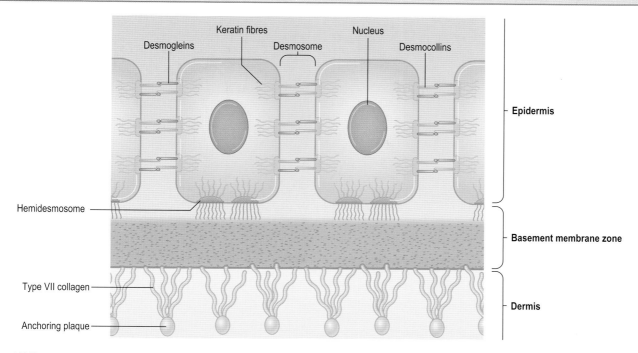

Fig. 17.2 **Cell adhesion in the skin.**

Table 17.1 Terms used in the description and diagnosis of skin disease

Term	Definition
Plaque	Elevated lesion with larger surface area in relation to height
Wheal	Elevation of skin caused by dermal oedema
Angio-oedema	Oedematous reaction in dermis, covering large skin area
Vesicle	Blister (<0.5 cm)
Bulla	Blister (>0.5 cm)
Erythema	Redness caused by vasodilatation

IgE-mediated (type I hypersensitivity) diseases, such as eczema, urticaria and angio-oedema; there is also the eczema generated in contact dermatitis, which is a result of a T cell-mediated process (previously called delayed or type IV hypersensitivity). In addition, skin disease may be a consequence of vessel inflammation (vasculitis). These disorders are discussed in other chapters (see Chs 12 and 16). The other main category of immune-mediated skin disease is termed the **vesiculo-bullous disorders**. In these diseases, fluid-filled vesicles and bullae appear as a result of damage to the mechanisms involved in the maintenance of cell–cell and cell–structure adhesion within the skin.

The main diagnostic tools for the diagnosis of immune-mediated skin disease are analysis by histology and immunofluorescence (p. 172). **Direct immunofluorescence** is carried out on skin biopsies taken from the patient and demonstrates immunoglobulin or complement deposition in his/her skin. Skin biopsies for these investigations should be taken from a perilesional site, since the skin components and architecture within a blister are disrupted. **Indirect immunofluorescence** can be carried out using patient serum and an appropriate skin/epithelial substrate obtained from elsewhere (e.g. monkey oesophageal mucosa) and demonstrates the presence of circulating autoantibodies in the patient against skin components. The pattern of the fluorescence is of considerable diagnostic help (e.g. antibodies against the BMZ), and in the vesiculo-bullous diseases it is generally agreed that the autoantibody itself is a major factor responsible for the tissue damage. In some disorders, antibodies are directed against components of the BMZ, at the dermal–epidermal junction. It can be of diagnostic help to establish whether the antibodies identify targets on the dermal or epidermal side of the BMZ. To investigate this, the skin biopsy can be split at the dermal–epidermal junction by treatment with a concentrated salt solution, and fluorescence studies then carried out to identify whether the site of antibody binding is on the dermal or epidermal side of the BMZ.

Psoriasis and vitiligo are also discussed. These diseases undoubtedly have an immune component, although the pathogenesis of psoriasis remains enigmatic.

Skin diseases

Pemphigus

Pemphigus is a group of disorders characterised by blister formation within the epidermis in association with auto-antibodies directed against constituents on the surface of squamous epithelial cells. There are two major types of pemphigus, divided according to whether the blisters form in the superficial epidermis (**pemphigus foliaceus**) or in the deep epidermis (**pemphigus vulgaris**).

Pemphigus vulgaris

This is the most common form of pemphigus; it principally affects the 40- to 60-year-old age group. Although pemphigus vulgaris (PV) may affect members of all races, it is classically seen in people of Mediterranean origin and especially Ashkenazi Jews. There is a strong association between PV and possession of the HLA genes *DRB1*0402* and *DQB1*0503*.

Pathology
Direct immunofluorescence reveals deposition of IgG, as well as the complement component C3, on the keratinocyte surface at all levels in the epidermis (Fig. 17.3). In indirect immunofluorescence, circulating IgG that binds to the surface of normal stratified squamous epithelium in the skin can be demonstrated in 80% of patients. Skin histology reveals acantholysis (separation of keratinocytes from each other). Typically, there is little in the way of inflammatory infiltrate and the dermis is intact. The antigen recognised by sera from patients with PV is the desmosomal cadherin **desmoglein 3** (Dsg 3). ELISA tests for Dsg 3 autoantibodies are positive.

Clinical features
Blisters typically appear first in the mouth and are also seen on the skin. Blisters are thin, flaccid and form on a base of normal or erythematous skin. Since the blisters form in the epidermis and have a thin ceiling, they are frequently rup-

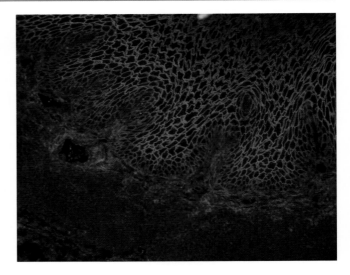

Fig. 17.3 Pemphigus vulgaris.
Indirect immunofluorescence analysis of a section of monkey oesophagus incubated with serum from a patient with pemphigus vulgaris, followed by a fluorescein-conjugated antihuman IgG antiserum raised in rabbits. Positive staining is seen as linear fluorescence around the perimeter of the keratinocytes in the intercellular space, producing a 'chicken wire' effect. The dermal–epidermal junction is not stained; this patient has circulating skin autoantibodies. (Courtesy of Dr Ted Davies, King's College Hospital.)

tured and replaced by large, superficial skin erosions. By the time a patient reaches the dermatologist, true blisters may be few and far between. There is increased skin fragility, such that rubbing apparently unaffected skin leads to removal of the epidermis (Nikolsky's sign). There is little tendency for PV to resolve spontaneously, and without treatment skin function is lost with severe clinical consequences.

Treatment
Largely fatal if untreated, the mainstay therapy consists of high-dose systemic steroids, frequently supplemented with azathioprine and cyclophosphamide. Treatment must be maintained for lengthy periods, and PV remains a potentially fatal disease with up to 25% of patients dying from the disease or the consequences of the therapy.

Pemphigus foliaceus

Pemphigus foliaceus (PF) is classically a rare and sporadic form of pemphigus in temperate climes, but is relatively common on the Indian subcontinent and in South America. It is more benign than PV. It is of interest because there is good evidence that an environmental insult provokes PF autoantibodies (see below).

Pathology
Immunofluorescence studies and histology are identical to those with PV. The antigen recognised by sera from patients with PF has also been identified as the desmosomal cadherin **desmoglein 1** (Dsg 1).

Endemic pemphigus foliaceus

Endemic pemphigus foliaceus (EPF), also known as fogo selvagem (which means literally 'wild fire' in Portuguese), is an autoimmune blistering disorder that is clinically identical to pemphigus foliaceus. Like PF, the autoantibodies generated are of the IgG4 subclass, bind desmoglein 1 and induce disease when transferred into neonatal mice. What makes EPF of great interest is that the epidemiology of this autoimmune disease strongly suggests involvement of bites by haematophagous (blood-sucking) insects. Descriptions of EPF first appeared in Brazil at the turn of the last century. During the 1980s, it became clear that the majority of cases occur within 15 km of several large rivers inland from Rio de Janeiro. This is the maximum flying distance of insects such as mosquitoes and the black flies known as simulium, which have the rivers as their main habitat. In endemic areas, the background level of anti-Dsg 1 autoantibodies in apparently unaffected individuals is >50%. Of the two potential vectors, the link with the black flies appears the strongest. One of the anecdotal pieces of evidence supporting simulium as the vector regards a local farmer moving to an area within the endemic zone of EPF. The people already in this locality complained bitterly of the constant irritation of bites from the black flies and had themselves already made the link between these and EPF. The newly arrived farmer decided to purchase a flock of canaries to try to reduce the number of black flies in the area. Amazingly, both the number of simulium and the incidence of EPF in his locality declined dramatically! What remains to be established in EPF is the nature of the stimulus for generating pathogenic antibodies to Dsg 1. A possible cross-reactive epitope in the insect's secretions, or in an organism carried by the vector, seems the most likely explanation and would shed light on the pathogenesis of other autoimmune skin diseases.

Table 17.2 Evidence that anti-desmoglein autoantibodies cause pemphigus

	Observations
Clinical studies	Antidesmoglein antibodies are detected in almost all patients
	Circulating levels of autoantibodies reflect disease severity, response to therapy and relapse
Animal studies	IgG from patients with PV, or from rabbits immunised with PV antigen, recreates clinical, histological and immunological features of PV after injection into neonatal mice
	IgG passing across the placenta from mothers with PV induces skin pathology (e.g. acantholysis) in the newborn
	Severe combined immunodeficient mice reconstituted with lymphocytes from patients with PV deposit human IgG in the skin and suffer PV-like lesions (see Clinical Box 17.1)
In vitro studies	IgG from PV patients causes loss of cell–cell adhesion in skin organ culture

Clinical features

PF is less severe than PV with oral lesions being rare and the disease controllable with topical steroid therapy. Drug-induced lesions similar to PF have been described, and an endemic form of the disease, termed fogo selvagem, is seen in Brazil (see Clinical Box 17.1). Separation between the keratinocytes takes place high in the epidermis so that the blister roof is relatively weak. As a consequence blisters rupture quickly leaving erosive surfaces.

Pathogenesis of pemphigus

A consensus view is that the autoantibodies generated in PV are pathogenic and cause the blistering. The accumulated body of evidence for this is given in Table 17.2.

The precise mechanism of tissue damage is not clear, however, and neither is there any explanation for the different patterns of superficial and deep blisters in PF and PV. Recruitment of complement is now considered an unlikely mechanism, since the autoantibodies in PV are predominantly of the IgG4 subclass, which fixes complement poorly. In addition, in vitro, the effect of IgG from PV patients in reducing cell–cell adhesion in skin organ culture does not require complement, and neither does the murine passive transfer model using IgG from affected patients. An alternative possibility is that PV autoantibody binding activates plasminogen activator. Plasminogen activator converts plasminogen to the active proteolytic enzyme plasmin, which could in turn digest the cadherins. In animal models of PV (see Science Box 17.1), disruption of cell–cell adhesion can be prevented by antibody that inhibits plasminogen activator.

Of course, for an autoimmune disease mediated by class-switched (IgG), high affinity antibodies it is likely that CD4 T cells are involved, since they would be required to direct the antibody production. Both T_H1 and T_H2 type responses against Dsg 3 have been detected and the consensus is that both are probably involved in the disease.

Immune-deficient mice as models for human autoimmune disease

Immune-deficient mice have become a much studied model of human disease. Mice can be genetically engineered so that they lack key components required for the development of the immune system. They thus become a 'living test tube' — since their own immune system is absent, they do not reject human immune cells that are transferred into them. The human immune cells thus artificially reconstitute the mouse immune system and, for their part, the human immune cells do not appear to generate a graft-versus-host disease. The human lymphocytes infused in appear reasonably healthy and functional, since human IgG is produced and it is even possible to demonstrate 'human' responses to immunisation and virus challenge.

This provides an ideal opportunity for studying the role of autoantibodies in disease. In a recent report, some 50 mice were reconstituted with peripheral blood lymphocytes from patients with pemphigus vulgaris. Approximately two thirds of the mice developed circulating PV antibodies of the IgG class, and half had deposits of IgG in the skin. In some mice, human skin had been grafted on before reconstitution. In almost all of these mice, PV-like blistering lesions containing human IgG developed in the human skin grafts. Immune-deficient mice, therefore, appear to be a powerful model for studying autoimmune diseases in which a circulating autoantibody has a pathogenetic role.

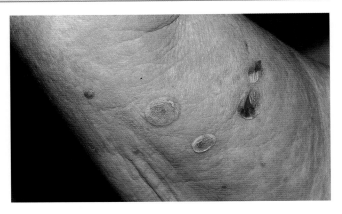

Fig. 17.4 Bullous skin disease.
(From White 2004 Color Atlas of Dermatology, 3rd edn, Mosby, with permission.)

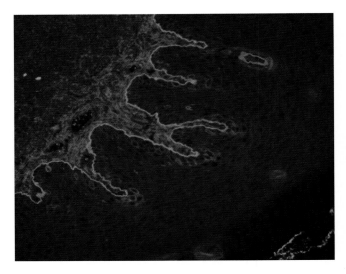

Fig. 17.5 Bullous pemphigoid.
Direct immunofluorescence analysis of a skin biopsy from a patient with bullous pemphigoid. The biopsy has been stained with a fluorescein-labelled antiserum raised in rabbits against human IgG. There is a linear fluorescence pattern along the dermal–epidermal junction, indicating deposition of IgG on the basement membrane. (Courtesy of Dr Ted Davies, King's College Hospital.)

Bullous pemphigoid

Bullous pemphigoid (BP) is a fairly common blistering disorder (6–7 per million of the population per year), especially in the elderly, in which bullae (Fig. 17.4) arise from the sub-epidermis in association with autoantibodies directed against constituents involved in the adhesion complex in the BMZ.

Pathology

Direct immunofluorescence reveals deposition of IgG and C3 in almost all patients, and the pattern is characteristically linear along the epidermal BMZ (Fig. 17.5). Circulating autoantibodies of the IgG class are found in the majority (approximately 80%) of patients on indirect immunofluorescence, but titres of the autoantibody correlate poorly with disease severity. Skin histology reveals blister formation in the BMZ and although there may be little inflammation, in some cases an extensive infiltrate including lymphocytes, macrophages and eosinophils is seen.

It is now established that the BMZ autoantibodies detected by immunofluorescence in BP bind to the non-collagenous 16A (NC16A) domain of type XVII collagen, often referred to as the BP antigen. Type XVII collagen is associated with the hemidesmosome structures in the adhesion complex. The targeting of skin molecules with such a key role in anchoring basal keratinocytes to the BMZ explains why the hallmark of the disease is a blister forming at this junction.

When the patient's biopsy is split along the BMZ using 1 molar sodium chloride, BP autoantibodies bind to the upper (epidermal) surface of the split.

Pathogenesis

The presence of lymphocytes, as well as mast cells, eosinophils and neutrophils around the BMZ in the skin of some patients argues for an immune pathogenesis to the blisters in BP. Initially, it was unclear whether BP autoantibodies cause blistering since their injection into mice generally failed to induce disease. However, it subsequently became clear that this was a result of differences in amino acid sequence in the major BP antibody epitope between mice and men. Once antibodies to the mouse sequence were used, then disease followed. Studies show that the disruption of the BMZ is optimal when complement is activated.

Clinical and immunological features

This is the most common bullous disorder, principally affecting those aged 50–80 years. Unlike PV, HLA associations with BP are weaker, with *DQB1*0301* the major susceptibility gene. Blisters may be generalised or localised on the skin (Fig. 17.4) and are also found on the mucous membrane in approximately one third of cases. The blisters, which are tense and typically occur on a base of erythematous skin, are often preceded by intense pruritus. The thicker capsule to these blisters means that they are usually intact and present on examination. There is a tendency for BP to resolve spontaneously and it is rarely fatal. Therapy is similar to pemphigus but requires less intensity and shorter maintenance.

Occasionally pemphigoid-like lesions are confined to the mucous membrane (**mucous membrane pemphigoid**). This may have serious consequences when the conjunctiva is involved (blindness secondary to scarring) and can also lead to hair loss when the scalp is affected.

Diseases related to pemphigoid

There are a number of conditions related to BP by the fact that they are characterised by blisters involving the subepidermal space. Some of the more interesting diseases are discussed here.

Pemphigoid gestationis (PG)

This is a rare bullous disorder associated with pregnancy (1 case in every 20 000 pregnancies). BMZ staining by immunofluorescence is similar to that for BP and autoantibodies against BP230 and BP180 are present. The disorder is characterised by an intense burning itchiness, with the appearance of blisters, usually in the second or third trimester of pregnancy, and usually resolves after delivery. An association with possession of HLA haplotypes containing *A*01* class I genes and *DRB1*03* and *DRB1*04* class II genes has been described. There are also rare reports of the newborn infant having transient skin blisters caused by placental transfer of maternal antibodies.

Dermatitis herpetiformis (DH)

This is characterised by small tense vesicles on an erythematous base, typically on the extensor surfaces (e.g. elbows and buttocks), and found in association with intense burning and itching. Direct skin immunofluorescence reveals a very characteristic deposition of IgA and complement in the dermal papillae (Fig. 17.6). The most striking clinical feature of DH is its association with an underlying gluten-sensitive enter-

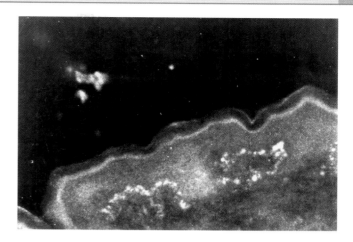

Fig. 17.6 Dermatitis herpetiformis.
Direct immunofluorescence analysis of a skin biopsy from a patient with dermatitis herpetiformis. The biopsy has been stained with a fluorescein-labelled antiserum raised in rabbits against human IgA. There is patchy, granular staining in the dermal papillae, indicating deposition of IgA at these sites. (Courtesy of Dr Ted Davies, King's College Hospital.)

opathy, with the same patchy villous atrophy as that seen in coeliac disease (see Ch. 15), although there may be no gastrointestinal symptoms. In addition, there is a strong association (95–100% of patients) with the HLA genotype *DQA1*0501, DQB1*0201*, the same as that found in coeliac disease, and with anti-tissue transglutaminase autoantibodies. The disease becomes even more intriguing when one considers that the same gluten-free diets used to treat coeliac disease cause the skin IgA deposits in DH to disappear, though they recur if gluten is reintroduced. Dapsone will also control the skin lesions.

Epidermolysis bullosa

This is a heterogeneous group of acquired and genetically determined bullous diseases, the hallmark of which is that the bullae are induced by mild mechanical trauma, reflecting an underlying weakness in skin adhesion. In the genetically determined EBs, disease results from mutations in genes encoding proteins involved in skin adhesion. In contrast, in acquired epidermolysis bullosa (**epidermolysis bullosa acquisita**; **EBA**) there is no family history. What makes EBA of interest is the similarity with BP. In EBA, the blisters are subepidermal, and there is linear IgG and C3 deposition along the BMZ indistinguishable from that in BP. However, split skin analysis shows that EBA sera bind to the dermal side of the BMZ, whilst BP sera bind to the epidermal side. The antigenic target of EBA sera is type VII collagen, an important component in anchoring the epidermis (Fig. 17.7).

Psoriasis

Psoriasis is a common, disfiguring, chronic skin disease, affecting some 2% of Caucasians. The onset is usually at puberty or menopause, and the characteristic skin lesion is a red plaque covered by silvery skin scales (Fig. 17.8). The

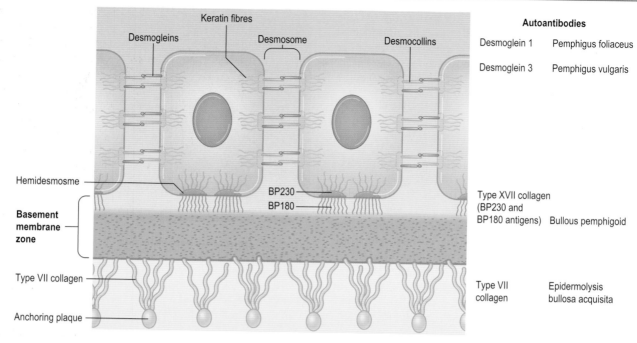

Fig. 17.7 Targets of skin autoantibodies. BP180 and BP230 are components of Type XVII collagen which forms the hemidesmosome. Type XVII collagen is the target of the autoantibodies found in bullous pemphigoid.

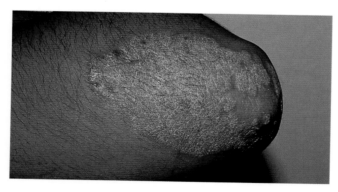

Fig. 17.8 Classic appearance of a silvery psoriatic skin plaque, with erythematous edge.
(From White 2004 Color Atlas of Dermatology, 3rd edn, Mosby, with permission.)

disease has a relapsing remitting course, and the typical sites affected are the elbows, knees, scalp and buttocks. A combination of genetic and environmental factors is at play. The onset or relapse of the disease may be provoked by a variety of stimuli including trauma, infection (particularly with β-haemolytic streptococci), drugs, UV radiation, alcohol, cigarette smoking and possibly stress. There is an association with the HLA alleles *Cw6* and *DR7*, the former giving a relative risk of 5–10 times the background population. Identical twins have a concordance rate for the disease of approximately 65%. Some 10% of patients may also be affected by an arthritis.

Pathogenesis

The underlying disease process giving rise to the skin manifestations of the disease is characterised by:

- an increase in the rate of skin turnover, in association with abnormal epidermal maturation
- dilatation and increased numbers of dermal blood vessels
- skin infiltration, mainly by neutrophils and T lymphocytes.

The epidermis usually turns over every 30–40 days, but the epithelial layer of the skin may turn over every 5 days. There is no single, accepted hypothesis as to the pathogenesis of psoriasis, but several immune abnormalities have been described, suggesting that at the very least the immune system makes a contribution. The pathology of the skin disease shows that early lesions are associated with peri-vessel dermal infiltrates of lymphocytes and macrophages. Neutrophils may appear within the epidermis to create microabscesses and can occasionally be seen leaving the vessels in the dermal peri-vascular unit. Epidermal hyperplasia is a characteristic feature and with the excessive keratinisation this gives rise to the micro- and macroscopic features of the skin. Even in uninvolved skin, cell cycling of keratinocytes may be abnormal. Any unifying hypothesis regarding the pathogenesis of psoriasis must combine the characteristic infiltrate, containing lymphocytes in the early lesions followed by neutrophils, with the apparent dysregulation of the keratinocyte life cycle.

Neutrophils in psoriasis

Neutrophils are a relatively late feature of psoriatic skin lesions. There is evidence that neutrophils are activated within the blood and skin of psoriatic patients, and mediators found within diseased skin (C5a, leukotriene B4, IL-8) are likely to be responsible for this. Interestingly, application of chemotactic factors to uninvolved skin in psoriatic patients induces microabscesses but not the typical skin lesions, suggesting that they contribute to persistence of the disease but are not primary factors.

Lymphocytes in psoriasis

As we have seen, in normal skin the great majority of T cells reside in the dermis, and most of these are in the dermal peri-vascular units. The CD4 : CD8 ratio amongst these cells is one, and over 80% of the resident cells are activated. In psoriasis, certain changes to these populations of T lymphocytes occur. A T lymphocyte infiltration is seen that is predominantly CD4$^+$, and the CD4 : CD8 ratio in psoriatic skin exceeds that in the patient's blood. This implies a selective accumulation, and most CD4 T cells present express CLA, as well as having a memory phenotype (CD45R0) and being polarised towards T$_H$1. Perhaps the strongest evidence that these activated CD4 T cells are involved in the pathogenesis of psoriasis comes from the powerful effect of drugs that block T cell activation or migration (e.g. ciclosporin A, or biologics such as anti-TNF-α, anti-LFA-1 and CTLA4-Ig (see Ch. 22). Psoriasis is also one of the inflammatory diseases in which the T$_H$17 pathway (see p. 102) is thought to play a role. Evidence for this comes from links between disease susceptibility and genes involved in the IL-23 pathway (IL-23 is involved in T$_H$17 development), as well as recent highly encouraging clinical trials in which an anti-IL-23 monoclonal antibody, Ustekinumab, has been used.

Antigen specificity

If these findings are accepted as strong evidence that activated CD4$^+$ memory T lymphocytes initiate/perpetuate the disease, two questions arise. What are the antigens against which the T cells are sensitised and how does their response result in profound changes in keratinocyte function? Little is known of the antigen specificity of skin T cells in psoriasis, but blood T cells from psoriatic patients proliferate to β-haemolytic streptococcal antigens, one of the better defined disease triggers, and there may be cross-reactivity between antigens from these bacteria and human skin components. Once activated, CD4 T cells could release a variety of cytokines that have been shown to act on keratinocytes to induce stimulation in vitro (IL-2, IL-3, GM-CSF) (Fig. 17.9).

One must also account for the role of HLA class I genes in this disease (see Science Box 17.2).

Vitiligo

Complete loss of skin pigment (depigmentation) in a patchy distribution is a common disorder, of which the best known cause is **vitiligo**. It is an acquired disorder, and the depigmentation results from destruction of melanocytes in the skin, which produce the pigment melanin. Affected patches appear totally white, whatever the racial origin, and hair affected typically grows white. Vitiligo is common, with an estimated incidence of up to 1%. Both sexes may be affected and, in a third of cases, there is a family history. The consensus view on the aetiology of vitiligo is that it is an auto-immune disease in which the immune system damages melanocytes irreparably. The evidence for this derives from:

- an association between vitiligo and the presence of other autoimmune disorders, notably thyroiditis, type 1

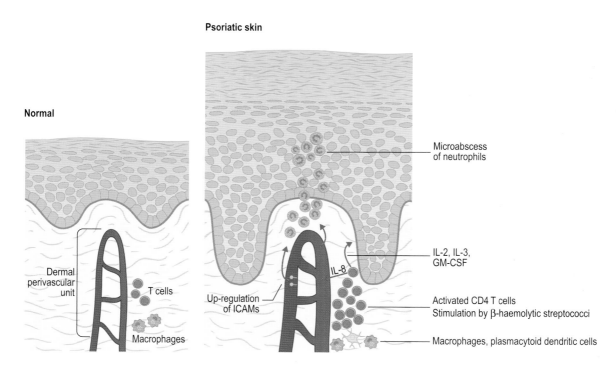

Fig. 17.9 **Possible immune mechanisms in the pathogenesis of psoriasis.**

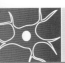

SCIENCE BOX 17.2

Psoriasis gene — the final word?

A final question relates to the complex genetics of this disease. There are at least 8 genetic loci in which polymorphisms are associated with psoriasis (*PSORS1–8*). *PSORS1* accounts for 30–50% of disease susceptibility and has therefore been the major focus of research in this area for many years. After it was localised to the MHC region, *PSORS1* was thought to be *HLA-Cw6*. However, doubts crept in when it became apparent that there were other genes in this region that could be involved in skin disease (e.g. the gene for corneodesmosin, a keratinocyte adhesion protein) and were in tight linkage disequilibrium with *Cw6*. It required a heroic sequencing effort, published in 2006, to have what appears to be the final word — it is *Cw6* after all. The only question remaining is how *HLA-Cw6* could be involved in psoriasis? Clearly, one obvious possibility is that HLA-Cw6 presents a critical disease-related peptide. This is supported by the fact that guttate psoriasis (small lesions all over the body) is strongly associated with *HLA-Cw6* and appears to be triggered by streptococcal throat infection. There is some evidence that skin-homing, CD8 T cells of *HLA-Cw6*-positive psoriatics respond more strongly to peptides found in a skin protein, keratin 17, and streptococcus than do CD8 T cells of *HLA-Cw6*-negative psoriatics. HLA class I molecules such as the C group are also responsible for interactions between self and natural killer cell receptors, and it is possible that regulation of activation of these cells is abnormal. It seems probable that confirmation of the nature of the major psoriasis susceptibility gene is just the beginning of our understanding of its pathogenic role.

recently, T_H1-type and CD8 T cell responses against the melanocyte antigen MART-1 have been detected in patients with progressive vitiligo. This is interesting since it resonates with some innovative studies in the use of immune-based therapies for the treatment of the skin cancer melanoma. In these studies, melanoma patient DCs were removed, activated and pulsed with antigens from their tumour to try and generate cytotoxic CD8 T cell responses against the melanoma. In some patients this was successful and there was evidence of tumour regression. However, patients also developed vitiligo, suggesting that the anti-melanoma T cells (which targeted MART-1, amongst other antigens) were also destroying healthy melanocytes in the skin.

SUMMARY BOX 17.2

Skin diseases

- In the blistering disorders, a variety of autoantibodies directed against components involved in cell adhesion appear to have pathogenic roles.
- The main blistering diseases are pemphiguS (remember the S for superficial lesions) and pemphigoiD (remember D for dermo-epidermal junction).
- In the main blistering disorders, an association with HLA genotypes is seen.
- Dermatitis herpetiformis is associated with pathology of the gastrointestinal tract (coeliac disease).
- In psoriasis, T lymphocyte recruitment and activation in the skin appears to be a key component in the dysregulation of keratinocyte function, which is central to the disease.
- In vitiligo anti-melanocyte autoantibodies indicate an autoimmune attack on melanocytes resulting in a loss of pigment. Tyrosinase, an enzyme involved in the synthesis and export of melanin, has been implicated as a target antigen.

diabetes, pernicious anaemia and adrenal insufficiency; vitiligo is commonly found in patients with autoimmune polyglandular syndromes

- autoantibodies to pigmented human melanocytes are detectable in the circulation of a high proportion of patients (see below)
- CD4 T cells bearing activation markers are seen in skin biopsies taken at the margins of new lesions
- the condition can be alleviated by topical use of glucocorticosteroids.

Vitiligo has a mixed prognosis. In some it may be very patchy and even resolve spontaneously. In others it is progressive; the social and psychological consequences, particularly in racially dark-skinned patients, can be devastating.

Autoantibodies against proteins in melanocytes have been detected, and molecular targets identified to date include tyrosinase and tyrosinase-related proteins. More

Further reading

Hertl M, Eming R, Veldman C 2006 T cell control in autoimmune bullous skin disorders. J Clin Invest 116(5): 1159–1166

Li N, Liu Z, Hilario-Vargas J, Diaz LA 2006 Bullous skin diseases: pemphigus pemphigoid. In: Rose NR, Mackay IR (eds) The autoimmune diseases, 2nd edn. Elsevier: London

Lowes MA, Bowcock AM, Krueger JG 2007 Pathogenesis and therapy of psoriasis. Nature 445(7130): 866–873

Worm M, Sterry W 2006 Non-bullous skin diseases: alopecia, psoriasis, vitiligo and urticaria. In: Rose NR, Mackay IR (eds) The autoimmune diseases, 2nd edn. Elsevier: London

Yancey KB 2005 The pathophysiology of autoimmune blistering diseases. J Clin Invest 115(4): 825–828

Immune-mediated diseases of the nervous system and eye

The key cells within the central nervous system (CNS) are the **neurons**, which initiate and conduct afferent and efferent electrical impulses for sensory and motor nerve functions. To enhance the speed of transmission, nerve fibres (axons) are insulated by a sphingolipid sheath, termed **myelin**, which is generated by **oligodendrocytes**. Loss of these sheaths in a pathological process termed **demyelination** leads to marked slowing of signal transmission and is one of the inflammatory/autoimmune processes to be discussed in this chapter. Other disorders of the nervous system arise when nerve conduction across the neuromuscular junction is disrupted. Finally, there are inflammatory and autoimmune conditions that affect visual processes.

Immune responses in the central nervous system

Primary immune responses may occur within the substance of the CNS (e.g. viral encephalitis) and the brain and periph-eral nervous system (PNS) may also become secondarily affected by systemic inflammatory processes (e.g. neurological complications of SLE). As far as the initiation of primary CNS immune responses are concerned, it is now clear that in normal brain white matter small numbers of lymphocytes are resident. In addition, a group of specialised cells, the **microglia**, display constitutive expression of class II MHC molecules and are the professional APCs of the CNS (Fig. 18.1). Microglia are capable of secretion of IL-1, IL-3, IL-6 and TNF-α in vitro. In inflammatory CNS diseases, MHC class I and II molecule expression may be present on a range of cell types, indicating that antigen presentation may occur more widely under the influence of cytokines. The **astrocyte** may be of particular importance in CNS inflammation; this is a cell with phagocytic properties and on which MHC expression is inducible. Astrocytes are support cells for the neurons, and in diseases in which there is neuronal death, astrocytes proliferate to form areas of scarring, in a process termed gliosis. In vitro, astrocytes are capable of secreting IL-1, IL-6 and TNF-α.

The **blood–brain barrier** is an ill-defined obstacle, originally invoked to account for differences in penetration of proteins, salts and drugs into the CNS. It applies equally to immunological proteins, such as immunoglobulin, and may also be an effective barrier to cell-mediated responses. Therefore, the extent to which primary brain immune responses recruit immune effector cells from the periphery, and the extent to which inflammatory processes in the periphery affect primary brain immune responses, are controversial. In no disease process is this controversy more hotly debated than in **multiple sclerosis**.

Multiple sclerosis

Multiple sclerosis (MS) is a disease of unknown aetiology, characterised by numerous, circumscribed areas of demyelination within the brain and spinal cord. It is the major form of the **demyelinating diseases**, a group of disorders in which loss of myelin occurs without axonal degeneration. The combination of intact axons and some capacity for myelin regeneration gives rise in approximately two thirds of patients to a repeated relapsing and remitting disease

Basic and clinical immunology

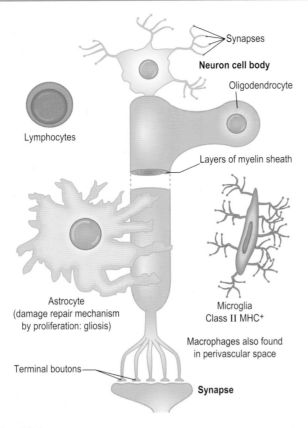

Fig. 18.1 Immunological cells and main components of the healthy CNS.
The axons are sheathed in myelin, generated by oligodendrocytes, to aid nerve conduction. Microglia are class II MHC-positive cells from the macrophage/monocyte lineage that act as the APCs for the CNS. Astrocytes are the support cells in the CNS and have phagocytic properties.

course, but with a general accumulation of disability over several years. In the remaining one third, the disease is slowly progressive. Considerable evidence has been amassed to suggest that MS is an autoimmune disease, arising on a distinct genetic background and influenced strongly by environmental factors.

The first evidence that MS is an immune-mediated disease derived from the finding that the cerebrospinal fluid (CSF) has abnormally high levels of immunoglobulin, which are demonstrated as 'oligoclonal bands' and appear to result from B cell activation. The concept that MS is an autoimmune disease is based on limited evidence, and derives from three principle facts. First, it has a strong association with HLA class II genetic polymorphisms, as do other autoimmune diseases (see Chs 5 & 9). Second, there is an animal model (extrinsic allergic encephalomyelitis, or EAE), which is induced by immunisation of animals with brain tissue or proteins and gives rise to a clinical and pathological appearance that is similar to human MS; EAE is most definitely autoimmune (see Science Box 18.1). Third, no microbe has been consistently isolated from MS patients, and, in its absence, an autoimmune explanation for the disease is invoked.

Epidemiology

MS is a common disorder, with a prevalence in the general population in Northern and Western Europe, the USA and Australia approaching 1 in 1000. The age of onset is usually between 10 and 60 years, with the median age between 25 and 30 years. It is more common amongst women, with estimates of the female:male ratio ranging between 2:1 and 7:1. Between 3 and 7 people develop the disease per

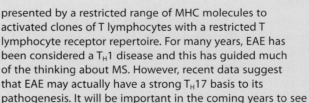

SCIENCE BOX 18.1

The experimental allergic encephalomyelitis model of MS

Experimental allergic encephalomyelitis (EAE) is induced by intravenous injection of constituents of brain, either from the same or another species. The inducing antigens may be crude brain homogenate, myelin sheath, myelin basic protein (MBP), myelin proteolipid protein (PLP) or shorter peptides from these myelin proteins. Within 2–3 weeks, the animals become lethargic, paralysed and lose sphincter control. In some immunising regimens in some strains, the disease has a relapsing remitting course, making it a particularly appropriate model for MS. However, in others, spontaneous recovery is the rule. The CNS pathological lesion in the animals is almost identical to that in MS. T lymphocytes, which proliferate when cultured with MBP or PLP, arise in the peripheral blood during the development of EAE and are capable of transferring the disease to unaffected animals. The disease is inducible in certain strains of mice, rats and guinea-pigs, with one of the determining factors in susceptibility being the MHC type. Therefore, EAE has the features of an autoimmune disease with well-defined autoantigens

presented by a restricted range of MHC molecules to activated clones of T lymphocytes with a restricted T lymphocyte receptor repertoire. For many years, EAE has been considered a T_H1 disease and this has guided much of the thinking about MS. However, recent data suggest that EAE may actually have a strong T_H17 basis to its pathogenesis. It will be important in the coming years to see whether T_H17 cells reactive with brain autoantigens are present in MS patients.

Many different manipulations of the animals can lead to permanent recovery from the demyelination (e.g. peptide and whole antigen immunotherapy, oral tolerance induction). The question of great importance is whether the immunological features of this model, induced by injection of autoantigen in the periphery, fit with those of the spontaneous human disease. Hence the search in MS for T lymphocyte reactivity, restriction of antigenic epitopes, T lymphocyte receptor usage and HLA restriction continues.

100 000 of the UK population per year. The epidemiology of MS is fascinating. The incidence is unevenly distributed within the same country and appears to be related to latitude, with higher numbers affected in populations nearer the poles. Therefore, in the southern states of the North American continent the prevalence of MS is 0.1 per 1000, rising to 1.3 per 1000 in northern Canada. Some have argued that these differences could relate to ethnic and, therefore, genetic differences between populations. Careful studies in Australia, however, where northern and southern populations have a similar ethnic composition, show the same relationship between disease incidence and latitude, though in this case MS is more common in the southern areas. In the UK, the prevalence is at its highest in Scotland, where cases number up to 3 per 1000. The relationship between latitude and risk of MS argues for an environmental agent, possibly a virus prevalent in temperate regions, acting as an important trigger for the disease. Moreover, the fact that the disease incidence peaks during the third decade argues for the main disease triggers operating during adolescence. Again, careful epidemiological studies have strengthened this concept. It appears, for example, that individuals migrating from a birthplace of relative high risk to one of low risk of MS, and vice versa, carry their level of disease susceptibility with them as long as they travel after the age of 15 years. In contrast, migration before the age of 15 incurs the level of susceptibility of the new environment.

What could the environmental factors be? Most would argue for a transmissible virus as one of the major triggers for the disease, although no single agent stands out. Common virus infections (e.g. measles, mumps, rubella) tend to affect MS patients at later ages than is typical; MS prevalence is greater in higher socioeconomic groups, who may be less likely to encounter common viruses until secondary school or university; and MS may occur in mini-epidemics in sheltered island populations (see Clinical Box 18.1). Infectious agents could also be important in disease exacerbations. Clinical observations indicate that relapses frequently follow upper respiratory tract infections, but that is likely to relate to the effects of systemic inflammation on ongoing immune processes.

Genetic factors are also important in susceptibility to MS. Caucasians are much more vulnerable than African blacks, American Indians (Mongolians) and some groups of mongoloid Asians, in whom the disease is extremely rare. Twin and HLA studies in MS have identified similar trends to those in type 1 diabetes (see p. 190), in that concordance for the disease is approximately 2.5% between dizygotic and 26% between monozygotic twins, who carry a relative risk for the disease 300–400 times that of the background population. Interestingly, though, some 70% of un-affected monozygotic twins of MS patients will have CNS lesions typical of MS detectable by magnetic resonance imaging (see below), implying that subclinical demyelination could occur on a wider scale. Some 50–70% of patients with MS have the HLA-DR15 allele (*B1*1501*; present in 20–30% of the normal population). This argues strongly

CLINICAL BOX 18.1

Lessons from an epidemiological study of the Faroe Islands

There have been several reports of epidemic outbreaks or large clusters of cases of MS, but none more convincing and intriguing than that in the Faroe Islands, a volcanic group in the north Atlantic Ocean and part of the state of Denmark. Between 1900 and the outbreak of the Second World War in 1939, there had been only two reported cases of MS amongst the 45,000 or so islanders. Both individuals affected had spent 3 or more years on mainland Denmark, where there is a high incidence of MS, some years prior to the onset of symptoms. However, between 1940 and 1979, 25 cases of MS were reported in islanders who were native born and had never lived anywhere else, and a further nine cases in islanders who had lived abroad for less than 2 years. What could have happened on the island during the war years to cause such a dramatic increase in incidence, which has now declined?

The answer appears to lie in the British Forces' occupation of the Faroe islands, which began on 13 April 1940 and ended 5 years later. At its peak, the British garrison had some 4000 soldiers in it, billeted on some 21 sites scattered throughout the islands. Of the 32 cases of MS occurring amongst the islanders over the next 40 years, only three occurred on sites where there were no troops, and only four occupation sites did not have a single case of MS on them.

This might argue for direct transmission of an agent from patient to patient. However, many studies have shown that the incidence of MS amongst spouses of affected patients is the same as in the background population, and the British Forces are unlikely to have contained large numbers of troops with significant neurological disease (i.e. potential carriers). What the Faroe Islanders' experience suggests is that the British Forces brought with them a transmissible agent not indigenous to the population but which is an important trigger in the train of events that leads to MS.

that the binding of an antigenic or autoantigenic peptide to this HLA-DR molecule is critical to the development of the disease.

Pathology

The typical pathological lesion of MS is a perivenous inflammatory infiltrate in the peri-ventricular white matter, composed of CD4 and CD8 T lymphocytes, B lymphocytes, plasma cells and macrophages. Most frequently affected regions of the CNS are the cerebrum, brain stem, spinal cord and optic nerve. Predominant in the infiltrate is the T lymphocyte, with CD4 T lymphocytes in the majority in early lesions and CD8 T lymphocytes in the later stages. Myelin and oligodendrocytes are destroyed and, depending on the age of the lesion, there may be variable evidence

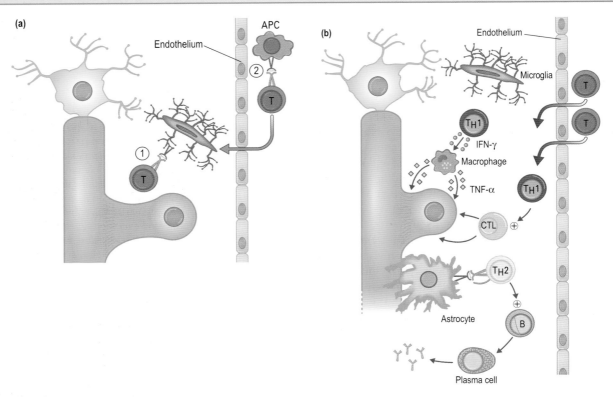

Fig. 18.2 Demyelination in MS.

(**a**) Mechanism of induction of demyelination. An antigen is presented to T lymphocytes. The peptide is possibly derived from a primary CNS autoantigen or from an infecting agent, and could have epitopes cross-reactive with myelin components. The activation of these autoreactive T lymphocytes may take place within the CNS (1), or is an external event (2) followed by migration through the brain endothelium. (**b**) Mechanisms of perpetuation of demyelinating plaques. Autoantigen-sensitised CD4 T_H1 cells arriving from the peripheral blood stimulate CD8 cytotoxic T lymphocytes or macrophages, resulting in damage to oligodendrocytes and myelin by direct cytotoxicity or through cytokines such as TNF-α. A range of myelin-derived peptides are presented by microglia and macrophages. Astrocytes, with their phagocytic properties and the capacity to express class II MHC molecules, may also become involved in antigen processing and presentation. Clones of B lymphocytes within the CNS may become activated as bystanders, producing the oligoclonal immunglobulin bands seen in the CSF.

of remyelination. There is localised oedema, and old lesions show evidence of gliosis. Demyelination appears to be closely related to the presence of macrophages, and at the sites of these lesions macrophages are actively endocytosing myelin, often through interaction between surface Fc receptors and IgG attached to the sphingolipid. MHC class I molecule expression is present on most cells, and class II molecules are expressed on microglia, B cells, macrophages and astrocytes in the lesions and on the surrounding endothelium. Interferon-γ is present in the CSF in MS patients and may be of importance in enhancing class II MHC expression. The ensuing inflammatory process appears to result in local breakdown of the blood–brain protein barrier, since complement proteins and immunoglobulins are found extensively in active lesions.

The picture is painted of a cell-mediated immune process, probably orchestrated by CD4 T lymphocytes (Fig. 18.2). The target is the oligodendrocyte or its important product myelin. Macrophages may be the final effectors of damage or may just be clearing the debris. The process could be initiated

from within the CNS, but evidence of the breakdown of the blood–brain barrier also suggests that exacerbations could be secondary to peripheral immune events.

Pathogenesis and immunological features

There is evidence in MS patients that small numbers of CD4 T lymphocytes in the peripheral blood and in the CSF react with myelin-derived autoantigens, mainly myelin basic protein (MBP), proteolipid protein (PLP) and myelin-oligodendrocyte glycoprotein (MOG). These results have been obtained through proliferation assays and T lymphocyte cloning studies, and the prevailing notion is that the cells are T_H1 in phenotype, although data on T_H17 subsets is awaited (see Science Box 18.1). Support for the concept that myelin-reactive T cells in the blood are important in the disease comes from the successful use of blockade of their migration into the CNS using a monoclonal antibody against the $\alpha4\beta7$ integrin VLA-4 (although unfortunate complications of the drug have prevented its adoption as a useful therapy). There are two main T lymphocyte epitopes in the centre of the MBP molecule, between amino acids 84 and 102, and 143 and 168. HLA-DR15 (B1*1501) molecules appear to be capable of presenting both of these and other MBP peptides. Using transgenic technology, it has now been possible to construct a mouse that expresses human HLA-DR15 and has T cells dominated by the TCR from a human T cell clone recognising the MBP84–102 epitope and under certain conditions develops severe demyelinating disease. Thus there is strong evidence overall that myelin-reactive T cells in the peripheral blood of patients can be pathogenic in this disease.

A major unanswered question is how these T cells become activated at the initiation of the disease. The epidemiology and genetics argues for a virus; the immunology and animal data indicate sensitisation against myelin components as being a critical feature. Bringing these together is evidence to support the possibility that a virus, acting through the mechanism of molecular mimicry, could induce an auto-immune response in the CNS. Several close homologies exist between short viral peptide sequences (e.g. measles, rubella and varicella) and myelin, and some myelin-reactive T cells can recognise mimicking microbial epitopes. Viruses have not been demonstrable in the CSF or in MS lesions, and injection of homogenates of affected brain into primates does not induce disease. However, the virus could be operating in the periphery and could also be long departed before the MS is revealed clinically. There is an intriguing parallel with the infection of mice with Theiler's virus, which leads to an autoimmune demyelinating disease with pathology not dissimilar to MS.

Clinical features

The initial clinical picture in patients presenting with MS is variable. Pyramidal tract features such as weakness and hyper-reflexia are common, and ataxia caused by cerebellar involvement may also be seen. When the brain stem is affected, there may be cranial nerve involvement. Blurred vision is also a frequent presenting symptom, indicating optic neuritis. Optic neuritis may also occur as a single entity, without evidence of dissemination of the demyelination, but it is estimated that 50–80% of such patients will ultimately develop MS. A relapsing remitting (RRMS) course is typical in 80% of patients after onset. Around half of these patients develop secondary progressive MS in which the relapses become more frequent and remissions less frequent. Around 10–15% of patients follow a more malignant primary progressive course from diagnosis.

The diagnosis of MS, at one time made on essentially clinical grounds, can now be supported by several investigations:

1. Measurement of IgG levels in CSF.
2. CSF electrophoresis for oligoclonal bands.
3. Visual evoked potentials.
4. Magnetic resonance imaging.

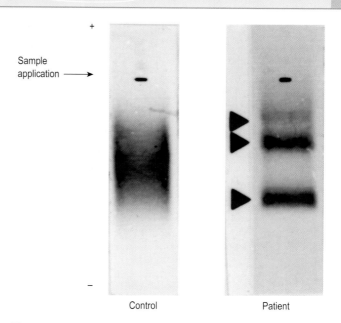

Fig. 18.3 Electrophoresis of cerebrospinal fluid from a healthy control and a patient with multiple sclerosis. In the control, immunoglobulins are diffusely stained, indicating polyclonality. In the patient, at least three discrete oligoclonal bands can be seen, indicating synthesis of immunoglobulins within the CNS by a small number of B cell clones (courtesy of Dr J. P. Frankel).

Examination of the CSF reveals an increased number of cells, predominantly lymphocytes, though this is not diagnostic. IgG levels in the CSF are modestly raised in MS. This could be the result of plasma cell secretion within the CNS, or in the periphery. To differentiate these two, the CSF IgG : albumin ratio can be compared with that in serum, since albumin is not synthesised in the CNS. A rise in the IgG : albumin ratio in CSF is a reasonably specific but not very sensitive test for MS. In contrast, CSF electrophoresis reveals **oligoclonal bands** in some 80–90% of MS patients (Fig. 18.3). Oligoclonal bands are not diagnostic of MS, since they may be seen transiently in other CNS inflammatory conditions (e.g. post-infectious encephalomyelitis), but persistence of the bands is a typical feature of this relapsing/remitting demyelinating disease. Despite intensive research, it is still not clear against what the IgG in the bands is directed. Anti-myelin antibodies form a small proportion (5%) and some 75% of MS patients have raised CSF titres of anti-measles antibody. The slowing of transmission of **visual evoked potentials** demonstrates the impairment of nerve function typically associated with demyelination. A relatively new but well-established examination for MS is the **magnetic resonance image** (MRI), which demonstrates plaques of demyelination, usually in several sites (Fig. 18.4).

Treatment

MS can be a devastating disease, and there has been no shortage of attempts to use immune modulating therapies as treatments and as 'proof-of-principle' for the autoimmune

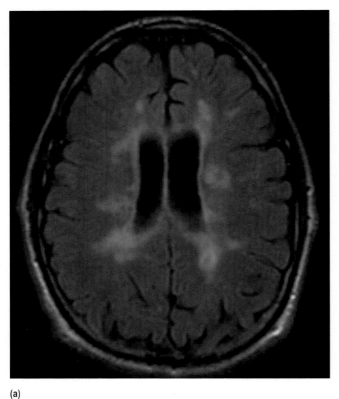

(a)

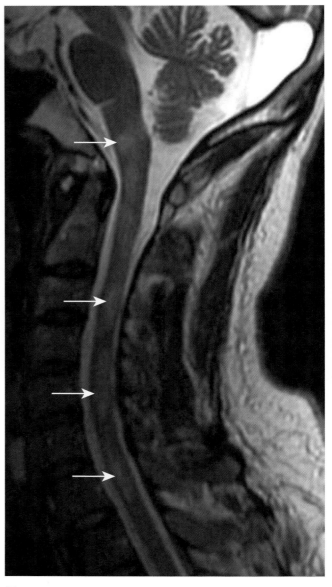

Fig. 18.4 Magnetic resonance images of the brain and spinal cord of a patient with MS, showing the typical peri-ventricular brain plaques of demyelination (a) and similar lesions in the cord (b).
The plaques appear as white regions (arrowed) (Courtesy of Dr E. J. Evanson).

(b)

theory. Apart from the anti-VLA-4 mentioned above, anti-T cell agents such as azathioprine, ciclosporin and depleting anti-CD4 monoclonal antibody therapy have not worked. In current clinical practice there is no specific therapy for MS and no entirely satisfactory non-specific therapy. The relapsing and remitting nature of the symptoms and signs has meant that clinical trials are difficult to perform and interpret. MS is a disease in which the requirements for randomisation, placebo and blindness of both patients and physicians to the treatment could not be greater. Corticosteroids may reduce the severity of acute exacerbations and speed their resolution, without having any effect on the course of the disease. In recent years, therapy with interferon β1b and β1a (synthetic analogues of IFN-β) has shown considerable

promise in clinical trials (having been tried in the first place to combat virus infections thought to be responsible for disease exacerbations). A reduction in the frequency of exacerbations of some 30% is achieved in some studies, and the treatment is well tolerated. However, there does not appear to be any effect on the presence of brain lesions detected by MRI, and the proscriptive cost (over $10 000 per patient per year) has led to some controversy over the use of β-interferons, with the UK National Institute for Health and Clinical Excellence (NICE) calling for careful clinical trials to establish the true value of this and other experimental therapies; the results of these are eagerly awaited. Another therapy for which NICE awaits definitive data is glatiramer acetate (GA, also called Copaxone®; see Clinical Box 18.2).

Demyelinating syndromes

- Multiple sclerosis is a demyelinating disease that results from a subtle interplay of genetic, e.g. HLA-DR15 (B1*1501), and environmental factors, e.g. a virus.

- The pathological lesion is one of plaques of CNS demyelination, infiltrated by T lymphocytes and with evidence of macrophages actively phagocytosing the myelin sheath.

- The presence of activated autoreactive T lymphocytes in the peripheral blood and CNS that recognise components of myelin suggests that these cells initiate and/or perpetuate the CNS lesions.

- Novel immune therapies are being devised based upon this knowledge and successful deployment in animal models.

The Guillain–Barré syndrome

The Guillain–Barré syndrome (GBS) is an acute, predominantly motor inflammatory peripheral polyneuropathy named after the two French Army neurologists who linked clinical and CSF findings in the early part of the twentieth century. It is preceded by a viral-like illness or gastrointestinal infection in some 60–80% of patients and has an acute onset, beginning with paraesthesiae affecting the toes and finger tips, and evolving into a global, symmetrical, motor neuropathy with weakness of the legs and subsequently of the muscles of the arms, face and pharynx. Frequently there is also some deep muscle pain, but, in general, sensory nerve loss is rare. The severity varies from mild weakness to quadriplegia and the need for supported mechanical ventilation for several months. The cause is unknown, but the consensus view is that there is immune system involvement in the destruction of myelin and nerve axons.

Criteria for diagnosis are:

- **Required**: progressive motor weakness of more than one limb and areflexia

- **Strongly supportive**: rapid progression of weakness that has ceased by 4 weeks; symmetrical development; mild sensory, cranial nerve and autonomic involvement; recovery starts 2–4 weeks after progression ends.

GBS has an annual incidence of 1–2/100 000 of the population. Although it may affect any age, there are two peaks of incidence, at 16–25 years and 45–60 years of age, and a slight male preponderance. No convincing genetic associations have been identified, and the disease has an essentially sporadic nature.

Approximately 25% of patients remain ambulant throughout the illness, 50% are chair- or bed-bound and 25% require cardiorespiratory support through mechanical ventilation, which carries a significant risk of morbidity and mortality.

Novel therapies for MS

There is no shortage of suggested approaches on the experimental front, as numerous successful therapies emerge from studies in the EAE model. These include antigen-specific and peptide immunotherapy. Such studies require careful planning, however. In 2000, two separate trials using peptides of MBP were terminated due to a combination of possible disease exacerbation and the development of hypersensitivity to the peptide. The peptides being used were altered from the native MBP sequence in an attempt to deviate the immune system towards T_H2. Since some of the patients developed allergic reactions to the peptides this may have been an approach that was too effective, leading to unwanted inflammatory responses.

Glatiramer acetate is a random sequence polypeptide consisting of four amino acids (alanine, lysine, glutamate and tyrosine) at a final molar ratio of 4.5 : 3.6 : 1.5 : 1. It has been designed to bind to multiple MHC class II molecules and, indeed, achieves this. There are many studies on its effects in MS, with some evidence for a T_H2-biasing effect, to counter the pathogenic T_H1 cells. It has now reached the stage of large phase III studies, and is claimed to reduce the rate of appearance of disease exacerbations.

Other therapies undergoing evaluation for MS include co-stimulation blockade and anti-CD20 to deplete B cells, which was recently reported to significantly reduce relapse rates (see p. 308).

One third of patients are left with significant disability and the mortality rate is around 3–8%. The diagnosis of GBS is essentially clinical. Protein levels in the CSF are raised, characteristically without the presence of cells; rarely there may be oligoclonal bands that are transient. In a typical case, the full syndrome takes some 4 weeks to develop, followed by a plateau of symptoms and neurological deficit lasting up to 1 month, and then recovery, which takes a median of some 9 months.

Pathology

A mononuclear cell infiltration, comprising lymphocytes and macrophages, is well established within days of the onset of symptoms. Such lesions are extremely unusual in the CNS, and signs of CNS involvement are rare. There is patchy myelin destruction and in some cases axonal destruction.

Pathogenesis and immunological features

Evidence of immune mechanisms in the pathogenesis of GBS are:

- mononuclear cell infiltration of affected peripheral nerves

- antibodies to myelin components

- peripheral T lymphocyte activation and reactivity to myelin components

SCIENCE BOX 18.2

Animal models of Guillain–Barré syndrome

There are two main animal models of GBS, which offer quite different perspectives on the disease. In one, rats and mice immunised with the P2 myelin protein develop a flaccid quadriplegia, from which there is recovery after 1–2 weeks. The animal disease can be transferred into virgin syngeneic recipients by T lymphocytes; the critical epitope on the P2 molecule capable of inducing the neuropathy is between amino acids 53 and 78. There has been some controversy as to how the P2-activated T lymphocytes mediate nerve damage and which cells in the peripheral nervous system present antigen, with some groups suggesting that the Schwann cell is important in APC function. This has been elegantly resolved in a series of experiments using the 'P2' animal model established in Lewis rats. T lymphocytes from this strain are unable to transfer the disease to another rat strain, DA, because of class II MHC incompatibility. However, if the recipient DA rats are irradiated to disable bone marrow

function and then reconstituted with bone marrow from the F_1 generation animals of a Lewis × DA cross, the disease is transferable using Lewis-derived T lymphocytes. This implies that bone marrow-derived APCs bearing Lewis rat class II MHC molecules emanate from the transplanted bone marrow to present antigen to the pathogenic T lymphocytes, and it confirms that cells of the monocyte/macrophage lineage are necessary for the induction of the nerve damage.

The second main animal model of GBS is induced in rabbits by injection of galactocerebroside, with resulting quadriplegia. Serum from the affected rabbits is able to transfer the disease into rats.

These animal models have directed research into the pathogenesis of GBS towards these two antigens, in much the same way that MBP- and PLP-induced EAE has in MS. It would appear, however, that immune reactivity to P2 and galactocerebroside is more difficult to pinpoint in GBS.

- two animal models in which T lymphocytes and antibody, respectively, may transfer disease
- the clinical efficacy of plasma exchange and intravenous immunoglobulin.

The major pathogenic element to the disease is damage to the myelin sheath around peripheral nerves, which is generated by Schwann cells. Myelin, or the Schwann cells themselves, could be the targets of the immune attack and there are several known target antigens. Two of these, the **P2 protein** component of myelin and **galactocerebroside** are implicated because of a clear role in animal models of inflammatory polyneuropathy (see Science Box 18.2). Evidence of T lymphocyte reactivity to these has now been gained. Other potential autoantigens include gangliosides, which are important components of lipid membranes particularly in the nervous system. Antibodies to the **gangliosides GM1** and **GM2** have been found and there is some evidence for cross-reactivity with putative pathogenic agents such as *Campylobacter jejuni* and cytomegalovirus.

This fits with some of the agents and events that appear to be capable of triggering GBS:

- viral-like illness in 60–70%
- immunisation in 5%
- pregnancy
- surgical procedure
- lymphoma.

The main viruses involved are cytomegalovirus and Epstein–Barr virus. One well-documented outbreak of GBS in 1976 following immunisation with an influenza vaccine has suggested that sporadic cases could follow immunisation, a recent history of which is found in 5% of patients. In pregnancy, GBS may occur in the third trimester, and the fact that the unborn foetus is not affected suggests that antibody-

mediated myelin damage is not a feature of this form. Up to 40% of GBS patients have evidence of recent infection with the intestinal pathogen *C. jejuni*.

Antibodies may well be involved in the pathological process, since there are elevated levels of intact membrane attack complexes (C5b6789) of the terminal complement pathway, peaking on the 4th day after admission to hospital and declining thereafter, to become undetectable by 1 month. A mechanism of antibody- and complement-mediated nerve damage (Fig. 18.5) would also explain why intravenous immunoglobulin is effective in the disease since it is known to 'mop up' complement components and reduce their availability to pathogenic antibodies.

Therapy for GBS

Both plasmapheresis (exchange of plasma from the patient for 'normal' plasma) and intravenous immunoglobulin (IVIG) (see p. 321) are accepted therapies and if applied within 2 weeks of the onset of symptoms shorten recovery time.

SUMMARY BOX 18.2

Guillain–Barré syndrome and other immune-mediated neuropathies

- Guillain–Barré syndrome is often preceded by a viral-like illness; the cause is unknown but myelin and nerve axons are destroyed.
- GBS may require cardiorespiratory support and carries a significant mortality risk.
- Other neuropathies may have immune components involved in nerve damage and different target antigens have been proposed.

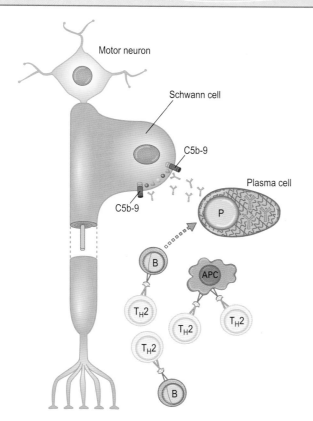

Fig. 18.5 **A putative mechanism of immune pathogenesis in Guillain–Barré syndrome.**
T_H2 lymphocytes are activated in response to antigens (possibly microbe-derived and cross-reactive with self antigens) presented by APCs within the peripheral nerve. The B lymphocytes activated as a result recognise myelin components (e.g. gangliosides, sulphatide) and recruit complement, with resulting nerve damage.

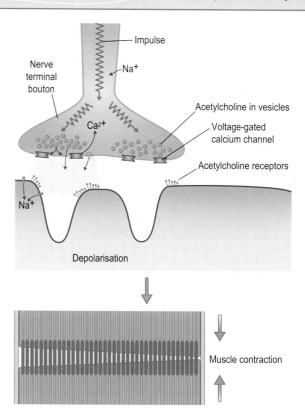

Fig. 18.6 **The ultrastructure of the neuromuscular junction.**
The depolarising action potential arriving in the nerve terminal causes voltage-gated calcium channels to open, with movement of acetylcholine-containing vesicles to the pre-synaptic membrane and release of the neurotransmitter into the synaptic cleft. Binding of acetylcholine to its receptor on the crests of the post-synaptic clefts causes opening of Na^+ channels and depolarisation of the muscle fibre, with subsequent contraction.

Myasthenic syndromes

Myasthenia is defined as a fatiguable weakness of striated muscle. It is the result of a defect of transmission of impulses from nerve to muscle at the neuromuscular junction (NMJ). The normal anatomy and physiology of the NMJ is shown in Figure 18.6. There are two clearly defined autoimmune disorders in which synaptic transmission at the NMJ is interfered with by an antibody-dependent mechanism. In **myasthenia gravis** (MG), an autoantibody is generated against the **acetylcholine receptor** (**AChR**), on the post-synaptic membrane. In the Lambert–Eaton **myasthenic syndrome** (**LEMS**), an autoantibody interferes with the pre-synaptic process of acetylcholine release by binding to **voltage-gated calcium channels** (**VGCC**). Of great interest in the pathogenesis of these disorders are the roles of the thymus and of neoplasia: MG is often associated with thymic hyperplasia and occasionally thymic neoplasia, whilst LEMS typically occurs in association with a small cell carcinoma of the lung.

Myasthenia gravis

The characteristic symptom of MG is muscle weakness arising with repeated usage. Any striated muscle may be affected, but those served by the cranial nerves, and especially the eye muscles, are affected in over 50% of patients. Patients often present after stressful events — infection or anaesthesia — with weakness that worsens as the day progresses, or after repeated usage of particular muscles. The characteristic laboratory finding is of a circulating antibody to the AChR, detectable in nearly 85–90% of patients. The prevalence of MG appears consistent throughout the world, at around 5–10 cases per 100 000 of the population.

Although there is an overall sexual bias in favour of women by 2 to 1 and the disease may occur at any age, distinctive clinical subgroups emerge when large numbers of patients with autoantibody-positive MG are pooled for analysis. In 'classical' MG, which accounts for 55% of patients and occurs between adolescence and the 20s, females predominate. In Caucasians, this group also has an excess of the HLA haplotype containing the *HLA-B*0801* class I allele and *HLA-DRB1*0301* class II allele; histological evidence of thymic hyperplasia is typically found in this group. Intriguingly, the hyperplastic thymus often contains cells (termed 'myoid'), which express AChR subunits (but not the whole receptor). In another subgroup (20% of patients), MG onset occurs equally in males and females over the age of 40 years. In these patients, there is an association with the class I molecule *HLA-B*07* and class II allele *HLA-DRB1*15*. In these cases the thymus is atrophic on histological analysis. Yet a third group of patients (10%) have a tumour of the thymus (thymoma); the sexes are equally affected and there is no genetic linkage.

In some 10–15% of patients with MG, autoantibodies to the AChR are not detectable. Of these patients, some 40% have autoantibodies against muscle specific kinase (MuSK) and have greater evidence of bulbar involvement (e.g. problems talking and eating).

There is a strong association of MG with other autoimmune disorders, notably type 1 diabetes, autoimmune thyroiditis and rheumatoid arthritis.

Pathology

Typically, there is a small collection of mononuclear inflammatory cells (lymphocytes, macrophages) near the NMJ, with occasional evidence of degeneration of the muscle fibres. Staining for IgG and complement components (C3, C5b6789 complexes) at the NMJ is positive. Electron microscopy reveals a widening of the post-synaptic cleft. The thymus is usually examined for enlargement radiologically since thymic hyperplasia is present in 60% of MG patients and is often associated with the existence of lymphoid germinal centres within the thymus, within which B cells and plasma cells make anti-AChR autoantibody. Thymectomy in 25% of such patients improves symptoms.

Pathogenesis and immunological features

MG is typified by the presence of anti-AChR antibodies and reduced numbers of AChRs at the motor end-plates. These two phenomena are most probably causally related (see Clinical Box 18.3). The AchR has four subunits forming a complex ($\alpha 2\beta\varepsilon\delta$). The α chain, which contains the binding site for ACh and the snake neurotoxin α-bungarotoxin (a venom that causes paralysis), is the target of the autoantibodies in MG. There are three mechanisms by which the presence of circulating anti-AChR antibodies results in loss of receptor (Fig. 18.7):

1. Complement-mediated damage to the end-plate with AChR loss (the main mechanism).

2. Decreased synthesis and increased degradation of AChRs.

3. Antagonist action by receptor blockade (rare).

The presence of IgG and complement C5b6789 (membrane attack complex) deposition at affected NMJs, with heaviest deposition at the NMJs with the least remaining AChRs, strongly supports the hypothesis of complement-mediated

Myasthenia gravis in a bone marrow-transplant recipient: a rare complication

Some convincing evidence for the hypothesis that MG arises from an immune response involving autoreactive B lymphocytes comes from a case report in 1983. A young girl with aplastic anaemia received bone marrow from her HLA-identical brother (*A3 B40 DR4/A2 B7 DR2*). Apart from the development of graft-versus-host disease, the transplant was a success. Some 2 years later, however, she developed ptosis and diplopia. The clinical diagnosis of MG was supported by a Tensilon test and the presence of anti-AChR antibodies. The existence of repeated serum samples dating from before the transplant allowed the clinicians in charge to establish that the anti-AChR antibodies had first appeared within 3 months of her receiving the bone marrow. Serum samples from the girl's brother and parents were negative for the autoantibodies. The first important question to answer was whether the clones of B lymphocytes producing the anti-AChR antibody were from the girl or her brother. Molecular techniques were not as advanced in the early 1980s as they are now, but the investigators were able to establish that all of the peripheral blood lymphocytes and bone marrow cells in her circulation carried a Y chromosome, which must have derived from her brother. The second question was why had the brother not developed the disease? It is conceivable that the presence of the autoreactive B cell clones alone is not sufficient to generate MG. MG in this age group is more common in females, as are several autoimmune diseases, and it may be that the manifestation of MG in members of this family required the presence of the 'female milieu'. Alternatively, it is possible that the autoreactive B lymphocytes in the brother were held in check by immunoregulatory T lymphocytes. These could have been inadequately represented in the bone marrow transplanted to his sister or were particularly sensitive to the methotrexate and steroids given to treat the graft-versus-host disease.

damage. Second, injection of MG sera into mice increases the daily turnover rate of AChRs by approximately threefold, with catabolism outstripping synthesis. Finally, serum from some patients is capable of blocking depolarisation of cultured muscle cell lines in vitro.

It is most likely that autoantibodies to the AChR are involved in the pathogenesis of myasthenia gravis:

- most patients (85–90%) have anti-AChR antibodies, which are undetectable in healthy controls

- one in eight babies born to mothers with MG have a transient myasthenic syndrome (neonatal MG), which lasts 2 to 3 weeks

- injection of MG sera into mice causes a myasthenic syndrome

- IgG and complement are seen at the NMJ in MG.

The explanation for the production of anti-AChR antibody by patients with MG remains elusive. No convincing cross-

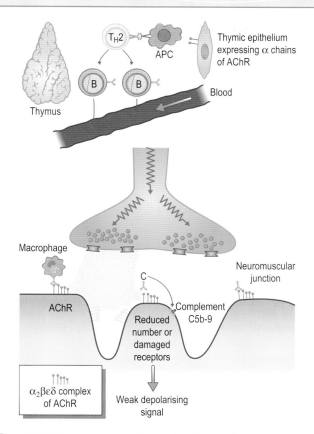

Fig. 18.7 Pathogenesis of myasthenia gravis.
Acetylcholine receptors (AChR) are damaged, reduced in number or blockaded by circulating anti-AChR antibodies. T_H2 lymphocytes are sensitised, possibly in the thymus, to the α subunit of the AChR. B lymphocytes become activated, leading to the generation of high-affinity, complement-fixing IgG autoantibodies to the AChR. These block binding of ACh, or damage the receptors and the motor end-plate by complement-mediated lysis or recruitment of Fc-receptor-bearing macrophages.

reactions between the receptor and microorganisms have been proposed to support a theory of molecular mimicry at the B cell level, and interest has concentrated more recently on the role of T helper cells in giving rise to these high affinity IgG autoantibodies. An intriguing association in this respect is the link between thymoma, thymic hyperplasia and MG. The presence of AChR subunits in the thymus suggests that intrathymic T cells become sensitised to the AChR α subunit due to its ectopic over-expression, possibly as part of an anti-tumour response. The histological appearance of hyperplastic thymus, found in the majority of patients with 'classical' MG, is of a gland largely taken over with germinal centres and surrounding T cell areas. When these glands are removed, dispersed and the cell suspensions cultured in vitro, there is spontaneous synthesis of anti-AChR antibodies, suggesting that this is the main site of antibody production in vivo. Studies in which clones of T cells have been generated from peripheral blood and the thymus of patients with MG have revealed that T_H2-like responses are directed against the α subunit of the AChR.

Clinical features

The diagnosis of MG is made on clinical grounds, along with autoantibody testing, single fibre electromyography and the Tensilon test. A suggestive history is supported by an examination, which may reveal fatiguability and weakness, particularly of muscles supplied by the cranial nerves (e.g. difficulty in holding a vertical gaze). Tendon reflexes are present. Anti-AChR autoantibodies, found in 85–90% of patients, are detected using a sensitive immunoassay in which purified human AChRs are labelled with radioactivity using ^{125}I-labelled α-bungarotoxin, which complexes with the AChR. In the Tensilon test, 5–10 mg edrophonium, a cholinesterase inhibitor, is given intravenously. It has the effect of making more ACh available at the NMJ and this can overcome the lack of functional AChRs, reversing the myasthenic symptoms temporarily for several minutes. Anti-AChR autoantibodies are an important diagnostic test.

Treatment

The treatment of MG is mainly based around the use of pyridostigmine, a long-acting cholinesterase inhibitor. Evidence of a thymoma should be sought with regular follow-up, and since local tumour spread may be life threatening, thymectomy is recommended even though improvement in the myasthenic symptoms is unusual. Thymectomy is beneficial if performed early in other cases, and in 35% of young patients with hyperplastic thymuses containing many germinal centres, it may induce a long period of remission, with a further 50% achieving a measurable but more limited benefit. Drugs such as corticosteroids, azathioprine, mycophenolate mofetil and ciclosporin A are all able to reduce anti-AChR levels with apparent benefit, and may be added as required. Plasmapheresis and intravenous gammaglobulin may also be used to remove or suppress autoantibodies to the AChR during acute MG exacerbations, prior to surgery or to achieve more rapid disease control.

SUMMARY BOX 18.3

Myasthenia gravis

- The presence of high-affinity, IgG autoantibodies to the acetylcholine receptor leads to myasthenia gravis, a syndrome of fatiguable weakness associated with loss of these receptors at the neuromuscular junction.

- The disease is multifactorial and has different subtypes; the most common form of the disease has many features typical of other autoimmune diseases (young, female predominance, HLA association).

- There is an intriguing link with events in the thymus: some patients have thymic neoplasia, others thymic hyperplasia; a protein homologous to the acetylcholine receptor, present in the gland, may be the focus of the initial immune response.

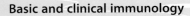
Lambert–Eaton syndrome and other antibody-mediated neuromuscular junction disorders

The Lambert–Eaton myasthenic syndrome (LEMS) is typified by proximal muscle weakness, increased muscle strength during isometric contraction (post-tetanic potentiation), loss of tendon reflexes and autonomic dysfunction. The onset is usually acute, and in roughly half the patients there is an associated malignancy. In about 50% of patients, the tumour is a small cell carcinoma of the lung (SCLC), with myasthenic symptoms preceding the detection of the cancer by up to 5 years. The LEMS is approximately 10 times less frequent than MG, although it may go undiagnosed in some patients with SCLC, and probably affects 3% of patients with this type of neoplasm.

The diagnosis of LEMS is made on electrophysiological tests, which include post-exercise recruitment, repetitive nerve stimulation and single fibre electromyography. Antibodies to the voltage-gated calcium channels (VGCC) are detected using a radioimmunoassay similar in principle to that used in the diagnosis of MG; here, VGCCs are solubilised and radioactively labelled using a different (snail) toxin, ^{125}I-labelled-ω-conotoxin. Anti-VGCC antibodies are present in approximately 65% of patients.

Pathology

The abnormality at the NMJ is best revealed by electron microscopy, which shows a reduction in the so-called 'active zones' on the presynaptic membrane that contain the VGCCs.

Pathogenesis and immunological features

The electrophysiological abnormalities seen in electromyography reflect a reduction in the pre-synaptic release of acetylcholine quanta. That this could be associated with autoantibodies was first suggested by the successful use of plasmapheresis, which gave clinical and electrophysiological improvement. Classical passive transfer experiments of a patient's IgG into mice then reproduced the syndrome, as well as the electrophysiological abnormalities. The reduction in VGCCs does not appear to be complement dependent, since the same changes were seen in mice genetically deficient in complement component C5 and, therefore, unable to construct the membrane attack complex, C5b6789. It appears that divalent antibody (as opposed to Fab fragments) is essential to recreate the lesion of LEMS in passive transfer models, indicating that the abnormality is not caused by blockade but may arise from cross-linking of VGCCs, with subsequent internalisation.

The remaining question is what initiates the production of anti-VGCC antibodies, most notably in patients with SCLC. There is evidence that VGCC-like molecules are present within the tumour. LEMS improves markedly when SCLC are removed surgically. These findings suggest that, like MG associated with a thymoma, LEMS associated with SCLC may arise as a result of an immune response to antigens expressed within the tumour.

Clinical features

Symptoms of fatiguability are similar to those in MG, but patients may get autonomic symptoms, with dry mouth, impotence and sphincter dysfunction.

Treatment with 3,4-diaminopyridine improves acetylcholine release and improves symptoms, as does any appropriate anti-tumour therapy. In LEMS not associated with cancer, prednisolone and azathioprine may give neurological improvement.

Additional, related syndromes have been described recently. In one syndrome of **acquired myotonia**, with muscle hyperactivity, there are autoantibodies against **voltage-gated potassium channels** (**VGKC**). The antibodies probably lead to reduced VGKC function leading to prolonged nerve action potentials. Another rare syndrome is **neuromyelitis optica**, which has features in common with MS and in which there are autoantibodies to a water channel, **aquaporin-4**.

SUMMARY BOX 18.4

Lambert–Eaton syndrome

- The Lambert–Eaton myasthenic syndrome is associated with antibodies to presynaptic structures, the voltage-gated calcium channels, which have a critical role in the release of the neurotransmitter acetylcholine.

- Some 50% of patients with this disorder have a tumour, small cell carcinoma of the lung, which has neuroendocrine origins.

- Calcium channels homologous to those seen on the pre-synaptic membrane may be expressed within the small cell carcinoma and could represent the autoantigenic targets involved in the initiation of this autoimmune disorder.

Stiff man syndrome

Stiff man syndrome (SMS) is characterised by symptoms of tightness and stiffness, with slowly progressive axial and abdominal wall rigidity. It is linked to the autoimmune disease type 1 diabetes (see p. 189), since both have in common autoantibodies to glutamic acid decarboxylase (GADA).

Pathology

Post-mortem studies in patients with SMS are rare and have not produced any clear pattern of pathological abnormalities.

Pathogenesis and immunological features

The most striking immunological feature is the presence of GADA in a high proportion (>60%) of SMS patients. Other autoantibodies (antithyroid microsomal, thyroglobulin, gastric parietal cell antibodies) are frequently found, making SMS one of the rarer components of polyendocrine disorders. GADA in SMS patients differ from those found in patients with type 1 diabetes since the titres (i.e. concentration) tend to be much higher in SMS patients. The causal relationship between GADA and SMS remains to be established, although therapeutic manoeuvres that impede autoantibodies (e.g. plasmapheresis) have been reported to be successful.

Clinical features

As a polyendocrine disorder, SMS is frequently associated with type 1 diabetes (60%) as well as thyroid autoimmune disease, pernicious anaemia and vitiligo. Initial treatment is usually with diazepam or baclofen, but steroids, with or without plasmapheresis, have been used successfully, as has intravenous immunoglobulin in anecdotal reports. Stronger immunosuppression (e.g. mycophenolate mofetil, rituximab; see Ch. 22) may also be required.

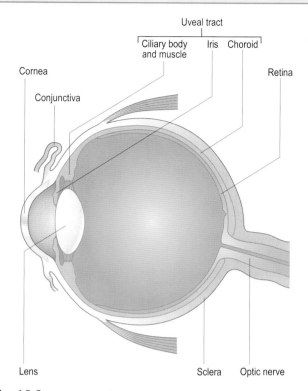

Fig. 18.8 **Anatomy of the eye.**

Immune-mediated eye disease

The eye is prone to involvement in immune-mediated disease, either secondarily as a result of systemic illness or as a primary event. Some special features of the eye are of importance in considering its involvement in disease. Microorganisms, allergens and other forms of antigens may enter the eye through the mucous membranes of the conjunctiva, or through the blood. Some structures (the conjunctiva, retina and uveal tract) are well vascularised, whilst others are normally avascular (cornea and sclera) and may only become vascular during inflammatory responses, with important consequences for visual acuity. Immune protection in the eye includes secreted proteins in tears, such as lysozyme and IgA, as well as the physical properties of the fluid itself. Diseases of the eye will be considered here according to the different anatomical locations affected (Fig. 18.8). Immune responses affecting the eye secondarily will be mentioned briefly, with full accounts of the underlying pathological processes (e.g. connective tissue disease) in the relevant chapters.

Skin and mucous membranes

Like other mucosal and skin surfaces, the eye may be affected by IgE-mediated allergic reactions (Ch. 10). Contact sensitivity (type IV hypersensitivity; p. 148) can arise in response to topical ocular medications and cleaning and preservation fluids used for contact lenses. Cicatricial pemphigoid, the term used to describe involvement of mucosal membranes in bullous pemphigoid (p. 244), can affect the conjunctiva as well as the oral cavity and is a difficult ophthalmic problem to treat. There may be extensive scarring of the conjunctiva and the formation of adhesions between its two surfaces, leading to distortion of the eye lids and lashes. In addition, the cornea may become secondarily vascularised, and blockage of lacrimal ducts leads to a dry-eye syndrome.

Cornea

Inflammation of the cornea, the avascular structure forming the anterior wall of the anterior chamber, is termed **keratitis**. Infective keratitis caused by herpes simplex infection may become recurrent, in a process that is believed to involve the generation of cellular immune responses to normal corneal components. **Keratoconjunctivitis sicca** is an inflammatory process involving the cornea and conjunctiva associated with lack of lacrimal secretions. The lacrimal glands are infiltrated with lymphocytes and plasma cells and become atrophic. The condition of dry eyes gives symptoms of grittiness, pain and dryness worsening as the day goes on and may be diagnosed formally using the **Schirmer test**, in which a thin strip of filter paper (0.5 × 3.5 cm) is inserted under the eyelid for 5 minutes. A positive test is one in which less than 10 mm of the paper has been moistened by tears. The triad of keratoconjunctivitis sicca plus a similar condition affecting the salivary glands resulting in a dry mouth and a connective tissue disease such as rheumatoid arthritis is **Sjögren's syndrome** (p. 185).

Sclera and episclera

The sclera is the tough, fibrous outer coat of the eye that has a white appearance and abuts the bony socket. It is nourished from a highly vascular coating, the episclera. **Episcleritis** results in pain, redness, photophobia and tenderness and is usually a benign, self-limiting condition of unknown aetiology. **Scleritis** is less common and is most frequently secondary to a chronic inflammatory process elsewhere in the body. Symptoms are similar to those of episcleritis, but usually more severe. A number of conditions give rise to this potentially blinding condition:

- Connective tissue diseases
  - ankylosing spondylitis
  - rheumatoid arthritis
  - Wegener's granulomatosis
  - polyarteritis nodosa
  - systemic lupus erythematosus.
- Type IV hypersensitivity states
  - tuberculosis
  - sarcoidosis
  - leprosy.

The underlying pathogenic processes leading to scleritis are likely to be the same as those of the primary condition (e.g. circulating immune complexes, vasculitis). In rheumatoid arthritis, the sclera may become thinned and ultimately perforate, a complication termed **scleromalacia perforans**.

Uveal tract and retina

Uveitis refers to inflammation of the uveal tract, a structure that includes the iris (coloured, circular membrane in front of the lens), ciliary body (ciliary processes and muscle suspending the lens) and choroid (vascular structure between the retina and sclera). Uveitis is generally divided into anterior (iritis and iridocyclitis) and posterior (choroiditis and choroidoretinitis). Uveitis is a relatively common condition, and in half the patients it arises either as a result of infection or secondary to a chronic, systemic illness, frequently a connective tissue disease. There is an unknown aetiology for 50% of cases, but there is considerable evidence to suggest that this 'idiopathic' form of uveitis is an autoimmune disease. Causes of immune-mediated uveitis include:

- Chronic inflammatory diseases
  - ankylosing spondylitis
  - autoimmune hepatitis
  - inflammatory bowel disease
  - juvenile rheumatoid arthritis
  - multiple sclerosis.
- Type IV hypersensitivity states
  - tuberculosis
  - sarcoidosis.
- Primary autoimmune (idiopathic) disease.

Uveitis usually presents with pain, photophobia and blurring of vision. There are several serious sequelae of the inflammatory process associated with this disorder, ranging from glaucoma precipitated by the formation of adhesions between the iris and lens, through cataract formation, to blindness caused by retinal detachment.

Idiopathic (autoimmune) uveitis typically affects the posterior segment of the uveal tract. On histological examination, there may be granulomatous lesions, containing macrophages, epithelioid cells and CD4 and CD8 T lymphocytes. Like other autoimmune diseases, this finding suggests a chronicity to the disease at presentation and makes it difficult to decipher the events and (auto)antigens that have incited the inflammation. Some of the best evidence for an autoimmune basis for uveitis, therefore, has come from an animal model, experimental autoimmune uveitis (EAU). Similar to EAE, the model of multiple sclerosis, EAU follows 9–10 days after systemic injection of animals with retinal photoreceptor-related antigens, the best known being retinal S-antigen. In the early phase, CD4 T cells accumulate around blood vessels in the retina and choroid, while macrophages infiltrate the same site. An abundance of local macrophages probably leads to efficient endocytosis and presentation of autoantigens within the posterior uveal tract. This phase is followed by a CD8 T cell-dominated infiltration. As in EAE, there is evidence of restricted T cell receptor Vβ chain usage, predominantly to Vβ8 and Vβ2. In addition, feeding animals retinal S-antigen orally provides protection from subsequent systemic injection of the same autoantigen.

Current conventional therapy for acute autoimmune uveitis involves the use of immunosuppressants such as corticosteroids and, more recently, ciclosporin A. Doses of these two drugs for chronic treatment may be reduced if azathioprine is added. Topical mydriatics are important to prevent adhesion of the iris.

Sympathetic ophthalmia

This is a potentially devastating condition following some weeks or months after an injury or perforation of one eye. A granulomatous, CD4 T cell-mediated inflammatory process is established in the uninjured eye (hence 'sympathetic'), leading to pan-uveitis, with the potential for loss of vision in both eyes. The condition is believed to result from the release of photoreceptor antigens (such as retinal S-antigen) and subsequent activation of sensitised CD4 T cells. CD4 T cells expressing the IL-2 receptor are seen in the infiltrate in the early phases of the disease. This implies that the state of tolerance to photoreceptor autoantigens is normally maintained by their being 'hidden' from the immune system, or present in only very small quantities. Release of large amounts

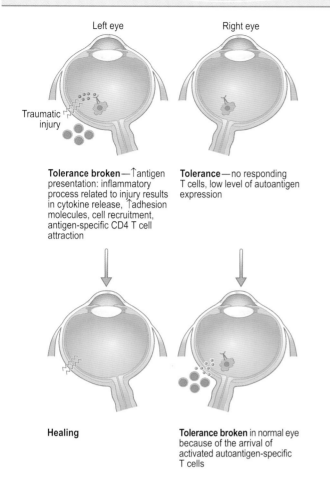

Left eye   Right eye

Traumatic injury

Tolerance broken—↑antigen presentation: inflammatory process related to injury results in cytokine release, ↑adhesion molecules, cell recruitment, antigen-specific CD4 T cell attraction

Tolerance—no responding T cells, low level of autoantigen expression

Healing

Tolerance broken in normal eye because of the arrival of activated autoantigen-specific T cells

Fig. 18.9 Possible sequence of events leading to sympathetic ophthalmia.
T cell tolerance to retinal photoreceptor proteins is maintained by lack of presentation of the autoantigens. Once released through trauma, autoantigen presentation leads to recruitment and activation of CD4$^+$ T cells. The mechanism by which the non-traumatised eye becomes sympathetically involved is not clear. Possibly low levels of retinal photoreceptor autoantigens are normally presented and tolerance is broken by the presence in the circulation of sensitised, activated T cells.

of the autoantigens, associated with a small, trauma-induced local inflammatory infiltration, cytokine release and up-regulation of endothelial adhesion molecules, is sufficient to lead to autoantigen-specific T cell activation (Fig. 18.9). Interestingly, the arrival of these T cells in the non-traumatised eye, where autoantigens are present at 'normal' levels, is then in turn sufficient to break local tolerance and lead to

ocular damage. Treatment is prophylactic in the first instance: sympathetic ophthalmia is very rare if the traumatised eye is removed within 10 days of injury. Once established, sympathetic ophthalmia should be treated vigorously with corticosteroids and/or ciclosporin A. Removal of the traumatised eye now is unwise: it may eventually prove to be the better of two damaged eyes.

A similar condition, termed **lens-induced uveitis**, may follow lens surgery. Leakage of 'hidden' lens proteins (remember the lens is avascular and, therefore, has no immune surveillance) leads to the establishment of an immune response, usually involving the formation of autoantibodies. Typically, it is the eye with the damaged lens that is affected, and sympathetic inflammation is rare.

SUMMARY BOX 18.5

Immune-mediated eye disease

- The skin and mucosa of the eye are frequently affected by hypersensitivity or autoimmune diseases such as perennial allergy and pemphigoid.

- Other disorders affect the eye secondarily to a systemic autoimmune disease, particularly the connective tissue diseases and vasculitic diseases.

- Uveitis may arise spontaneously as an autoimmune disease, or in response to trauma and release of 'hidden' autoantigens.

Further reading

Hafler DA, Slavik JM, Anderson DE, O'Connor KC, De Jager P, Baecher-Allan C 2005 Multiple sclerosis. Immunol Rev 204: 208–231

Vincent A, Lang B, Kleopa KA 2006 Autoimmune channelopathies and related neurological disorders. Neuron 52: 123–138

Vincent A, Rothwell P 2004 Myasthenia gravis. Autoimmunity 37: 317–319

Immunodeficiency

This chapter focuses on immune deficiency — what happens when the immune system fails, how this comes about and what therapies are effective. The consequences of a failure in the immune system, or immunodeficiency, should now be apparent: most obvious is an increased risk of infection, but cancer, autoimmune disease and hypersensitivity are also seen. These are the clinical features of immunodeficiency, which will be discussed first. Next, the role of the diagnostic immunology laboratory in distinguishing the underlying cause of, for example, an increased frequency of infection, will be highlighted, before individual defects in immune function are discussed in detail.

Immunodeficiency may arise either as a primary event, through congenital or genetic abnormality, or secondary to another condition or therapy. Secondary immunodeficiency is by far the more common, particularly now that steroids, cytotoxic agents for cancer treatment and immunosuppression for organ and bone marrow transplantation and autoimmune disease are so widely used. One should not forget either that the acquired immunodeficiency syndrome (AIDS) epidemic is an immunodeficiency state secondary to a virus infection (see Ch. 20). In stark contrast to these common conditions, a primary immunodeficiency, such as congenital absence of the thymus (the DiGeorge syndrome), may only be encountered every 100 000 births, so that an average hospital might only see a case every 25 years! Although rare, these conditions are natural 'gene knock-outs' and can be enormously instructive about the physiological roles of different components of the human immune system. This is an expanding area of clinical activity and research, with more than 100 primary immunodeficiency syndromes now described. And, since the technology exists to correct gene defects, some of these conditions are discussed here to introduce gene therapy as an exciting new therapeutic modality.

Classification and clinical features

The easiest way to classify the immune deficiency disorders is on the basis of which part of the immune system is primarily affected. It should be noted, though, that some defects may affect more than one cell type, or more than one arm of the immune response, so strict compartmentalisation is often difficult. Table 19.1 gives a working classification, and identifies some of the main diseases. These diseases will be used as the prototypes for discussing specific lesions in immune function (Fig. 19.1).

Immunodeficiencies may arise at any age, but the infections associated with them have several typical features:

● they are often chronic, severe or recurrent

● they may resolve only partially with antibiotic therapy

● the organisms involved may be unusual ('opportunistic' or 'atypical').

Opportunistic organisms are often involved. These are pathogens of low virulence that are easily held in check by an intact immune system but that take their moment to invade when the host's guard is lowered.

Patterns of infection may be typical of certain immune deficiencies (Table 19.2). B lymphocyte and antibody defects, for example, result in infections with pyogenic ('pus-forming') organisms. T lymphocyte deficiency is associated with infection with fungi, protozoa and intracellular microorganisms, such as viruses and mycobacteria, whilst deep skin infections, abscesses and osteomyelitis are seen in patients with phagocyte defects. Other features relate more specifically to particular syndromes. Congenital or genetic deficiencies of antibody production are typically not revealed for several months after birth, for example, since the half-life of IgG is 28 days and maternal antibody remains at protective levels for only 5–6 months.

A family history, possibly of unexplained infant death, may be helpful in indicating a heritable disorder that has affected other siblings, whilst the sex of affected children gives a clue to the mode of inheritance. Consanguinity is a predisposing factor to any disorder with an autosomal recessive inheritance pattern. Finally, autoimmunity is inextricably linked to immunodeficiency, and autoimmune disease is occasionally the mode of presentation.

Graft-versus-host disease (GVHD; p. 156) is a frequent complication of both primary and secondary T cell immunodeficiency. For GVHD to arise, the prerequisites are impaired T cell function in the recipient and the transfer of immunocompetent T lymphocytes from an HLA non-identical donor. In patients with T cell immunodeficiency, GVHD usually arises from therapeutic interventions such as

Table 19.1 Classification of immunodeficiencies and the main diseases in each category

Immune component	Examples of diseases
T lymphocyte deficiency	DiGeorge syndrome Acquired immunodeficiency syndrome (see Ch. 20) T cell activation defects (e.g. CD3γ chain mutation) X-linked hyper-IgM syndrome (XHIM)
B lymphocyte deficiency	X-linked agammaglobulinaemia (XLA) Common variable immunodeficiency (CVID) Selective IgA deficiency (IgAD) IgG subclass deficiency
Combined T and B cell defects	Severe combined immunodeficiency (SCID) (e.g. due to defects in common γ chain receptor for IL-2, 4, 7, 9, 15)
T cell–APC interactions	IFN-γ receptor deficiency IL-12 and IL-12 receptor deficiency
Neutrophil defects	Chronic granulomatous disease (CGD) Leukocyte adhesion deficiency (LAD)
Deficiency of complement components	Classical pathway Alternative pathway Common pathway Regulatory proteins Mannan binding lectin

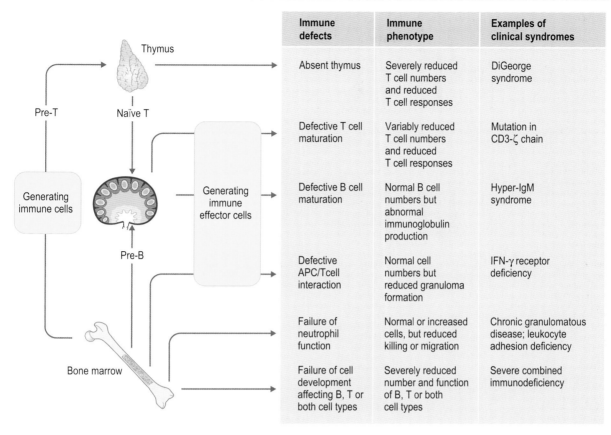

Immune defects	Immune phenotype	Examples of clinical syndromes
Absent thymus	Severely reduced T cell numbers and reduced T cell responses	DiGeorge syndrome
Defective T cell maturation	Variably reduced T cell numbers and reduced T cell responses	Mutation in CD3-ζ chain
Defective B cell maturation	Normal B cell numbers but abnormal immunoglobulin production	Hyper-IgM syndrome
Defective APC/Tcell interaction	Normal cell numbers but reduced granuloma formation	IFN-γ receptor deficiency
Failure of neutrophil function	Normal or increased cells, but reduced killing or migration	Chronic granulomatous disease; leukocyte adhesion deficiency
Failure of cell development affecting B, T or both cell types	Severely reduced number and function of B, T or both cell types	Severe combined immunodeficiency

Fig. 19.1 **Sites at which immune cell defects may occur.**

transfusion of red blood cells or platelets, or transplantation of bone marrow. In new-born babies with T cell deficiency, GVHD may arise through trans-placental transfer of maternal T cells. Transfusions destined for patients with suspected T cell deficiency should first be irradiated to inactivate donor T lymphocytes. GVHD has also been described in association with solid organ transplants during which the recipient is immunosuppressed to avoid graft rejection.

Assessing immune function

The clinical features described above are important pointers to the presence of an immune deficiency. In order to make the diagnosis firm, the immune system must also be examined: an obvious point, you may think. Yet our access to the sites of active immunity — lymph nodes, spleen, infected tissues — is severely limited and almost all tests must be performed on blood samples (Table 19.3). These represent the main screening tests, and they serve two main purposes — first to provide 'hard' evidence that there is indeed an immune defect, and, second, to give some insight into the arm of the immune system that is affected. If these tests confirm that there is a problem, then a more specific battery of assays can be applied. Frequently, this may involve screen-

ing for the specific gene or protein defect that might underlie the particular clinical picture (Fig. 19.2).

T lymphocytes

Counting the numbers of circulating cells is a useful initial test. T lymphocytes and their subsets are identified with monoclonal antibodies directed against relevant CD markers: CD3, CD4, CD8, as the main functional subsets. The percentages of T lymphocytes or subsets can be measured using flow cytometry (p. 89) and converted to a cell concentration (cells/mm^3) using a full blood count and white cell differential and these are the parameters of most use in the diagnosis and monitoring of lymphocyte immunodeficiency. It is important to note that lymphocyte numbers are generally much higher in cord blood and in early infancy; therefore what appears a normal count for an adult is actually abnormally low for a baby.

Tests of T lymphocyte function, however, are a bit more difficult to perform and standardise. The best known is stimulation of T lymphocytes with **mitogens** (i.e. compounds capable of inducing mitosis). Three to five days after stimulation, cell proliferation is measured. The lectin **phytohaemagglutinin** (**PHA**) is a potent and commonly used mitogen. The T cell growth factor IL-2 and a stimulatory monoclonal

Table 19.2 Patterns of infectious organisms encountered in immunodeficiency

Infective agent	Location of defect					
	T cell	B cell	T cell–APC interaction	Neutrophil	Complement classical pathway	Complement membrane attack complex
Bacteria		*Haemophilus influenzae, Strep. pneumoniae, Staph. aureus*	Low virulence *Salmonella* spp. (e.g. non-typhi)	*Staph. aureus, Staph. epidermidis, Pseudomonas aeruginosa*	*Haemophilus influenzae, Strep. pneumoniae, Staph. aureus*	*Neisseria meningitidis, N. gonorrhoeae*
Viruses	*Cytomegalovirus, Herpes zoster*	*Echoviruses*				
Flagellate parasites	*Giardia lamblia*					
Fungi	*Candida albicans*			*Candida albicans*		
Intracellular microorganisms	*Mycobacterium tuberculosis*		Low virulence mycobacteria (e.g. BCG)			
Protozoa	*Pneumocystis carinii, Toxoplasma gondii*					

Table 19.3 Useful screening tests for the assessment of immune function in the investigation of immunodeficiency

Tests	T lymphocytes	B lymphocytes	Phagocytes	Complement
Enumeration	CD3$^+$ lymphocytes CD4$^+$, CD8$^+$ subsets	CD20$^+$ lymphocytes Ig$^+$ cells Immunoglobulin levels IgG subclass levels	Neutrophil count	
Assessment of in vitro functioning	PHA stimulation Antigen-specific stimulation IL-2 production		NBT test (nitroblue tetrazolium)	Haemolysis assay
Assessment of in vivo functioning	Delayed hypersensitivity reaction to purified protein derivative (PPD) of *M. tuberculosis*	Specific antibody levels: isohaemagglutinins; anti-*E. coli*; anti-tetanus, anti-diphtheria toxins (with booster injections if necessary)		

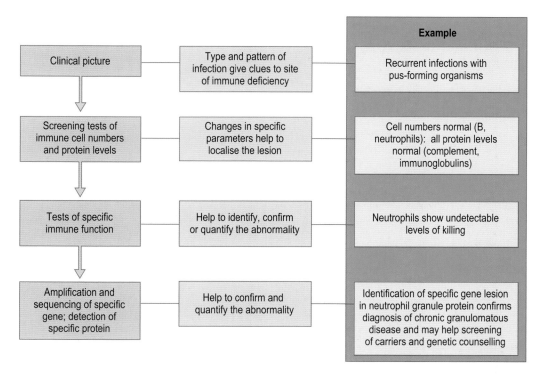

Fig. 19.2 **Strategy for pinpointing a specific immunodeficiency syndrome.**

antibody against CD3 can also be used. Each of these reagents is capable of stimulating all T lymphocytes through a mechanism independent of TCR recognition and, therefore, these tests are not antigen specific. In general, impaired proliferation to mitogens is only detectable in relatively severe T lymphocyte deficiencies. An alternative 'read-out' for T cell function is detection of secreted cytokines, such as IFN-γ and IL-2.

Assessment of the integrity of T lymphocyte functions in vivo can be performed using intradermal injection of an antigen and measurement of the degree of swelling and redness after 48–72 hours caused by a **delayed hypersensitivity** reaction (p. 148). This is exemplified by tests that can be used to assess immunity to *Mycobacterium tuberculosis* by injection of mycobacterial extracts (the Heaf or tuberculin reaction).

B lymphocytes

Measurement of the levels of circulating IgG, IgA and IgM and the number of circulating B lymphocytes are the most apt screening tests for B cell dysfunction. Immunoglobulin levels are best measured directly by a technique called nephelometry (see Science Box 19.1 and Fig. 19.3). In the investigation of immunodeficiency in childhood, it is important to note the age dependence of immunoglobulin levels;

SCIENCE BOX 19.1

Detection of serum levels of immunoglobulin, complement and other immune mediators

The commonest and most accurate automated way to measure serum immunoglobulins and complement components is based upon the principle of nephelometry: the measurement of light scattering immune complexes (Fig. 19.3). Here, a specific antiserum (e.g. anti-IgG antiserum raised in an animal by injection of human IgG) is added to the patient's serum and incubated in a cuvette to allow antigen/antibody complexes to form. A laser light source is passed through, and the light scatter detected depends upon the density of complexes, which depends in turn upon the concentration of the serum protein being measured.

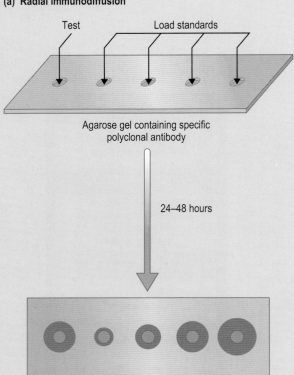

Fig. 19.3 **Measurement of immune-related proteins by (a) radial immunodiffusion and (b) nephelometry.**

Serum immunoglobulin
levels (% adult values)

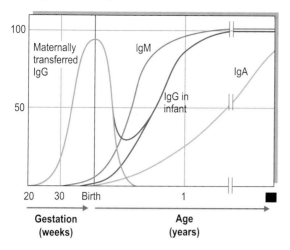

Fig. 19.4 **Serum immunoglobulin levels in the fetus during the last trimester and in the newborn period.**

maternal IgG is present at moderate levels at birth and declines over 5–6 months (see Fig. 19.4). IgA and IgM levels are very low at birth. From infancy onwards, levels of all immunoglobulin classes tend to increase with age until the late teenage, when they plateau. B lymphocytes are counted by flow cytometry using monoclonal antibodies to CD19, CD20 or surface immunoglobulin (sIg).

As for T lymphocytes, there are few antigen-specific tests of B lymphocyte function. Levels of specific antibody can be measured to assess whether the individual has (or has ever had) the ability to mount a directed immune response. The blood group antigens of the ABO system are a good starting point — individuals with A, B and O blood groups (about 97% of the population of the UK) should have IgM class anti-A and/or anti-B antibodies (the **isohaemagglutinins**). Anti-tetanus or anti-diphtheria antibodies are found in recently immunised individuals. Booster injections may be required, therefore, bearing in mind that live vaccines should never be given to individuals with suspected primary immunodeficiency.

Phagocytes

The number of circulating neutrophils is usually available from the full blood count and should be interpreted in the light of any concurrent illness that would normally induce a high neutrophil count. Neutrophil functions that can be tested in the laboratory include phagocytosis, killing of microorganisms and chemotaxis. The most common screening test performed is for killing. When a killing defect is suspected, an assay that assesses the integrity of the respiratory burst is required. Several assay types exist, the simplest being the **nitroblue tetrazolium** (**NBT**) test. NBT is a yellow

dye that is added to a culture of neutrophils (pre-activated with bacterial cell wall endotoxin) along with an appropriate target, usually species of the fungal genus *Candida*. Healthy, activated neutrophils engulf and kill the *Candida*, employing toxic metabolites generated by the respiratory burst (p. 31). As a direct result of this metabolic burst, NBT is converted to a blue/black precipitate, formazan, which can be viewed by light microscopy within the neutrophil cytoplasm. Newer assays measure the respiratory burst using flow cytometry.

A number of cases have been described in which recurrent infection arises because neutrophil migration to the relevant tissues is defective, due to mutations in specific adhesion molecules. The integrity of these molecules can be examined using specific monoclonal antibodies and flow cytometry.

Complement

Complement is a series of approximately 40 serum and membrane-bound proteins, and there are numerous, well-described deficiency syndromes. Levels of individual complement components can be measured directly, but often a screening assay is used first to assess the overall functioning of the whole cascade, from attachment of C1qrs to antibody through to insertion of the membrane attack complex. The typical **complement haemolysis assay** comprises (i) antibody against red blood cells; (ii) the patient's serum as a source of complement; and (iii) some healthy human serum as a positive control. When the antibody and test serum are mixed, there should be red cell lysis, as long as the classical pathway is intact. If lysis is reduced or absent, individual complement components can be measured directly.

Deficiency of regulatory proteins in the cascade may lead to uncontrolled complement activation, resulting in disease. When such a condition is suspected, individual proteins should be measured directly.

Tests for specific immune abnormalities

As shown in Figure 19.2, at the end of the diagnostic trail, there will often be a requirement for a specific genetic or molecular diagnosis. This not only completes the assessment of the patient, but provides the necessary information for genetic counselling and screening of other, potentially affected family members. In the case of the monogenic primary immune deficiencies, this will typically involve a screening test for abnormalities in selected chromosomal regions (e.g. sequence-specific conformational polymorphism; SSCP) followed by sequencing of the candidate gene.

In some cases, where genetic mutations lead to the deletion of a protein, the screening can be more easily performed by looking for the absence of the protein using monoclonal antibodies. This can be carried out as a flow cytometry assay, or by Western blotting.

SUMMARY BOX 19.1

Assessing immune function

- Primary immunodeficiency is rare but instructive.
- Secondary immunodeficiency is far commoner, and is either secondary to infection (HIV/AIDS) or immune-suppressive drugs.
- The clinical features of an immune deficiency state conform to patterns that guide laboratory investigations.
- Laboratory tests screen for activity in the different immune system components.

T lymphocyte deficiencies

Thymic hypoplasia/DiGeorge syndrome

Clinical and immunological features

In this congenital abnormality, there is failure of development during the 12th week of gestation of the third and fourth pharyngeal arches, which normally give rise to the parathyroid glands and the thymus (see Clinical Box 19.1). More common than a complete defect is **partial DiGeorge syndrome**, in which the features are variably less severe. In

---

CLINICAL BOX 19.1

The DiGeorge syndrome: an experiment of nature

By a coincidence, Angelo DiGeorge, a paediatrician in Philadelphia, attended a scientific meeting in 1965 in which the results of seminal studies on the origins of immune cells were presented. A series of experiments had examined the effect on the chicken immune system of removal of either a lymphoid organ (called the bursa) or the thymus. Chickens from which the bursa was removed were unable to produce immunoglobulins, whilst thymectomy rendered the birds incapable of rejecting grafts but immunoglobulin levels remained normal. Through his interest in hypoparathyroidism, DiGeorge had seen four children with low calcium associated with absence of parathyroid glands and thymus. He was able to relate his own observations on this experiment of nature in which, as in the thymectomised chicken, immunoglobulin levels were indeed normal in the absence of a thymus gland.

---

most cases, deletions on chromosome 22q11.2 have been identified.

Typical diagnostic features are absence of the thymus and neonatal hypocalcaemia with low levels of parathormone. Children with DiGeorge syndrome often also have other defects, particularly developmental abnormalities of the aortic arch. The frequency of the DiGeorge syndrome is somewhere between 1 and 5 per 100 000 of the population. It is usual for the syndrome to present in the newborn period as a result of hypocalcaemic tetany or cardiac defects rather than with episodes of infection, which may take several months to appear. Viral, protozoal, fungal and bacterial infections are typically found and infants fail to thrive.

The laboratory findings depend on the severity of the loss of thymic function, and can therefore be variable. Severely affected children have reduced T lymphocyte number and make reduced T cell proliferation responses. Paradoxically, immunoglobulin levels are often normal.

Management

Calcium supplements and vitamin D, correction of cardiac abnormalities and prophylactic antibiotic treatment (e.g. with sulphonamides to avoid *Pneumocystis carinii* pneumonia) may be required once the diagnosis is made, depending on severity of the T lymphopenia. There have been three different therapies used in an attempt to reverse the immunodeficiency and each can claim some success. Early therapy centred upon thymic transplants using fetal tissue and it is also reported that bone marrow transplant from HLA identical siblings can be successful; the bone marrow should be unfractionated (i.e. should contain mature effector T cells). More recently, transplant of cultured, mature thymus tissue has emerged as perhaps the most effective therapy, in most cases leading to reconstitution of antigen-specific T cell function and a reasonable prognosis.

Deficiency in T cell surface molecules, signalling pathway or cytokine

A variety of T cell deficiencies have been described and for many of these the defective gene/molecule has been characterised. These primary immunodeficiencies tend to present soon after birth in much the same way that severe combined immunodeficiency (SCID) does (see below), and the management is very similar to that of SCID. Examples of T cell deficiencies include deficiency of CD3 itself; defects in signal transduction pathways; and even deficiency of IL-2, the T cell growth factor (Fig. 19.5).

It is unusual for B lymphocytes to be able to function normally when T cells are so abnormal. However, in the case of one disease, the T cell abnormality is sufficiently mild, that the B cell abnormality becomes the dominant presenting feature. This is a disorder called Hyper IgM syndrome (HIGM). At the molecular level, it is due to an X-linked defect in the CD40 ligand (CD40L; CD154) gene. Signalling between CD40 on B cells and CD40L on T cells has two important outcomes — first is B cell activation, with generation of mature, class switched B cells bearing high affinity immunoglobulin. Second is activation and maturation of the T cell response. In CD40L deficiency, B cells cannot progress through their life cycle and stack up at the immature level, where they can only produce IgM (Fig. 19.6). The HIGM of the syndrome is accompanied by low levels of IgG, A and E, and mild T cell defects.

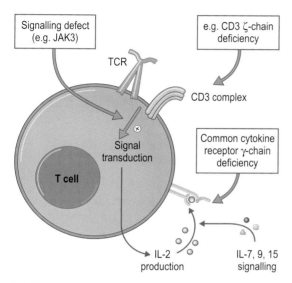

Fig. 19.5 T cell primary immunodeficiency states can occur as a result of defective molecules involved at different stages of the cell activation process.

SUMMARY BOX 19.2

T lymphocyte deficiencies

■ Isolated T cell deficiency, as in the DiGeorge syndrome, is rare but has devastating consequences.

■ T cell deficiencies are likely to have knock-on consequences for B cell antibody production.

■ The molecular basis for severe T cell deficiencies includes defects in cytokines, surface molecules and activation pathways.

■ Bone marrow transplantation from an HLA identical donor can reconstitute T cell immunity.

B lymphocyte deficiencies

Deficiencies in B lymphocyte function can result from lesions occurring at multiple sites in the pathway of production of mature active B cells (Fig. 19.6).

X-linked agammaglobulinaemia (XLA)

Clinical and immunological features

In X-linked agammaglobulinaemia (XLA; also known as Bruton's syndrome), affected males have IgG levels less than 2.0 g/l and all five classes of immunoglobulins are affected,

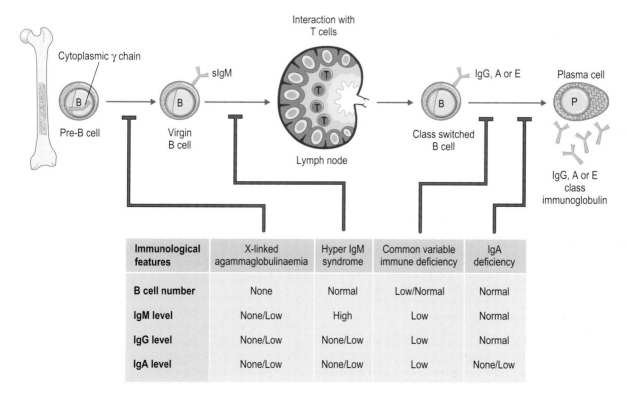

Fig. 19.6 Scheme of the major lesion sites leading to B cell immunodeficiency.

Immunological features	X-linked agammaglobulinaemia	Hyper IgM syndrome	Common variable immune deficiency	IgA deficiency
B cell number	None	Normal	Low/Normal	Normal
IgM level	None/Low	High	Low	Normal
IgG level	None/Low	None/Low	Low	Normal
IgA level	None/Low	None/Low	Low	None/Low

with total levels of less than 2.5 g/l. Specific antibody is undetectable. Pre-B cells staining positive for cytoplasmic μ chains are present in normal/reduced numbers in the bone marrow, although these IgM heavy chain molecules lack the variable region segment (this is a marker that the B cell development is arrested). There are no subsequent members of the B cell lineage, however, and B lymphocytes detected using the CD19 or CD20 markers by flow cytometry are absent from the peripheral blood and lymph nodes. In 1993 the gene defect responsible for XLA was identified as a loss of function mutation on chromosome Xq22 affecting the gene for a tyrosine kinase (Bruton's tyrosine kinase; BTK). The function of BTK remains unclear, except to say that it is phosphorylated after activation of B cells via the BCR and may be involved in cell activation and maturation. BTK can be detected by flow cytometry or Western blotting, and if absent the *BTK* gene should be analysed.

Children present after the age of 5–6 months, when the protective benefits of placentally transferred maternal IgG have worn off (see Fig. 19.4). Recurrent infections of the upper and lower respiratory tract with pyogenic organisms are typical, whilst enteritis and malabsorption are frequently associated with the presence of *Giardia lamblia* in the gut. Morbidity and mortality are related mainly to chronic lung disease and occasional CNS infections with enteroviruses.

T lymphocyte function is normal, although recent evidence suggests that BTK has a role in neutrophil function, which may be abnormal in XLA.

Treatment

The major threat from the disease is chronic lung damage; the major goal is replacement of circulating Ig to a level that controls infections (intravenous administration of immunoglobulins; IVIG). Home treatment with IVIG after proper training in hospital is widely used, as well as subcutaneous administration by pump. The aim of therapy is that the trough IgG concentration, taken just before the next infusion, remains within the normal range (i.e. >5–6 g/l). Administration of IVIG appears to improve lung function, and use of preparations with high antiviral titres may control enterovirus infections. Prophylactic antibiotics may also be required, along with chest physiotherapy in established lung disease. Prognosis has improved in recent years as more patients survive into adulthood, but chronic lung disease and lymphomas are life-threatening complications.

Selective IgA deficiency

Clinical and immunological features

Serum IgA levels of <0.05 g/l, with normal levels of IgG and IgM, is termed selective IgA deficiency (IgAD). IgAD is found in approximately 1/600 northern Europeans, making it the most common primary immunodeficiency. B lymphocytes bearing surface IgA are present in the circulation, but

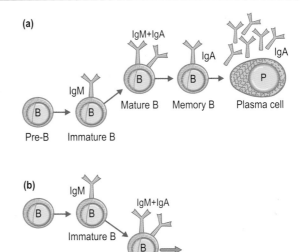

Fig. 19.7 Selective IgA deficiency: (a) in normal individuals; (b) in IgA deficiency.

IgA-producing plasma cells are markedly reduced in number or absent. The underlying defect in IgAD remains unknown. (Fig. 19.7).

Approximately 85% of IgAD patients present to their doctors with infections. Typically, these are recurrent, caused by pyogenic organisms and affect mucosal sites, usually the upper respiratory tract. Other symptoms at presentation reflect an association between IgAD and other disorders, including allergy and autoimmune diseases (rheumatoid arthritis, haemolytic anaemia, autoimmune hepatitis, type 1 diabetes and coeliac disease are the commonest). It is also true to say that IgAD can be an incidental finding and that some people are entirely asymptomatic.

Both IgA1 and IgA2 subclasses are reduced or absent, as is secretory IgA. B and T lymphocyte numbers are normal and function normally.

Treatment

Treatment mainly comprises antibiotics as required and therapy for any associated disease. However, of great clinical importance is the tendency of some patients to produce anti-IgA antibodies of the IgG and IgE class. Infusion of exogenous IgA, as would occur in blood transfusion, can result in anaphylaxis. All IgA-deficient patients should be screened for anti-IgA antibodies, and, if necessary, transfused with washed red cells, blood from an IgA-deficient donor or with their own blood, which has been stored. IVIG is of little value in IgA deficiency: preparations contain little IgA, will not benefit secretory IgA levels and what little IgA there is may be sufficient to provoke adverse reactions in sensitised individuals. The rare exceptions to this rule may be patients with an associated IgG class or subclass deficiency in whom the therapy gives demonstrable benefit. The prognosis is reasonably good as long as the diagnosis is made before life-threatening complications such as chronic lung disease have become established.

IgG subclass deficiency

Clinical and immunological features

It was noted several years ago that antibody responses to certain bacterial antigens may preferentially belong to a particular IgG subclass. An example of this is the restriction of antibody response to some bacterial coat polysaccharides to the IgG2 subclass. It seemed logical, then, to suppose that some recurrent infections could be due to an underlying deficiency in a particular IgG subclass.

Despite much research, the field of IgG subclass deficiency remains controversial. Perhaps the exception is selective absence of IgG2 associated with increased susceptibility to infection with organisms such as *Streptococcus pneumoniae* and *Haemophilus influenzae* type b, which do, indeed, have distinctive bacterial coat polysaccharides. IgG2 subclass deficiency may often be found in association with IgAD, and probably represents part of a clinical spectrum along with CVID.

When investigating the patient with a suspected antibody deficiency, IgG subclass levels can be measured if indicated, but should be interpreted in the light of the appropriate normal ranges, particularly taking age into consideration, as different subclass levels mature at different rates. A firm diagnosis of antibody deficiency should be backed by marked deficiency of one or other subclass. Therapy is mainly dependent on antibiotics; IVIG may be used when there is a demonstrable subclass or specific antibody defect and conventional treatment fails.

Common variable immunodeficiency (CVID)

Clinical and immunological features

Hypogammaglobulinaemia (IgG <0.5 g/l) that typically arises during late childhood and early adulthood, in association with progressively worsening infections, is termed common variable immunodeficiency (CVID), and is the second most common primary immunodeficiency after IgAD (although much rarer at 1/50 000). It is a label that is used after all other firm diagnoses have been excluded and at present the diagnosis of CVID represents a heterogeneous collection of disorders with the common feature of low immunoglobulin levels. CVID shares features in common with IgAD, suggesting that these might be different components of a spectrum of immunoglobulin deficiencies.

The dominant feature of CVID is antibody deficiency and, for this reason, it is considered here rather than in the section on combined T and B cell defects. However, T cell defects do occasionally occur and, when severe, give a clinical picture in which T cell deficiency may even be dominant. A variety of ill-defined cellular immune defects have so far been described in CVID. It is likely that in the coming years a number of distinct syndromes under this umbrella will be described. Indeed, this has already begun; several individuals with a diagnosis of CVID were recently shown to

CLINICAL BOX 19.2

Common variable immunodeficiency: viruses and co-stimulators

Common variable immunodeficiency is an intriguing condition. One of its more peculiar features has been described by several groups, and gives some hope that a cure could be found. It has been noted that rarely, after a severe viral illness, there is a sudden reversal of the immunodeficiency, with progressive increase in IgG and IgM levels, sustained over a considerable period. This has been noted after both hepatitis B virus and human immunodeficiency virus (HIV) infection. It is known that HIV infection induces a general increase in immunoglobulins, possibly through effects on T cell regulation of B cell function. Perhaps this paradoxical effect of virus infection on CVID implies that the T cell regulation, rather than B cell function, is the defective mechanism underlying the disease. Some support for that concept comes from the recent identification that a small subset of patients with the diagnosis of CVID have a defect in ICOS, the 'inducible co-stimulator' on activated T cells. These patients had fairly normal T cells by all possible tests. The suggestion is that ICOS is an important molecule when it comes to T cells helping B cells to differentiate into class-switched, antibody producing memory cells.

have a defect in the gene encoding ICOS-L (see Clinical Box 19.2).

Clinically, patients present with recurrent upper and lower respiratory tract infections with organisms typical of antibody deficiency, chronic bronchiectatic lung disease, and malabsorption and diarrhoea often secondary to giardiasis. Malignancy in patients with CVID has a high incidence, as do autoimmune diseases, particularly pernicious anaemia and autoimmune cytopenia. Rarely, patients present with features of a T cell immunodeficiency.

Total immunoglobulin levels are less than 3 g/l and the concentration of IgG is less than 2.5 g/l. Specific antibody production is impaired, but circulating B cell numbers are usually normal.

Treatment

Appropriate antibiotic therapy, including metronidazole for giardiasis, should be readily available. Replacement therapy with IVIG should also be employed if the severity of the immunodeficiency warrants it. In the absence of complications such as chronic lung disease and haematological malignancy, the prognosis remains good.

Transient hypogammaglobulinaemia of infancy

Clinical and immunological features

An abnormally low level of IgG (e.g. below the 5th centile) occurring after maternal IgG has disappeared and persisting

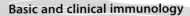
for up to 2 years is known as transient hypogammaglobulinaemia of infancy (THI). Transfer of maternal IgG begins at around the 16th week of gestation but is maximal during the 3rd trimester (Fig. 19.4). Maternal IgG has a half-life of 4 weeks and the majority has been catabolised by 5–6 months, before the infant's own IgG synthesis is fully under way. The resulting trough, which is found in all healthy babies, is a period of **physiological hypogammaglobulinaemia**. It may be of importance clinically when it is prolonged, as in THI, or when maternal transfer is incomplete, as in prematurity.

In THI, recurrent, severe respiratory tract infections after 5–6 months of age produce a clinical picture similar to XLA and IgG levels remain in the trough (Fig. 19.4). Other causes of primary antibody deficiency should be excluded. Typically, IgA and IgM levels begin to rise as expected and circulating B lymphocyte numbers are normal, making this easily differentiated from XLA.

As far as treatment is concerned, infections should be treated as appropriate, but generally IVIG therapy can be avoided.

SUMMARY BOX 19.3

B lymphocyte deficiencies

- ■ Life-threatening agammaglobulinaemia can be treated with intravenous gammaglobulins (IVIG) to reduce infections.
- ■ IgA deficiency (IgAD) is the most common primary immunodeficiency.
- ■ Anti-IgA antibodies in the circulation of IgAD patients can give rise to potentially lethal reactions.
- ■ Common variable immunodeficiency (CVID), is a heterogeneous group of disorders, for which the molecular bases are only just beginning to be unravelled.

Combined T and B lymphocyte deficiencies

Severe combined immunodeficiency

Severe combined immunodeficiencies (SCID) are a heterogeneous group of rare, genetically determined disorders resulting from impaired T, NK and B cell immunity (Table 19.4). The condition is diagnosed in 1–2 live births per 100 000. The combined cell deficiency gives rise to the early onset of susceptibility to infection by virtually all types of microorganism.

Because this condition is rare and may arise from many different underlying genetic defects, for the sake of clarity this section will focus on the most common form of SCID.

Approximately 50% of SCID results from an X-linked, lymphopaenic disorder with low T and NK cells but normal B cell numbers. The genetic basis for this is a defect in the IL-2 receptor γ chain. The IL-2 receptor γ chain was the last component of the receptor to be identified. Once its gene was known to be located on the X chromosome, an immediate examination of IL-2 receptor γ chain genes in patients with X-linked SCID was prompted, revealing that each had a mutation at this site. However, one puzzle remained. Why was the defect in X-linked SCID so severe, in comparison, say, to children with an isolated deficiency of IL-2 itself, in whom T lymphocyte numbers may be normal? It was reasoned that the IL-2 receptor γ chain might have other functions; one obvious possibility was that it acts as a receptor for other cytokines. This was soon shown to be the case, with receptors for IL-4, IL-7, IL-9 and IL-15 requiring the γ chain for normal function. With each of these important cytokines unable to function normally, it is not surprising that the T cell abnormalities seen are profound.

Clinical and immunological features

In SCID of whatever form, persistent infections usually develop by the age of 3 months. Candidal infections of the mouth and skin, protracted diarrhoea, fever and failure to thrive are typical presenting features; if the underlying condition is left untreated, *Pneumocystis carinii* pneumonia is one of the most frequent causes of death.

The results of B and T lymphocyte phenotype analysis in peripheral blood are variable, according to the type of SCID. In γ-chain deficiency, for example, T and NK cells are lacking. B cell numbers may be normal, but when sufficient lymphocytes are available for analysis, both T and B lymphocyte functions are severely impaired. Once the diagnosis is suspected, molecular and genetic diagnosis of the underlying defect is undertaken.

Treatment

The most successful treatment for all forms of SCID has been bone marrow transplantation (BMT). Using marrow from HLA-identical donors, such as siblings, can result in rapid T cell reconstitution. B cell reconstitution is more variable, and even when present B cells may not make immunoglobulin: for this reason IVIG infusions may be required. Figures obtained in recent European studies indicate that success rates for such BMT in SCID are typically >90%. Only 40% of affected children will have a related, matched donor, however, and haploidentical donors, usually a parent, are the next best option. In this case, the donated marrow is purged of T lymphocytes using monoclonal antibodies to avoid GVHD, with success rates as high as 80%. Other treatment issues are worthy of note; before BMT, SCID patients requiring blood transfusion must have the blood packs irradiated first to avoid GVHD. Live vaccines (e.g. for viruses or BCG) should be avoided at all costs.

Table 19.4 Severe combined immunodeficiency and related forms of combined immunodeficiency

Designation	Cell numbers	Inheritance
X-linked SCID	T lymphocytes ↓ B lymphocytes normal	X-linked
Autosomal recessive SCID	T lymphocytes ↓ B lymphocytes ↓	Autosomal recessive
Adenosine deaminase deficiency	Progressive T lymphocytes ↓ Progressive B lymphocytes ↓	Autosomal recessive
Purine nucleoside phosphorylase deficiency	Progressive T lymphocytes ↓ B lymphocytes normal	Autosomal recessive
TCR immunodeficiency	CD2⁺ T lymphocytes normal B lymphocytes normal	Autosomal recessive
MHC class II deficiency	T lymphocytes normal B lymphocytes normal	Autosomal recessive
Defective IL-2 production	T lymphocytes normal B lymphocytes normal	Not known

A new, exciting, 'Brave New World' form of treatment has been pioneered recently, that of gene therapy for SCID (see Clinical Box 19.3).

SUMMARY BOX 19.4

Combined lymphocyte defects

- Severe combined immune deficiencies (SCID) are usually fatal without bone marrow transplantation.
- Combined deficiencies may affect predominantly T or B cell immunity.
- Ex vivo gene therapy shows great promise in the future treatment of single gene defect immunodeficiency.

Defects in antigen presenting cell function

This has been one of the more interesting areas of immunodeficiency research in recent years. A series of genetic defects have been uncovered in which antigen presenting cell function is impaired. The defect manifests as an inability to protect the host from intracellular bacteria, particularly low virulence mycobacteria and salmonella. The main axis that gets disrupted and gives rise to these syndromes is between the T cell and the APC (see Fig. 19.8). Apart from powerful antimicrobial drugs, other therapeutic options include giving recombinant IFN-γ or IL-12, depending upon the nature of the lesion.

Neutrophil defects

Chronic granulomatous disease

Clinical and immunological features

Chronic granulomatous disease (CGD) is a rare (1/250 000) immunodeficiency that results from a defect in neutrophil killing. Granulomata (swollen, organised and inflamed collections of cells) form, representing the chronic struggle between the defective host cells and the invading pathogen. The functional defect lies in being unable to generate antibacterial superoxides through the action of the phagocyte NADPH oxidase (see p. 31). This enzyme complex has

Gene therapy for severe immunodeficiency

There is a fantastic logic to the concept that an immunodeficiency, identified to result from a single gene defect, could be corrected by re-insertion of a correct version of the gene. This type of 'molecular surgery', called ex vivo gene therapy, has now become reality. The first landmark study involved a retroviral vector modified to encode the common cytokine γ chain. A defect in this chain leads to X-linked SCID, commonly known as the 'baby in the bubble' syndrome. The retrovirus was used to transduce stem cells (CD34⁺) taken from the bone marrow of the immunodeficient child. This was done in the laboratory and the cells reinfused. Two weeks later, NK cells started to appear in the blood, followed by T cells some 10 weeks later. Astonishingly, the T cells had normal function when stimulated with mitogens or appropriate antigens. B cell function became sufficiently good that IVIG supplements could be stopped.

Not all of the news has been good, however. In two of the 14 boys treated there was an unexpected complication, with inappropriate insertion of the retroviral vector near the proto-oncogene *LMO2* promoter, leading to uncontrolled clonal proliferation of mature T cells (i.e. leukaemia). A new generation of viral vectors has been designed to avoid this problem in the future.

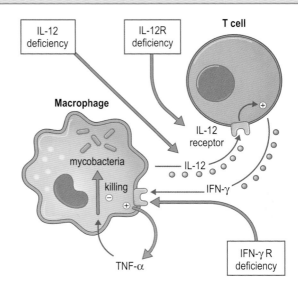

Fig. 19.8 **Control of intracellular bacteria by APC–T cell interactions. Molecular defects that give rise to immunodeficiency states are shown.**

multiple components; roughly two thirds of cases of CGD are X-linked and due to loss of gp91^PHOX function.

By the age of 2 years, children with chronic granulomatous disease will have begun to experience infections; these typically affect the deep tissues (lymphadenitis, osteomyelitis and skin abscesses) as well as causing pneumonia and periodontitis. Neutrophil numbers are either normal or increased in response to intercurrent infection. The qualitative NBT test reveals a complete deficiency of neutrophils capable of undergoing a respiratory burst.

Treatment

Aggressive treatment of infections, with surgical drainage of deep abscesses, enhances survival. Antibiotic and antifungal therapy should be prolonged for 5–6 weeks or given prophylactically. Immunotherapy with interferons may have a role in patients with intractable infections, and in some cases BMT may be required.

Leukocyte adhesion deficiency

Clinical and immunological features

Leukocyte adhesion deficiency (LAD) results from defects in the family of immune cell surface glycoproteins, termed the integrins (see p. 27). The β₂ integrin family has a common β

chain, CD18, which combines with different α chains (CD11a, CD11b and CD11c) to form heterodimers including the complement receptor 3 (CD11b/CD18, receptor for the opsonin iC3b) and LFA-1 (CD11a/CD18), which is important in lymphocyte, monocyte and phagocyte adherence. Over 200 cases of leukocyte adhesion deficiency type I, or LAD-I, have been described, in which CD18 is non-functional. This leads to decreased adherence, phagocytosis and chemotaxis by neutrophils, and impaired T cell-mediated cytotoxicity. Other, rarer forms of LAD (LAD-II and III) result from other defects elsewhere in the integrin recognition and post-receptor signalling pathways.

LAD-I has autosomal recessive inheritance and may present almost immediately after birth, with delayed umbilical cord separation. Recurrent infections similar to those in chronic granulomatous disease appear during the first decade of life. In LAD-I, monoclonal antibodies directed against CR-3 and LFA-1 demonstrate their absence on neutrophils, monocytes and lymphocytes.

Treatment

Patients require aggressive treatment with antimicrobial and antifungal agents, with BMT offering the prospect of cure.

Deficiency of complement and mannan binding lectin components

The consequences of deficiency of complement proteins, whether pro-inflammatory or regulatory components, can be predicted from knowledge of their functions (Table 19.5).

Table 19.5 Deficiencies of the complement cascade and associated syndromes

Deficiency	Number of cases/prevalence	Associated features
Classical pathway		
C1q, C1r/C1s	>50	SLE-like syndrome; pyogenic infections
C4	17	SLE-like syndrome
C2	>100	SLE-like syndrome; vasculitis
C3	16	Pyogenic infections
Alternative pathway		
Factor D	1	Neisserial infection
Properdin	>50	Neisserial infection
Membrane attack pathway		
C5, 6, 7, 8	>130	Neisserial infection, SLE
C9	Common in Japan (1/1000)	None/neisserial infection
Regulatory proteins		
Factors H, I	27	Pyogenic infections, SLE
C1 inhibitor	Prevalence of 1/150 000	Hereditary angio-oedema

Broadly speaking, the main physiological roles of complement are in enhancing neutrophil-mediated lysis of bacteria and in solubilising and removing immune complexes. Failures in these will lead to impaired non-specific immunity with an increase in bacterial infections, and a tendency towards diseases in which immune complex deposition causes inflammation, such as SLE. Whilst it is easy to accept that complement deficiency predisposes to infection with pyogenic bacteria, it is somewhat unexpected to find that neisserial infections are often encountered in patients with complement defects, particularly defects of the membrane attack complex. Therefore, complement deficiency reveals a function of the cascade that might not otherwise have been uncovered, to mediate lysis of *Neisseria* directly.

This section mainly deals with complete complement deficiency, but it should not be forgotten that partial deficiency provides an underlying genetic predisposition to SLE. As a general principle, defects in the classical pathway are more associated with autoimmune disease than infection; in contrast, defects in the MBL and alternative pathways are associated more with infection.

Most complement deficiencies are inherited in an autosomal recessive pattern with two notable exceptions: properdin deficiency is X-linked and C1 inhibitor deficiency has an autosomal dominant inheritance. Deficiencies may also be acquired. For example, levels can decline during increased consumption: loss of C2 and C4 resulting from uncontrolled classical pathway activation in C1 inhibitor deficiency can result in immune complex disease.

Classical pathway

Classical pathway defects are often associated with an increased risk of immune complex disease, because of their critical role in the solubilisation of antigen–antibody complexes. Infection may also be a feature. Defects of C1r and C1s occur together, probably as a consequence of their close genetic linkage on chromosome 12. Complete C4 deficiency requires the inheritance of non-functional ('null') alleles at all four *C4A* and *C4B* loci. More than two thirds of patients with C4 deficiency will have an autoimmune disease, and it has the highest incidence proportionally of

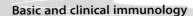

SLE amongst the complement deficiencies. C2 is the most common homozygous complement deficiency in northern Europeans, with a prevalence of between 10 and 30 per 100 000 of the population.

Alternative pathway

Defects in alternative pathway components are mainly associated with increased susceptibility to infection, notably with *Neisseria*, reflecting the role of this part of the cascade in immediate and innate responses to microorganisms.

Mannan binding lectin (MBL)

Genetically determined low levels of MBL are associated with a number of inflammatory and infectious diseases. It is also clear that MBL deficiency lowers the threshold at which infectious complications become dangerous. For example, in intensive care units, sepsis is much commoner in children who have low levels of MBL. Clinical trials are planned to see whether screening for MBL levels would enable such at-risk children to be protected with antibiotics, or with recombinant MBL itself.

Common pathway

The component C3 lies at the convergence of the classical and alternative pathways, has a major role in opsonisation and must be activated before the membrane attack pathway can proceed. Given its pivotal role, therefore, it is not surprising that no homozygous C3-deficient patient has been reported who is disease free. Approximately one fifth of C3-deficient patients will have a disorder that is usually attributed to damage mediated by circulating immune complexes: SLE, vasculitis or glomerulonephritis.

Absence of any one of the components between C5 and C8 in the membrane attack complex results in a significantly increased risk of infection with *Neisseria meningitidis*.

Complement regulatory proteins

Amongst the complement regulatory proteins deficiency of **C1 inhibitor** (also termed C1 esterase deficiency) was first described in 1881 and is relatively common. This enzyme is involved in regulation of several plasma enzyme systems (e.g. the kinin system) and is continuously consumed. This means that a single parental chromosome defect, which results in 50% of normal production, barely copes with the demand (hence the autosomal dominance). Under minimal stress, therefore, uncontrolled activation of complement and the kinins may occur. The clinical picture is then one of progressive oedema of the deep tissues affecting the face, trunk, viscera and the airway, hence the name **hereditary angio-oedema** (HAE). Laryngeal oedema may be fatal unless the acute attack fades or is treated. The increase in fluid loss into the tissues may be a result of bradykinin release or C2 kinin

derived from complement. Uncontrolled classical pathway activation leads to reductions in C2 and C4, but controls at the C3 level are intact and other pathways are not affected. Treatment of acute attacks previously relied upon fresh frozen plasma as a source of C1 inhibitor, but purified preparations are now available. Plasmin inhibitors (tranexamic acid, ε-aminocaproic acid) may control C1 inhibitor consumption and can be used prophylactically to cover surgical procedures. Prophylactic therapy centres upon drugs belonging to a class called **impeded androgens** or **anabolic steroids**, of which the most commonly used is danazol, which increases C1 inhibitor levels by an unknown mechanism.

Some 85% of patients with HAE have symptoms resulting from an absence of C1 inhibitor (type 1 HAE) and in the remainder the protein is present but non-functional (type 2 HAE). An acquired version of the syndrome (AAE) is described in association with B cell lymphoproliferative disorders (type 1 AAE) or an autoantibody to C1 inhibitor (Table 19.6).

SUMMARY BOX 19.5

Defects of the innate immune system

- Recently defined immune defects in the interaction between APCs and T cells have major consequences for mycobacterial immunity.
- Primary defects of neutrophils leading to failure to kill or migrate severely compromise host immunity.
- Complement defects are associated with an increased risk of bacterial infections and immune complex-mediated diseases such as SLE.
- C1 inhibitor deficiency is relatively common and can result in life-threatening laryngeal oedema.

Secondary immunodeficiency

As stated in the introduction, secondary causes of immune deficiency, particularly of neutrophil and antibody function, are relatively common. These may arise secondary to treatment, neoplasia or viral infection. Steroids are widely used as immunosuppressants in autoimmune and other inflammatory conditions and have a range of deleterious effects on most parts of the immune system. Immunosuppressive agents that inhibit T cell activation are widely used in transplantation to control graft rejection and have direct inhibitory effects on T cell function. Infections with *Candida albicans*, *Pneumocystis carinii*, herpes zoster and cytomegalovirus are relatively common sequelae, therefore. Cytotoxic drugs and radiotherapy are used to treat leukaemia and lymphoma, either directly or as part of the marrow ablation required before bone marrow transplantation. Prolonged states of lymphopenia and neutropenia may follow, during which patients are acutely susceptible to infection. Finally, lymphoproliferative disorders, particularly those affecting

Table 19.6 Function and presence of C1 inhibitor and classical pathway components in hereditary and acquired angio-oedema

	C1 inhibitor function	C1 inhibitor antigen	C1q	C2	C4
Hereditary angio-oedema					
Type 1	↓	↓	N	↓	↓
Type 2	↓	N or ↑	N	↓	↓
Acquired angio-oedema					
Type 1	↓	N or ↓	↓	↓	↓
Type 2	↓	N or ↓	↓	↓	↓

Note: N normal; ↓ reduced levels; ↑ raised levels.

the B cell compartment, such as B cell chronic lymphatic leukaemia (CLL) and multiple myeloma, can result in functional antibody deficiency.

Further reading

Bacchelli C, Buckridge S, Thrasher AJ, Gaspar HB 2007 Translational mini-review series on immunodeficiency: molecular defects in common variable immunodeficiency. Clin Exp Immunol 149: 401–409

Casanova JL, Abel L 2007 Primary immunodeficiencies: a field in its infancy. Science 317(5838): 617–619

Cunningham-Rundles C 2005 Molecular defects in T- and B-cell primary immunodeficiency diseases. Nat Rev Immunol 5: 880–892

de Vries E 2006 Patient-centred screening for primary immunodeficiency: a multi-stage diagnostic protocol designed for non-immunologists. Clin Exp Immunol 145: 204–214

Fischer A 2007 Human primary immunodeficiency diseases. Immunity 27: 835–845

Wood P, Stanworth S, Burton J, Jones A, Peckham DG, Green T et al 2007 Recognition, clinical diagnosis and management of patients with primary antibody deficiencies: a systematic review. Clin Exp Immunol 149: 410–423

Human immunodeficiency virus and AIDS

The epidemic that is represented by the terms AIDS (for Acquired Immune Deficiency Syndrome) and HIV (for Human Immunodeficiency Virus) has generated many statistics. It has resulted in the death of 2–3 million people per year during the early part of the twenty-first century, with an estimated 40 million currently infected worldwide, 25 million of whom are in sub-Saharan Africa (Fig. 20.1). During the period 1981–91 some $5–10 billion were spent worldwide on research funding and the publication of tens of thousands of research papers. It has captured public, media and scientific attention for a host of different reasons. For the immunologist, HIV is of interest because of its ability to directly infect CD4 T cells and in doing so give rise to a profound level of acquired immunodeficiency. In this chapter the underlying basis for this process is considered, along with the future possibilities for prevention or cure.

First of all, it is worth considering HIV from a historical perspective, since its rapid emergence as a new infectious disease represents a unique experience in modern times. In June 1981, the US public health agency (Centers for Disease Control; CDC) reported an unexplained cluster of five cases of an unusual pneumonia caused by the parasite *Pneumocystis carinii* in Los Angeles, all in homosexual men. Until then, this infection was typically seen in immunocompromised individuals, most frequently in immunosuppressed transplant recipients and patients with haematological malignancies undergoing cytotoxic therapy. The report resonated throughout America, where physicians began to recognise that for up to 2 years they had been witnessing unusual disorders in young men: CNS infection with the protozoal parasite *Toxoplasma gondii*, severe herpes skin infections, widespread infection with the common fungus *Candida albicans*, as well as manifestations unrelated to infections, such as extreme weight loss, fevers, lymphadenopathy and the appearance of a tumour, Kaposi's sarcoma, previously associated with elderly men. The disease was labelled the acquired immunodeficiency syndrome (AIDS) and was destined to engender not only a mini-revolution in social behaviour but also an unprecedented level of international scientific interest and controversy.

A novel retrovirus, now named HIV-1, was isolated from a patient in 1983. For this major breakthrough in our understanding of the cause of AIDS, Luc Montagnier and Françoise Barré-Sinoussi were jointly awarded the Nobel Prize in Physiology or Medicine in 2008. In 1985, another retrovirus (HIV-2) associated with a clinical immunodeficiency syndrome resembling AIDS was isolated from patients in West Africa. The dominant immunopathogenic feature of the syndrome is an absolute deficiency of circulating CD4 T lymphocytes, leading to a profound secondary immune deficiency state.

HIV may be considered as an infectious disease like any other, in that transmission is largely related to behaviour: changes in sexual and social behaviour, therefore, offer the best hope of controlling the disease. In addition, the early part of the twenty-first century has witnessed the development of viral inhibitors with dramatic effects on the clinical progression of disease. Although highly effective, these ultimately fall short of a cure, and a safe and effective vaccine will be required before there is hope of eradicating the virus.

Epidemiology

Modes and risk of transmission of HIV

HIV has been isolated from virtually all body fluids, including blood, semen, vaginal secretions, tears, urine, saliva and breast-milk. The most common form of transmission worldwide is through sexual contact. In the developed nations, needle-sharing by intravenous drug users remains an important cause of transmission. Successful programmes of blood, blood-product and organ-donor screening have minimised the risk from transfusion and transplantation. Other

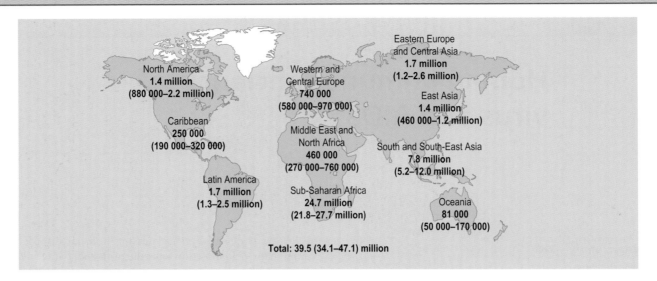

Fig. 20.1 The global burden of HIV infection.
Adults and children estimated to be living with HIV, 2006. Data from UNAIDS — AIDS Epidemic Update (online at
http://www.searo.who.int/).

recognised transmissions are maternal–fetal and mother–baby at birth and during breast-feeding. Extremely rarely, HIV has been acquired following skin or mucous membrane exposure to contaminated blood. The risk of transmission after such exposure is estimated at about 1/300, although the risk is negligible if standard barrier precautions in the handling of bodily fluids are taken. There are no reported cases of transmission via kissing or food, drink or casual contact, from infected doctors to their patients, or from mosquito bites.

Epidemiology of HIV infection and AIDS

The number of people living with HIV continues to grow, as does the number of deaths due to AIDS. A total of 40–45 million people were living with HIV in 2006 — 2.6 million more than in 2004. Sub-Saharan Africa is the worst affected region: two thirds of HIV infected individuals live there as do more than three quarters (76%) of all women with HIV infection. Three quarters of all deaths due to AIDS in 2006 occurred in sub-Saharan Africa, where in 2005, there were 12.0 million AIDS orphans. South and South East Asia represent the second worst affected region with 15% of all cases. India has two thirds of HIV/AIDS infections in Asia (estimated 5.7 million infections), the highest number of HIV infections for a single country.

Data obtained between 2004 and 2006 show that the number of people living with HIV increased in every region in the world. The most striking increases have occurred in East Asia, in Eastern Europe and Central Asia, where the number of people with HIV increased by 20% in the 2004–2006 period. Globally more adult women than ever before are HIV positive.

In countries with low-level epidemics, most HIV infections occur in groups of the population with high-risk behaviours, including female sex workers and their clients, injecting drug users, and men who have sex with men.

In the UK, at the end of 2005 some 63 000 adults (15–59 years) were HIV positive, a third of whom were unaware of their infection. The number of documented HIV-infected individuals keeps rising, the main contributors to this increase being male homosexual intercourse, acquisition of the virus in Africa by heterosexual men and women; and earlier and more widespread HIV testing.

In the USA, the total number of people living with HIV (estimated at 1.2 million in 2005) also continues to increase, in great part due to the life-prolonging effects of anti-retroviral therapy. Risk factors included unsafe sex between men (44%), unprotected heterosexual intercourse (34%) and the use of non-sterile drug injecting equipment (17%)

Table 20.1 Rate of transmission of HIV according to risk behaviour

Risk behaviour	Rate of transmission
Receptive anal intercourse with infected partner	1/100–1/500 contacts
Heterosexual intercourse (infected male partner)	1/500–1/1000 contacts
Heterosexual intercourse (infected female partner)	1/1000–1/2000 contacts
Needlestick injury	Approximately 1/250
Child delivered of infected mother	1/3–1/8

(Table 20.1). The proportion of women among new HIV or AIDS diagnoses has increased dramatically — from 15% before 1995 to 27% in 2004. Racial and ethnic minorities continue to be disproportionately affected by the HIV epidemic. In the period spanning 2001–2004, 50% of AIDS diagnoses were among African Americans who constitute only 12% of the US population. An estimated one quarter are unaware of their HIV-infected status: they are thought to account for 54–70% of all new sexually transmitted HIV infections in the USA.

SUMMARY BOX 20.1

Epidemiology

- HIV causes an acquired immunodeficiency syndrome in which CD4 T helper cells are severely depleted.
- There are 35–45 million cases of HIV infection in the world at present and 2–3 million die each year from AIDS worldwide.
- Transmission of the virus is mainly sexual, with some disease acquired parenterally by intravenous drug abusers in the developed world.

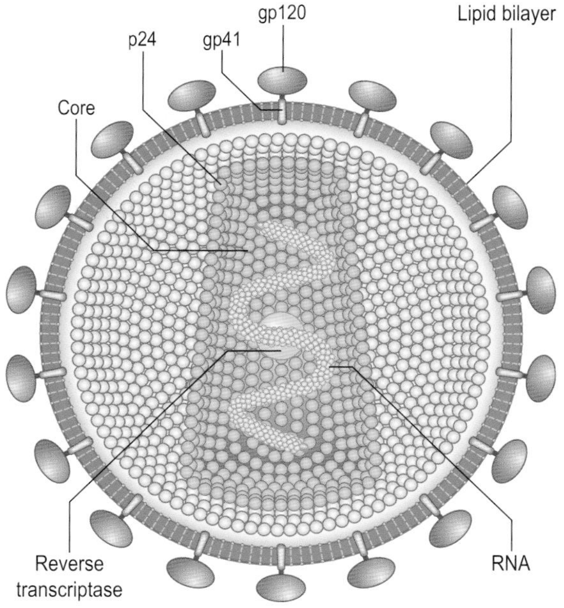

Fig. 20.2 The human immunodeficiency virus.
The envelope is made up of glycoproteins (gp) of 120 kDa and 41 kDa. The main core protein is p24. As an RNA virus, it relies on reverse transcriptase to produce complementary DNA for transcription and translation.

The human immunodeficiency virus

Detection of virus in blood samples stored in the USA from the mid-1970s, coupled with descriptions of AIDS-like illnesses in Africa during the same decade, suggest this, or closely preceding decades, as the period during which HIV began to appear in humans. It is now widely thought that HIV evolved from multiple cross-species transmission events from African non-human primates (mainly chimpanzees and sooty mangabeys) into humans. A similar type of agent, termed SIV (for simian immunodeficiency virus, which is most closely related to HIV-2), is a natural but non-lethal infection in African green monkeys. SIV causes an AIDS-like disease in captive rhesus monkeys and this is a useful model for evaluating vaccine strategies.

HIV is a member of the retrovirus family, which are small enveloped viruses containing a single-stranded RNA genome. Retroviruses are so named because their genomes encode the enzyme reverse transcriptase, capable of transcribing viral RNA into DNA, and thus allowing the virus to integrate into the host cell genome. Viral nucleic acid and replication enzymes are contained within a core surrounded by capsid proteins (Fig. 20.2). This in turn is enveloped by a lipid membrane, which is anchored internally to viral matrix proteins and crossed by integral envelope glycoproteins that protrude into the external milieu. The constituents of the virus are denoted by a p (for protein) or gp (for glycoprotein) followed by their molecular weight. Antibody responses to capsid, matrix and envelope proteins are detectable in the serum of infected

patients. For the most part, responses such as these, mainly to p24, are sufficient for diagnosis of infection. In the early primary HIV infection stage, before seroconversion and when free p24 in the blood is at levels below detection, very sensitive polymerase chain reaction amplification of viral transcripts may be used diagnostically. Most cases of infection with HIV will follow the pattern shown in Figure 20.3, in which p24 and anti-p24 antibody run a reciprocal course.

The HIV genome may be divided into three regions: one encoding the capsid and matrix proteins (*gag*), one the reverse transcriptase, a protease and an integrase (*pol*) and one the envelope proteins (*env*). Various other genes, including *tat*, *rev* and *nef*, have been identified as having regulatory effects on viral assembly, and drugs that modulate these functions are actively being sought. An understanding of the virus life cycle has been critical in informing inhibitory drug design. Key stages include attachment, fusion with the target cell membrane, reverse transcription to make viral DNA, followed by integration into the host DNA. It is noteworthy that the HIV reverse transcriptase is almost 'hard-wired' to make mistakes. It has no proof-reading capacity, and therefore gives rise to frequent mutations. This has probably been an important component of its successful transition across species of hosts, but also has grave implications for the mounting of a cell-mediated immune response (which is based on recognition of short viral peptides by T cells) and for the development of drug resistance. After transcription and translation, virus proteins are assembled into virions and the virus leaves the cell by budding through the host cell membrane. Some of the key viral proteins involved

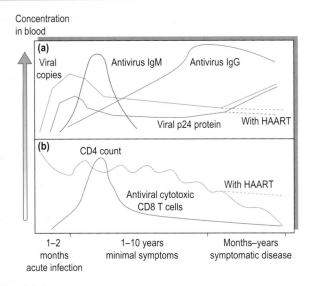

Fig. 20.3 **Pattern of virus replication and immune responses in acute, chronic and late stages of HIV infection.** (**a**) The graph shows the acute rise in concentration of viral RNA and p24 protein in the blood followed by a stabilisation of levels, presumably as a result of the actions of cytotoxic CD8 T cells and other elements of the immune response. Antibody levels (IgM then IgG) rise acutely and in the case of IgG remain high throughout disease. (**b**) The graph shows the early and catastrophic loss of CD4 cells in the circulation. The loss stabilises in association with the antiviral CD8 response emerging, but both decline during the asymptomatic period, until the CD4 count reaches 2–400 cells/µl of blood. At this point AIDS-defining illnesses are seen, unless HAART is commenced, in which case an amelioration of viral load and CD4 cell number is seen.

in these processes (reverse transcriptase, integrase and protease) are targets for highly successful anti-retroviral drug therapy.

Clinical aspects of HIV infection

There are three important aspects to clinical management of patients with suspected HIV/AIDS, namely the testing for evidence of HIV infection, the diagnosis of AIDS and the staging of disease.

HIV infection is diagnosed by testing serum for (i) the presence of anti-HIV antibodies or (ii) the presence of the virus protein called p24 antigen (see previous section on virus structure). Either of these appearing in the serum for the first time is evidence of HIV infection. Antibodies typically appear at detectable levels 3–4 weeks after virus exposure. UK guidelines stipulate that HIV testing should only be carried out with consent and that a confirmatory test is performed at least 14 days later.

After infection with HIV, different disease phases can be observed, related to the progressive pathogenic effects of the virus, and these have been moulded by the Center for Disease

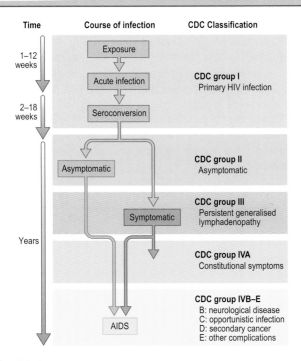

Fig. 20.4 **The CDC classification used to define stages of HIV-related illness.**

Control into a CDC classification (see Fig. 20.4). For patients in whom the time of virus exposure can be clearly documented, each of these phases may be observed progressively. More often, patients will present at later stages, as symptoms emerge (typically Group III and beyond). Primary HIV infection is very similar to a glandular-fever-like syndrome, with symptoms such as lymphadenopathy, fever, malaise, rash, sore throat and joint pains. Seroconversion after exposure is the point at which anti-HIV antibodies become detectable. It is now clear that this early phase of the illness is associated with large-scale loss of CD4 T cells as massive viral replication takes place (see p. 289). Viral load rises (measured by amplifying viral RNA from plasma and quantified as copies of virus per ml), and then falls as antibody levels increase (see Fig. 20.3). Patients at the asymptomatic Group II stage have low virus load, high circulating anti-HIV antibodies and a CD4 T cell count in the normal range. This phase may persist for many years (e.g. 10 or more), and is the period during which anti-retroviral drug therapy (ART) may be initiated (see p. 287). The decision to start ART is made on the basis of a change in the balance of CD4 count and viral load. Typically, ART is initiated as the CD4 count dwindles to $\sim350 \times 10^6$ cells/l of blood and the virus load begins to increase. Some patients also pass into, or are diagnosed at, the Group III stage of infection, with swelling of at least two extra-inguinal nodes in the absence of other cause. As disease progresses, patients enter the Group IV stage. Initially, this may involve constitutional symptoms and blood abnormalities (weight loss, mouth ulcers, disturbances in full blood count) but if untreated will progress to include disorders that define the illness as AIDS. The most widely accepted definition of AIDS, used in the UK, Europe and by the World

Table 20.2 Examples of commonly recognised AIDS-defining conditions

Disseminated *Mycobacterium avium* or *kansasii* infection
Pneumonia caused by *Pneumocystis carinii*
Cerebral toxoplasmosis
Progressive multifocal leukoencephalopathy
Kaposi's sarcoma in a patient under 60 years old
Candidiasis (affecting oesophagus, trachea, bronchi or lungs)
Cryptosporidiosis with diarrhoea persisting >1 month
Cytomegalovirus infection (at sites other than liver, spleen and lymph nodes)
Severe forms of herpes simplex infection

Health Organization, is that of an illness characterised by the presence of one or more indicator diseases, arising in the absence of another cause of immune deficiency. Some of the more commonly recognised indicator diseases are listed in Table 20.2. Most of these are opportunistic infections, arising as the cell-mediated immune response becomes impaired. In the USA, there has been a move to quantify this by using a definition of AIDS that includes severe immunosuppression, defined as a CD4 T cell count of $<200 \times 10^6$ cells/l of blood.

Laboratory immunological abnormalities in HIV infection

The absolute number of CD4 T lymphocytes in the peripheral blood has proved the most useful laboratory index of disease severity in HIV infection. The CD4 T cell count is measured by flow cytometry directly on whole blood (see p. 89) and is widely used clinically. Levels in asymptomatic patients are lower than in matched controls and there is progressive decline through the CDC stages of disease unless checked by introduction of highly active ART (Fig. 20.4). In contrast, CD8 T lymphocyte numbers are unaffected (normal value approximately 600×10^6 cells/l) in the early stages of HIV infection, or may be observed to rise, presumably as part of the antiviral response. Towards the end of the disease process the absolute CD8 count begins a precipitous decline, but it is not considered a useful laboratory marker. It is not just the absolute count of CD4 T cells that is diminished post-HIV infection. The CD4 T cells that are present are less able to respond functionally (e.g. by proliferation or

cytokine production, see p. 290) to recall antigens such as tetanus toxoid or mycobacterial extracts.

A host of other virus effects can be observed on cells of the innate and adaptive immune system, but they have little utility in disease management. CD4 and CD8 T lymphocytes often bear markers of chronic cellular activation (which may have important consequences, as this is a trigger of viral replication in CD4 cells). B cell number is unchanged, but there is a generalised, polyclonal increase in immunoglobulin levels (hypergammaglobulinaemia) with progressing disease affecting the IgG and IgA classes predominantly. The precise aetiology of this B cell abnormality is not known, but the excess Ig produced is not pathogen-specific and patients become at increasing risk of functional antibody deficiency. This may lead to infection with pyogenic organisms such as *Streptococcus pneumoniae*, against which antibodies would normally be protective. Response to immunisation tends to be poor, presumably due to a lack of CD4 T cell help.

Management of HIV infection

There is as yet no cure for HIV infection, but the advent of virus-retarding drugs and appropriate treatment of the complications of the disease has transformed life expectancy and quality of life. As discussed, the timing of initiation of therapy is a critical decision, based on clinical and laboratory evaluations. An increasingly better understanding of the components of HIV and its biology has allowed the development of therapies targeted at different stages of the virus life cycle. The first ART was azidothymidine (AZT), a reverse transcriptase inhibitor, introduced in 1995. It has been followed in subsequent years by similar drugs and others acting at different stages of virus replication (see Science Box 20.1). In current practice, it is typical to administer drugs in combination, leading to the term 'highly active' ART, or HAART. These drugs will usually target HIV reverse transcriptase and HIV protease. The different drugs are classified as nucleoside and non-nucleoside reverse transcriptase inhibitors (NRTI and NNRTI); protease inhibitors and boosted protease inhibitors (PI and BPI). Typical regimens are 3-drug combinations comprising NRTIs, NNRTIs and a PI/BPI. Recent evidence has suggested that those combinations that include an NNRTI and BPI offer improved reductions in viral load and infectious complications as well as increasing survival. Typically, HAART is accompanied by a dramatic improvement in laboratory parameters. More than 80% of patients have reduction in viral load to <50 copies/ml, and also see dramatic improvements in CD4 counts and other blood parameters. The initial expansion is of memory CD4 T cells and subsequently there is a repopulation of the blood with naïve, lymph-node homing CD4 T cells (see Clinical Box 20.1). Other studies suggest that the functional polarisation of the repopulating cells is also different, with a T_H1 bias that may have greater antiviral activity.

SCIENCE BOX 20.1

The cost of treating HIV infection

The introduction of HAART has been an important part of the battle against HIV, and its effect on survival times has been dramatic. In 1993 it was estimated that the average life expectancy of an adult with a CD4 count of $500 \times 10^6/l$ was 6–7 years. The introduction of AZT added 4 years onto this figure, and HAART has increased it by perhaps a further 15 years, on average. It is estimated that introduction of HAART in the UK has brought about a two thirds reduction of death from AIDS. This unprecedented enhancement of survival is most welcome in such a devastating disease, but does not come without a price. The first is economic. When this increased survival time and use of drug combinations is factored together, it is estimated that the lifetime cost of HAART is approximately £250,000. The total drug bill in the UK, then, might be £10 billion for the currently diagnosed 40,000 cases. Clearly, this is not a drug bill that non-developed countries, with much greater HIV burdens, can sustain. The second cost is that drug resistance is becoming an important consideration. None of the drugs or combinations achieve HIV eradication; rather they retard viral replication and select resistant strains. Typically the resistance gained by the virus is at some cost to its fitness, but it remains an important consideration that HAART is essentially enabling the longer survival of carriers of more and more resistant HIV strains.

CLINICAL BOX 20.1

The immune reconstitution inflammatory syndrome (IRIS)

The advent of HAART and its highly desirable effects on the immune system, in terms of enhancing lymphocyte counts, has brought with it a rare but interesting and novel set of diseases. These come under the umbrella term of IRIS, the immune reconstitution inflammatory syndrome. It is the 'paradoxical deterioration of the clinical status of a patient attributable to the recovery of the immune system following HAART'. Essentially it appears that the re-emergence of competent cellular immunity, in an individual that had become progressively more immune compromised, can give rise to the sudden appearance of disease. The most frequent occurrences of IRIS relate to infections present in a patient at the time of initiating HAART. For example, a patient with severe immune deficiency may not make an inflammatory immune response to *Mycobacterium avium* complex, *Cryptococcus neoformans*, or cytomegalovirus. However, shortly after receiving HAART, the re-acquisition of immune cell function that follows allows a sudden inflammatory response to the infection, which can lead to severe symptoms as tissues are infiltrated and become swollen. This can be particularly true in CNS infections, with sudden increases in intracranial pressure resulting in florid symptoms.

SUMMARY BOX 20.2

Clinical aspects

- The severity of HIV infection is indicated by the balance of CD4 T cell count and the number of viral copies in the blood; a clinical staging system (the 'CDC classification') is also widely used.
- Reduction in the absolute numbers of circulating CD4 T lymphocytes is the most striking laboratory abnormality, and the best monitor of disease severity.
- Management centres upon treatment of, and prophylaxis against, infectious complications, plus antiviral therapy with agents used in combination that target different stages of the virus life cycle.

The immunopathogenesis of HIV infection

In the early stages of infection some 10^9 virions are generated each day, and the circulating concentration of virus may be as high as 10^7 virions per ml of plasma.

Steady progress has been made in understanding how HIV causes AIDS. Undoubtedly the main component of the immunodeficiency is the CD4 T lymphopenia, and various mechanisms for this component of the pathogenesis have been invoked. A recent breakthrough in understanding has made it clear that this happens much earlier in the disease course than previously thought. Additional effects of the virus on other components of the innate and adaptive immune system are also undoubtedly important in the clinical outcome, and where relevant are discussed here.

CD4 is the HIV receptor; chemokine receptors form viral co-receptors

As soon as HIV had been isolated, the recognition that marked depletion of CD4 T lymphocytes was the hallmark of AIDS led to the identification of CD4 as the viral receptor (Fig. 20.5a). HIV has a tropism for cells bearing CD4, the accessory molecule that stabilises interactions with class II MHC in antigen recognition (p. 63). The envelope protein gp120 binds CD4 with a high affinity constant (K_d 10^{-9} M). HIV entry into the CD4 T cell is then facilitated by interaction with a surface chemokine receptor (Fig. 20.5b; usually CCR5 and CXCR4, see p. 26). In fact, during early infection the predominant cellular targets are T cells expressing CD4 and CCR5. Both molecules can also be found on monocytes, macrophages and dendritic cells (CD4 is present on these cells at low levels), and thus HIV is capable of infecting the major antigen presenting cells.

The envelope gp120 and gp41 anchor proteins exist as trimers on the HIV surface membrane. Interaction of a single gp120 in the trimer induces a change in conformation of the envelope protein and exposure of the V3 loop that interacts with CCR5. This further exposes a domain at the stalk of

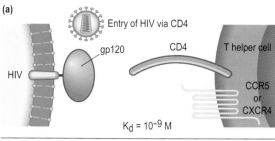

(a)

Entry of HIV via CD4

gp120

CD4

T helper cell

HIV

CCR5
or
CXCR4

$K_d = 10^{-9}$ M

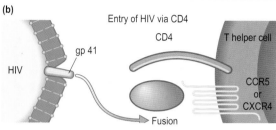

(b)

Entry of HIV via CD4

CD4

T helper cell

gp 41

HIV

CCR5
or
CXCR4

Fusion

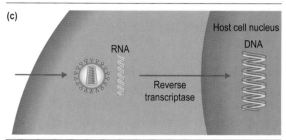

(c)

Host cell nucleus

RNA

DNA

Reverse
transcriptase

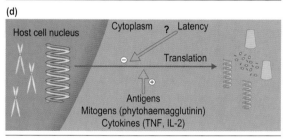

(d)

Host cell nucleus

Cytoplasm   ?   Latency

Translation

Antigens
Mitogens (phytohaemagglutinin)
Cytokines (TNF, IL-2)

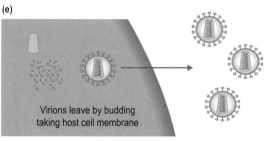

(e)

Virions leave by budding
taking host cell membrane

Fig. 20.5 HIV infection of a cell, from binding to the CD4 molecule to viral budding.
See text for details.

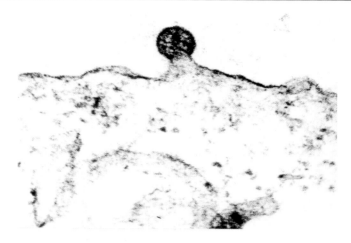

Fig. 20.6 Electron micrograph of HIV fusing with cell membrane of a CD4 T lymphocyte.
(From Stein et al. Cell 49: 659–668, with permission.)

gp41 that facilitates fusion with the target cell membrane (Figs 20.5b & 20.6). HIV is so dependent upon the interaction with CCR5 as the co-receptor that homozygosity for a naturally arising 32 base pair deletion in the CCR5 gene (called the CCR5-delta 32 mutation) affords complete protection from HIV infection. It is also significant to note that the gp120–CD4 interaction is very high affinity and that binding to CCR5 requires a conformation change. These features have meant that natural, and indeed artificial, neutralising anti-HIV antibodies do not exist, further hampering host immunity and vaccine development. Indeed, one of the earliest vaccine trials, conducted in 2005, was of a gp120 subunit, which had worked well in chimpanzee studies. However, it failed to provide protection among gay men and intravenous drug users, despite inducing antibodies in 90% of those vaccinated.

In response to HIV infection, the host mounts an adaptive immune response, including the co-ordinated effects of CD4 and CD8 T lymphocytes and antibodies. This response, however, is ineffective in adequately controlling infection. The ultimate consequences of unhindered viral replication are immune suppression and AIDS. A very small percentage of infected individuals are thought to control infection (so-called long-term non-progressors or LTNPs) and there is currently active research studying their anti-HIV immune response to decipher possible correlates of virus protection.

Once inside the CD4 T cell, the virus is uncoated and viral RNA transcribed to double-stranded DNA using the enzyme reverse transcriptase. The DNA is then circularised and inserted into the host cell genome. The fate of the infected cell may follow different courses. Active viral replication may lead to cell death, and many CD4 T cells are lost in this way (see below). The virus may also remain relatively non-replicative. What controls these two extremes is unknown, although the HIV genome has sequences within the 5′ region known as the long terminal repeats (LTRs) that are capable of binding host cell transcription factors. Thus, activation of the host CD4 T cell may activate viral replication (Fig. 20.5d). When the virus is assembled and leaves the cell, it does so by budding, incorporating host cell membrane into its coat (Figs 20.5e & 20.7).

Virus-mediated depletion of CD4 T cells

During the CDC group I, primary HIV infection stage, there is highly active viral replication. It is estimated that

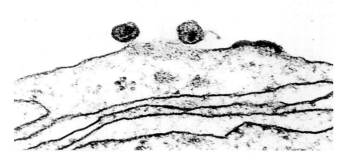

Fig. 20.7 **Electron micrograph of HIV virions budding from the cytoplasm of a CD4 T lymphocyte.**
(From Stein et al. Cell 49: 659–668, with permission.)

the viral copy number can rise as high as 10^8/ml. During this period the virus population may double every 6–10 hours and each infected cell can in turn infect 20 new cells. During this period, it is thought that there is mass destruction of the CD4$^+$ CCR5$^+$ T cell pool. These are memory cells, and many reside within the gut. The immune system never quite recovers from this loss, which accounts for many of the subtle functional defects that have been observed, such as the loss of recall responses. The virus-mediated death is relentless until, after a few weeks, viral load declines as the immune response kicks in, with production of antibodies and virus-specific CD4 T_H1 cells and cytotoxic CD8 T cells. A semblance of host–pathogen balance is established that may continue for years or decades. During this period, loss of CD4 T cells is slow and attritional, until symptoms of immune deficiency begin to arise at CDC group III–IV stages. Some studies suggest that during this period there is preferential loss of T_H1 responses, and default T_H2 dominance arises that is less effectively antiviral.

The molecular mechanisms through which HIV mediates cellular loss are not known with confidence. Some loss of infected CD4 T cells is attributable to the CD8 T cell response (see below). In vitro, HIV infection of CD4 T lymphocytes can lead to cell death in the absence of CD8 T cells, and three mechanisms have been observed. In the first, large numbers of viral particles budding simultaneously from the cell fuse with CD4 on the same cell's surface, destroying membrane integrity in an 'auto-fusion' process (Figs 20.7 & 20.8a). This mechanism is dependent upon a high concentration of surface CD4, as seen on T lymphocytes but not on macrophages and DCs, which could explain why they form an effective reservoir without being depleted. The second mechanism centres upon the observation in vitro that infected cells fuse to form large, multinucleate giant cell syncytia that have a markedly reduced half-life compared with intact cells (Figs 20.8b & 20.9). Finally, HIV-induced apoptosis can also be observed in vitro, as have other cytotoxic processes such as antibody-dependent cell cytotoxicity (ADCC) reactions (Fig. 20.8d; and see p. 113) in the presence of serum from HIV-infected patients.

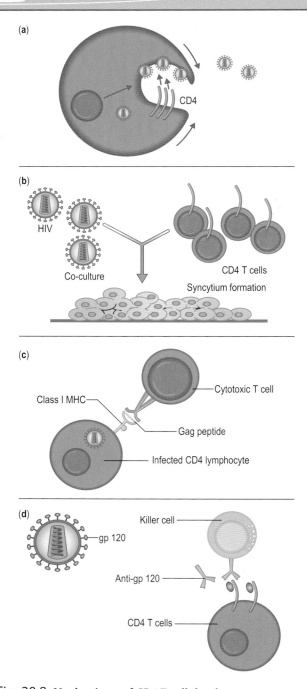

Fig. 20.8 **Mechanisms of CD4 T cell death.**
(**a**) Large-scale viral budding leads to 'auto-fusion'. (**b**) Cell death caused by fusion of cells to form giant cell syncytia. (**c**) Cytotoxic T cells can destroy target cells expressing class I MHC molecules presenting viral peptides (gag). (**d**) Antibody-dependent cell toxicity.

CD8 responses to HIV

As discussed, CD8 cytotoxic T lymphocyte (CTL) responses to HIV are early and robust. An indication of the importance of the CD8 response is given by the fact that certain HLA class I types (HLA-B*27, B*51 and B*57) are associated with slow progression of disease and others (HLA-B*35) with more rapid progression. Individuals who are homozygous

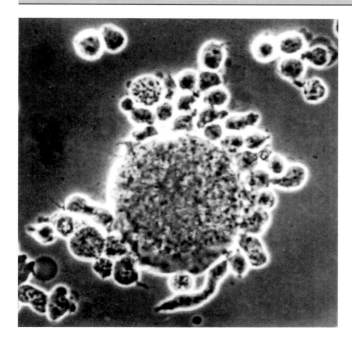

Fig. 20.9 CD4 T lymphocytes cultured with HIV forming a large syncytium by repeated cell–cell fusions.
(From Stein et al. Cell 49: 659–668, with permission.)

for any of the HLA class I alleles also progress more rapidly. How are these data to be explained? It is thought that the CTL response is largely responsible for arresting and controlling viral replication. HLA class I allele homozygosity is thought to be bad simply because it compromises the ability to mount a broad response to multiple epitopes. The fact that some HLA class I molecules are 'good' or 'bad' for protection from HIV suggests that they present a critical epitope. What might constitute a critical epitope? One strong possibility is that a key epitope is one that the virus cannot mutate without catastrophic loss of function. Remember, HIV is highly mutable because of its 'faulty' reverse transcriptase. It is estimated that at the peak of infection, $\sim 10^9$ new virions are produced each day. HIV reverse transcriptase induces a mutation every 10^5 base pairs, and in a virus of 10^4 bases, every possible mutation could be made each day. This allows CTL escape — mutation of critical peptide sequences presented by HLA class I molecules and targeted by CTLs. As long as the virus can adapt to the change in structure, the mutated form will acquire a survival advantage. It is plausible that HLA-class I molecules encoded by B*27, B*51 and B*57 genes present peptides that HIV cannot afford to alter, accounting for the survival advantage they confer. CTL escape, of course, has important implications for vaccine design.

Antigen presenting cells and HIV

As stated, dendritic cells and macrophages express low levels of CD4 and CCR5, and therefore represent possible targets of HIV infection. Moreover, these cells are present at the major sites of viral entry (mucosal surfaces). Some studies have estimated that up to 90% of initial HIV dissemination

after virus introduction at the mucosa is attributable to DCs. There is, indeed, strong evidence that DCs are capable of ingesting HIV particles. In addition to CD4 and CCR5, DC-SIGN (for DC-specific, ICAM-3-grabbing non-integrin, CD209) binds HIV directly to facilitate viral entry. Actual infection of DCs by HIV is probably 10 to 100-fold less efficient than for CD4 T cells. However, DCs may play an important role in bringing virus from the periphery to the local lymph node. DCs can transfer HIV to T cells without even being infected (so-called *trans*-infection), possibly via surface molecules such as DC-SIGN, or be productively infected and release virions into the local nodes (*cis*-infection).

SUMMARY BOX 20.3

HIV immunopathogenesis

- HIV is an RNA retrovirus, relying upon a reverse transcriptase to translate its genome into DNA: this and other essential enzymes are potential drug targets.
- The key event is an early, catastrophic loss of memory CD4 T cells from gut and peripheral lymph nodes.
- A strong tendency to mutate is an important feature of virus pathogenicity, giving it an ability to become drug resistant and avoid CTL responses.
- The predominant effect of HIV infection is depletion of CD4 T lymphocytes, but B cell and DC/macrophage immunity is also compromised.
- The precise mechanism by which HIV mediates destruction of CD4 T lymphocytes is unknown.

Vaccines

While a vaccine remains the best hope of controlling HIV infection, there are numerous issues that overshadow the quest for an effective, inexpensive and safe immunisation regimen to protect against HIV infection.

The challenges:

1. Virus can survive and be transmitted within a host and between hosts both in extracellular (i.e. blood-borne virus particles) and intracellular (hidden within infected host cells) forms.

2. HIV copies its genome into the host cell. This means that any form of live attenuated virus vaccine (one of the most successful approaches to vaccine development) is fraught with a key safety issue, namely could the virus in the vaccine revert to wild type?

3. The virus has multiple strains and a very high mutability, which is challenging for a vaccine using fixed virus sequences. The question is, can one vaccine fit all?

4. No small animal model of HIV infection exists; efficacy studies are therefore often carried out in non-human primates, which are expensive and require the use of surrogates for HIV.

5. The nature of protective immunity against HIV is not known. The study of long-term non-progressors has yet to provide clear answers as to how their healthy status is maintained.

6. Neutralising antibodies do not exist, and to achieve them may be an unrealistic goal.

7. The virus may be able to escape CTL killing.

The possible options:

1. Sterile immunity would be a vaccine approach that prevents viral entry or the early transmission phase. As discussed, this is complicated by the inability to find neutralising antibodies against HIV that would protect mucosal and other entry sites. There is the added problem of *trans-* and *cis*-infection.

2. Protective immunity (in which the infection is allowed but controlled) is countered by the argument that, thus far, infection always seems to lead to disease.

Protective immunity will also require very high vaccination levels in the population, since infected, protected individuals will remain able to pass on the virus, at least theoretically. Another option is to prevent infection completely, so-called 'sterile immunity'. This requires a constant, high level of protection, which may be difficult to maintain.

Despite these potential blocks to translation of the basic science discoveries, there is a considerable drive to test vaccine approaches and see whether any of them induce a glimmer of hope in terms of a therapeutic effect. A vaccine based on gp120, that was initially disappointing in early human trials (see above), is the focus of a large study (16 000 participants) in Thailand, on the basis of some evidence of a preferential effect in Asians. Another large study (6000 volunteers) is using a recombinant adenovirus, genetically engineered to carry HIV genes (*gag, pol* and *nef*). Of course, the scale of the HIV problem is such that even a small effect could protect many individuals. With 14 000 people infected each day worldwide, even a 10% effective vaccine would make a substantial difference to the global disease burden.

Up-to-date information on these and other clinical trials of HIV vaccines can be obtained from the International AIDS Vaccine Initiative (www.iavi.org) and the Center for HIV-AIDS Vaccine Immunology (www.chavi.org).

SUMMARY BOX 20.4

Vaccines

- The biology of HIV and the complexity of the host response make this a challenging scientific and clinical arena.
- Nonetheless, large-scale therapeutic trials are in progress, and even small measures of successful vaccination will provide an important platform for future success.

Further reading

Adler MW (ed) 2001 ABC of AIDS, 5th edn. BMJ Books: London

Devadas K, Lal RB, Dhawan S 2005 Immunology of HIV-1. In: Gendelman HE, Grant I, Everall IP, Lipton SA, Swindells S (eds) The neurology of AIDS, 2nd edn. Oxford University Press: Oxford

Goulder PJ, Watkins DI 2004 HIV and SIV CTL escape: implications for vaccine design. Nat Rev Immunol 4(8): 630–640

Hel Z, McGhee JR, Mestecky J 2006 HIV infection: first battle decides the war. Trends Immunol 27: 274–281

Letvin NL 2006 Progress and obstacles in the development of an AIDS vaccine. Nat Rev Immunol 6(12): 930–939

Rogstad K, Palfreeman A, Rooney G, Hart GJ, Lowbury R, Mortimer P et al 2006 UK national guidelines on HIV testing 2006. Int J STD AIDS 17: 668–676

Veazey RS, Lackner AA 2005 HIV swiftly guts the immune system. Nat Med 11: 469–470

Weiss RA 2008 Speical anniversary review: twenty-five years of human immunodeficiency virus research: successes and challenges. Clin Exp Immunol 152: 201–210

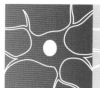

Immunological manifestations of haematological disease

Malignant neoplastic expansions of red and white blood cells give rise to diseases such as leukaemia, lymphoma and myeloma. The diagnosis and management of the neoplastic diseases of blood are largely the realm of the haematologist, and these aspects are not covered in any depth in this chapter. The effects of such diseases on the functioning of immune cells are several. First, marrow replacement by malignant cells and suppression of normal haemopoiesis may result in reduced or defective generation of healthy immune effectors, such as neutrophils, leading to **secondary immunodeficiency**. Second, a malignant neoplastic expansion of cells of the B lymphocyte lineage can lead to disease as a result of an inability to regulate normal antibody production (i.e. **secondary antibody deficiency**).

Finally, **autoimmune disorders** may arise, either as a consequence of the nature of antibody produced by a neoplastic clone or as a result of defective immune regulation. These are secondary immune manifestations of malignant haematological cancers.

Autoimmune diseases affecting white and red blood cells result in shortening of cell survival and cytopenias (reduction in cell numbers) if production cannot compensate. These conditions may arise as primary disorders, or as complications of haematological malignancies, autoimmune disease, infections or drug therapy.

Autoimmune diseases of the blood

Autoimmune haemolytic anaemia

Autoimmune haemolytic anaemia (AHA) is a relatively uncommon disease, which, in its mildest form, may manifest as a compensated normochromic normocytic anaemia but may rarely present acutely as a life-threatening haemolytic disease. It may arise as a primary condition, or secondary to a range of other malignant, autoimmune or inflammatory diseases (Fig. 21.1). The cause of the haemolysis is the presence of circulating autoantibodies to red blood cell surface antigens, which reduces the survival of red blood cells. The bone marrow compensates for the reduced survival by increasing cell production. It is the combination of reduced survival, increased production and increased metabolism of haem that makes up the clinical and laboratory manifestations of haemolytic anaemia.

One of the features of these disorders is the distinctive physicochemical nature of some of the autoantibodies. The majority (80–90%) of anti-red blood cell autoantibodies react optimally with their targets at physiological temperatures (i.e. 37°C) and are termed **warm** autoantibodies. The remainder (**cold** autoantibodies, ~13%) react best with their targets at temperatures below 37°C.

Warm autoimmune haemolytic anaemia

The so-called warm AHAs are a result of circulating red blood cells becoming coated with IgG. Complement components are also frequently deposited on the red blood cell surface and, when present, are associated with more severe haemolysis. Warm autoantibodies are usually directed against rhesus (Rh) antigens — or rhesus associated antigens — but

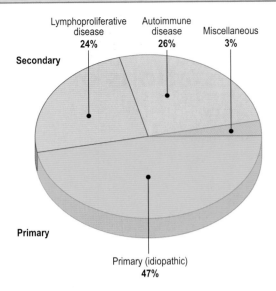

Fig. 21.1 **Causes of autoimmune haemolytic anaemia.**

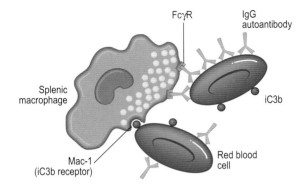

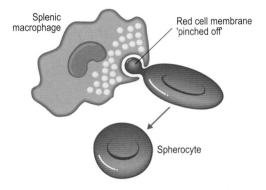

Fig. 21.2 **Development of spherocytes in warm AHA.**
IgG- and complement iC3b-coated red blood cell membranes are 'pinched off' by splenic macrophages, resulting in spherocytes that are more susceptible to mechanical stress and haemolysis.

the exact autoantibody specificity is not frequently identified, since it adds little to the management of the condition. Typically, the red blood cells become sequestered in the spleen and, occasionally, the liver, where macrophage-derived cells express receptors for IgG (FcγRI and FcγRIII) and for C3b, iC3b and C4. Here, phagocytosis either results in the engulfment of whole red blood cells, or 'pinching off' of segments of membrane (Fig. 21.2). The loss of membrane leads to development of spherical-shaped cells (spherocytes), which are more susceptible to further damage from mechanical stress.

There are a number of causes of warm AHA:

- idiopathic warm AHA
- secondary types:
  - connective tissue disease, e.g. SLE, rheumatoid arthritis
  - autoimmune disease, e.g. autoimmune hepatitis
  - lymphoproliferative disorders, e.g. chronic lymphocytic leukaemia, non-Hodgkin's lymphoma
  - viral infections, e.g. hepatitis B virus infection
  - drugs.

Patients with warm AHA may be asymptomatic or present with the symptoms and signs of the anaemia or of the underlying disorder. On examination, there may be an enlarged spleen. Typical laboratory findings are of a normochromic normocytic anaemia. On the blood film, there may be polychromasia (an indication of increased red blood cell production) and spherocytosis, reticulocytosis (increased immature red blood cells), a raised serum bilirubin and urinary urobilinogen. Investigation of the bone marrow reveals hyperplasia of the erythroid lineage. The key laboratory assay is the **Coombs'** or **antiglobulin test**. The Coombs' reagent is an animal antiserum raised against human globulins (sometimes termed antiglobulin) and, therefore, it contains antibodies to immunoglobulins (mainly IgG, IgA, IgM) and complement components. When incubated with the patient's washed red blood cells, in the **direct Coombs' test**, the Coombs' reagent causes agglutination (Fig. 21.3). This screening test can be followed by one using more selective antisera to IgG or complement components to establish the nature of the immune coating on the red blood cell surface. Typically, red blood cells are found to be coated with IgG alone (30% of patients), complement alone (20%) or both (50%).

The approach to therapy in warm AHA includes the diagnosis and appropriate management of any underlying diseases. In addition, warm AHA can be treated with immunosuppression (e.g. corticosteroids, antimetabolites such as methotrexate, and ciclosporin). These usually have a beneficial effect in 90% of patients, but greater levels of immunosuppression or splenectomy may be required in chronic or intractable disease (Fig. 21.4). In a small proportion, splenectomy may not help as red blood cell destruction may relocalise to the liver.

Cold autoimmune haemolytic anaemia

Cold AHA can arise from a number of causes:

- idiopathic cold AHA
- secondary types:

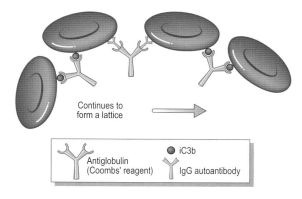

Fig. 21.3 Direct Coombs' test.
The antiglobulin, added to red blood cells coated with IgG autoantibodies and deposited complement components (e.g. iC3b), causes cross-linking of red blood cells, to give a lattice; agglutination is apparent to the naked eye.

— lymphoproliferative disorders, e.g. chronic lymphocytic leukaemia

— infections, e.g. *Mycoplasma pneumoniae*, Epstein–Barr virus.

In cold AHA the autoantibodies are typically optimal in their reactivity at between 0 and +5°C. Cold AHA may be a chronic condition, in which case it arises most frequently as an idiopathic disease. Alternatively it may be a transient, self-limiting complication of an infection with agents such as *Mycoplasma pneumoniae* or Epstein–Barr virus. The antibodies giving rise to cold AHA are termed **cold agglutinins** (hence the other term, **cold haemagglutinin disease** or CHAD for this syndrome). The agglutinins are usually of the IgM class and directed against red blood cell antigens of the I/i system. In vivo, the cold agglutinins combine with their targets when the circulation is exposed to slightly lower temperatures, as in the fingers, ear lobes and nose. Under these circumstances of a transient vascular 'window' in which agglutination may occur, extensive haemolysis is rare. More typically, the complement classical pathway is activated to a limited degree with deposition of the opsonins C3b, iC3b and C4b on the red blood cell surface, in addition to the IgM autoantibody. This is an important point, since macrophages do not have receptors for IgM, and in cold AHA these phagocytes will only clear cells coated with complement. Clearance of opsonised red blood cells in cold agglutinin disease typically occurs in the liver.

Clinically, patients with cold AHA may be asymptomatic, having a mild haemolytic anaemia with or without evidence of vaso-occlusion in the periphery, which leads to a bluish skin tinge termed acrocyanosis. Indeed, one of the most frequent presentations is associated with red blood cell indices analysed on automated cell counters. Agglutinating red blood cells give a spuriously high mean cell volume and mean cell haemoglobin, which return to normal if the sample is warmed to 37°C and reanalysed. In the laboratory tests, the direct Coombs' test is usually positive for complement only: IgM is loosely bound on the red blood cell surface and tends to be lost in the washing steps. Treatment of the idiopathic disease

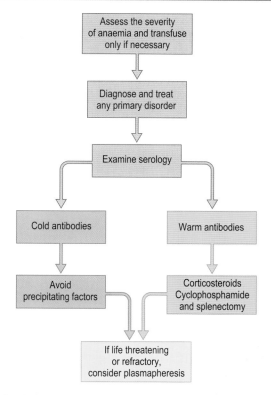

Fig. 21.4 Management of autoimmune haemolytic anaemia.

is centred around avoidance of the cold, though immunosuppression may also be required. Removal of the spleen is ineffective, since it is not the main site of haemolysis. Cold AHA secondary to infections is self-limiting and rarely causes significant haemolysis.

Paroxysmal cold haemoglobinuria (PCH)

This is a complication of infections. Congenital and tertiary syphilis were the most common causes, but the decline in that infection means that PCH is exceedingly rare, although it can occur in a chronic idiopathic form or transiently, and especially in children, as a complication of viral infections (notably with Epstein–Barr virus). The IgG autoantibody involved is unusual (termed the Donath–Landsteiner antibody) since it binds to the P antigen on red blood cells in the cold but dissociates in the warm. In a typical paroxysm occurring in the cold or in an exposed limb, the IgG autoantibody binds, recruiting classical pathway complement components, which are deposited on the red blood cell surface. As the red blood cells warm, the lytic membrane attack complex becomes activated, and a brief episode of intravascular haemolysis, with resulting haemoglobinuria, takes place.

Drug-induced haemolysis

Drug-induced haemolysis may arise as an immune-mediated process with certain therapeutic agents. At least three well-defined mechanisms have been described (Fig. 21.5). The most common results in a haemolytic syndrome indistinguishable from warm AHA, in which IgG autoantibodies to Rh antigens are formed. This form of drug-induced haemolysis has been most frequently associated with α-methyldopa, a drug formerly used in hypertension but now rarely prescribed. Some 20% of patients on treatment developed a positive direct Coombs' test, and 1% had clinically relevant haemolysis. The precise mechanism by which anti-Rh autoantibodies develop secondary to such drug therapy is unclear. The most plausible theory is that the drug binds to red blood cell surface antigens, rendering them immunogenic in the process. This may operate through a T cell bypass mechanism (see Ch. 9) in which the drug provides a new T cell epitope on the red blood cell surface antigen, to bypass the existing control of potentially autoreactive anti-rhesus B lymphocytes.

In the second and third mechanisms, it has been postulated that the drugs act as haptens: in other words they need to bind to a macromolecule in order to become immunogenic. In one process (typically associated with penicillin and the cephalosporins), the drug requires attachment to a

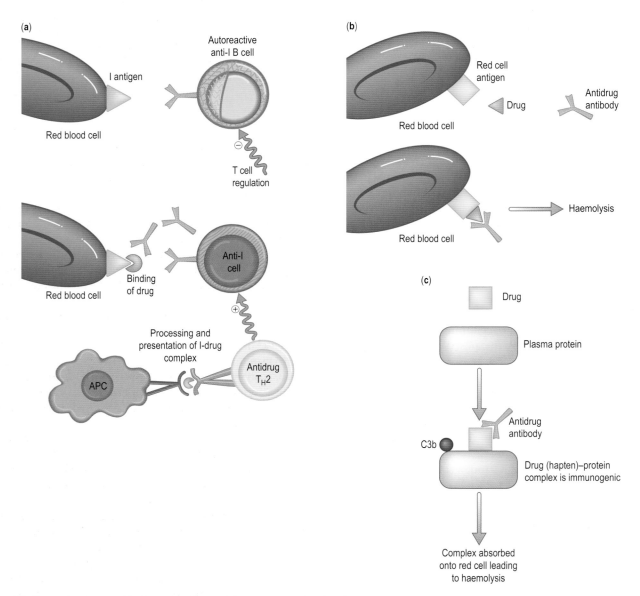

Fig. 21.5 Mechanisms of induction of haemolytic autoantibodies by drugs.
(a) In healthy individuals, anti-I antibodies are not produced because autoreactive B cells are controlled by regulatory T cells. Binding of drug to the I antigen may lead to processing and presentation of the complex, which behaves as a novel antigen. A T$_H$2 lymphocyte reactive with epitopes on the I-drug antigen promotes autoantibody production, bypassing the T cell control. (b) The drug, behaving like a hapten, is not antigenic until bound to a macromolecule, in this case a red blood cell surface protein. The drug now induces antibody production, indirectly targeting the red blood cell. (c) The haptenic drug complexes with a plasma protein to induce antidrug antibodies. The immune complex formed is adsorbed onto the red blood cell, which is now prone to phagocytosis in the spleen.

What is the explanation for drug-induced haemolysis?

Although the three explanations given in the text are popular accounts for drug-induced direct Coombs' test-positive haemolysis, there are several flaws in the argument. First, two of the mechanisms rely upon drug binding to the red blood cell surface, yet this is very difficult to demonstrate convincingly. Second, two of the mechanisms rely upon the drug becoming a hapten after binding to the red blood cell surface or plasma-derived proteins. However, according to the classical theory (see p. 296) a hapten becomes the target of the antibody. Therefore, it should be possible to adsorb out antidrug antibodies from a patient's serum using the free drug; again, this has not been demonstrable.

An explanation, which unites all of the theories as well as their flaws, is as follows. The drug, or its metabolite, binds to

the red blood cell surface and creates a complex termed a 'neoantigen'. For example, an epitope on the neoantigen might be composed of part of the drug and part of a red blood cell protein. Antibodies to the neoantigen lead to haemolysis. Since it is a neoantigen, pure drug alone will not adsorb out the antibodies. In addition, the generation of an immune response to the neoantigen on the red blood cell allows the production of true 'auto' antibodies, through T cell bypass. These autoantibodies could target the Rh system, a group of red blood cell surface antigens frequently involved in Coombs' test-positive drug-induced haemolysis. Understandably, the 'neoantigen' theory is difficult to prove, but it remains an attractive compromise.

protein molecule on the erythrocyte surface before antibodies are generated. These then bind drug–cell complexes and the cells are open to immune damage. In the final proposed mechanism, used to account for haemolysis associated with quinine-based drugs, the hapten (drug) binds to a soluble plasma protein to become immunogenic. The immune complex subsequently formed is adsorbed onto the red blood cell surface through recruitment of classical complement components, and haemolysis results (see Science Box 21.1).

Autoimmune thrombocytopenia

Destruction of platelets by immune mechanisms is a much more common clinical problem than autoimmune haemolysis. Again, the syndrome may be primary (**idiopathic thrombocytopenic purpura; ITP**) or occur as an **autoimmune thrombocytopenia** (**ATP**) secondary to a range of disorders:

- Virus infection: occurs frequently in childhood with common viruses, usually follows acute infection by 3 weeks; HIV.

- Autoimmune disease: SLE; rheumatoid arthritis; autoimmune hepatitis.

- Lymphoproliferative disorders: chronic lymphocytic leukaemia; non-Hodgkin's lymphoma.

- Drugs: similar mechanisms to haemolytic syndromes are presumed.

Purpura in ITP refers to the purple skin rash that typically appears in any form of thrombocytopenia, resulting from subcutaneous haemorrhages. Other clinical presentations include bruising and, in severe disease, active mucosal bleeding (bleeding gums or nose, melaena, bleeding per rectum, haematuria, fundal haemorrhage). Any secondary disease or associated cytopenia may also be apparent.

The laboratory diagnosis is made on the platelet count (usually $<80 \times 10^9/l$). Bone marrow response to thrombo-

cytopenia, in the form of increased production, may be detected on a bone marrow aspiration as elevated numbers of megakaryocytes or in the blood as an increase in the mean platelet volume, since immature platelets are large. Various assays for the detection of platelet-bound and circulating anti-platelet autoantibodies may be performed, all based on the principle of the Coombs' test. Typically bound or circulating autoantibody of the IgG class is detected (>90%) but IgM and IgA autoantibodies may also be detected in up to half the patients. In some 70% of patients the autoantibodies are directed against the platelet glycoprotein complexes IIb–IIIa or Ib–IX.

The pathogenesis of autoimmune platelet destruction revolves around the presence of surface-bound autoantibody. IgG autoantibodies probably lead to platelet loss in the spleen, in a process analogous to that of warm AHA. IgM anti-platelet autoantibodies are presumed to operate through the recruitment of complement. Autoantibodies may interfere with the role of platelets in haemostasis, leading to platelet dysfunction.

In secondary autoimmune thrombocytopenia, the management of the primary disease should be addressed. In autoimmune thrombocytopenia, through whatever cause, the platelet count can be increased in 80% of patients by the administration of corticosteroids. Intravenous immunoglobulin (IVIG) may be used, either to enhance the response rate to steroids or as a means of elevating the platelet count immediately prior to surgery (e.g. splenectomy). IVIG is thought to operate through blockade of splenic Fc receptors, halting the phagocytic destruction of platelets. As such, it has also been used in haemolytic anaemia. However, it provides a transient respite in the disease, is relatively expensive to administer and offers no long-term cure in either condition. When reduced levels of platelets lead to evidence of mucosal blood loss, there is a real risk of intracranial haemorrhage. This life-threatening complication should be treated with platelet infusions and high-dose corticosteroids combined with IVIG. In refractory ATP there have been reports of successful use of the anti-CD 20 monoclonal antibody (Rituximab).

Autoimmune neutropenia

Primary autoimmune neutropenia (AIN) is a rare disease typically affecting infants. The low neutrophil concentrations in the blood and tissues gives rise to infectious diseases typical of this type of immune deficiency (see p. 277). A large series of patients indicated that the neutropenia arises as a primary disease in some two thirds of patients and secondary to other diseases in the remainder.

Primary AIN is typically a disease of infancy, arising within the first 3 years of life. Children usually present in the first year of life with infections of moderate severity (impetigo, folliculitis, otitis media), although pneumonia, meningitis and septicaemia may also be seen. The leukocyte count is usually normal or decreased, with an absolute neutrophil count less than 0.5×10^9/l. IgG anti-neutrophil antibodies are detectable in more than 90% of patients using assays akin to the Coombs' test for agglutination or by direct immunofluorescence to demonstrate IgG bound to the neutrophil surface. Several target antigens on the neutrophil surface have been identified, including one associated with the $Fc\gamma$RIII. The aetiology of primary AIN is still debated. An association with recent viral infection has not been demonstrated, but a higher incidence in individuals carrying *HLA-DR15* (*DR2*) has been reported. The early age of onset supports one hypothesis, namely that in these infants there is a relative immaturity of immune regulation, allowing autoantibodies to develop. However, whilst this explanation is plausible, one would expect that if such a mechanism operates many other autoimmune diseases would also be more common in this age group. The disease is usually self-limiting with spontaneous recovery by the age of 3 years in the majority, and therapy may be restricted to therapeutic or prophylactic use of antibiotics.

Secondary AIN arises in adulthood in the context of other autoimmune blood cytopenias, lymphoproliferative disorders, other autoimmune diseases (typically SLE and rheumatoid arthritis) and in association with some infections such as those caused by Epstein–Barr virus and HIV. Some patients with secondary AIN have anti-neutrophil cytoplasmic antibody (ANCA) in their circulation.

SUMMARY BOX 21.1

Autoimmune diseases of the blood

- Autoimmunity leading to antibody coating of circulating blood cells and platelets, frequently resulting in a reduction in cell or platelet survival with consequent clinical symptoms and signs, is a common problem in clinical haematology.
- A variety of underlying conditions, ranging from infective and inflammatory disorders to haematological

---

SUMMARY BOX 21.1

Autoimmune diseases of the blood—cont'd

malignancies, as well as the administration of numerous drugs, are associated with development of the autoimmune cytopenias.

- Autoantibodies in autoimmune haemolytic anaemias are detected by the Coombs' test and have distinctive physicochemical (warm- versus cold-reacting) properties.
- The disorders may be self-limiting or may require immunosuppression and splenectomy.

Alloimmune diseases of the blood

Haemolytic disease of the newborn

Haemolytic disease of the newborn (HDN) results from maternal IgG directed against antigens on the fetal red blood cell surface crossing the placenta and mediating immune destruction of erythrocytes. Transfer of antibody across the placenta is limited in the first 22 weeks of pregnancy but increases rapidly thereafter. The red blood cell antigens targeted in over 90% of patients are those of the Rh D system. Alloantibodies to fetal red blood cell antigens typically arise in the mother following sensitisation resulting from fetal haemorrhage into the maternal circulation following delivery, spontaneous or therapeutic abortion, or invasive procedures (e.g. chorionic villus sampling). In the late 1960s, human anti-D antiserum was introduced as a prophylactic measure and has been a successful means of reducing the incidence of HDN caused by such fetal–maternal haemorrhage. Not all such 'spontaneous' HDN has been eradicated, however, as other blood group mismatches occur (e.g. the ABO and Kell systems).

HDN arises when fetal red blood cells bear red blood cell antigens not present on maternal cells. For example, the mother may be negative for a Rh antigen such as D and the fetus positive. The Rh D⁻ phenotype is present in 17% of the Caucasian population. Antigens of the Rh blood system are particularly immunogenic, since an injection of as little as 0.03 ml of D⁺ red blood cells is capable of inducing antibody production, and approximately 0.5 ml will induce antibodies in 50% of Rh D⁻ recipients. Transfer of fetal red blood cells into the maternal circulation is rare until the third trimester, but by term between 5 and 10% of women carry more than 0.5 ml of fetal blood in their circulation. This opportunity for sensitisation, therefore, usually occurs too late in the first pregnancy to be of clinical importance but may establish anti-D production in the mother as a threat to subsequent pregnancies. Clinically, HDN varies in severity from death of the fetus in utero to oedema, with cardiac failure, bilirubinaemia and anaemia, all of varying severity, at birth.

The incidence of HDN in the past 50 years has fallen, both as family sizes have contracted and following the introduction of anti-D antiserum. Current practice is that pregnant women are blood group typed and screened for alloantibodies, and Rh D⁻ mothers are identified. Anti-D antiserum is then administered as an intramuscular injection within 72 hours of the birth of a Rh D⁺ baby, at a dose of 100 µg (500 iu). This will compensate for fetal–maternal haemorrhage of up to 4 ml. Larger doses are needed for bleeding in excess of this, which occurs only rarely (<1% deliveries) and can be assessed by examining the maternal circulation for fetal red blood cells (the Kleihauer technique identifies red blood cells bearing fetal haemoglobin). Mothers undergoing spontaneous or therapeutic abortion who are Rh D⁻ should be given 50 µg anti-D. For routine antenatal prophylaxis, two doses of at least 100 µg should be given at 28 and then at 34 weeks' gestation.

How successful is the anti-D prophylaxis and how does it work? Sensitisation to fetal red blood cell antigens is avoided if the mother and fetus are incompatible for the ABO blood system (anti-A and anti-B antibodies in the mother remove the fetal cells) (Fig. 21.6). In pregnancy involving Rh D⁻ mothers, carrying an ABO compatible Rh D⁺ fetus, it is estimated that a sensitisation rate of 17% is reduced to 1.5% with anti-D prophylaxis. The mortality in the UK resulting from HDN is approximately 4 per 100 000 births per year. In these cases sensitisation of the mother to D or other antigens has either occurred early in the first pregnancy, through transfusion mismatch, or because an insufficient dose of anti-D antiserum was given. It is presumed that prophylactic anti-D antibodies mediate their beneficial effect by coating any fetal cells transferred and that these are then removed in the spleen rapidly, with destruction of the D antigen and no opportunity for antigen persistence and sensitisation.

Once the diagnosis of HDN is established, treatment may commence in utero or after birth, with exchange transfusion. This corrects the anaemia, removes bilirubin and circulating antibodies and can enhance red blood cell life if Rh D⁻ cells are given to replace the susceptible Rh D⁺ ones.

Other alloimmune diseases of the blood

Red blood cells are not the only cells that bear surface alloantigens and may cross into the maternal circulation to generate alloresponsiveness of potential danger to the fetus. Neonatal alloimmune thrombocytopenia is now more recognised as the incidence of HDN has waned. In addition, transfusion-related alloantibodies against targets on red blood cells and platelets may give rise to clinically relevant cytopenias.

SUMMARY BOX 21.2

Alloimmune diseases of the blood

■ The production of antibodies directed against alloantigens encountered on the surface of circulating blood cells and platelets can have potentially serious consequences. This is best exemplified by the production of IgG antibodies to red blood cell rhesus antigens in a rhesus-negative mother bearing a rhesus-positive fetus, giving rise to intrauterine death or haemolytic disease of the newborn.

■ Possibly one of the earliest examples of immunotherapy in the era of modern immunology is the administration of anti-rhesus D antigen antiserum prophylactically to pregnant women at risk of allosensitisation.

■ Allosensitisation remains a real risk in pregnancy and in the post-transfusion period.

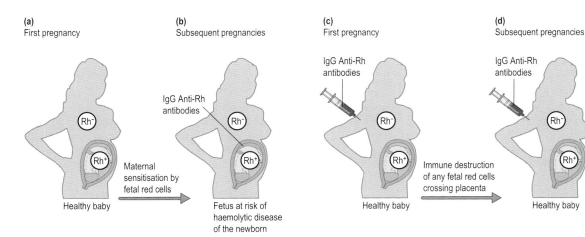

Fig. 21.6 Immunoprevention of haemolytic disease of newborn.
(**a**) In the first pregnancy of an Rh-negative mother, the baby is normal but Rh positive, and at some point (e.g. during delivery) fetal red blood cells cross into the maternal circulation, giving rise to production of IgG anti-Rhesus antibodies. (**b**) During subsequent pregnancies, the IgG antibodies cross the placenta and cause fetal anaemia and heart failure. (**c**) Prevention relies on removing the red cells as they cross the placenta by administering anti-Rhesus antibody to the mother, e.g. at delivery. (**d**) This prevents sensitisation but must be given in all subsequent pregnancies as well.

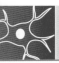

Neoplastic disease of cells of the B lymphocyte lineage

Malignant monoclonal proliferations of cells of the B lymphocyte lineage lead to numerous different clinical manifestations, largely dependent upon the stage of maturation of the B cell at the time of malignant transformation. Neoplastic expansions of mature antibody-secreting plasma cells give rise to multiple myeloma, Waldenström's macroglobulinaemia, monoclonal gammopathy of unknown significance, and heavy chain disease. Tumours affecting plasma cells are often also referred to as **plasma cell dyscrasias** and are associated, to a greater or lesser extent, with complications related to immunoglobulin produced by the abnormal clone:

- hyperviscosity syndromes
- secondary antibody deficiency
- autoimmune phenomena.

Disease can, therefore, arise secondary to the excessive production of an immunoglobulin (e.g. a hyperviscosity syndrome); reduced production of protective immunoglobulins (e.g. secondary antibody deficiency, with poor response to polysaccharide antigens present in bacterial cell wall); or as a result of the nature of the target of the antibody produced by the neoplastic clone (e.g. autoimmune cytopenias).

Multiple myeloma

Multiple myeloma is an abnormal proliferation of malignant plasma cells typically characterised by the excessive production of an immunoglobulin molecule of single heavy and light chain type (termed **paraprotein**). It is the most prevalent and clinically important plasma cell neoplasm and accounts for 10% of all haematological malignancies. Approximately 4 per 100 000 of Western Europeans and North Americans are diagnosed per year and multiple myeloma is twice as common in Black Americans than in their White compatriots. Median age of onset is 68 years, men and women are equally affected, and the median survival from diagnosis is 3 years, with a range up to 10 years. Environmental factors are presumed to have an influence on the development of this, as of other neoplasms, and some have been identified (see Science Box 21.2). Agricultural workers and those exposed to benzene and radiation have a higher incidence, but the major factors have yet to be identified.

Patients typically present with symptoms arising from lytic bone disease (Fig. 21.7), anaemia, renal failure or secondary antibody deficiency. Approximately 20% of patients with multiple myeloma are diagnosed by chance, usually when liver function tests on a blood sample reveal an excessive concentration of total protein or gammaglobulins, caused by excessive immunoglobulin production. The criteria for the diagnosis of multiple myeloma have been recently simplified. These include paraprotein in the serum equalling or exceeding 30 g/l and bone marrow clonal plasma cells equalling or exceeding 10%. A diagnosis of asymptomatic myeloma is made in the absence of organ or tissue impairment (no end organ damage, including bone lesions) or symptoms. In the presence of clinical manifestations — gathered under the acronym CRAB that stands for increased calcium, renal insufficiency, anaemia, or bone lesions — the diagnosis is of symptomatic myeloma. Some 3% of the patients with symptomatic myeloma have a non-secretory form of the disease with no monoclonal protein in either the serum or the urine. In such cases, the monoclonal protein should be identified in the plasma cells by immunoperoxidase or immunofluorescence. Tests important for diagnosis and management are summarised in Table 21.1.

Once the diagnosis is made, it is generally accepted that patients with symptoms should commence treatment. In asymptomatic patients, treatment is started in the presence

---

Growth factors in multiple myeloma

Although there is an association between the development of multiple myeloma and radiation, the effect is weak and only demonstrable in individuals exposed to high doses or for long periods. The trigger(s) for the disease in the vast majority of patients remains unknown. However, recent studies have increased our knowledge about some of the factors that influence malignant plasma cell growth and have offered the potential for new therapies.

Several strands of evidence have implicated IL-6 as a growth factor for healthy plasma cells. Mice transgenic for IL-6 have a massive polyclonal increase in plasma cells, many of which enter the circulation. There is also a human condition, cardiac myxoma, in which high levels of IL-6 are associated with a plasma cell expansion. When attempts are made to grow plasma cells from such patients in vitro, the resulting cultures are dependent upon the addition of supplements of IL-6. This led several groups to look at the role of IL-6 in the growth of malignant plasma cells. High levels of IL-6 are found in the circulation of approximately one third of patients with multiple myeloma. When the plasma cells from these patients are cultured in vitro, they only grow in the presence of stromal support cells (e.g. macrophage-like cells and fibroblasts from the bone marrow). It has been shown that, in these culture systems, IL-6 is secreted into the supernatant by the stromal cells: more importantly, antibodies to IL-6 added to the culture completely inhibit the growth of the plasma cell clone. These exciting findings suggest that IL-6, and possibly other cytokines that synergise with it (IL-3, IL-5 and GM-CSF), promote plasma cell growth in vitro; interfering with these factors in vivo is currently being explored as a new therapy for myeloma.

of a large tumour burden or may be delayed until symptoms arise.

There is a popular misconception that the finding of a paraprotein or **M band** (M for myeloma) makes the diagnosis of multiple myeloma. As we will see later (see monoclonal gammopathy of unknown significance), this is not the case: the presence of an M band alone is not diagnostic of myeloma and neither is it an absolute requirement to make the diagnosis. In the majority of patients, there is excessive production of free immunoglobulin light chains (κ or λ) by the malignant plasma cell, and these are of a sufficiently low molecular weight to be excreted in the urine (termed **Bence Jones proteinuria**). The measure of light chains in the serum has been recently shown to act as a sensitive marker of response to treatment, an early marker of relapse and a useful tool for monitoring patients with the oligosecretory and non-secretory forms of the disease. New markers of poor prognosis have also been recently defined and include the complete deletion of chromosome 13 or of its long arm, detected by karyotyping; the t(4,14) and t(4,16) translocations; and an increased density of bone marrow microvessels.

Immunological features

The hallmark of multiple myeloma is the overproduction of a single immunoglobulin by a malignant plasma cell clone. More than 95% of patients will have evidence of this in the serum or urine (Fig. 21.8). The $\kappa:\lambda$ light chain ratio of paraproteins in patients reflects that of normal immunoglobulin (2 : 1). In the majority of patients (>50%), the malignant clone produces IgG, with 20% secreting IgA and a small proportion IgD (2%) (Fig. 21.9). IgE myeloma is exceedingly rare. **Immune paresis**, i.e. a drastically reduced production of normal immunoglobulins, is frequently seen.

In some patients (15%), only free light chains are secreted. In a small proportion (0.5%), the neoplastic expansion is present (with depression of normal immunoglobulin production) but no paraprotein is detected. Bone marrow examination reveals an excess of plasma cells by conventional staining techniques. If necessary, these can be stained using immunofluorescence with specific antisera to κ or λ light chains, revealing the monoclonality of the plasma cell expansion.

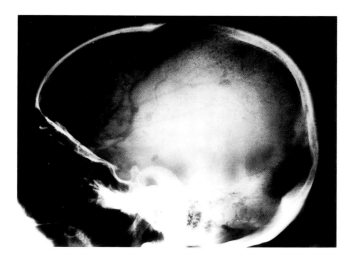

Fig. 21.7 X-ray demonstrating the typical 'punched out' appearance of lytic bone lesions in a patient with multiple myeloma.
(Courtesy of Dr E. J. Evanson.)

Table 21.1 Tests in the diagnosis and management of myeloma

Test	Interpretation
Serum immunoglobulin levels	Evidence of immune paresis
Serum electrophoresis	Identify and quantify paraprotein; paresis of other Ig isotypes
Immunofixation	Paraprotein type
Urine electrophoresis	Bence Jones proteinuria
Bone marrow examination	Percentage plasma cells; plasma cell clonality
Skeletal radiology	Lytic bone lesions
Calcium, urea and electrolytes	Hypercalcaemia; renal function
Levels of β_2-microglobulin	Prognostic marker
Full blood count	Anaemia; leukopenia; thrombocytopenia; rouleaux; increased background staining

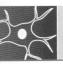

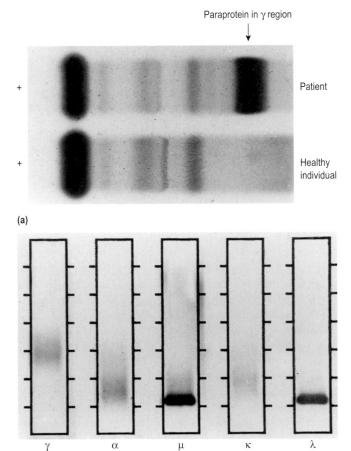

(a)

(b)

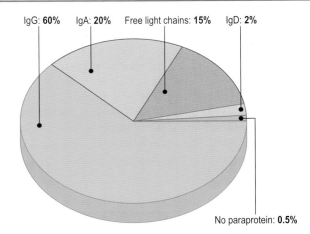

Fig. 21.9 **Distribution of immunoglobulin isotypes among paraproteins in multiple myeloma.**

Fig. 21.8 Immunoglobulin overproduction in multiple myeloma.

(**a**) Serum electrophoresis in a patient with suspected myeloma demonstrates a paraprotein in the γ region, revealed as a discrete, densely stained band. This represents the monoclonal immunoglobulin being produced by the plasma cell tumour. (**b**) Immunofixation is used to identify the heavy and light chain class of the monoclonal paraprotein. Here the serum is separated in five separate lanes in an electrophoretic field, as for serum electrophoresis. Then, each lane is overlain with a different specific antiserum, raised in animals against human γ, α and μ heavy chains and κ and λ light chains. The specific antiserum binds where it finds the appropriate antigen, and the binding is revealed with a protein dye. Diffuse binding (as seen here for γ, α and κ chains) indicates that immunoglobulins bearing these chains are polyclonal in nature. The monoclonal immunoglobulin is revealed in the lanes representing μ and λ chains. Therefore, this patient has an IgM, λ monoclonal paraprotein.

Paraproteins are identified by **serum electrophoresis** (see p. 37 and Fig. 21.8). The immunoglobulin molecules of single heavy and light chain type have identical charge characteristics and migrate to form a single discrete band on the electrophoretic strip. Urine electrophoresis should always be performed in parallel, to identify light chains being excreted, which are found in some 50% of patients. These free light chains, termed Bence Jones proteins, are not detected by

routine assays for urinary protein and must be specifically sought in a concentrated (up to 200-fold) urine sample. The heavy and light chain type of a paraprotein are identified by **immunofixation** (Fig. 21.8). The amount of paraprotein in the serum is a useful measurement, since reductions indicate the beneficial effects of therapy, whilst increases indicate relapse.

Another measurement of value in the management of multiple myeloma is the serum level of β_2-microglobulin (the invariant part of the class I HLA molecule). This is a low-molecular-weight protein that rises in concentration when cell turnover is high and, thus, acts as an independent prognostic indicator in myeloma. Since it is typically excreted in the kidney, a rising level in myeloma is also an index of deteriorating renal function. As severe renal failure is frequently a fatal complication of multiple myeloma, serum β_2-microglobulin is one of the best prognostic markers in this condition.

Clinical features

Once the diagnosis and decision to treat have been made, the question is whether the patient is suitable or not for autologous haematopoietic stem cell transplantation. A recommended approach to treatment is summarised in Figure 21.10. For the patient non-eligible for transplantation, because of age, poor physical condition or co-existing pathologies, intermittent courses of alkylating agents (e.g. melphalan, cyclophosphamide) and a corticosteroid such as prednisolone remain the mainstays of therapy. For those eligible for transplantation, an induction phase is followed by autologous transplantation and then by maintenance therapy (Fig. 21.10). It must be remembered that there remain two limitations to this approach: the conditioning regimens are still inadequate and the re-infused stem cells contain tumour cells. Treatment of myeloma achieves remission in 50% of patients. Remission is maintained for a median of 2 years, with some patients remaining disease free for 10 years or more. A complete response is rare (less than

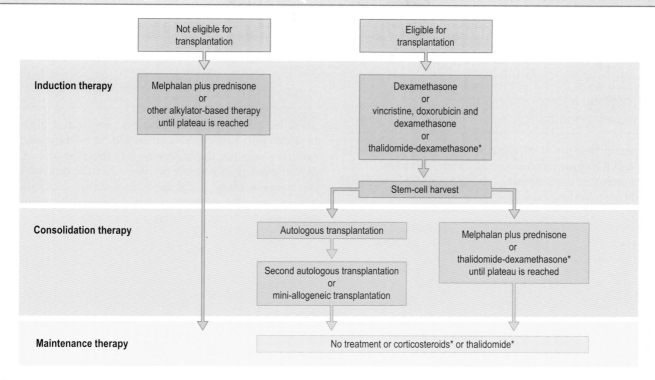

Fig. 21.10 Newly diagnosed myeloma: possible modes of treatment.
In patients non-eligible to autologous haematopoietic stem cell transplantation, the conventional treatment with alkylating agents and corticosteroids is offered. In those eligible to tranplantation an induction course is followed by stem cell harvesting. Plateau refers to stable disease. Those treatments under current investigation are indicated by a star.

10%). In relapsed or refractory myeloma, thalidomide is used either alone or in combination with other drugs in view of its anti-angiogenic effect. Lenalidomide, an amino acid substituted variant of thalidomide with a more powerful activity, is currently under investigation. Clinical trials are also underway with bortezomib, a proteasome inhibitor, with preliminary encouraging results in refractory patients. This drug not only targets the tumour but also the tumour–cell bone marrow interaction.

There are several important, life-threatening complications of multiple myeloma. First, the lytic lesions seen in 60% of patients at some stage are painful and may give rise to vertebral collapse, with spinal cord damage or pathological fractures (Fig. 21.7). Bone disease, probably caused by the osteoclast-activating activity of cytokines such as IL-6, IL-1β and TNF-α, gives rise secondarily to hypercalcaemia, which results in nausea, constipation, fatigue, confusion and poly-uria. Secondary antibody deficiency is common and gives rise to recurrent bacterial infections. Prompt and prolonged use of antibiotics is the treatment of choice, although for recurrent serious infections associated with hypogamma-globulinaemia IVIG should be used.

Waldenström's macroglobulinaemia

This condition is a malignant expansion of mature B cells at the stage of IgM secretion and can also be described as a slow-growing small-cell lymphocytic lymphoma. Its median age of onset is 60 years and it has a better prognosis than myeloma, with median survival of 5–10 years. Typically, small lymphocytes that stain IgM positive and express only a single light chain type are seen infiltrating the bone marrow, lymph nodes and spleen. Distinctive clinical features in Waldenström's macroglobulinaemia are the result of the nature of the IgM paraprotein produced. Being a pentamer, IgM has a high molecular weight, and high levels of circulating paraprotein produce a **hyperviscosity syndrome**. This manifests itself as fatigue, headaches, dizziness, visual disturbance and confusion. Hyperviscosity is treated by removal of the patient's plasma and replacement with donor plasma or albumin (**plasmapheresis**). Plasmapheresis may also be required if the paraprotein has the physico-chemical properties of a cryoglobulin (see p. 233) or cold agglutinin (see p. 295). The high levels of paraprotein can also interfere with the function of other plasma proteins, such as those of the clotting cascade, producing a coagulopathy, with nose bleeds and bruising being common signs at presentation. Anaemia is typically present and often more severe than in multiple myeloma. Bence Jones proteinuria is only found in 10% of patients, and bone lesions are rare.

Therapy for Waldenström's macroglobulinaemia involves the use of highly effective single agents such as the adenosine analogues fludarabine and cladribine, giving a response in some 80% of patients and over 3 years' survival. Anti-CD20 monoclonal antibody (Rituximab) has also been used successfully either alone or combined with chemotherapy.

Younger patients may be suitable for more aggressive therapy, with autologous or allogeneic bone marrow transplantation.

Monoclonal gammopathy of unknown significance

Frequently, high levels of gammaglobulins or total protein detected in routine screening result in the identification of a paraprotein, but the diagnostic criteria for multiple myeloma are not met. In these cases, a diagnosis of monoclonal gammopathy of unknown significance (MGUS) may be made if the patient is asymptomatic and the paraprotein levels are below 30 g/l for IgG and 20 g/l for IgA; there are no Bence Jones proteins in the urine (<1 g/24 hours free light chains); there are <10% plasma cells in the bone marrow; and there are no bone lesions. Estimates of the frequency of MGUS are of 1% in the population over the age of 50 years, rising to 10% in the over 75. In some cases, the condition is premalignant and the conversion rate to frank myeloma is of the order of 1% of patients per year. Approximately 50% of the patients have translocations that involve the heavy-chain locus on chromosome 14q32. A similar proportion of MGUS patients will progress to Waldenström's macroglobulinaemia or amyloidosis (see below). For this reason, regular monitoring of these patients for evidence of marrow suppression, increasing level of paraprotein and depression of normal immunoglobulin production is advisable. Disease progression to myeloma is illustrated in Figure 21.11.

One interesting complication of MGUS is the presence of a monoclonal paraprotein with specificity for the peripheral nerve component **myelin-associated glycoprotein**, giving rise to peripheral neuropathy.

Heavy chain disease

There are rare B lymphocyte lymphoproliferative disorders in which only heavy chains are produced by the malignant cells. Typically it is the Fc region alone that is produced, and in the majority of patients described to date, this has been the α heavy chain. There are approximately 100 reported patients with γ heavy chain disease and even fewer involving production of μ chains. In most patients, the level of paraprotein is very low and the diagnosis difficult to make. The α heavy chain disease is the best characterised and appears to be a premalignant syndrome in which young patients of Mediterranean origin present with gastrointestinal symptoms (pain, diarrhoea, fever and weight loss). The condition occasionally responds to antibiotics or may progress to a lymphomatous condition. Response to antibiotics is in keeping with an aetiological role of chronic antigenic stimulation: a high degree of intestinal infestation with microorganisms has been suggested as the causative factor in this condition, though no single organism has been identified to date.

Amyloidosis

Amyloidosis is a descriptive pathological term, reserved for conditions in which there is a tissue accumulation of

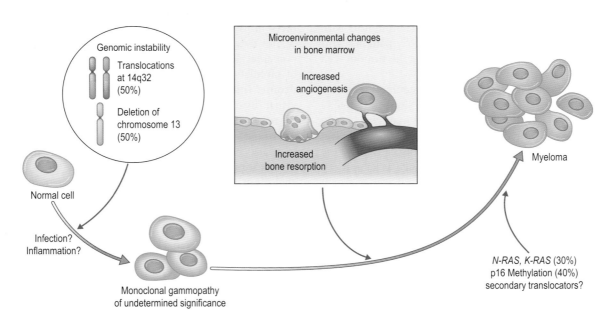

Fig. 21.11 **Factors influencing the development of myeloma.**
Chromosomal abnormalities in concert with environmental stimuli such as inflammation and infection lead to the development of a monoclonal gammopathy of unknown significance. Progression to myeloma is promoted by a series of changes in the bone marrow microenvironment, that include bone resorption, angiogenesis, increased levels of interleukin 6 and vascular endothelial growth factor and impaired immune surveillance. From Kyle & Rajkumar 2004 N Engl J Med 351: 1860–1873, with permission.

insoluble fibrillar proteins, arranging themselves as non-branching β-pleated sheets that are resistant to proteolysis and phagocytosis. Deposition in the kidneys, heart, adrenal glands, spleen, liver, peripheral nerves and joints give rise to the multi-organ failure seen in the disease, most frequently typified by renal failure and cardiomyopathy.

There are several different forms of amyloidosis, two of which are pertinent to a discussion of immune-mediated disease. **Primary amyloidosis** is the most common form of amyloidosis. Light chains of immunoglobulin molecules are excessively produced by a neoplastic clone of plasma cells, either as an idiopathic disease or as part of frank multiple myeloma. The particular nature of these light chains is presumed to favour the production of the insoluble fibrillar proteins characteristic of the disease. Of relevance here may be the fact that the κ:λ ratio is reversed in primary amyloidosis in favour of λ chains.

In the other immunological form of the condition, termed **secondary amyloidosis**, there is deposition of a serum protein (serum amyloid A). Serum amyloid A is an acute-phase reactant, and this condition is usually seen in chronic infectious (e.g. tuberculosis) or inflammatory (e.g. rheumatoid arthritis) diseases characterised by prolonged acute-phase responses.

Patients with amyloidosis usually present with multisystem symptoms and signs and the diagnosis is easily made from tissue (e.g. rectal) biopsies: the abnormal proteins stain distinctively with Congo red. Up to 80% of patients with primary amyloidosis may have a low-level paraprotein in the serum or urine. Reversal of the tissue deposition is difficult to achieve, and management may rest upon cessation of further light chain production using stem cell transplantation and melphalan or, in the case of secondary amyloidosis, abrogation of the acute-phase response by treatment of the underlying condition.

Chronic lymphocytic leukaemia and non-Hodgkin's lymphoma

Although these tumours are not discussed here, it is important to note that such malignancies of mature circulating or lymph node B lymphocytes may manifest immune complications. Autoimmune phenomena are more commonly seen than paraproteinaemias, which accompany less than 5% of cases. In both disorders, paraproteins with the properties of cryoglobulins or cold agglutinins are occasionally found, giving rise to vasculitic lesions and cold autoimmune haemolysis, respectively.

SUMMARY BOX 21.3

Neoplastic disease of B cells

- Autoimmune disease and immunodeficiency states are the major complications of malignancies of cells of the B cell lineage. By far the most common malignancy is multiple myeloma.

- A distinctive feature of myeloma is the production of a monoclonal antibody by the malignant clone.

- A greater understanding of the cell biology of mature B cell malignancies may lead to harnessing immune-based therapies in haematological malignancies, such as myeloma and non-Hodgkin's lymphoma.

Further reading

Gilliland BC 2006 Hemolytic anemia. In: Rose NR, Mackay IR, eds. The autoimmune diseases. 4th edn. Amsterdam: Elsevier; 557–574

Green D, Karpatkin S 2006 Thrombocytopenic purpura. In: Rose NR, Mackay IR, eds. The autoimmune diseases. 4th edn. Amsterdam: Elsevier; 575–584

Kyle RA, Rajkumar SV 2004 Multiple myeloma. N Engl J Med 351: 1860–1873

Kyle RA, Rajkumar SV 2008 Multiple myeloma. Blood 111: 2962–2972

Immune-based therapies

Harnessing the immune system for therapeutic means has been one of the major research goals since the 1980s, and the subject of this chapter. Therapies might be directed at dampening excessive or unwanted immune responses that cause spontaneous disorders such as allergy and autoimmune disease. Equally, immune responses against tumour cells might be encouraged, or those against transplanted allogeneic tissues switched off. Perhaps the greatest stimulus for realising the potential offered by immune-based therapies has been the advent of monoclonal antibody technology. Monoclonal antibodies offer the opportunity to neutralise the unwanted effects of cytokines, or to direct immune responses, drugs, toxins or irradiation against a specific target, possibly a tumour or even an immune cell involved in a damaging autoimmune or rejection response. Also of importance has been the identification of naturally occurring antiviral molecules, such as the interferons. The role of cytokines in modulating immune responses has offered hope for the treatment of conditions, such as autoimmune diseases, arising from disturbances of immune regulation.

Finally, our increased understanding of immune responses has enabled targeting of particular components for interference or enhancement.

Monoclonal antibody therapy

Since the advent of monoclonal antibody technology in the mid-1970s, efforts to harness their power for the treatment of disease have been intense, but numerous issues remain to be addressed. First, the optimal therapeutic antibody must be of human origin, since xenogeneic (i.e. non-human) proteins induce immune responses that negate the effect of the treatment. Second, the attributes of the antibody must be selected. For example, is the isotype one that recruits complement or is effective in antibody-dependent cell-mediated cytotoxicity (ADCC)? Finally, can any other accessory, such as toxins, drugs or radiolabels, be attached to the antibody to provide a 'magic bullet'? Not all monoclonal antibody-targeting strategies are directly therapeutic, however. In some cases, monoclonal antibodies directed against tumour antigens and conjugated to radiolabels are under development for imaging tumour metastases. The monoclonal antibodies in current clinical use, their antigenic target and their clinical indications are summarised in Table 22.1.

Generations of antibodies

Initially, hybridoma technology allowed the generation of rodent monoclonal antibodies alone. Reagents made in mice have several drawbacks: they have a short half-life in the human circulation; they are variable in their ability to recruit human complement or ADCC as an effector mechanism; and they behave as foreign proteins, resulting in human anti-murine antibodies that block function, shorten the half-life and may lead to hypersensitivity reactions. More recently, it has been possible to engineer antibodies combining the attributes of mice and humans. The main advantage of rodent-derived monoclonal antibodies is the ability to immunise with a specific target and to raise high-affinity antibodies.

Table 22.1 Monoclonal antibodies in current therapeutic use

Type	Name	Target	Indication
Murine	OKT3	CD3	Graft rejection
Chimaeric	Abciximab	Platelet gpIIb/IIIa	Adjunct to percutaneous transluminal coronary angioplasty
Chimaeric	Rituximab	CD20	Non Hodgkin's lymphoma (NHL)
Chimaeric	Basiliximab	IL-2R	Organ rejection prophylaxis
Chimaeric	Infliximab	TNF-α	RA, Crohn's
CDR-grafted	Daclizumab	IL-2R	Organ rejection prophylaxis
CDR-grafted	Palivizumab	RSV	Respiratory syncytial virus infection
CDR-grafted	Trastuzumab	HER2	Metastatic breast cancer
CDR-grafted	Gemtuzumab	CD33	Acute myeloid leukaemia
CDR-grafted	Alemtuzumab	CD52	Chronic lymphocytic leukaemia
Murine radio-labelled	Ibritumomab	CD20	NHL
Phage display	Adalimumab	TNF-α	RA
CDR-grafted	Omalizumab	IgE	Asthma
Murine radio-labelled	Tositumomab	CD20	NHL
CDR-grafted	Efalizumab	CD11a (block binding of LFA-1 to ICAM-1)	Psoriasis
CDR-grafted	Cetuximab	EGFR (epidermal growth factor receptor)	Colorectal cancer
CDR-grafted	Bevacizumab	VGEG (vascular endothelial growth factor — prevents angioneogenesis)	Colorectal cancer
CDR-grafted	Natalizumab	VLA-4 (very late antigen 4 — blocks transmigration)	Multiple sclerosis

This attribute is confined to the antibody-binding Fab region. The advantage of using human antibodies would be the lack of inherent immunogenicity in the antibody proteins themselves and the ability to optimise recruitment of effectors. These characteristics reside in the Fc region. A newer approach, therefore, is protein engineering, to combine the Fab region of a murine monoclonal antibody with a human Fc region and produce a **chimaeric humanised rodent monoclonal antibody** (Fig. 22.1).

Originally, humanised rodent monoclonal antibodies were generated by transplanting the murine variable chains onto the human constant chains. Subsequently, so-called

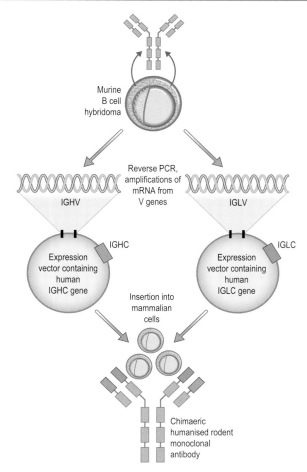

Fig. 22.1 **Generation of chimaeric, humanised monoclonal antibody.** PCR, polymerase chain reaction; IGHV, immunoglobulin heavy chain variable region gene; IGLV, immunoglobulin light chain variable region gene; IGHC, immunoglobulin heavy chain constant region gene; IGLC, immunoglobulin light chain variable region gene.

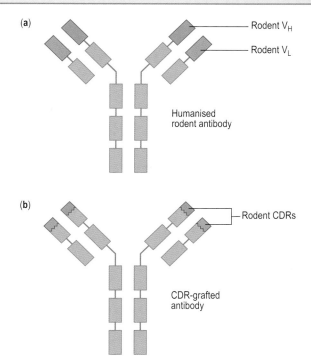

Fig. 22.2 **Antibody engineering.** Rodent monoclonal antibodies can be humanised by combining immunoglobulin heavy chain variable (V_H) and light chain variable (V_L) regions from the monoclonal antibody with human immunoglobulin G heavy chain constant ($C\gamma$) and light chain constant (C_L) chains (**a**) or by grafting the CDR regions of the monoclonal antibody, which carry the antigen-binding function, onto a human framework, that carries the effector functions (**b**).

CDR-grafted antibodies were constructed (Fig. 22.2). Here the antigen-binding loops of the rodent antibody, determined by the complementarity-determining regions (CDRs; see p. 39) were built onto human antibodies. Usually, direct transplantation of the murine CDR onto a human framework results in some degree of loss of affinity. However, minor alterations in the amino acid sequence of the framework can counter this. One advantage is that the same successful framework can be used for carrying numerous different CDRs. CDR-grafted antibodies do elicit some xenoresponse, directed against the antigen-binding site. This may be less of a problem when a 'one-shot' therapy (as in the treatment of acute transplant rejection) is needed. Several such successfully engineered antibodies are in current therapeutic use (see Table 22.1).

Another strategy in antibody engineering technology is the use of **bacteriophage antibody libraries** (Fig. 22.3). Animals are immunised against a protein (e.g. a tumour antigen) and B lymphocytes obtained from the spleen (an alternative would be to take human B cells from peripheral blood or lymph nodes). mRNA for the variable region genes of the antibodies is purified and the complementary DNA made. This provides a 'library' of immunoglobulin heavy chain variable region (IGHV) and immunoglobulin light chain variable region (IGLV) genes, which can be screened for the ones with the highest affinity for the target. A further advantage is that the genes are already cloned and available for development as human chimaeric molecules for therapeutic use.

A novel approach, harnessing this technology in a double dose, is the production of **bi-specific antibodies**. These have two different antigen-binding arms, with different specificities. Bi-specific antibodies can be used in at least two different therapeutic approaches. First, each of the two antigen-binding sites could target two different tumour antigens. Since some tumour antigens are also expressed on normal tissues, doubling the number that need to be recognised before antibody binding occurs should enhance the specificity of the targeting (Fig. 22.4). Another use of bi-specific antibodies is to combine an antigen-binding site specific for a cytotoxic effector cell with another antigen-binding site specific for the tumour. These antibodies can then bring cytotoxic T cells with potential anti-tumour function directly onto the surface of the tumour cell (Fig. 22.5). Currently there is one bi-specific construct directed against CD19 and CD3 in a clinical phase I safety trial for the treatment of non-Hodgkin's lymphoma (the lymphomatous B cells express CD19 and the anti-CD3 should draw in and activate tumour-specific T cells). This antibody has been shown to be very potent in destroying CD19-expressing tumour cells in vitro and in vivo.

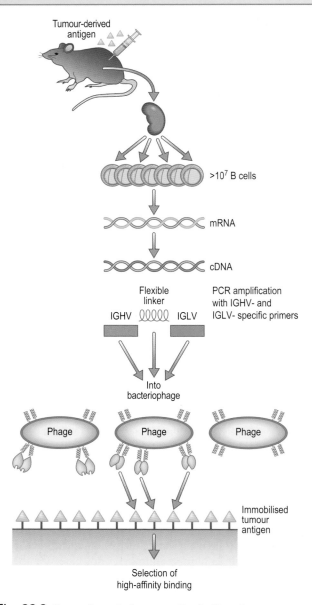

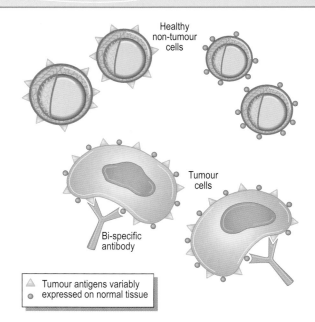

Fig. 22.4 **Use of bi-specific antibodies targeting two tumour antigens as a means of reducing binding to normal tissues expressing one or other of the antigens.**

Fig. 22.3 **Screening of phage antibody libraries to generate DNA encoding high-affinity antigen-binding proteins.** (See text for details.) IGHV, immunoglobulin heavy chain variable region gene; IGLV, immunoglobulin light chain variable region gene.

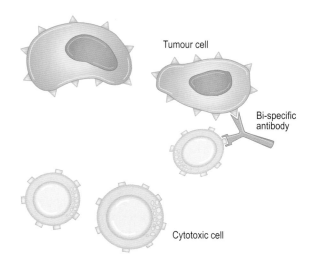

Fig. 22.5 **Use of bi-specific antibodies simultaneously targeting tumour antigens and effector cells to recruit cytotoxic lymphocytes to the tumour site and to distant metastases.**

A promising recent technological development has been the production of **fully human** monoclonal antibodies. This has previously been a challenge since it is hard (because of immunological self tolerance) to generate a human antibody response to a normal human cellular target such as CD3. To get around this, scientists have generated transgenic mice in which the germline mouse genes encoding immunoglobulin light and heavy chains are silenced and replaced by the human counterparts. These mice, when immunised with foreign antigen (e.g. human CD3), produce human antibodies. Boosting the animals leads to production of high affinity antibodies, which can be harnessed as monoclonal antibodies using hybridoma techniques (see p. 45). The

human monoclonal antibodies from transgenic mice in current clinical trial are summarised in Table 22.2. A surprising feature of administering these monoclonal antibodies, which are fully humanised and therefore theoretically non-immunogenic, has been the finding that they can induce human antihuman antibodies (HAHAs). This has raised theoretical concerns that the HAHAs could result in untoward reactions to these drugs on re-administration, or a reduction in their efficacy because of a neutralising effect.

Table 22.2 Human monoclonal antibodies derived from transgenic mice in clinical testing

Target	Indication	Company	Clinical trial phase
EGFR	Colorectal cancer and non-small cell lung cancer, renal cell carcinoma	Amgen/Abgenix	2/3
EGFR	Head and neck cancer	Genmab	3
CTLA-4	Melanoma and various other cancers	Medarex, Pfizer	2/3
Prostate-specific membrane antigen	Prostate cancer	Medarex	2
Alpha v integrins	Solid tumours	Johnson & Johnson	1
CD89*	Solid tumours	Medarex	1
TRAIL-R2	Solid tumours	Human Genome Sciences	1
Dendritic cell mannose receptor**	Human gonadotropin-positive cancers	Medarex	1
CD4	Lymphoma	Genmab	3
CD30	Lymphoma	Medarex	2
CD20	Non-Hodgkin's lymphoma	Genmab	3
CD40	Chronic lymphocytic leukaemia	Chiron	1
Interleukin-15	Rheumatoid arthritis	Amgen/Genmab	2
Tumour necrosis factor-α	Inflammatory disease	Johnson & Johnson	2
Interleukin-12	Psoriasis and multiple sclerosis	Johnson & Johnson	2
CXCL10	Ulcerative colitis	Medarex	2
Platelet-derived growth factor-D	Inflammatory kidney disease	Curagen	1
Connective tissue growth factor	Pulmonary fibrosis	Fibrogen	1

(continued)

Table 22.2 Human monoclonal antibodies derived from transgenic mice in clinical testing—cont'd

Target	Indication	Company	Clinical trial phase
RANKL	Osteoporosis and treatment-induced bone loss	Amgen	2/3
Parathyroid hormone	Hyperparathyroidism	Abgenix	1
Clostridium difficile toxin A	*C. difficile* infection (frequent hospital-acquired infection)	MBL/Medarex	2
CC chemokine receptor 5	HIV infection	Human Genome Sciences	1

EGFR = epithelial growth factor; TRAIL-R2 = a receptor expressed on a number of solid tumours and tumours of haematopoietic origin; CXCL10 = CXC chemokine ligand 10; RANKL = receptor activator of NFκB ligand; *Human antigen-binding fragment (Fab) fused to epidermal growth factor; **Human Fab fused to b-hCG.

'Magic bullet' therapy

As discussed above, one strategy in using monoclonal antibody therapy is to exploit natural effectors, such as Fc receptor-bearing cells for ADCC or complement, and deplete the target cell population (e.g. tumour cells, autoreactive T cells). Another approach is to modulate the immune response. For example, some forms of anti-CD3 antibody therapy do not actually deplete T cells, yet have an effect on T cell-mediated immune responses. In animal models of autoimmune disease, administration of these so-called 'non-depleting' anti-CD3 monoclonal antibodies appears to arrest the autoimmune process, and restore tolerance, which is long lived and can be transferred from one animal to another (Fig. 22.6). An anti-CD3 monoclonal antibody with these properties has now been used successfully to arrest beta cell loss in human type 1 diabetes (see p. 192), without causing immune suppression.

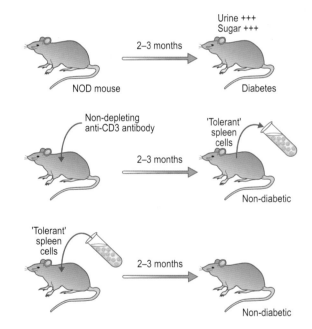

Fig. 22.6 **Use of non-depleting antibodies to modulate damaging autoantigen-specific immune responses in the non-obese diabetic (NOD) mouse, a close animal model of human type 1 diabetes.**

SUMMARY BOX 22.1

Monoclonal antibody therapy

- Monoclonal antibodies allow immune responses to be directed against a specific target.
- Accessories, such as toxins, drugs or radioisotopes, can be linked to monoclonal antibodies.
- Monoclonal antibodies therapy has established itself as a powerful new mode of treatment in conditions ranging from rejection to cancer.
- Advances in technology have produced completely human monoclonal antibodies now in clinical trials.

Immunosuppressive drugs

Corticosteroids

Glucocorticosteroids (cortisone, hydrocortisone, prednisone and prednisolone) are the most commonly used steroids. They have been used extensively to control damaging inflammatory immune responses in clinical practice for many years and appear to have a variety of effects on immune function

SCIENCE BOX 22.1

TeDegenero

On the evening of 13 March 2006 six seriously ill patients were admitted to the Critical Care Unit at Northwick Park Hospital in London. Together with two other volunteers who were given placebo, they were part of a trial on the humanised monoclonal antibody TGN1412 (also known as CD28-SuperMAB®), produced by TeGenero Immuno Therapeutics, Germany. This is a monoclonal antibody that mimics a second T cell activation signal and acts without the need of T cell receptor engagement (superagonist). The antibody reacts with a specific part of the CD28 molecule called the C'D loop. The antibody was developed to fight autoimmune disease and leukaemia.

Five minutes after the last volunteer received his intravenous dose, the first started complaining of a severe headache, fever and pain. He took his shirt off, since he felt like he was burning. The remaining participants who received the actual drug became ill as well, vomiting and complaining of severe pain. The two who received placebo watched aghast. A patient was described as having suffered a ballooned head similar to the 'Elephant Man' (TeDegenero).

Within 12 hours all six receiving the antibody had collapsed. At least one participant begged the doctors to put him to sleep. By the end of May 2006, however, all patients had been discharged.

The effect observed is most likely due to a cytokine storm following uncontrolled activation of T cells. Other cells activated by CD28 ligation in humans include eosinophils and granulocytes. They can release potent neurotoxins, INF-γ as well as IL-2, IL-4 and IL-13.

In the aftermath, bioethicists, public prosecutors and immunologists entered an animated debate. An immunologist noted, 'You are going beyond the regulatory network, so all hell can break loose', and a second, 'You don't need to be a rocket scientist to work out what will happen if you non-specifically activate every T cell in the body'. Apparently, preliminary studies in non-human primates had failed to show this type of side-effect however. In Würzburg the public prosecutor launched an investigation to see whether there was any criminal wrongdoing, while the president of a scientific institute wondered, 'Why do you treat six people at the same time? Why don't you start with one?' and a bioethicist in New York noted that, 'There is going to be a lot of soul searching'. How much of that went on is difficult to say when a scientist leading a Clinical Trials Unit of the UK Medical Research Council reported that, 'Paradoxically, there has been an upsurge in interest in these healthy volunteer studies'. The men enrolled in the TeGenero trials had been paid £2000 (US$3500) to enter the trial.

Table 22.3 Major mechanisms of steroid anti-inflammatory actions

Target cell	Effect	Consequences
Monocyte	Block IL-1 production	Inhibition of T cell activation
	Block TNF-α production	Inhibition of activation and recruitment of monocytes, endothelial cells, neutrophils
	Reduced chemotaxis	Inhibition of migration to inflammation
T lymphocyte	Block IL-2 production	Inhibit T cell activation
	Block IFN-α production	Inhibit monocyte activation, reduce antiviral effect
	Redistribution out of circulation	Reduced migration of lymphocytes (especially CD4⁺) to inflammation

(Table 22.3). Hydrocortisone succinate is water soluble and may be given intravenously; prednisone is given orally and is metabolised to prednisolone by liver enzymes. Endogenous glucocorticoid concentrations in plasma vary five-fold diurnally and may rise by up to 20 times in stressful situations, such as surgery (in the patient, not the surgeon). Therapeutic doses of steroids may increase plasma concentrations by up to 100 times.

Steroid effects are mediated through cytoplasmic receptors that translocate to the nucleus and modify gene expression. The recorded effects of steroids on immune function are legion. Difficulties in interpreting many of these data centre around the relevance of in vitro studies, while species differences in steroid physiology call into question data from many animal studies. What is clear is that steroid-mediated immune effects do not relate to a single mechanism. The major effects of steroids on immune function can be divided into effects on cytokine networks, direct effects on cells and effects on compartmentalisation within the immune system.

At pharmacological doses, glucocorticoids inhibit release of TNF-α and IL-1 from monocytes and reduce production of IFN-γ and IL-2 by T lymphocytes. These effects are apparent when monocytes or T cells are maximally stimulated, for example by incubation with bacterial lipopolysaccharide or with allogeneic lymphocytes in a mixed lymphocyte reaction. Overall, the summated effect of such reductions in cytokine secretion would be to inhibit monocyte and T cell activation. This is likely to have a profound effect on antigen-specific T cell responses, particularly those mediated by T_H1 cells.

Direct effects of steroids on lymphocytes and monocytes are more difficult to assess. In general, suprapharmacological doses will inhibit T cell proliferation in vitro. B cell activity appears to be enhanced, in that immunoglobulin secretion rises in the presence of steroids. This is probably the result of an inhibitory effect on the T cells controlling B cell function. Direct effects on monocyte function are difficult to assess. In vitro, pharmacological doses of steroids inhibit monocyte chemotaxis, but monocytes from patients on long-term high-dose therapy have normal chemotactic responses. Suprapharmacological doses are required to demonstrate inhibitory effects on monocyte phagocytosis and bacterial killing in vitro. Equally, most neutrophil functions appear steroid resistant.

An observation was made in the 1970s regarding the effects of steroids on circulating immune cell populations. Quite small doses of glucocorticoids reduce the circulating white blood cell count within 6 hours: CD4 T lymphocytes are particularly affected. Similar effects in animals are accompanied by redistribution of cells to the bone marrow and spleen. In contrast, circulating monocyte and neutrophil numbers appear to increase.

The side-effects of steroid therapy should not be forgotten. Some of these are predictable from the mode of action (e.g. increased susceptibility to infection) but equally important are impaired wound healing, growth suppression in children, depression, hyperglycaemia and hypertension.

Ciclosporin, tacrolimus and sirolimus

In view of their shared mode of action, i.e. the ability to block calcineurin (see below), two major immunosuppressive drugs, ciclosporin and tacrolimus, are referred to as calcineurin inhibitors (CNI). Ciclosporin is the product of the fungus *Tolypocladium inflatum* and was first identified in 1976 during screening for novel antibiotic agents. It was adopted widely in clinical practice in the mid-1980s and has revolutionised many areas of medical and surgical practice. Much is now known about its mode of action, and within the last decade a drug of completely different structure, but similar *modus operandi*, has also entered clinical practice. This is tacrolimus (previously called FK506), which is derived from the fungus *Streptomyces tsukubaensis*.

Ciclosporin is an undecapeptide containing one unique amino acid, whilst tacrolimus is a macrolide lactone antibiotic. Therefore, they have quite different structures, but both act as pro-drugs, only becoming active when complexed to intracellular binding proteins termed **immunophilins**. In early in vitro studies, ciclosporin was noted to have a profound effect on T cell activation, inhibiting it with a high degree of specificity and potency. Initially its use was restricted to prophylaxis against graft rejection, but it has undergone trials in autoimmune diseases, asthma and psoriasis. It is indicated as a potential therapy in any disease in which activation of T cells has a pathogenic role, though toxicity is a major drawback. Ciclosporin therapy not only results in a propensity to opportunistic infections but also has major toxic effects on the kidney (reduced glomerular filtration and tubular interstitial fibrosis). In the transplantation setting, tacrolimus has been found to be superior to ciclosporin in improving graft survival and preventing acute rejection, but it increases post-transplant diabetes, and is associated with gastrointestinal side-effects.

Initial studies on the mode of action of ciclosporin revealed that it enters T cells and binds to an intracellular protein. The cytosolic binding protein for ciclosporin was originally called **cyclophilin** and has subsequently been identified as the enzyme **peptidyl prolyl *cis–trans* isomerase** or **rotamase**. First discovered in 1984, rotamase accelerates the interconversion of *cis* and *trans* rotamers of proline-containing peptides or proteins, which is believed to be the rate-limiting step during protein folding. The binding protein for tacrolimus is termed just that (TBP) or also FKBP12 and collectively this and cyclophilin go under the term immunophilins.

Intriguingly, the drug-binding protein complex in both cases (tacrolimus–TBP and ciclosporin–cyclophilin) has affinity for the same target, a Ca^{2+}-dependent protein phosphatase called **calcineurin**. Calcineurin receives the second messenger signal generated by the rise in intracellular Ca^{2+} concentration after TCR-mediated activation. Calcineurin then dephosphorylates a nuclear transcription factor present in the cytoplasm NF-AT$_c$ (for nuclear factor of activated T cells$_{cytoplasm}$, see p. 106), which is thus enabled to translocate from the cytoplasm to the nucleus and there initiate transcription of the IL-2 gene in concert with a similar nuclear transcription factor (NF-AT$_n$) (Fig. 22.7). Blocking of calcineurin function within the T cell by the complex of drug and binding protein has obvious consequences for TCR-mediated T cell activation.

Rapamycin is a macrolide antibiotic with a structure similar to tacrolimus. It was first discovered as a product of the bacterium *Streptomyces hygroscopicus* in a soil sample from the island of Rapa Nui, better known as Easter Island. **Sirolimus**, as rapamycin is also known, binds FKBP12, and this feature was thought to prevent the simultaneous use of tacrolimus and sirolimus. Clinical practice has, however, shown this not to be the case, the reason for this being that pharmacological levels of both drugs are well below the capacity of FKBP12. It is the combined use of sirolimus and ciclosporin that is impractical since both drugs are metabo-

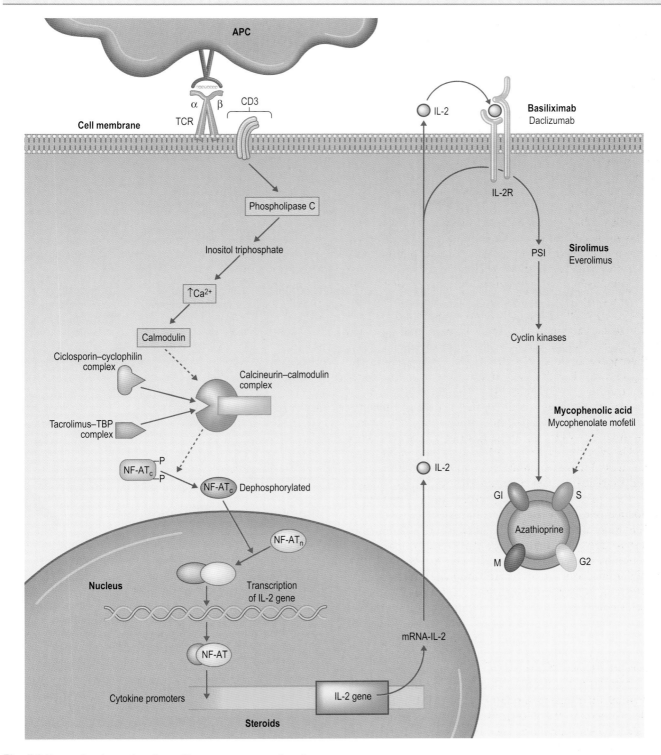

Fig. 22.7 **Mechanism of action of immunosuppressive drugs.**

lised by the same enzymes and addition of sirolimus increases ciclosporin nephrotoxicity.

In contrast to CNI that act early in the T-cell activation pathway, sirolimus acts at a late stage, inhibiting an enzyme called **mTor** (**mammalian target of rapamycin**). mTor acts as a checkpoint by sensing cell status and regulates cell progress through G1-S phase following changes in local cytokine concentration. Sirolimus uncouples these regulatory activities, negatively affecting T cell proliferation and survival.

Used alone or in combination with CNI, sirolimus is associated with a lower risk of acute rejection and a higher glomerular filtration rate but also with bone marrow suppression and lipid disturbance (Table 22.4).

Table 22.4 Ciclosporin, tacrolimus and sirolimus

Name	Structure	Mode of action	Clinical indications	Side-effects	Possible combinations
Ciclosporin	Cyclic non-ribosomal polypeptide of 11 aa	Prevents production of IL-2 via calcineurin inhibition	Anti-rejection	Nephrotoxicity, hyperkalaemia, hypomagnesaemia, hirsutism, gingival hyperplasia	Corticosteroids, azathioprine, mycophenolate mofetil
Tacrolimus	Macrolide antibiotic	Prevents production of IL-2 via calcineurin inhibition	Anti-rejection	Nephrotoxicity, neurotoxicity, glucose intolerance	Corticosteroids, mycophenolate mofetil, sirolimus
Sirolimus	Macrolide antibiotic	Inhibits G1-to S-phase cell division, hence cell proliferation	Anti-rejection	Hyperlipidaemia, impaired wound healing	Tacrolimus, ciclosporin, mycophenolate mofetil

Other anti-inflammatory agents

In an attempt to limit the dangers of toxicity caused by use of high doses of a single agent, combined anti-inflammatory therapy is often used and may be particularly important in reducing the side-effects of steroids.

Purine analogues such as **azathioprine** are frequently used as anti-inflammatory drugs in conjunction with steroids. They inhibit DNA synthesis and in vitro suppress antigen-specific T cell proliferation. In vivo, they have an effect on numbers of circulating cells, most notably inducing a reduction in T and B lymphocyte numbers, and natural killer cell number and activity. Azathioprine also appears to inhibit antibody production. Similar to azathioprine but more powerful is **mycophenolate mofetil** (**MMF**). This drug is metabolised in the liver to mycophenolic acid, which inhibits inosine monophosphate dehydrogenase, the enzyme controlling the de novo pathway of purine synthesis used by proliferating lymphocytes. It is frequently used as a CNI/steroid sparing agent.

Alkylating agents, such as cyclophosphamide and chlorambucil, are also used for immunosuppression. Their activity is dependent upon the alkylation of purine bases, interfering with DNA production and killing cells in mitosis. Alkylating agents induce a small reduction in circulating T and B cell numbers. More importantly, they suppress antibody production very effectively, and reduce antigen-specific T cell responses.

SUMMARY BOX 22.2

Immunosuppressive drugs

- Immunosuppressive drugs remain powerful agents in immune-mediated disease, but their side-effects still limit their use.

- Ciclosporin, tacrolimus and sirolimus inhibit T cell activation; this has therapeutic potential where this is pathogenic, e.g. graft rejection. Major side-effects include vulnerability to opportunistic infections, tumours, renal toxicity and dyslipidaemia.

Cytokines and anticytokines

Cytokines are pleiotropic agents with powerful pro-inflammatory and immunosuppressive effects. Manipulation of their actions could be aimed at inhibiting the function of a cytokine that has a key role in promoting a disease, or enhancing the activity of a cytokine that has a potentially beneficial effect. In general terms, there are four major strategies for reducing the effects of a cytokine. First, production can be blocked; second, intracellular processing, which produces the active protein, can be inhibited; third, the cytokine can be neutralised in the circulation; and, finally, specific

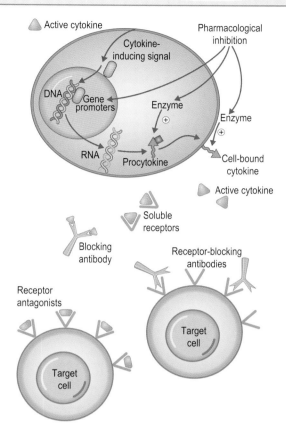

Fig. 22.8 Mechanisms by which cytokine functions may be blocked.

to qualify the results obtained in a trial with the more powerful of the two drugs, Anakinra appears to be safe but its therapeutic effect modest.

Tumour necrosis factor-α

Tumour necrosis factor is a multipotent cytokine that occurs in soluble and transmembrane form, the soluble form binding to both TNF receptors (p55 and p75), the transmembrane form predominantly to NFRp75. In view of its pivotal role in inflammation, TNF-α has become the focus of biotechnology efforts with three biological agents antagonising the action of the cytokine available for clinical use. These include: Etanercept, a construct of two p75 TNF receptors linked by the Fc portion of human IgG1; Infliximab, a mouse/human chimaeric monoclonal antibody and Adalimumab, a completely human monoclonal antibody. All three agents have proved their efficacy in clinical trials. Blocking TNF-α has been shown to produce significant improvement in RA, ankylosing spondylitis, psoriatic arthritis, psoriasis and Crohn's disease, all conditions for which this biological therapy is approved. There is evidence, however, of an increased risk of serious infections and a dose-dependent increased risk of malignancies in patients treated with anti-TNF antibody therapy. The US Food and Drug Administration sums up: 'As a class, anti-TNF-α drugs have demonstrated both efficacy and a number of serious adverse events including infections (TB, fungal), congestive heart failure, neurologic events including demyelination, lymphomas and autoimmunity including lupus-like syndromes. The decision to use these drugs — as with all other immunosuppressives — should consider both their efficacy and potential side-effects'.

receptors can be blocked (Fig. 22.8). Cytokine-based therapies either in clinical use or in clinical trial are summarised in Table 22.5.

Interleukin-1

The interleukin (IL)-1 family comprises the well defined proinflammatory cytokines IL-1α, IL-1β and IL-18. In general, manipulation of IL-1 is aimed at blocking its function in inflammatory diseases, and several strategies are available. The administration of antibodies to IL-1 and soluble forms of the receptor will neutralise excessive IL-1 in the circulation or, for example, in the joints of patients with rheumatoid arthritis. Antibodies to the receptors and use of recombinant interleukin 1 receptor antagonist (IL-1ra) will blockade the reception of IL-1-mediated pro-inflammatory signals. Although some agents clearly reduce IL-1 production (corticosteroids, non-steroidal anti-inflammatory drugs), they lack specificity for IL-1 alone.

The results of clinical trials with interleukin-1 receptor antagonists such as Anakinra and the high-affinity IL1-Trap in rheumatoid arthritis were eagerly awaited. Though 'disappointing' and 'dismal' were the words used by the editorialist

Interleukin-2

Since IL-2 has a key role in T cell activation, it is an important target of therapeutic interventions in T cell-mediated diseases. These include autoimmune disorders and transplant rejection. In addition, many T cell malignancies overexpress the IL-2 receptor and may be reliant upon IL-2 as a growth factor. In contrast, promotion of IL-2 function has been used as a strategy to enhance immune responses, most notably against tumours.

For blocking the involvement of IL-2 in immune responses, there are again several strategies available. IL-2 receptors are not expressed on quiescent effector T cells, but rapid induction takes place within hours after stimulation. In terms of targeting this process, enormous success has been achieved with ciclosporin and tacrolimus in controlling IL-2-mediated T cell activation. Antibodies against the IL-2 receptor α chain (CD25) have been available for some years, and in vitro studies indicate that these can block T cell activation.

Table 22.5 Cytokine-based therapies

Cytokine	Drug	Name/code	Application	Clinical trial	Company
IL-1Rα	Recombinant IL-1Rα antagonist	Kineret®/Anakinra	Rheumatoid arthritis (RA)	Approved	Amgen
			Sepsis	Approved	
			Osteoarthritis	Phase II	
IL-2	Recombinant IL-2	Proleukin	Metastatic renal cell carcinoma	Approved	Chiron
			Metastatic melanoma	Approved	
			Non-Hodgkin's lymphoma	Phase II	
IL-11	Recombinant IL-11	Oprelvekin/Neumega®	Chemotherapy-induced thrombocytopenia	Approved	Genetics Institute, Inc./Wyeth
			Crohn's disease	Phase III	
			RA	Phase II	
			Psoriasis	Phase II	
			Colitis	Phase I	
IFN-γ	Bioengineered IFN-γ-1b	Actimmune	Chronic granulomatous disease	Approved	Intermune Pharma
			Osteoporosis	Approved	
			Idiopathic pulmonary fibrosis	Phase III	
			Ovarian cancer	Phase III	
IFN-α	IFN-α-con-1	Infergen®	Hepatitis C	Approved	Intermune Pharma
IFN-α	IFN-α-n3 leukocyte derived	Alferon-N®	HPV genital warts	Approved	Hemi sperx Biopharma
			Hepatitis C	Phase II/III	
			West Nile virus	Phase II/III	
			HIV	Phase I/II	

IFN-α	Pegylated IFN-α-2a	Pegasys®	Hepatitis C Hepatitis B	Approved Phase III/filed	Roche
IFN-α	Recombinant IFN-α-2a	Roferon-A®	Hairy cell leukaemia Kaposi's sarcoma Chronic myeloid leukaemia Chronic hepatitis C	Approved Approved Approved Approved	Roche
IFN-α	Recombinant IFN-α-2b	Intron-A®	Hairy cell leukaemia Kaposi's sarcoma Chronic hepatitis B/C Malignant melanoma Follicular lymphoma Condylomata acuminata	Approved Approved Approved Approved Approved Approved	Schering-Plough
IFN-α	PEG recombinant IFN-α-2b	PegIntron®	Hepatitis C Malignant melanoma	Approved Phase III	Schering-Plough
IFN-β	IFN-β-1a	Avonex®	Relapsing multiple sclerosis	Approved	Biogen Idec
IFN-β	IFN-β-1a	Rebiferon®	Relapsing multiple sclerosis Hepatitis C	Approved Phase III	Serono
IFN-β	IFN-β-1b	Betaseron®	Early/relapsing multiple sclerosis	Approved	Berlex
GM-SF	Recombinant GM-CSF	Leukine®/Sargramostim®	Leukaemia Bone marrow/stem cell transplants Crohn's disease	Approved Approved Phase III	Schering-AG

Basic and clinical immunology

A murine antibody to the IL-2 receptor α chain (anti-CD25, known as anti-Tac antibody) was used in original clinical trials for the treatment of severe graft-versus-host disease and in rejection of renal transplants. Although it has undoubted efficacy in these circumstances, anti-Tac was too immunogenic to be of value itself. However, it has provided the impetus for the development of humanised anti-CD25 antibodies, which are in current clinical use such as Basiliximab and Daclizumab (see Table 22.1).

Promoting IL-2-mediated activation of immune effector cells has been most widely applied in cancer immunotherapy. An approach pioneered by Steven Rosenberg, in the USA, was to take peripheral blood lymphocytes from patients with tumours and activate and expand these in vitro with IL-2 over several days. Under these conditions, there is a preferential expansion of non-T lymphocytes with a large granular lymphocyte (LGL) morphology. In animal experiments, these cells have greatly enhanced cytotoxic potential against experimental tumours, and are termed lymphokine-activated killer (LAK) cells. Initial results showed that LAK cell therapy could induce partial and complete remissions in up to 20% of patients with certain tumours, notably malignant melanoma and renal cell carcinoma. It was then observed that intravenous infusion of IL-2 gives results similar to those obtained with the direct use of LAK cells, hence IL-2 is generally now used alone. Partial and complete remission rates of 10–20% are found in malignant melanoma and renal cell carcinoma, which remain the most responsive tumours, and for which IL-2 is licensed both in the UK and USA. Side-effects are considerable and similar to those of IL-1, with a capillary leak syndrome and cardiac failure being the major clinical problems. Therefore, therapy is advised for relatively fit patients and must take place in adequate facilities.

Interferon-α

IFN-α has been one of the most successful therapeutic cytokines in clinical practice. It has activity against chronic viral infections and certain haematological malignancies. Whilst natural leukocyte-derived IFN-α is actually a cocktail of interferon proteins (there are multiple genes for this cytokine), human recombinant proteins from the IFN-α2 gene are available commercially (IFN-α-2a and IFN-α-2b, which differ at amino acid position 23).

Over half of the patients acquiring acute hepatitis C virus infection will develop a chronic illness, of whom 20% will become cirrhotic. Trials with IFN-α in chronic hepatitis C infection have demonstrated an objective remission (e.g. biochemical evidence of improved liver function, sustained viral remission) in 40–50% of patients. In a similar vein, IFN-α treatment in chronic hepatitis B virus infection is effective in a third of patients. **Pegylated interferon** is currently used for both types of chronic viral hepatitis, since its link to polyethylene glycol extends its half life and therapeutic effect. Pegylated interferon is frequently used in combination with nucleoside/nucleotide analogues that impair virus replicative

machineries in both infections. Adverse effects are not as severe as for IL-1 and IL-2, centring on the induction of a 'flu-like' illness.

SUMMARY BOX 22.3

Cytokines and anticytokines

- Cytokines can have both beneficial effects and pathogenic effects: anticytokines can reduce the latter.
- Reducing levels of TNF-α can reduce its inflammatory action, e.g. in rheumatoid arthritis and Crohn's disease.
- IL-2 is involved in T cell activation and antibodies blocking IL-2 action are effectively used in combating graft rejection.
- IL-2 is also used to enhance immune responses against malignant melanoma and renal cell carcinoma.
- IFN-α is used in therapy against viral infections, especially hepatitis B and C.
- IFN-α is currently used in a pegylated form that has a much longer half-life than standard interferon.

Other therapeutic approaches

Using antigens to control unwanted immune responses

One of the major goals for immune-based therapies designed for autoimmune disease is to restrict the immunosuppressive elements of the treatment so that they act upon the relevant autoimmune response without producing a state of generalised immunosuppression. It was noted several decades ago that simply giving a protein antigen in sufficient quantity through selected routes (oral, intranasal, intradermal, intravenous) could inhibit subsequent attempts to generate an immune response to the same antigen. As animal models of autoimmune disease were devised over subsequent years, the effect of administering the key autoantigens in a simple form was explored, and, seemingly without exception, this strategy has resulted in protection from disease in a large range of animal models tested.

Refinements of the approach include giving key peptide epitopes (**peptide immunotherapy**), rather than whole protein autoantigens (**antigen-specific immunotherapy**); giving the epitope or antigen not as a protein but in the form of naked DNA; and giving multiple antigens/epitopes. These strategies are almost always successful in animal models — there have been very few failures (or perhaps they don't get reported) and very few examples of this manipulation making the disease worse.

How does it work? There are plenty of possibilities. Giving antigen without co-stimulation (usually no adjuvant is used) could provide excessive amounts of TCR-dependent signal 1

Biologics

A large number of the items discussed in the present chapters falls under the label of **biologics**. A biologic is defined as a preparation, such as a drug, a vaccine or an antitoxin, that is synthesised from living organisms or their products and used as a diagnostic, preventive or therapeutic agent. In addition to monoclonal antibodies and cytokines, the biologics comprise other compounds such as fusion proteins.

The CTL4Ig is a fusion protein that has reached approval for clinical use. You will remember that following T cell receptor recognition of an antigenic peptide, T cells need a second signal to become activated. This second signal results from the binding of a co-stimulatory receptor on the T cell to a ligand on the APC; the interaction of CD28 on T cells with CD80 or CD86 on APCs is a key example of a co-stimulatory signal (see p. 99). CTLA4 (CD152) is a CD28 homologue, which provides down-regulation instead of stimulation.

The possibility for CTLA4 to interrupt the delivery of the second signal required for full T cell activation was exploited by fusing the extracellular domain of human CTLA4 to the modified Fc (hinge, CH2 and CH3 domains) portion of human immunoglobulin G1 (IgG1), resulting in a soluble fusion protein, CTLA4Ig, which is now known as **Abatacept.**

CTLA4Ig has proved its therapeutic efficacy in rheumatoid arthritis when all disease-modifying drugs, including the biologics blocking TNF-α (see p. 317), have failed. Both clinically and radiologically the disease was significantly slowed down in patients receiving the drug as opposed to those receiving a placebo.

in the absence of signal 2, leading to anergy. There could also be activation-induced cell death. Finally, many believe that giving simple antigens leads to presentation to T cells by immature DCs, which probably biases T cells towards a regulatory phenotype.

The diseases that have the most advanced clinical data are in the field of allergy. For example, administration of cocktails of peptides of the cat allergen Fel d 1 has led to a reduction in detectable skin-prick responses and improved clinical scores. Clinical trials of antigen-specific and peptide immunotherapy are now planned in the autoimmune diseases type 1 diabetes and multiple sclerosis. Although it sounds like 'treating fire with fire', the approach has great promise.

Intravenous immunoglobulin

IVIG is a therapeutic preparation of poly-specific IgG chemically purified from plasma pools of large numbers (approximately 20 000) of healthy donors. With such a large donor number, IVIG represents a wide spectrum of the expressed normal human IgG repertoire, including antibodies to external agents, as well as autoantibodies (see p. 234, Science Box 16.2). IgG subclasses are present in physiological proportions, and the IgG has an approximate half-life of 3 weeks (compared with 4 weeks for physiological IgG). IgA and IgM are present only in trace amounts.

IVIG therapy can be viewed as a replacement strategy for primary and secondary antibody deficiencies; as a blocking agent, to prevent Fc-mediated effector mechanisms, such as destruction of IgG-coated erythrocytes; or as a therapy that has subtle effects on the balance of an immune response: so-called **immunomodulation**. In replacement IVIG, the rationale and the indications for use are straightforward and have been dealt with elsewhere (see Ch. 19). Similarly, the use of IVIG in preventing splenic and hepatic destruction of antibody-coated blood cells in the circulation has been discussed (see Ch. 21). In contrast, use of IVIG as an immunomodulator is controversial. Many therapeutic benefits are claimed: few are backed up with randomised double-blind controlled clinical trials. To examine and pronounce on this area of controversy, the US National Institutes of Health have attempted to produce some guidelines for therapeutic use of IVIG (Table 22.6).

Proposed mechanisms of action of IVIG include:

- blockade of Fc receptors on mononuclear or polymorphonuclear phagocytes
- feedback inhibition of autoantibody synthesis by autoreactive B cells
- inhibition of complement consumption by pathogenic autoantibodies
- interference with T cell regulation and cytokine release.

Table 22.6 Guidelines on the use of intravenous immunoglobulin

Primary immunodeficiencies
Immune-mediated thrombocytopenia
Kawasaki syndrome
Recent bone marrow transplantation
Chronic B cell lymphocytic leukaemia
Paediatric HIV infection
Chronic inflammatory demyelinating polyneuropathy
Post-transfusion purpura
Recommendations of Food and Drug Administration, National Institute of Health and University Hospital Consortium.

However, the actual mechanism by which IVIG works in most autoimmune and inflammatory conditions, apart from the immune cytopenias, is still unclear and its benefit in inflammatory polyneuropathy and vasculitis remains to be established. One theory is that large doses of extrinsic antibody block endogenous autoantibody production, which would be beneficial in inflammatory polyneuropathy and vasculitis. IVIG could also interfere with complement-mediated tissue damage, by providing excess Fc regions to 'soak up' complement components. Effects on regulatory T cells and cytokine-releasing mechanisms have been proposed, but with little corroborative data. A final possibility is that IVIG contains neutralising IgG antibodies directed against the autoantigen-binding site of autoantibodies: so-called anti-idiotypic antibodies.

SUMMARY BOX 22.4

Other immunotherapies

- IVIG therapy can be used in primary and secondary immunodeficiencies and in inflammatory conditions.

Further reading

Liu XY, Pop LM, Vitetta ES 2008 Engineering therapeutic monoclonal antibodies. Immunol Rev 222: 9–27

Lonberg N 2005 Human antibodies from transgenic animals. Nat Biotechnol 23: 1117–1125

Wark KL, Hudson PJ 2006 Latest technologies for the enhancement of antibody affinity. Adv Drug Deliv Rev 58: 657–670

Adams GP, Weiner LM 2005 Monoclonal antibody therapy of cancer. Nat Biotechnol 23: 1147–1157

Cutler A, Brombacher F 2005 Cytokine therapy. Ann N Y Acad Sci 1056: 16–29

Scott DL, Kingsley GH 2006 Tumor necrosis factor inhibitors for rheumatoid arthritis. N Engl J Med 355: 704–712

Immunisation

There can be little doubting the fact that immunisation has been a major public health success story. Achievements include the eradication of smallpox from the globe and the near elimination of wild poliovirus. In the developed world the number of individuals experiencing the devastating effects of measles, pertussis and other infections has been vastly reduced, at a considerable saving on death, disability and health cost.

The term 'immunisation' can be used to denote an artificial process whereby an individual is rendered immune. There are two broad categories of immunisation: active and passive (or adoptive). **Active immunisation** implies that a non-immune individual acquires long-lasting ability to respond to an organism or its toxic products by generating his or her own protective mechanisms. Active immunisation is largely synonymous with 'vaccination'. **Vaccination** (from the Latin *vacca*, meaning a cow) was the term originally used to describe the process of generating immunity to the lethal smallpox virus by injecting, under the skin, extracts from lesions of the cowpox virus, cause of a relatively harmless infection in humans. **Passive immunisation** denotes the process of conferring protective immunity without the need for an immune response on the part of the recipient, for example by giving injections of antibodies.

Active immunisation, or vaccination, is based upon exploitation of the characteristics of primary (slow, low-affinity, low-capacity IgM produced in antibody responses) and secondary (fast, high-affinity, high-capacity IgG and IgA) immune responses (see p. 44). The vaccine itself is an attenuated or inactivated infective agent, disabled toxin, or an inert subunit of an infective agent. It is introduced, usually by intradermal or intramuscular injection, or sometimes orally, to a non-immune individual. The characteristic of this process is that it is a *safe* encounter with an agent that mimics the natural primary infection. Immunity is acquired, and when the 'wild-type' agent is confronted, either protective immunity is in place (e.g. circulating neutralising antibody) or a rapid, high-affinity secondary response can be mobilised.

The history of immunisation begins in the eighteenth century. The observation had been made that individuals who recovered from certain diseases were protected from recurrences. This led to the introduction of a process known as variolation (*Variola major* is the smallpox virus), in which fluid extracts from the pustules caused by the smallpox virus were obtained from individuals who appeared to have recovered from the infection and injected under the skin of uninfected individuals. The procedure was hazardous but occasionally successful. There is a famous letter from Lady Mary Wortley Montagu, wife of the British Ambassador in Turkey in 1717, who is largely credited with introducing variolation to England, in which she wrote that, 'The smallpox so fatal and so general among us, is here entirely harmless by the invention of ingrafting, which is the term they give it'. On her return, Lady Montagu had her daughters 'ingrafted', but only after it had been tried first on six condemned criminals in the local prison!

In a distinct approach, Edward Jenner, a country doctor with a practice in the West Country in England, made the observation that milkmaids, who frequently suffered with disfiguring cowpox lesions, rarely contracted smallpox. He used extracts from the cowpox lesions to protect successfully against smallpox, and the science of immunisation was born. Many spectacular successes were witnessed in the twentieth century, but see Clinical Box 23.1.

The introduction of modified toxins (toxoids) from *Corynebacterium diphtheriae* and *Clostridium tetani* had a dramatic effect on the incidence of these infections. Polio vaccine, produced as a killed virus by Salk in 1954 or as a live but attenuated virus by Sabin in 1956, rapidly eradicated the scourge that was poliomyelitis in many countries (Fig. 23.1). Hepatitis B vaccine, introduced in 1975 as a viral surface antigen (HBsAg) purified from the plasma of patients

Need for regulatory bodies: the lesson from Jim

In his career Jim — a former milk wagon horse — had produced some 30 litres of diphtheria antitoxin: he undoubtedly saved many lives. On 2 October 1901 Jim was discovered to have contracted tetanus and was killed. Following the death in St Louis of a girl who had received diphtheria antitoxin, it was soon clear that she had received Jim's contaminated serum. The contaminated sample was obtained on 30 September, while the sample of 24 August was not contaminated. Unfortunately, samples from 30 September had also been used to fill bottles labelled 24 August. The result is that 12 more children died. This incident, and a similar one involving contaminated smallpox vaccine, led to the passage by the US Congress of the Biologics Control Act of 1902, which established the Center for Biologics Evaluation and Research and anticipated the formation of the US Food and Drug Administration (FDA) and similar control bodies.

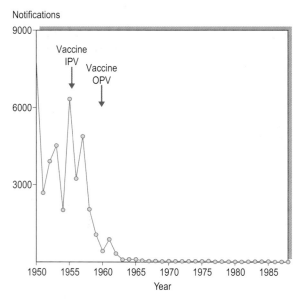

Fig. 23.1 Annual notifications of polio infection in the UK between 1950 and 1987.
Demonstrating the powerful effect of the introduction of the injected (IPV) and oral (OPV) polio vaccines.

with chronic infection, was the first subunit vaccine and, subsequently, the first recombinant vaccine in 1986. It is chastening for modern immunologists to remember that the vast majority of the highly successful vaccines in current use were all developed before 1970.

Anything new and exciting for the future? The recently developed vaccine against the human papilloma virus, cause of cervix cancer, is destined to drastically reduce this type of tumour in the future (see Science Box 23.1). Also promising is the inclusion of pathogen associated molecular patterns (PAMPS) into newly devised adjuvants. These are capable of making vaccine-induced antimicrobial immune responses

Harald zur Hausen and the prevention of cervical cancer

When the virologist Harald zur Hausen first reported in 1975 that human papilloma virus (HPV) may be associated with cervical cancer, the scientific world reacted with scepticism. A quarter of a century later, thanks to the availability of PCR, it was found that practically 100% of cervical cancers contained papilloma viral DNA — and zur Hausen was fully vindicated. The development of HPV vaccines received an enormous boost: by June 2006 one vaccine had received FDA approval and a second was approved in September 2007 by European regulatory bodies. Tested on more than 3000 participants, the two vaccines have given similarly spectacular results preventing persistent HPV infection in 100% of the vaccinated women and reducing cervical abnormalities by more than 90%. Both vaccines contain HPV 16 and 18, the types most frequently encountered in cervical cancer.

Who should receive the vaccine? Cervical cancer is the second most common tumour in women from less-developed countries. Surely these women should represent the key target population. But, will they be able to afford the vaccine?

Leaving ethical concerns aside, the HPV story shows that a vaccine is able to prevent cancer, echoing the success of hepatitis B virus vaccine in preventing hepatocellular carcinoma. A lesson also for the clinical scientist: have confidence in your own data, as the now Heidelberg Professor Emeritus Harald zur Hausen had in his. You may be in the running for a Nobel Prize: HzH became Nobel Laureate on 7 October, 2008.

stronger and longer lasting. Last, but not least, is the real possibility of success with therapeutic anti-tumour vaccines. Recently two patients with end-stage melanoma have been successfully treated with a genetically engineered melanoma vaccine (see Science Box 23.2).

Vaccines

General principles

Vaccines in current use are either whole or subunit. Whole vaccines may have been inactivated (attenuated) or killed, and each of these has relative advantages and disadvantages (Table 23.1).

Not surprisingly, the choice of vaccine type involves trading off the advantages against the disadvantages. Administration of live, attenuated vaccines by their natural route is perhaps the optimal approach for the induction of immunity, but the least safe since there is a possibility of reversion of the organism to its pathogenic wild type. Choice of route is important: an agent typically encountered at a mucosal site (e.g. the enterovirus polio) requires good levels of specific secretory IgA for protection. This may not be generated as

SCIENCE BOX 23.2

Cancer immunotherapy

To educate the immune system to fight cancer has been an immunologist's dream for a long time and several avenues have been explored. In 2006, Steve Rosenberg and his group at the National Institute of Health (NIH) reported a success combining a variety of previously attempted modes of treatment: vaccination, genetic engineering, adoptive cell transfer and cytokine treatment.

Two patients with metastatic melanoma who had failed all previous treatments underwent long-lasting remission following this new immunotherapy. The approach is schematically shown in Figure 23.2.

Cytotoxic T lymphocytes are harvested from the patient with melanoma, engineered to express a melanoma-specific T cell receptor, expanded in vitro, re-infused in the lympho-depleted patient who also receives interleukin 2 to boost the re-infused cells. Lymphodepletion is used to reduce the number of regulatory cells that may counteract the action of the engineered cytotoxic T cells.

The undeniable success of the NIH group is somewhat lessened by the fact that the treatment was not successful in another 13 simultaneously treated patients. Why was it unsuccessful? The pessimistic view is that the results we have seen are a measure of the maximal potency of cancer immunotherapy. A more positive view is that there is scope for further development. The genetic engineering of anti-tumour T cells used in the NIH study, for example, can be improved. Vectors used to transfer transgenes can be optimised to prevent silencing of the transgenes over time. The transgene itself may be modified to reduce the risk of mispairing with endogenous genes, with the resultant decrease in expression of the tumour-specific T cell receptor. The possibility to expand and infuse high affinity tumour-specific helper T cells, in addition to tumour-specific cytotoxic T cells, is also being considered. Vaccination with tumour antigen is an allied strategy for expanding the pool of tumour-specific effector immune cells, but the vaccination strategies are being revisited. The frequent use of a small tumour peptide loaded onto dendritic cells, while leading to anti-tumour immunity in some cases, may lead to tolerance in others, especially if the exogenously loaded dendritic cells lack stimulatory molecules. The replacement of the small peptide with larger tumour antigens, taken up and processed by dendritic cells, should obviate this problem. In the experimental protocol of the American scientists, interleukin 2 was used to stimulate the adoptively transferred cells: the less toxic interleukin 15 may be considered instead. In a nutshell, the NIH study prolongs the immunologist's dream of curing cancer.

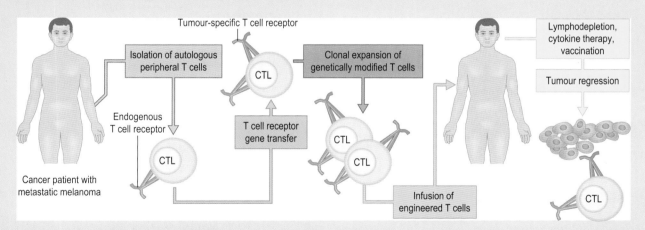

Fig. 23.2 **An immunotherapeutic regimen.**
Lymphocytes taken from a cancer patient are engineered to express a T cell receptor that recognises a melanoma-specific molecule. Once expanded, these anti-tumour lymphocytes are transferred back into the patient to destroy cancer cells (from Science, with permission).

effectively when the killed vaccine is given by injection as when the attenuated virus is given by the natural, oral route.

Reversion to virulence is an important consideration. In the UK, almost all cases of polio infection acquired within this country were the result of reversion to virulence of an attenuated virus. This is one of the reasons why the attenuated vaccine has now been discontinued and replaced by the killed form of the vaccine. The potential advantages of using an attenuated vaccine is the increase in so-called **herd immunity**. For example, with the Sabin live attenuated polio vaccine, even now used in several countries, the virus is still able to replicate, and some person–person passage takes place, increasing immunity even amongst non-immunised individuals. Therefore to achieve protection of the whole population, immunisation rates need not be 100%. This is in contrast with killed vaccines, which can only protect the recipient and for which immunisation rates must be nearer

Table 23.1 Advantages and disadvantages of live and killed vaccines

Vaccine type	Advantages	Disadvantages
Live attenuated vaccine		
	Reproduces natural infection	Possible reversion to virulent wild type
	Provides good level of protection, especially if Sabin (polio vaccine)	Limited shelf-life and requires refrigeration for storage in tropics
	Usually only one dose required	Presence of viral growth media or culture cells produces adverse effects
	Person–person passage of attenuated virus enhances herd immunity: uptake levels need not be 100%	Contraindicated in T cell immunodeficiency states, pregnancy
Killed vaccine		
	Safe from reversion to virulence	Less effective than live vaccines
	More stable for transport and storage	More than one dose required
	Acceptable for immunocompromised recipients	No herd immunity induced: uptake levels must approximate 100%

100% to achieve population immunity. Legislative measures are usually required for such a high level of uptake, and in the USA, for example, school entry is often conditional upon production of the appropriate documentation to prove that immunisations have been carried out.

Vaccine constituents

Vaccines include the antigen, against which adaptive immune responses are elicited; immune potentiators to stimulate the innate immune system; and delivery systems to ensure that the vaccine is delivered to the right place.

Antigens

- Whole inactivated or attenuated organisms or a mixture of various strains.
- Isolated and purified proteins, glycoproteins and carbohydrates.
- Recombinant proteins and glycoproteins.

Adjuvants — immune potentiators

- Bacterial products.
- Toxins and lipids.

- Nucleic acids.
- Peptidoglycans.
- Carbohydrates, peptides.
- Cytokines and hormones.

Delivery systems

- Mineral salts.
- Surface active agents.
- Synthetic microparticles.
- Oil-in-water emulsions.
- Liposomes.

Adjuvants and immune potentiators

The response to immunisation can be enhanced by a number of agents, and collectively these are termed adjuvants. These are a heterogeneous group of compounds, with several different mechanisms of action. In the history of immunisation, many compounds have been used empirically, with little knowledge about how they may work.

Several vaccines are composed of proteins that have been precipitated with **alum**, and others are **emulsified** in oil-based compounds. One of the best known emulsifying agents in vaccine studies is **Freund's complete adjuvant** (FCA), which contains mycobacterial derivatives. Amongst these, bacterial cell wall components such as lipopolysaccharide (LPS) are powerful immune stimulants, having a mitogenic and activating effect on antigen presenting cells and T cells (FCA produces such a vigorous local inflammatory response, however, that it cannot be used clinically). Manoeuvres such as the use of alum and oils are thought to retain antigen at the site of injection, prolonging the immune response, as well as providing relatively 'indigestible' antigenic compounds. This leads to chronic stimulation of APCs, which is likely in turn to enhance co-stimulation of T cells.

Knowledge about the nature of immune responses can now be put to use to design specific new adjuvants for particular types of immunopotentiation. An important goal is to identify adjuvants that specifically enhance cytotoxic T cell generation, or those that alter the T_H1/T_H2 balance in favour of the subset known to confer protection in a particular disease. For example, mice immunised with the same vaccine precipitated in alum, or emulsified in an oil-based adjuvant produce differing responses: alum mainly induces an antibody response (T_H2), whilst emulsification induces a cell-mediated response (T_H1). In addition, many of the potential vaccines produced during the current molecular biology revolution are protein subunits or even short peptides, which, on their own, are not inherently immunogenic. A new generation of adjuvants and immune potentiators is being sought to complement the activity of the new vaccines.

Since cytokines were found to be the effector molecules for any adjuvant effects, there has been an attempt to build the optimal vaccine adjuvant effect using one cytokine at a time. This approach, however, underestimated the complexity of events necessary to augment immune responses. Currently, efforts are focused on how to stimulate the innate immune system, since its key role in the evolution of the adaptive immune response is increasingly appreciated. This requires the inclusion in vaccines of immune potentiators that trigger early innate immune responses to aid in the generation of robust and long-lasting adaptive immune responses. This approach was promoted by the discovery of Toll-like receptors (TLRs), which recognise pathogen associated molecular patterns (PAMPS), see Chapter 6. The addition of such microbial components to experimental vaccines favours the development of durable adaptive immune responses. The engagement of TLRs leads to secretion of cytokines and chemokines, as well as maturation and migration of immune cells. TLR signalling results mainly in the activation of transcription factors such as NF-κB and IRF3 (interferon regulatory factor 3), which provide the inflammatory milieu for the rapid activation of host defences. The NF-κB pathway controls the expression of pro-inflammatory cytokines such as IL-1β and tumour necrosis factor-α, whereas the IRF3 pathway leads to the production of antiviral type I interferons. This results in the formation of a cellular infiltrate consisting of activated dendritic cells, neutrophils, basophils, eosinophils and natural killer cells. Within this inflammatory microenvironment, monocytes differentiate into macrophages and dendritic cells, which are pivotal to the initiation of adaptive immune responses.

Virus vaccines

Virus vaccines have been produced that are live attenuated, killed or represent subunits:

- Live-attenuated vaccines: measles, mumps, rubella, varicella zoster.
- Inactivated (killed) vaccines: polio (Salk), influenza, rabies.
- Subunit vaccines: hepatitis B, influenza.

Attenuation is applicable only to viruses that are easily and reliably inactivated. In general, RNA viruses are easier to attenuate than DNA viruses, since RNA is more susceptible to inactivation. Countries differ in their choice of killed or attenuated vaccine for polio. The live attenuated type (Sabin) has been discontinued in the USA, UK and several other European countries, but it is still used in endemic areas.

For the generation of subunit vaccines, some knowledge about the part of the virus that induces T cell responses and the targets of the most effective neutralising antibodies is required. As a generalisation, neutralising antibodies tend to target surface proteins, whilst T cell responses are directed against internal components. The other major consideration in the construction of viral subunit vaccines is to ensure that the subunit is represented in all strains of the virus (i.e. using group-specific rather than strain-specific subunits). T cell epitopes are likely to differ between different individuals in an HLA-dependent fashion, and the size of subunit should also take this constraint into consideration.

Influenza outbreaks occur as pandemics, with an unpredictable, periodic frequency. Four such pandemics occurred during the twentieth century, and during the 1918–19 outbreak, more people died within a few months than in the whole of the First World War. The pandemics result from antigenic shift in the influenza A strain, giving rise to virus with a previously unseen or resurgent haemagglutinin or neuraminidase subtype. Children and the elderly are at risk, along with those with known chronic respiratory or cardiac disease, diabetes, and immune suppression caused by disease or therapy. Each year, the Department of Health in the UK issues guidelines as to the use of the vaccines. Long-stay facilities, particularly nursing homes for the elderly, should also be targeted. Although annual vaccination is recommended for those at risk, there is some controversy as to whether this offers optimal protection. Keen public health surveillance is constantly in place to recognise outbreaks early. The antigenic composition of the vaccines available is also under constant review, and typically these contain haemagglutinin and neuraminidase from at least two influenza A subtypes and influenza B (see Science Box 23.3).

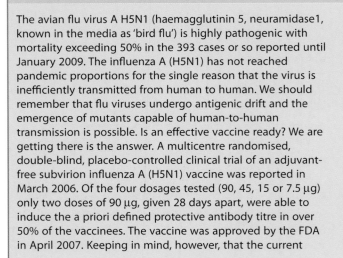

SCIENCE BOX 23.3

Avian flu vaccination

The avian flu virus A H5N1 (haemagglutinin 5, neuramidase1, known in the media as 'bird flu') is highly pathogenic with mortality exceeding 50% in the 393 cases or so reported until January 2009. The influenza A (H5N1) has not reached pandemic proportions for the single reason that the virus is inefficiently transmitted from human to human. We should remember that flu viruses undergo antigenic drift and the emergence of mutants capable of human-to-human transmission is possible. Is an effective vaccine ready? We are getting there is the answer. A multicentre randomised, double-blind, placebo-controlled clinical trial of an adjuvant-free subvirion influenza A (H5N1) vaccine was reported in March 2006. Of the four dosages tested (90, 45, 15 or 7.5 µg) only two doses of 90 µg, given 28 days apart, were able to induce the a priori defined protective antibody titre in over 50% of the vaccinees. The vaccine was approved by the FDA in April 2007. Keeping in mind, however, that the current

worldwide manufacturing capacity for influenza vaccine is estimated at 900 million doses (at the dose level of 15 µg), a two-dose vaccination per person with 90 µg would mean that only 75 million persons (1.25% of the world's population) could have the vaccination. It is clear from these data that there is an urgent need for a better vaccine. Efforts are being made in that direction with small vaccine doses coupled to adjuvants. What happens if the virus gets there before a sufficient supply of vaccine is obtained? A tentative answer comes from a US Congressional office. Their calculations indicate that a severe pandemic infection would, in the United States, affect 200 million people, with 90 million being clinically ill, and 2 million dying. This estimate should provide politicians with a reasonable argument for allocating finances to vaccine development programmes, also in view of the rather devastating economic blow anticipated by the report alluded to above.

Bacterial vaccines

As for viral vaccines, bacteria may be rendered as useful immunogens by killing or inactivation. Both of these approaches require the bacteria to be cultured in vitro, which is not possible with some organisms (e.g. *Treponema pallidum*, the cause of syphilis). Bacterial vaccines in common use include:

Live-attenuated vaccine

- Bacille Calmette–Guérin for tuberculosis.

Inactivated (killed) vaccine

- *Bordetella pertussis* for whooping cough.
- *Salmonella typhi* and *S. paratyphi* for typhoid.

Subunit/toxin vaccine

- Chemically inactivated *Clostridium tetani* neurotoxin.
- Chemically inactivated *Corynebacterium diphtheriae* toxin.
- Cell wall polysaccharide from *Haemophilus influenzae* type b.
- Cell wall polysaccharides from *Neisseria meningitidis* A and C.

In general, bacterial vaccines are killed using heat treatment or agents such as formaldehyde and phenol. One of the best examples of an attenuated vaccine is that for tuberculosis, the bacille Calmette–Guérin. This was originally *Mycobacterium bovis* isolated from a cow, which through repeated culture passages (231 times in 3 years) lost its virulence and has now been administered to over 10^9 people worldwide.

Whole cell bacterial vaccines can be associated with problems related to production in cell culture, as well as with side-effects that have made their use controversial. This has led to a shift towards the development of subunit vaccines, often termed **acellular vaccines**. For example, *Bordetella pertussis*, the aetiological agent in whooping cough, has a toxin and a surface fimbrial haemagglutinin that is thought to be important in attachment to host epithelial cells. A combined vaccine, based on purified, inactivated forms of these proteins was developed and represented a step forward in bacterial vaccine design. Similarly, the traditional killed whole-cell typhoid vaccine is associated with unpleasant side-effects, and an acellular vaccine based on the Vi capsular polysaccharide confers adequate protection without this drawback. A live oral vaccine — Ty2la — has also been developed, which is effective and administered in an enteric-coated or liquid formulation.

A success in the generation of acellular vaccines includes the **Hib vaccine** for *Haemophilus influenzae* type b. This is composed of capsular polysaccharide coupled to tetanus protein and has dramatically reduced the incidence of *Haemophilus* meningitis (which carried a mortality of almost 8%) since its introduction.

Parasite vaccines

Parasites pose some difficult problems for vaccine development. They are multicellular, frequently have more than one host organism and also colonise more than one organ during their life cycle. In addition, many of them have evolved some sophisticated mechanisms for evading host immune responses. Despite these problems, there is no doubting the need for parasite vaccines. Malaria (caused by *Plasmodium* spp.) kills 1.2 million people per year and annually infects an estimated 800 million worldwide. Other infections that cause considerable morbidity and for which vaccines are urgently sought are schistosomiasis (*Schistosoma* spp.; 200 million infected), Chagas' disease (*Trypanosoma cruzi*; 12 million), leishmaniasis (*Leishmania* spp.; 12 million) and sleeping sickness (*Trypanosoma gambiense/rhodesiense*; 1 million).

There are several well-documented immune-evasion mechanisms exploited by the organisms causing these infections. Organisms may vary the antigens they present (e.g. *Plasmodium* spp., trypanosomes). The mastigote stage of trypanosomes can escape from macrophage lysosomes, negating attempts to kill them or establish an immune response. Schistosomes are able to camouflage their surface using host-derived antigens. An additional problem for the vaccinologist is the difficulty in culturing the organisms, which reduces the opportunity to study the life cycle and purify relevant antigens.

Nonetheless, certain facts indicate that immunisation against parasites is an achievable goal. First, for some of the infections (e.g. malaria) it is clear that individuals in endemic areas have some resistance to the parasite, indicating a state of protection. Second, passive immunisation of experimental animals with antibodies against the circumsporozoite antigens of malaria offers protection from challenge with the whole organism.

Immunisation protocols: protection for life

The current UK immunisation programme is shown in Table 23.2, and the US program in Figure 23.3. Diphtheria, tetanus and pertussis immunisation within the first 6 months of life is an important public health priority. Whooping cough is most dangerous when acquired at this age and early immunisation for *Haemophilus influenzae* type b is an

Vaccine	Birth	1 month	2 months	4 months	6 months	12 months	15 months	18 months	19-23 months	2-3 years	4-6 years	7-10 years	11-12 years	13-18 years
Hepatitis B	HepB	HepB			HepB						Hep B series			
Rotavirus			Rota	Rota	Rota									
Diphtheria, Tetanus, Pertussis			DTaP	DTaP	DTaP		DTaP				DTaP		Tdap	Tdap
Haemophilus influenzae type b			Hib	Hib	Hib	Hib								
Pneumococcal			PCV	PCV	PCV	PCV				PPSV				
Inactivated poliovirus			IPV	IPV	IPV						IPV	IPV Series		
Influenza					Influenza (yearly)						Influenza (yearly)			
Measles, mumps, rubella						MMR					MMR	MMR Series		
Varicella						Varicella					Varicella	Varicella series		
Hepatitis A						HepA (2 doses)				HepA series				
Meningococcal										MCV		MCV	MCV	
Human Papillomavirus													HPV 3 doses	HPV Series

Hepatitis B vaccine. *AT BIRTH*; All newborns should receive HepB soon after birth. Infants born to mothers who are HBsAg-positive should receive HepB and 0.5mL of hepatitis B immune globulin (HBIG) within 12 hours of birth and should be tested for HBsAg and antibody to HBsAg after completion of the HepB series, at age 9-18 months.
Human papilloma virus vaccine. First dose to females of age 11-12

Influenza vaccine. Influenza vaccine is recommended annually for children aged > 6 months with certain risk factors such as asthma, cardiac disease, sickle cell disease, human immunodeficiency virus [HIV] infection, diabetes and conditions that can compromise respiratory function.

    Range of recommended ages   Catch-up immunization   Certain high risk groups

HepB = Hepatitis B vaccine; **Rota** = Rotavirus vaccine; **DTaP** = Diphtheria and tetanus toxoids and acellular pertussis vaccine; **Hib** = Haemophilus influenzae type b conjugate vaccine; **MMR** = Measles, mumps and rubella vaccine; **Tdap** = Tetanus and diptheria toxoids and acellular pertussis vaccine; **HPV** = human papillomavirus vaccine; **MCV** = Meningococcal vaccine; **PPSV** = Pneumococcal polysaccharide vaccine; **IPV** = Inactivated poliovirus vaccine.

Fig. 23.3 Recommended childhood and adolescent immunisation schedule, by vaccine and age — United States 2009. (Modified from Department of Health and Human Services, Centers for Disease Control and Prevention, USA. www.cdc.gov/vaccines/recs/schedules.)

Table 23.2 UK routine childhood immunisation programme 2008

When to immunise	Diseases protected against	Vaccine given
Two months old	Diphtheria, tetanus, pertussis (whooping cough), polio and *Haemophilus influenzae* type b (Hib) Pneumococcal infection	DTaP/IPV/Hib + Pneumococcal conjugate vaccine (PCV)
Three months old	Diphtheria, tetanus, pertussis, polio and *Haemophilus influenzae* type b (Hib) Meningitis C	DTaP/IPV/Hib + MenC
Four months old	Diphtheria, tetanus, pertussis, polio and *Haemophilus influenzae* type b (Hib) Meningitis C Pneumococcal infection	DTaP/IPV/Hib + MenC + PCV
Around 12 months	*Haemophilus influenzae* type b (Hib) Meningitis C	Hib/MenC
Around 13 months	Measles, mumps and rubella Pneumococcal infection	MMR + PCV
Three years four months to five years old	Diphtheria, tetanus, pertussis and polio Measles, mumps and rubella	DTaP/IPV or dTaP/IPV + MMR
Thirteen to eighteen years old	Tetanus, diphtheria and polio	Td/IPV

Non routine immunisations

When to immunise	Diseases protected against	Vaccine given
At birth (to babies who are more likely to come into contact with TB than the general population)	Tuberculosis	BCG
At birth (to babies whose mothers are hepatitis B positive)	Hepatitis B	Hep B

important addition to the protocol. The MMR triple vaccine was phased in during the late 1980s, and once uptake is complete, immunisation of schoolgirls with rubella will no longer be required as a routine practice.

Despite the existence of such a rigid programme, there is considerable flexibility within the public health systems of developed countries for rapid responses to real or potential risks. For example, the upsurge in reported diphtheria cases outside Western Europe and America has seen the adoption of a diphtheria booster at school-leaving age in these countries. Tetanus and inactivated poliomyelitis are frequently added to the low-dose diphtheria booster.

Future approaches

The use of recombinant DNA technology to generate vaccines has several obvious advantages. First it is safe in terms of viral virulence. For example, recombinant subunit vaccines are greatly preferred over attenuated viruses in potential vaccination programmes for HIV infection (Science Box 23.4), since they carry no risk of viral pathogenicity. Second, it can be applied to the generation of subunit vaccines for agents (e.g. malaria and some hepatitis viruses) that cannot be grown easily in culture. Third, it can be used to combine selected subunits in a single vaccine, so that more than one

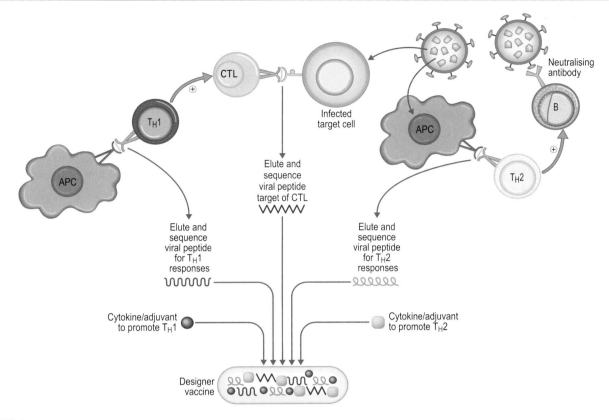

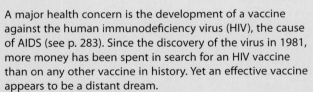

Fig. 23.4 **Designer vaccines.**

SCIENCE BOX 23.4

A distant dream?

A major health concern is the development of a vaccine against the human immunodeficiency virus (HIV), the cause of AIDS (see p. 283). Since the discovery of the virus in 1981, more money has been spent in search for an HIV vaccine than on any other vaccine in history. Yet an effective vaccine appears to be a distant dream.

While scientists have discovered how the virus cripples the immune system, they have not yet found an answer on how to protect against the infection. As acknowledged over 10 years ago by an AIDS vaccine scientist, in this field we are 'Flying without a compass'.

Will we ever get there? The sceptics argue that the virus replicates so quickly and makes so many mistakes during the process that vaccines cannot possibly control all types of HIV that exist. Moreover, HIV has evolved mechanisms to evade the immune attack, covering itself in sugars to fend off antibodies directed to vulnerable protein regions and

producing proteins that frustrate engagement of other immune effectors.

Nonetheless, experiments on monkeys have shown that vaccines can protect animals from SIV, the simian equivalent of HIV. It is also documented that there are people who repeatedly expose themselves to HIV but remain uninfected: there must be something that stops the virus. A small percentage of people who do become infected never seem to suffer any harm, and others hold the virus at bay for a decade or more before showing damage to their immune systems.

The vaccine perhaps is not such a distant dream. Some figures highlight how badly needed the vaccine is: over 25 million people have died since the virus discovery and over 45 million are currently infected, with populations in sub-Saharan Africa remaining by far the worst affected.

immunodominant epitope can be employed. Finally, DNA technology avoids some of the problems associated with large-scale culture of viruses. These include the question of safety and the fact that some culture systems are disadvantageous. For example, cells of neurological origin are used to culture the rabies virus and inevitably some components of the neuronal cells are incorporated in the vaccine. These have been implicated in an autoimmune polyneuropathy syndrome that has been associated with administration of the rabies vaccine. While waiting for a DNA technology vaccine, this serious neurological side-effect has been successfully tackled by the development of a vaccine in cell-lines of non-neurological origin.

Recombinant DNA technology, coupled with the identification of viral and bacterial epitopes for T and B cell responses will result in the ultimate in reductionist, 'designer' vaccines (Fig. 23.4). The vaccine of the future may contain a combination of short peptide sequences known to bind to a majority of class II MHC allotypes to stimulate T helper cell responses. These may be combined with peptides known to bind class I MHC molecules as targets of CD8 cytotoxic T cells, and with a variety of B cell epitopes known to induce neutralising antibodies. These peptides will be packaged appropriately and 'garnished' with a suitable adjuvant (Fig. 23.4).

SUMMARY BOX 23.1

Immunisation

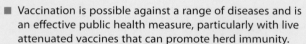

- Vaccination is possible against a range of diseases and is an effective public health measure, particularly with live attenuated vaccines that can promote herd immunity.

- Adjuvants enhance the response to immunisation; alums, oils and bacterial cell wall components are used.

- Future adjuvants will be devised to stimulate innate immunity pattern-recognition receptors, such as Toll-like

receptors, which are key to a vigorous and long-lasting immunity.

- Vaccines can be live attenuated, inactivated (killed) or subunit based.

- Challenges for the future include the provision of vaccines for parasites and viruses and the generation of 'designer vaccines'.

Further reading

Pulendran B, Ahmed R 2006 Translating innate immunity into immunological memory: implications for vaccine development. Cell 124: 849–863

Pashine A, Valiante NM, Ulmer JB 2005 Targeting the innate immune response with improved vaccine adjuvants. Nature Medicine 11(4 Suppl): S63–68

Esser MT, Marchese RD, Kierstead LS et al 2003 Memory T cells and vaccines. Vaccine 21: 419–430

Steinbrook R 2006 The potential of human papillomavirus vaccines. N Engl J Med 354: 1109–1112

Poland GA 2006 Vaccines against avian influenza—a race against time. N Engl J Med 354: 1411–1413

Morgan RA, Dudley ME, Wunderlich JR et al 2006 Cancer regression in patients after transfer of genetically engineered lymphocytes. Science (New York, NY) 314: 126–129

Appendices

Appendix 1   Commonly encountered CD molecules

CD designation	Other names	Molecular structure	Main cellular expression	Function(s)
CD1a	T6	49 kDa IgSF, MHC-like	Cortical thymocytes, Langerhans cells, DC	Antigen presentation, with β2m
CD1b	T6	45 kDa IgSF, MHC-like	Cortical thymocytes, Langerhans cells, DC	Antigen presentation, with β2m
CD1c	T6	43 kDa IgSF, MHC-like	Cortical thymocytes, Langerhans cells, DC, B cell subset	Antigen presentation, with β2m
CD1d		49 kDa IgSF, MHC-like	Intestinal epith., B cell subset, monocytes (low), DC	Antigen presentation, with β2m
CD1e		28 kDa IgSF, MHC-like	DC	Antigen presentation, with β2m
CD2	LFA-2; sheep red blood cell receptor	50 kDa	T cells, NK cells	Adhesion molecule (binds LFA-3); T cell activation
CD3		Composed of five chains (see Ch. 7)	T cells	Signal transduction as a result of antigen recognition by T cells
CD4		55 kDa	Class II MHC-restricted T cells	Adhesion molecule (binds to class II MHC); signal transduction
CD5		67 kDa	T cells; B cell subset	T–B cell interaction
CD8		Composed of two 34 kDa chains; expressed as αα or αβ dimer	Class I MHC-restricted T cells	Adhesion (binds to class I MHC); signal transduction

CD designation	Other names	Molecular structure	Main cellular expression	Function(s)
CD11a*	LFA-1 α chain	180 kDa; associates with CD18 to form LFA-1 integrin	Leukocytes	Adhesion (binds to ICAM-1)
CD11b	Mac-1; CR3 (iC3b receptor) α chain	165 kDa; associates with CD18 to from Mac-1 integrin	Granulocytes, monocytes, NK cells	Adhesion; phagocytosis of iC3b-coated (opsonised) particles
CD11c	p150,95; CR-4 α chain	150 kDa; associates with CD18 to form p150,95 integrin	Monocytes, granulocytes, NK cells	Adhesion; chemotaxis; receptor for fibrinogen
CD14		55 kDa; PI-linked	Monocytes	LPS receptor; role in oxidative burst
CD15	Lewis X	Carbohydrate epitope	Granulocytes	Sialylated form (CD15s) is a ligand for selectins
CD16	FcγRIII	50–70 kDa; PI-linked and trans-membrane	NK cells, granulocytes, macrophages	Low-affinity Fcγ receptor: ADCC, activation of NK cells
CD18	β chain of LFA-1 family (β_2 integrins)	95 kDa; non-covalently linked to CD11a, CD11b or CD11c	Leukocytes	See CD11a, CD11b, CD11c
CD19		90 kDa	B cells	Complex with CD21 and CD81, BCR co-receptor, B cell activation/differentiation
CD20		Heterodimer: 35 and 37 kDa chains	B cells	Role in B cell activation
CD21	CR2; C3d receptor	145 kDa	Mature B cells	Receptor for C3d, Epstein–Barr virus; B cell activation; complex with CD19 and CD81, BCR co-receptor
CD22		135 kDa	B cells	Role in cell adhesion and B cell activation
CD23	FcεRIIb	45–50 kDa	Activated B cells, macrophages	Low-affinity Fcε receptor, induced by IL-4

335

CD designation	Other names	Molecular structure	Main cellular expression	Function(s)
CD25	IL-2 receptor α chain; TAC	55 kDa	Activated T and B cells; Regulatory CD4 T cells, activated macrophages	Complexes with IL-2Rβγ to form high-affinity IL-2 receptor; T cell growth
CD28		Homodimer of 44 kDa chains	T cells (most CD4$^+$, some CD8$^+$ cells)	T cell receptor for co-stimulator molecules CD80 (B7-1), CD86 (B7-2)
CD29	β chain of VLA antigens (β$_1$ integrins)	130 kDa; non-covalently associated with VLA α chains (CD49)	Broad	Adhesion to extracellular matrix proteins, cell–cell adhesion (see CD49)
CD30	Ki-1	105 kDa	Activated T and B cells; Reed–Sternberg cells in Hodgkin's disease	Receptor for CD153 (CD30L), regulation of cellular growth and transformation of activated lymphoblasts
CD31	PECAM-1	140 kDa	Platelets, monocytes, granulocytes, B cells, endothelial cells	Role in leukocyte–endothelial adhesion
CD32	FcγRII	40 kDa	Macrophages, granulocytes, B cells, eosinophils	Low affinity Fc receptor, binds aggregated IgG; role in phagocytosis, ADCC; feedback inhibition of B cells
CD34		105–120 kDa	Precursors of haematopoietic cells	Stem cell marker, CD62L receptor
CD35	CR1; C3b receptor	Polymorphic; 190–280 kDa	Granulocytes, monocytes, erythrocytes, B cells	Binding and phagocytosis of C3b-coated particles and immune complexes
CD40		Heterodimer of 44 and 48 kDa chains	B cells	Receptor for CD154 (CD40L), role in B cell activation induced by T cell contact, isotype-switching, rescues B cells from apoptosis
CD44	Pgp-1, HERMES	80–100 kDa, highly glycosylated	Leukocytes, erythrocytes	May function as homing receptor; receptor for matrix components (e.g. hyaluronate)

CD designation	Other names	Molecular structure	Main cellular expression	Function(s)
CD45	T200; leukocyte common antigen	Multiple isoforms, 180–220 kDa	Leukocytes	Role in signal transduction (tyrosine phosphatase)
CD45R	Forms of CD45 with restricted cellular expression	CD45R0: 180 kDa CD45RA: 220 kDa CD45RB and CD45RC: 190, 205 and 220 kDa isoforms	CD45R0: memory T cells CD45RA: virgin T cells CD45RB: B cells, subset of T cells CD45RC: subset of T cells	See CD45, adhesion
CD49a	VLA α1 chain	210 kDa; associates with CD29 to form VLA-1 (β_1 integrin)	T cells, monocytes	Adhesion to collagen, laminin
CD49b	VLA α2 chain; platelet gpla	170 kDa; associated with CD29 to form VLA-2 (β_1 integrin)	Platelets, activated T cells, monocytes, some B cells	Adhesion to extracellular matrix: receptor for collagen
CD49c	VLA α3 chain	Dimer of 130 and 25 kDa; associates with CD29 to form VLA-3 (β_1 integrin)	T cells; some B cells, monocytes	Adhesion to fibronectin, laminin
CD49d	VLA α4 chain	150 kDa; associates with CD29 to form VLA-4 (β_1 integrin)	T cells, monocytes, B cells	Peyer's patch homing receptor, binds to VCAM-1; adhesion to fibronectin
CD49e	VLA α5 chain	Dimer of 135 and 25 kDa; associates with CD29 to form VLA-5 (β_1 integrin)	T cells; few B cells and monocytes	Adhesion to fibronectin
CD49f	VLA α6 chain	150 kDa; associates with CD29 to form VLA-6 (β_1 integrin)	Platelets, megakaryocytes; activated T cells	Adhesion to extracellular matrix receptor for laminin
CD52	CAMPATH-1	21–28 kDa	Thymocytes, T, B (not plasma cells), monocytes	Unknown
CD54	ICAM-1	80–114 kDa	Broad; many activated cells (cytokine-inducible)	Adhesion: ligand for LFA-1, Mac-1

CD designation	Other names	Molecular structure	Main cellular expression	Function(s)
CD55	Decay accelerating factor (DAF)	70 kDa; PI-linked	Broad	Regulation of complement activation
CD56	N-CAM	Heterodimer of 135 and 220 kDa chains	NK cells, NKT cells	Homotypic adhesion; isoform of neural cell adhesion molecule (N-CAM)
CD57	HNK-1	110 kDa	NK cell subset, subset of T cells	Unknown
CD58	LFA-3	55–57 kDa; PI-linked or integral membrane protein	Broad	Adhesion: ligand for CD2
CD62E	E-selectin, ELAM-1	115 kDa	Endothelial cells	Leukocyte–endothelial adhesion
CD62L	L-selectin, LAM-1	75–80 kDa	T lymphocytes, other leukocytes	Leukocyte–endothelial adhesion; homing of virgin T cells to peripheral lymph nodes
CD62P	P-selectin, GMP 140, PADGEM	130–150 kDa	Platelets, endothelial cells	Leukocyte adhesion to endothelium, platelets
CD64	FcγRI	75 kDa	Monocytes, macrophages	High-affinity Fcγ receptor: role in phagocytosis, ADCC, macrophage activation
CD71	Transferrin receptor	95 kDa homodimer	Activated T and B cells, macrophages, proliferating cells	Receptor for transferrin: role in iron metabolism, cell growth
CD74	Class II MHC invariant (γ) chain; I$_i$	Three protein species: 35, 41 and 53 kDa	B cells, monocytes, macrophages; other MHC class II$^+$ cells	Associates with newly synthesised class II MHC molecules
CD79a	Igα, MB1	32–33 kDa	Mature B cells	Component of B cell antigen receptor
CD79b	Igβ, B29	37–39 kDa	Mature B cells	Component of B cell antigen receptor

CD designation	Other names	Molecular structure	Main cellular expression	Function(s)
CD80	B7-1, BB1	50–60 kDa	Dendritic cells, activated B and T cells and macrophages	Co-stimulator for T lymphocyte activation; ligand for CD28 and CTLA-4
CD81	TAPA-1	22 kDa	Broad	Associated with CD19 and CD21; role in B cell activation; hepatitis C virus receptor
CD86	B7-2	50–60 kDa	Dendritic cells, activated B cells and macrophages	Co-stimulator for T lymphocyte activation; ligand for CD28 and CTLA-4
CD88	C5a receptor	40 kDa	Neutrophils, macrophages, mast cells, eosinophils	Receptor for complement component: role in complement-induced inflammation
CD89	Fcα receptor	55–70 kDa	Neutrophils, monocytes	IgA-dependent cytotoxicity
CD95	Fas antigen, APO-1	42 kDa	Multiple cell types	Role in programmed cell death
CD102	ICAM-2	55–65 kDa	Endothelial cells, monocytes, other leukocytes	Ligand for LFA-1 integrin
CD106	VCAM-1	90–95 kDa	Endothelial cells, macrophages, follicular dendritic cells, marrow stromal cells	Receptor for VLA-4 integrin; role in cell adhesion, lymphocyte activation, haematopoiesis
CD122	IL-2Rβ	75 kDa	NK, T and B cells, monocytes	IL-2Rβ and IL-15Rβ, signal transduction
CDw123	IL-3R	70 kDa	Lymphocyte subset, basophils, haematopoietic progenitors, mac, DC, megakaryocytes	IL-3Rα, with CDw131
CD127	IL-7R	65–75 kDa	T, pro-B cells	IL-7Rα, with CD132, B and T cell development

CD designation	Other names	Molecular structure	Main cellular expression	Function(s)
CD132	Common γ	64 kDa	T, B, NK cells, monocytes, granulocytes	Subunit of IL-2R, IL-4R, IL-7R, IL-9R, and IL-15R, signal transduction
CD152	CTLA-4	33 kDa	Activated T and B cells	CD80 and CD86 receptor, negative regulation of T cell co-stimulation
CD154	CD40L, gp39, TRAP	32–39 kDa	Activated T cells	CD40 ligand, B and DC co-stimulation
CD159a	NKG2A	43 kDa	T cell subset, NK cells	Binds to CD94, NK cell receptor
CD159c	NKG2C	40 kDa	NK cells	Binds to MHC class I HLA-E molecules, forms heterodimer with CD94
CD161	NKR-P1A	40 kDa	T cell subset, NK cells	NK cell-mediated cytotoxicity
CD179a	V pre B	16–18 kDa	Pro- and Pre-B cells	B cell differentiation/ signalling, pseudo light chain, associates with Igμ chain
CD179b	Lambda 5	22 kDa	Pro- and Pre-B cells	B cell differentiation/ signalling, pseudo light chain, associates with Igμ chain
CD205	DEC-205	205 kDa	DC, thymic epithelial cells	Endocytic receptor directing captured antigens from the extracellular space to a specialised antigen-processing compartment
CD207	Langerin	40 kDa	Langerhans cells	Endocytic receptor
CD208	DC-LAMP	70–90 kDa	Activated DC, interdigitating DC	Unknown
CD209	DC-SIGN	44 kDa	DC subset	ICAM-3 receptor, HIV-1 binding protein
CD252	OX-40 Ligand, gp34	34 kDa	Activated B cells, cardiac myocytes	T co-stimulation

CD designation	Other names	Molecular structure	Main cellular expression	Function(s)
CD253	TRAIL, Apo-2L, TL2, TNFSF10		Activated T cells, broad expression	Induces apoptosis
CD254	TRANCE, RANKL, OPGL	35 kDa	Lymph node & BM stroma activated T cells	Binds OPG[1] and RANK[2], osteoclast differentiation, enhances DC to stimulate naïve-T proliferation
CD281	TLR1	90 kDa	Low levels in PBMC, monocytes and possibly DC	Innate immunity, co-operates with TLR2 and modulates the response to microbial constituents
CD282	TLR2	90 kDa	Monocytes, neutrophils, up-regulated in macrophages	Binds dsRNA, response to bacterial lipoproteins, innate immunity
CD283	TLR3	100 kDa	Derived moDC (may be intracellular)	Binds dsRNA, innate immunity
CD284	TLR4	100 kDa	PBMC (weak in monocytes, immature DC and neutrophils)	Binds LPS, innate immunity
CD289	TLR9	120 kDa	pDC (intracellular)	Binds CpG-DNA, innate immunity
CD314	NKG2D, KLR	42 kDa	NK, activated CD8 T cells, NK1.1+ T, some myeloid cells	Binds MHC class I, MICA, MICB, activates cytolysis and cytokine production, co-stimulation

Notes: [1]OPG = Osteoprotegerin, [2]RANK = receptor activator of nuclear factor-κB; *CD11a, CD11b and CD11c are three α chains that can non-covalently associate with the same β chain (CD18) to form three different integrins, all of which are members of the 'CD11CD18' family (also called the 'LFA-1 family' or the 'β2 integrins'). See also CD29 and CD49a–f.

Related websites

http://www.ebioscience.com/ebioscience/whatsnew/humancdchart.htm
http://pathologyoutlines.com/cdmarkers.html

Appendix 2 Major cytokines, cells releasing them, targets and functions

Name	Cell releasing	Cell targeted	Effect	Other functions/comments
Interferons (IFN)				
Type I IFN				
α (13 subtypes)	Plasmacytoid DC, most cells at lower levels	All	Anti-viral, $\uparrow$ MHC expression	Bind to type I interferon receptor
β (2 subtypes)	Fibroblasts	All	Anti-viral, $\uparrow$ MHC expression	
Type II IFN				
γ	T cell	Macrophages	Activation	Bind to type II interferon receptor
		B cells	Ig class selection	
		T cells	Activate and influence T_H type	
		NK	Activation	
Tumour necrosis factor-α (TNF)	Macrophage	Macrophages Neutrophils	Activation $\uparrow$ cytotoxicity	Acts on hypothalamus to $\uparrow$ temp.; acts on liver to $\uparrow$ acute phase response. Physiologically important in anti-microbial responses. Pathologically has major role in shock syndromes secondary to Gram-negative bacterial infection
		All cells	$\uparrow$ MHC expression	
		Endothelium	$\uparrow$ adhesion molecules	
	T cells	T cells	Co-signal for activation	

Name	Cell releasing	Cell targeted	Effect	Other functions/ comments
Interleukin-1 (IL-1α, IL-1β)	Macrophages, monocytes, DC	Endothelium	↑ adhesion molecules; pro-coagulant	Also ↑ acute phase response (via IL-6) and induces fever
		T cells	Co-signal for T cell activation	
Interleukin-2	T cells (mainly T_H1)	T cells	The major autocrine and paracrine T cell growth factor; activates CTLs	Also activates NK cells and increases their cytotoxicity
		B cells	Growth and differentiation factor	
		NK cells	Growth and differentiation factor	
Interleukin-3	T cells (T_H1 and T_H2)	Immature bone marrow progenitor cells; plasmacytoid DCs	Promotes growth and differentiation	
Interleukin-4	T cells (T_H2)	T cells	Growth factor (for T_H2 cells); inhibitory (for T_H1)	Promotes IgE production; inhibitory effects on macrophages
		B cells	Activator and growth factor	
Interleukin-5	T cells (T_H2), mast cells	Eosinophils	Growth and differentiation; promote killing of helminths	
		B cells	Growth and differentiation; enhances Ig production	
Interleukin-6	T cells, macrophages	B cells	Growth and differentiation factor	Very important mediator of acute phase response by action on liver
	MPS	Liver	Acute phase	In conjunction with TGF-β promotes T_H17 cell differentiation
Interleukin-7	Marrow stromal cells	Developing B cells, T and NK cell survival	Growth and differentiation	

Name	Cell releasing	Cell targeted	Effect	Other functions/ comments
Interleukin-8	Monocyte lineage cells, T cells, endothelium	Neutrophils	Activation	Reclassified as the chemokine CXCL8
Interleukin-10	T cells (T_H2, Tr1[1]) Macrophages, DCs	T lymphocytes	Immunosuppressant effect: inhibits cytokine release and proliferation of T cells; with IL-4 influences differentiation of T_H1 to T_H2	Antagonises synthesis of IFN-γ and TNF-α
		B lymphocytes	Promotes differentiation	
Interleukin-12	DCs	Naïve T cells	Potent polarising agent along with IFN-γ; influences T_H cells along the T_H1 lineage	
		CD8 T cells	Activation of CTLs	
Interleukin-13	T cells (T_H2)	T cells	Growth factor (for T_H2 cells); inhibitory (for T_H1)	Function similar to IL-4
		B cells	Activator and growth factor	
Interleukin-15	mRNA expressed in multiple tissues but not T cells	T cells, B cells, NK cells	Similar effects to IL-2	Uses IL-2 Rβ and IL-2Rγ receptors on T cells
Interleukin-17	T_H17 cells. Generated from naïve CD4 T cells in the presence of IL-6 and TGF-β	Fibroblasts, endothelial cells, epithelial cells, keratinocytes and macrophages	Induces production of cytokines, chemokines and prostaglandins	Induces and mediates inflammatory responses. Believed to have key role in some autoimmune diseases
IL-28A, IL-28B, IL-29 (collectively type III interferons)	Most cells	All	Antiviral	Bind to type III interferon receptor
Transforming growth factor-β	CD4 T cells, monocyte lineage cells	Inhibits proliferation	Has the generalised immunosuppressive effect of an 'anticytokine'	Acting on naïve CD4 T cells promotes development of CD4+, CD25+ regulatory T cells. In concert with IL-6 induces T_H17 cells

Name	Cell releasing	Cell targeted	Effect	Other functions/ comments
Granulocyte-CSF[2]	CD4 T cells, MPS cells, endothelium	Granulocyte lineage	Promotes growth and differentiation	Extensive clinical use to restore white blood cell counts after use of marrow-toxic treatment (e.g. antileukaemic chemotherapy, or following haemopoietic stem cell transplant)
Granulocyte-macrophage-CSF	CD4 T cells, monocyte lineage cells, endothelium	Granulocyte/ monocyte lineage	Promotes growth and differentiation, activates mature forms	Also used to enhance the pool of peripheral blood progenitor cells in normal donors
Monocyte-CSF-macrophage	Monocyte lineage cells	Monocyte lineage cells	Promotes growth and differentiation	

Notes: [1]T-regulatory 1 cells. [2]Colony-stimulating factor.

Related website

http://www.copewithcytokines.de/cope.cgi

Appendix 3 List of class II human leukocyte antigen alleles

Gene locus	HLA molecules as defined by serology	Number of alleles at locus	New nomenclature for alleles
DRB1	DR1	3	DRB1*0101–0103
	DR15 (DR2)	3	DRB1*1501–1503
	DR16 (DR2)	2	DRB1*1601, 1602
	DR3	3	DRB1*0301–0303
	DR4	14	DRB1*0401–0414
	DR11 (DR5)	6	DRB1*11011–11016
	DR12	2	DRB1*1201, 1202
	DR13 (DR6)	6	DRB1*1301–1306
	DR14 (DR6)	10	DRB1*1401–1410
	DR7	2	DRB1*0701, 0702
	DR8	7	DRB1*0801–0807
	DR9	1	DRB1*09011
	DR10	1	DRB1*1001
DRB3	DR52	4	DRB3*0101–0104
DRB4	DR53	1	DRB3*0101
DRB5	DR51	4	DRB5*0101–0104
DQA1	No molecules defined serologically	13	DQA1*0101–0113
DQB1	DQ5 (DQ1)	5	DQB1*0501–0505
	DQ6 (DQ1)	6	DQB1*0601–0606
	DQ2	1	DQB1*0201
	DQ3	5	DQB1*0301–0305
	DQ4	2	DQB1*0401, 0402
DPA1		8	DPA1*0101–0108
DPB1		32	DPB1*0101–0132

Molecules in parentheses denote 'parent' antigens, from which the new specificities have 'split' (e.g. DR15 and DR16 used to be defined by the same antiserum and were called DR2, but have recently been split into two new specificities).

Related website

http://www.ebi.ac.uk/imgt/hla/

Appendix 4 Abbreviations used for amino acids

A	alanine	M	methionine
C	cysteine	N	asparagine
D	aspartic acid	P	proline
E	glutamic acid	Q	glutamine
F	phenylalanine	R	arginine
G	glycine	S	serine
H	histidine	T	threonine
I	isoleucine	V	valine
K	lysine	W	tryptophan
L	leucine	Y	tyrosine

Index

Note: This index is in word-by-word order whereby spaces between words are recognised in the alphabetization, so that, for example, B cell comes before bacterial infections.

Abbreviations:
CVID — common variable immunodeficiency
HSCT — haematopoietic stem cell transplantation
SCID — severe combined immunodeficiency